Atlas of Nuclear Cardiology
Third Edition

Editors

Vasken Dilsizian, MD
Professor
Department of Medicine and Radiology
University of Maryland School of Medicine
Director, Cardiovascular Nuclear Medicine and PET Imaging
Chief, Division of Nuclear Medicine
University of Maryland Medical Center
Baltimore, Maryland

Jagat Narula, MD, PhD
Professor of Medicine
Chief, Division of Cardiology
University of California, Irvine School of Medicine
Orange, California

Series Editor

Eugene Braunwald, MD, MD (Hon), ScD (Hon)
Distinguished Hersey Professor of Medicine
Harvard Medical School
Chairman, TIMI Study Group
Brigham and Women's Hospital
Boston, Massachusetts

With 24 Contributors
Developed by Current Medicine Group, Inc.
Philadelphia

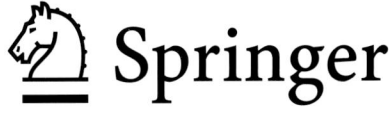

CURRENT MEDICINE GROUP LLC, PART OF SPRINGER SCIENCE+BUSINESS MEDIA LLC

400 Market Street, Suite 700 • Philadelphia, PA 19106

Senior Developmental Editor	Elizabeth Orthmann
Editorial Assistant	Juleen Deaner
Design and Layout	Daniel Britt and William Whitman
Illustrator	Wieslawa Langenfeld
Production Coordinator	Carolyn Naylor
Indexer	Holly Lukens

Library of Congress Cataloging-in-Publication Data

Atlas of nuclear cardiology / editors, Vasken Dilsizian, Jagat Narula. -- 3rd ed.
   p. ; cm.
 Includes bibliographical references and index.
 ISBN 978-1-57340-310-8 (alk. paper)
 1. Cardiovascular system--Radionuclide imaging--Atlases. I. Dilsizian, Vasken. II. Narula, Jagat.
 [DNLM: 1. Heart--radionuclide imaging--Atlases. 2. Cardiovascular Diseases--radionuclide imaging--Atlases. WG 17 A884394 2009]

RC670.5.R32A86 2009
616.1'07575--dc22

ISBN 978-1-57340-310-8
ISBN 1-57340-310-5

Although every effort has been made to ensure that drug doses and other information are presented accurately in this publication, the ultimate responsibility rests with the prescribing physician. Neither the publishers nor the authors can be held responsible for errors or for any consequences arising from the use of information contained herein. Products mentioned in this publication should be used in accordance with the prescribing information prepared by the manufacturers. No claims or endorsements are made for any drug or compound at present under clinical investigation.

© 2009 Current Medicine Group LLC, part of Springer Science+Business Media LLC.

All rights reserved. This work may not be translated or copied in whole or in part without the written permission of the publisher (Springer Science+Business Media, LLC., 233 Spring Street, New York, NY 10013, USA), except for brief excerpts in connection with reviews or scholarly analysis. Use in connection with any form of information storage and retrieval, electronic adaptation, computer software, or by similar or dissimilar methodology now known or hereafter developed is forbidden. The use in this publication of trade names, trademarks, service marks, and similar terms, even if they are not identified as such, is not to be taken as an expression of opinion as to whether or not they are subject to proprietary rights.

www.springer.com

For more information, please call 1 (800) 777-4643 or email us at orders-ny@springer.com

www.currentmedicinegroup.com

10 9 8 7 6 5 4 3 2 1

Printed in China by L. Rex Printing Company Limited

This book was printed on acid-free paper

Preface

Over the past three decades, nuclear cardiology has evolved from a research tool into a well-established clinical discipline. Approximately 9 million nuclear cardiology procedures are performed annually in the United States. The field has excelled in the noninvasive evaluation and quantification of myocardial perfusion, function, and metabolism. Unlike anatomically oriented approaches to diagnostic medicine, the strengths of nuclear techniques are based on physiologic, biochemical, and molecular properties. The ability to define myocardial perfusion, viability, and ventricular function from a single study has become a powerful diagnostic and prognostic tool. As a result of its important contribution to the management and care of cardiac patients, nuclear cardiology is now recognized as a distinct clinical entity.

Nuclear cardiology first originated as a discipline in the early 1970s. A major breakthrough in the field came with the development of myocardial perfusion radiotracers, such as ^{201}Tl, which permitted noninvasive detection and physiologic characterization of anatomic coronary artery lesions. First-pass and equilibrium radionuclide angiography allowed for the noninvasive assessment of regional and global left ventricular function. The field blossomed further with incorporation of the concepts of exercise physiology, demand-supply mismatch, coronary vasodilator reserve, and systolic and diastolic left ventricular dysfunction in nuclear testing. Pharmacologic vasodilators, such as dipyridamole and adenosine, widened the application of myocardial perfusion studies to patients who were unable to exercise, had uncomplicated acute coronary syndromes, or were undergoing intermediate- to high-risk noncardiac surgical procedures. Subsequently, the field advances from detection of coronary artery disease to risk stratification and prognosis. As such, nuclear cardiology procedures have become the cornerstone of the decision-making process to appropriately select patients for medical or interventional therapy, as well as monitoring the effectiveness of that therapy.

Parallel advances in both radiopharmaceuticals and instrumentation have further fostered the growth of nuclear cardiology. The introduction of ^{99m}Tc-labeled perfusion tracers in the 1990s improved the count rate and image quality of myocardial perfusion studies, which allowed for electrocardiogram-gated acquisition and simultaneous assessment of regional myocardial perfusion and function with a single radiotracer. Because ^{99m}Tc-labeled perfusion tracers demonstrate minimal redistribution over time after injection, they have been used in the emergency room and in the early hours of an infarct to estimate the extent of myocardium in jeopardy. A follow-up study, performed several days later, provides information on final infarct size and myocardial salvage. PET has broadened the scope of the cardiac examination from perfusion and function alone to assessment of metabolic substrate utilization, cardiac receptor occupancy, and adrenergic neuronal function. The ability to image the shift in the primary source of myocardial energy production from fatty acids toward glucose utilization in the setting of reduced blood flow has helped explain the pathophysiology of hibernation and myocardial viability, as well as management of patients with chronic ischemic left ventricular dysfunction and heart failure for the assessment of myocardial viability.

The aim of the third edition of the *Atlas of Nuclear Cardiology* is to elucidate the role of cardiovascular nuclear procedures in the clinical practice of cardiology. Diagnostic algorithms and schematic diagrams integrated with nuclear cardiology procedures are generously interspersed with color illustrations to emphasize key concepts in cardiovascular physiology, pathology, and metabolism. In the first chapter, the principles of nuclear cardiology imaging along with an introduction to instrumentation and image acquisition are presented. The next three chapters (chapters 2–4) detail SPECT and PET myocardial perfusion radiotracers and techniques for the detection of coronary artery disease as well as quantification of myocardial blood flow during exercise and pharmacologic stress. In chapter 5, the techniques of first-pass and equilibrium radionuclide angiography and gated myocardial perfusion SPECT are reviewed for assessment of cardiac function. Chapters 6 and 7 detail current evidence for the use of myocardial perfusion imaging for risk stratification in patients with chronic coronary artery disease; in special populations such as women, diabetics, the elderly, and patients of diverse ethnicity; and for identifying survival benefits with revascularization versus medical therapy. The next two chapters (chapters 8 and 9) focus on the role of imaging cardiac metabolism for identifying ischemic and viable myocardium, as well as new neurohumoral targets for prevention of heart failure and left ventricular remodeling. Chapter 10 addresses the role of left ventricular radionuclide imaging in the diagnosis and risk stratification of patients suffering from acute coronary syndromes. The last two chapters (chapters 11 and 12) examine the latest approaches of radionuclide techniques for advancement of cardiovascular research, myocardial innervation, and molecular imaging of atherosclerosis.

In the next century, innovative imaging strategies in nuclear cardiology will propel the field into molecular imaging while it continues to build on its already well-defined strengths of myocardial perfusion, function, and metabolism. Realization of these ideas and progress in the diagnosis, treatment, and prevention of cardiovascular disease will depend not only on new discoveries but also on meaningful interaction between clinicians and investigators. It is our hope that the third edition of the *Atlas of Nuclear Cardiology* will serve as a foundation for clinicians and a reference guide for scientists within and outside the field.

Vasken Dilsizian, MD
Jagat Narula, MD, PhD

Contributors

Stephen L. Bacharach, PhD
Professor
Department of Radiology
University of California, San Francisco
San Francisco, California

Frank M. Bengel, MD
Associate Professor of Radiology and Medicine
Russell H. Morgan Department of
 Radiology and Radiological Sciences
Division of Nuclear Medicine
Johns Hopkins School of Medicine
Baltimore, Maryland

Daniel S. Berman, MD
Professor of Medicine
David Geffen School of Medicine at UCLA
Director, Nuclear Cardiology/Cardiac Imaging
Cedars-Sinai Medical Center
Los Angeles, California

Elias H. Botvinick, MD
Professor
Department of Radiology and Medicine
University of California, San Francisco
San Francisco, California

Ji Chen, PhD
Assistant Professor
Department of Radiology
Emory University
Atlanta, Georgia

Nick G. Costouros, MD
Clinical Fellow
Department of Radiology and
 Biomedical Imaging
University of California, San Francisco
San Francisco, California

Vasken Dilsizian, MD
Professor
Department of Medicine and Radiology
University of Maryland School of Medicine
Director, Cardiovascular Nuclear Medicine
 and PET Imaging
Chief, Division of Nuclear Medicine
University of Maryland Medical Center
Baltimore, Maryland

Tracy L. Faber, PhD
Associate Professor
Department of Radiology
Emory University
Atlanta, Georgia

James R. Galt, PhD
Assistant Professor
Department of Radiology
Emory University School of Medicine
Director, Nuclear Medicine Physics
Emory University Hospital
Atlanta, Georgia

Ernest V. Garcia, PhD
Professor
Department of Radiology
Emory University
Atlanta, Georgia

Guido Germano, PhD
Professor of Medicine
Department of Medicine
UCLA School of Medicine
Director, Artificial Intelligence Program
Cedars-Sinai Medical Center
Los Angeles, California

Rory Hachamovitch, MD, MSc
Cardiac Imaging Associates
Los Angeles, California

Farouc A. Jaffer, MD, PhD
Assistant Professor
Department of Medicine
Harvard Medical School
Attending International Cardiologist
Cardiology Division
Massachusetts General Hospital
Boston, Massachusetts

Jennifer H. Mieres, MD
Associate Professor of Medicine
Department of Medicine/Cardiology
New York University School of Medicine
Director of Nuclear Cardiology
Department of Medicine-Division of Cardiology
New York University Medical Center
New York, New York

D. Douglas Miller, MD
Regents' Professor
Department of Medicine
Dean, School of Medicine
Senior Vice President for Health Affairs
Medical College of Georgia
Augusta, Georgia

Jagat Narula, MD, PhD
Professor of Medicine
Chief, Division of Cardiology
University of California,
 Irvine School of Medicine
Orange, California

J. William O'Connell, MS
University of California, San Francisco
San Francisco, California

Antti Saraste, MD, PhD
Research Fellow
Nuklearmedizinische Klinik Der Tu Munchen
Klinkum Rechts Der Isar Munchen
Munich, Germany

Leslee J. Shaw, PhD
Professor
Department of Cardiology
Emory University School of Medicine
Atlanta, Georgia

Heinrich R. Schelbert, MD, PhD
George V. Taplin Professor
Department of Molecular and
 Medical Pharmacology
David Geffen School of Medicine at UCLA
Los Angeles, California

Thomas H. Schindler, MD
Assistant Professor
Department of Medicine and Cardiology
Director, Nuclear Cardiology
School of Medicine at the
 University Hospitals of Geneva
Geneva, Switzerland

Markus Schwaiger, MD
Professor and Chairman
Department of Nuclear Medicine
Technical University of Munich
Munich, Germany

Heinrich Taegtmeyer, MD
Professor of Medicine
Department of Internal Medicine
Division of Cardiology
University of Texas Medical School-Houston
Houston, Texas

James E. Udelson, MD
Associate Professor of Medicine
Department of Medicine
Tufts University School of Medicine
Chief, Division of Cardiology
Tufts Medical Center
Boston, Massachusetts

Contents

Chapter 1
Principles of Nuclear Cardiology Imaging 1
Ernest V. Garcia, James R. Galt, Tracy L. Faber, and Ji Chen

Chapter 2
SPECT and PET Myocardial Perfusion Imaging: Tracers and Techniques 37
Vasken Dilsizian

Chapter 3
Pharmacologic Stressors in Coronary Artery Disease 61
D. Douglas Miller

Chapter 4
PET Perfusion Tracers: Quantitation of Myocardial Blood Flow 79
Thomas H. Schindler and Heinrich R. Schelbert

Chapter 5
Assessment of Cardiac Function:
First-Pass, Equilibrium Blood Pool, and Gated Myocardial SPECT 109
Elias H. Botvinick, Nick G. Costouros, Stephen L. Bacharach, and J. William O'Connell

Chapter 6
Risk Stratification and Patient Management 141
Daniel S. Berman, Rory Hachamovitch, and Guido Germano

Chapter 7
The Role of Stress Myocardial Perfusion Imaging in Special Populations 169
Leslee J. Shaw and Jennifer H. Mieres

Chapter 8
Imaging Cardiac Metabolism 181
Heinrich Taegtmeyer and Vasken Dilsizian

Chapter 9
Nuclear Investigation in Heart Failure and Myocardial Viability 201
Vasken Dilsizian and Jagat Narula

Chapter 10
Diagnosis and Risk Stratification in Acute Coronary Syndromes 225
James E. Udelson

Chapter 11
Myocardial Innervation 243
Markus Schwaiger, Antti Saraste, and Frank M. Bengel

Chapter 12
Molecular Imaging of Atherosclerosis: A Biological Roadmap 257
Farouc A. Jaffer and Jagat Narula

Index 279

Principles of Nuclear Cardiology Imaging

Ernest V. Garcia, James R. Galt, Tracy L. Faber, and Ji Chen

Nuclear cardiology imaging is solidly based on many branches of science and engineering, including nuclear, optical, and mathematical physics; electrical and mechanical engineering; chemistry; and biology. This chapter uses principles from these scientific fields to provide an understanding of both the signals used and the imaging system that captures these signals. These principles have been simplified to fit the scope of this atlas.

Nuclear cardiology's signal is a radioactive tracer, and its imaging systems are either single-photon emission CT or positron emission tomography cameras. This combination has met with remarkable success in clinical cardiology. This success is the result of the combination of sophisticated electronic nuclear instruments and a highly specific signal. The signal is as important as or more important than the imaging system, which can be explained with the following analogy.

When we look at the heavens on a clear night, our naked eye can see stars, objects that are millions of miles away, yet when we look into our patients just a few feet away, even with sophisticated systems, we can sometimes miss a signal associated with cardiac disease. The reason is that a star generates an incredibly powerful signal surrounded by a dark background, a signal much more powerful than the signals we currently use. This analogy provides several lessons. First, it illustrates the need to keep improving our signals. Second, it provides a motivation: by improving our signal, we have the capacity to detect anything. Finally, it explains the success of nuclear cardiology imaging over cardiovascular MRI, echocardiography, or CT for detecting perfusion abnormalities.

There is a misconception that MRI, echocardiogram, and CT are superior to nuclear cardiology imaging because of their superior spatial resolution. Yet, for detecting perfusion defects, what is really necessary is superior contrast resolution. It is this superior contrast resolution that allows us to differentiate between normal and hypoperfused myocardium, facilitating the visual analysis of nuclear cardiology perfusion images. Because these objects are bright compared with the background, we have been able to develop computer algorithms to totally, automatically, and objectively process and quantify our images, a feat yet to be successfully performed by other modalities.

This chapter explains the many important scientific principles necessary to understand this analogy, as well as nuclear cardiology imaging in general, starting from how radiation is emitted from a nucleus to how these sophisticated imaging systems detect this radiation. These principles are explained at a simple but highly applied level, so the nuclear cardiologist can understand them and apply them in routine clinical practice. The better one's understanding of how images are formed and what can go wrong in their formation, the higher one's accuracy in interpreting studies and the more successful one's practice should be.

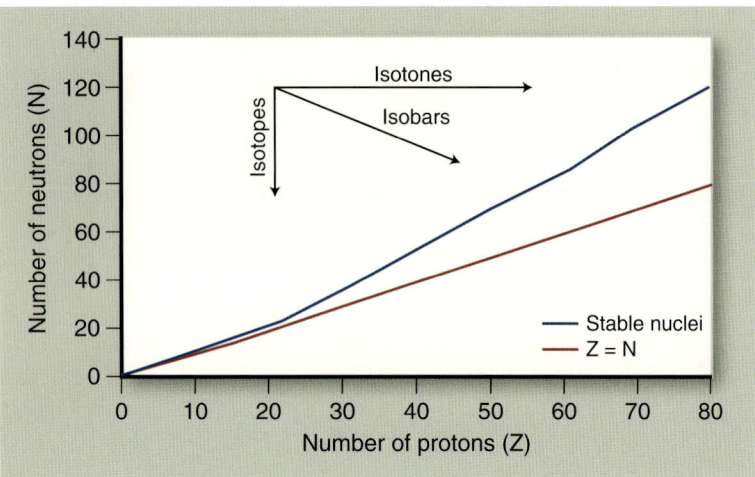

Figure 1-1. Stability of the nucleus. The graph plots as a *blue line* the number of neutrons versus the number of protons for stable nuclei. The *red line* indicates a neutron–proton ratio of 1. Only nuclides with low proton numbers fall on this line. Note in the *blue line* that as the number of protons increases, more neutrons are required to keep the nucleus stable. Nuclides with neutron–proton ratios that are not on the *blue line* of stable nuclei are unstable and thus radioactive. These radioactive nuclides are known as radionuclides. The type of radioactivity emitted depends on which side of the line the radionuclide is found. Isotopes are a family of nuclides that all have the same number of protons, or atomic number (Z), and are not necessarily radioactive. Isotones are nuclides with the same number of neutrons (N), and isobars have the same mass number (A) or number of mass particles in the nucleus (A = Z + N).

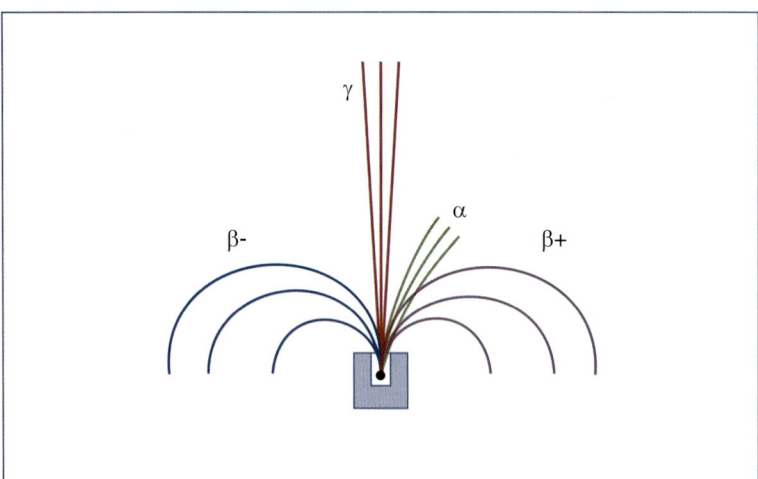

Figure 1-2. Types of radiation. The diagram represents the path deviation of different types of radiation from nuclei by a magnetic field perpendicular to the page. The direction of the deflection depends on the charge of the radioactive particle. The least penetrating radiation is deflected to the right and corresponds to the heaviest radiation, called an alpha particle (α). An alpha particle is actually the nuclei of a helium atom (two protons plus two neutrons) with a positive charge. The moderately penetrating radiation deflected in the direction opposite to an alpha particle consists of negative particles called beta particles (β). Because these particles are more strongly bent, they are lighter than the alpha particles. Beta particles are actually electrons emitted from the nucleus. Showing the same degree of penetration but bending in the direction opposite to the beta particles are positron particles, or positive electrons (β+). These are particles made of antimatter and emitted by positron tracers. The radioactive particles that go straight and are not deflected do not consist of charged particles. They are called gamma (γ)-rays and have been shown to be identical to particles emitted from an x-ray tube [1]. Both x- and γ-rays are called photons and are used in nuclear cardiology imaging.

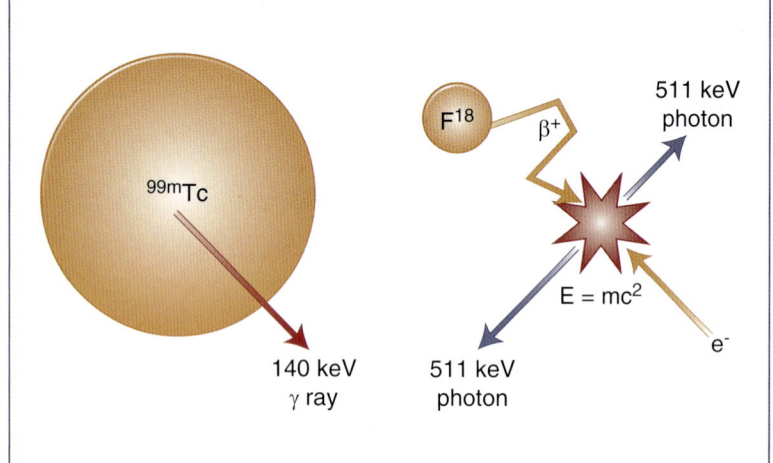

Figure 1-3. Single-photon emission CT (SPECT) versus positron emission tomography (PET) radionuclides. The figure shows two very different types of radionuclides, technetium-99m (^{99m}Tc) and fluorine-18 (^{18}F). ^{99m}Tc is a large radionuclide that emits a single photon or γ-ray per radioactive decay that is used in SPECT to create images. The energy of the emitted photon is 140 keV. The m in ^{99m}Tc means that the nucleus is meta-stable (almost stable but really unstable). ^{18}F is a much smaller radionuclide that emits a positron (β+) antiparticle. This ionized antiparticle travels through a medium interacting with it, losing energy and slowing down until it interacts with an electron, usually from some atom. Because the electron and the positron are antiparticles of each other (ie, same mass but opposite charge), they undergo a phenomenon called *pair annihilation*. In pair annihilation, the mass of both particles disintegrates and is converted into energy as explained by Einstein's famous equation, $E = mc^2$, where E is the emitted energy, m is the mass of the two particles, and c is the speed of light in a vacuum. Because of the nature of the interaction, most of the time the energy is emitted in the form of two photons traveling in exactly opposite directions from each other and each having the same energy, 511 keV, which is the energy equivalent to the rest mass of an electron. It is these two photons that are used to create images in PET.

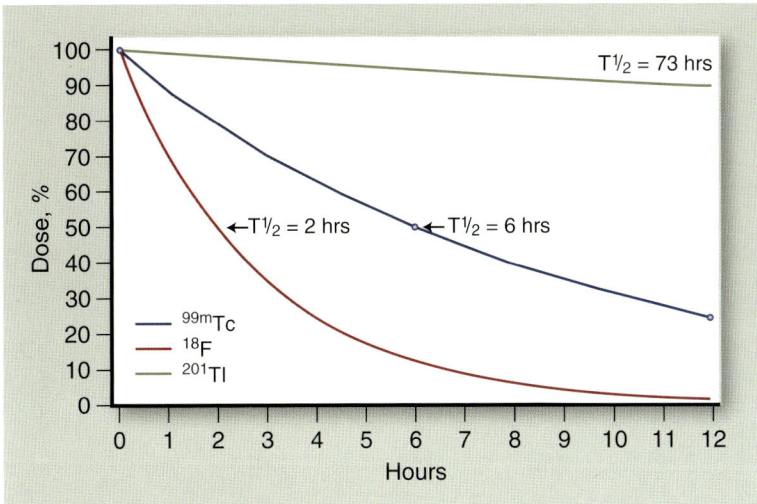
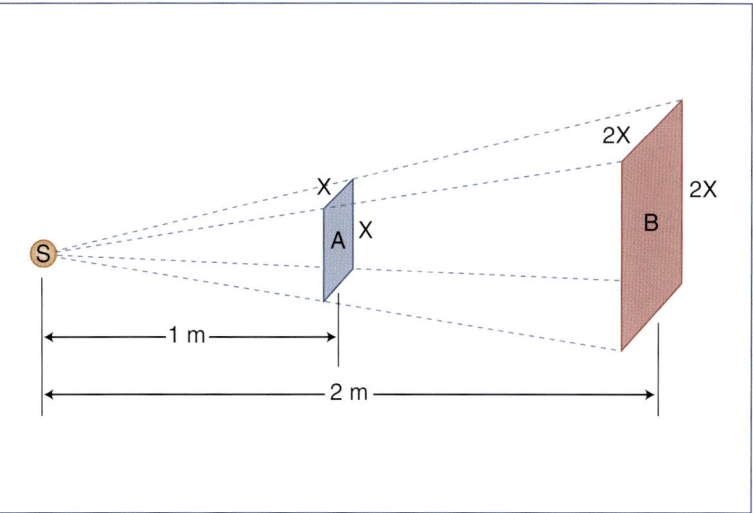

Figure 1-4. Radioactive decay law: concept of half-life. The diagram shows decay curves for three different radionuclides: technetium-99m (^{99m}Tc), fluorine-18 (^{18}F), and thallium-201 (^{201}Tl). The decay curves express the amount of radioactive nuclides that have not decayed as a function of time. The shorter the interval between emissions for a specific radionuclide, the faster the radioactivity is depleted. It is practical to express the rate of radioactive transformations (disintegrations) by specifying the period during which half of all the atoms initially present will disintegrate. This period of time is known as the half-life, or T½. Note from the graph that the ^{18}F curve is disintegrating the fastest of the three radionuclides and that it reaches a level of 50% of original at 2 hours; therefore, the half-life of ^{18}F is 2 hours. Compare this with the half-life of ^{201}Tl, which is 73 hours, and the half-life of ^{99m}Tc, which is 6 hours. The amount of radioactive nuclide is specified in terms of disintegration rate or its activity. This relationship is provided by the radioactive decay law:

$$A(t) = A_0 e^{-(0.693t)/T½}$$

In this equation, $A(t)$ is the radioactivity remaining at time t, A_0 is the activity at time 0, and T½ is the half-life of the radionuclide.

A common unit of radioactivity is the curie (Ci), which is 3.7×10^{10} disintegrations per second. Another common unit of radioactivity used is the becquerel (Bq), which is one disintegration per second. One thousandth of a curie is a millicurie (mCi), which corresponds to 3.7×10^7 disintegrations per second. Note from the graph that if a 40-mCi dose of a ^{99m}Tc radiopharmaceutical (radioactive pharmaceutical) is delivered to an imaging clinic at 6 AM, 6 hours later, at noon, only half—or 20 mCi—remains, and at 6 PM, only half of that—or 10 mCi—remains.

Figure 1-5. Inverse square law. The diagram illustrates the concept of the inverse square law for radioactivity. The intensity of a radioactive point source at a distance from the source obeys the same law as for visible light. If the amount of radioactivity at the point source (S) remains constant, then the intensity of the radioactivity (number of photons) passing through a flat surface is inversely proportional to the square of the distance from the source. At a distance of 1 m, the diverging radioactive beam covers an area (A, small square), with each side of dimension x, or an area of x^2. At 2 m, the diverging beam covers an area (B, large square) in which each side is now twice as long as A (2x) and the area is $4x^2$, which is four times the area at 1 m. Because the amount of radioactivity remains constant, the number of photons falling on square A must spread out over four times as large by the time it reaches square B. Thus the activity per unit area at B, which is twice as far as A from the source, is one fourth of the activity passing through A [2]. The value of this principle to radiation workers is that they can significantly reduce their radiation burden just by increasing their distance between themselves and a radioactive source, such as a patient already injected with a radioactive dose.

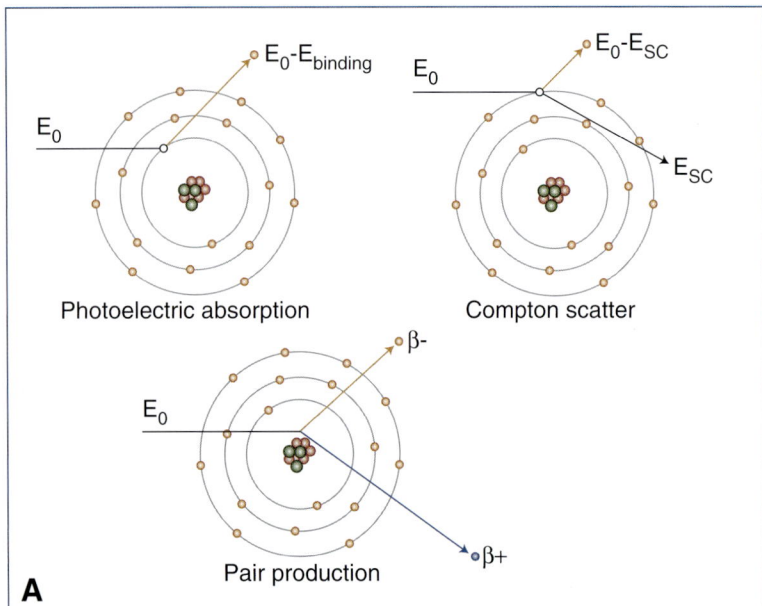
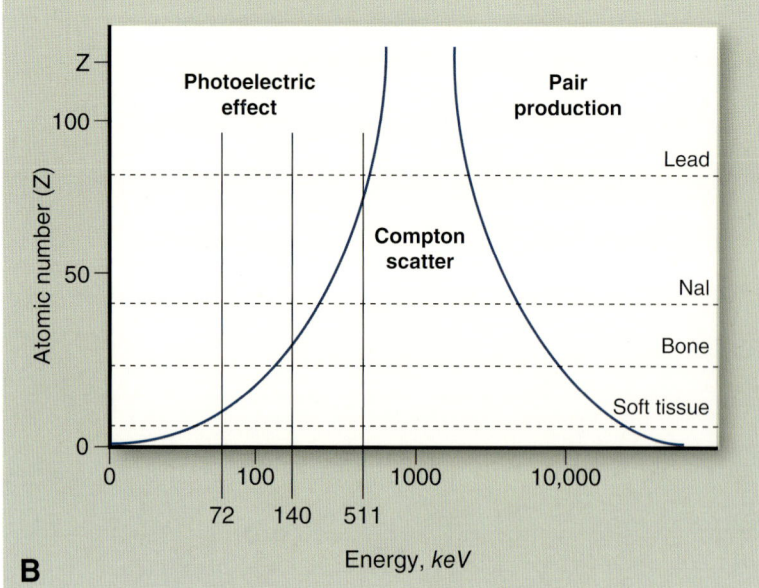

Figure 1-6. Interaction of radiation with matter: photons. High-energy photons, such as γ- and x-rays, interact with matter in three ways that are relevant to nuclear medicine: photoelectric effect, Compton scatter, and pair production [3]. Each of these processes results in the emission of charged particles (electrons or positrons) that produce much more ionization than the original event. Thus high-energy photons are classified as secondary ionizing radiation.

A, The photoelectric effect (or photoelectric absorption) occurs when a photon (γ- or x-ray) is completely absorbed as it interacts with an inner-shell electron. All the energy is lost to the electron, now called a photoelectron, which is emitted from the atom with an energy equivalent to the photon energy (E_0) less the binding energy of the electron ($E_{Binding}$). After photoelectric absorption, the atom has a vacancy in an inner electron shell that will be filled by an outer-shell electron, resulting in the emission of characteristic x-rays and possibly auger electrons.

Compton scattering occurs when a photon interacts with an outer-shell electron, changing direction and losing some energy. The amount of energy of the photon after scattering depends on the angle of scatter (Θ) according to the following formula:

$E_{sc} = E_0/1 + (E_0/511\ keV) \times (1 - \cos(\Theta))$

In this formula, E_0 is the energy of the photon before scattering, E_{sc} is the energy of the photon after scattering, and Θ is the angle between the photon's original path and its new one. The larger the angle, the more energy lost. Maximum energy is lost when the photon reverses course (Θ = 180°) and backscatters. All the energy lost to the γ-ray ($E_0 - E_{sc}$) is transferred to the electron, which on ejection from the atom is called a *recoil electron* (the binding energy of the outer-shell electron is negligible). Energies of Compton-scattered photons as a function of angle are given in Figure 1-7.

Pair production occurs when a photon passes near a charged particle (usually the nucleus of an atom). The photon is destroyed, and a positron–electron pair (β+, β-) is created. According to the formula $E = mc^2$, the mass of the electron is equivalent to 511 keV, thus the photon has to have at least 1022 keV for pair production to occur. Energy in excess of 1022 keV is shared by the positron and the electron as kinetic energy. Because of the high energy required for the process, it is of little importance in clinical nuclear medicine laboratories.

B, The most probable interactions between high-energy photons and matter depend on the energy of the photons and the density of the material. Compton scatter is by far the most common interaction within the patient from the photons produced by clinical radiopharmaceuticals. The photoelectric effect is more likely to take place in the lead shielding of the collimator.

Energies of Compton-Scattered Photons in Kiloelectron Volts

		Scattering angle			
Radionuclide	E_0, keV	30°	60°	90°	180°
Thallium-201	72	71	67	63	56
Technetium-99m	140	135	123	110	90
Positron annihilation	511	451	341	256	170

Figure 1-7. Energies of Compton-scattered photons (E_0) in kiloelectron volts. The table shows the relationship between the photopeak energy of common radionuclides used in nuclear cardiology, the scattering angle of the Compton-scattered photon, and the resulting energy of that photon. Note that in many instances, the original emitted photon may undergo a large scatter angle and still be counted by a 20% energy window in a camera's pulse height analyzer.

Figure 1-8. Photon attenuation. As photons are absorbed through the photoelectric effect or scattered away from the detector through Compton scatter, their loss is called *attenuation*. The percentage of photons lost depends on the energy of the photons, the density of the material, and the material's thickness. The dependence on thickness is straightforward: the thicker the material, the more photons will be absorbed. The thickness at which half of the photons are absorbed is called the half-value layer (HVL). In the example, N_0 photons pass through a material after 1 HVL, one half of photons, has been lost; after 2 HVLs, only one fourth of the photons is left. In practice, the attenuation of a beam of photons is usually calculated using the linear attenuation coefficient ($\mu = \ln 2 / HVL$) in the following equation:

$$I = I_0 \, e^{-\mu x}$$

In this equation, I_0 is the initial beam intensity and I is the intensity after traveling through thickness x. The values of linear attenuation coefficients depend on the energy of the photon and the composition of the material. The denser the material and the higher the energy of the photon, the less attenuation and the lower the value of μ. Linear attenuation coefficients and HVLs for radionuclides and materials of interest to nuclear cardiology are given in Figure 1-9.

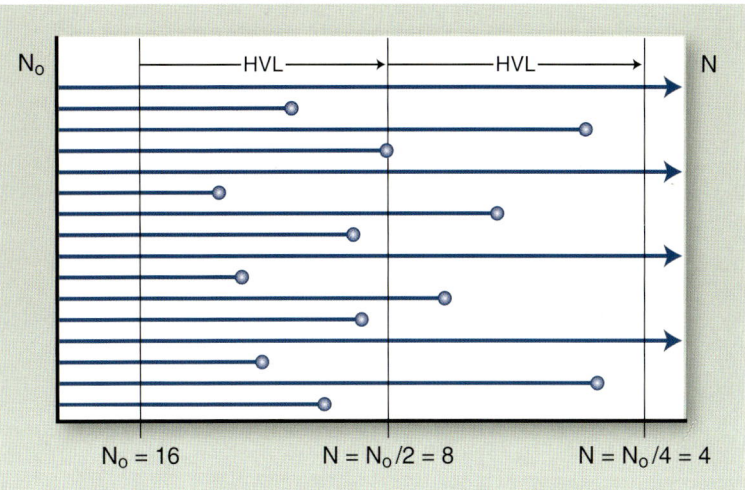

Linear Attenuation Coefficients and Half-Value Layers

Radionuclide	Energy, keV	Soft tissue (1.0 g/cm³) μ, 1/cm	HVL, cm	Bone (1.9 g/cm³) μ, 1/cm	HVL, cm	Lead (11.3 g/cm³) μ, 1/cm	HVL, cm
Thallium-201	72	0.191	3.62	0.493	1.40	39.1	0.018
Technetium-99m	140	0.153	4.52	0.295	2.35	30.7	0.023
Positron annihilation	511	0.095	7.28	0.170	4.08	1.78	0.390

Figure 1-9. Linear attenuation coefficients and half-value layers (HVL). The table shows the relationship between the photopeak energy of common radionuclides used in nuclear cardiology and their corresponding linear attenuation coefficient (μ) and HVL in soft tissue, bone, and lead. Note that the denser the material, the smaller the HVL has to be in order to reduce the photon beam by 50%. The values in the table were calculated from data obtained from Hubble and Seltzer [4].

Principles of Nuclear Cardiology Imaging

Figure 1-10. Interaction of radiation with matter: charged particles. High-energy charged particles such as alpha particles (α), beta particles (β), and the photoelectrons and recoil electrons discussed earlier slow down and lose energy as they pass through matter. This loss is a result of the forces their charge exerts on the electrons (and to a lesser extent, on the nuclei) of the material. These interactions are called *collisions*. The loss of energy is termed *collisional losses* (even though it does not actually involve a collision between the two particles) or *radiation losses*, depending on the nature of the encounter.

Beta particles have the same mass as electrons, and as they pass through material, the electrical forces of the electrons (attractive for β+ and repulsive for β-) cause them to change course with each interaction. These collisions transfer some of the beta particles' energy to the orbital electrons, causing them to escape orbit (the ejected electron is called a delta ray) or to be raised to a higher energy state (excitation). Because of their tortuous path, the depth that beta particles will penetrate a material (range) varies between different beta particles of the same energy, a process called *straggling*. Two measures of the depth of penetration of beta particles are the extrapolated range (an estimation of the maximum positron penetration) and the average range (the mean penetration). A short positron range is desirable for positron emission tomography (PET) imaging because PET determines the origin of the electron–positron annihilation event, not the actual site of the positron emission. Figure 1-11 presents extrapolated and average ranges for several PET radionuclides.

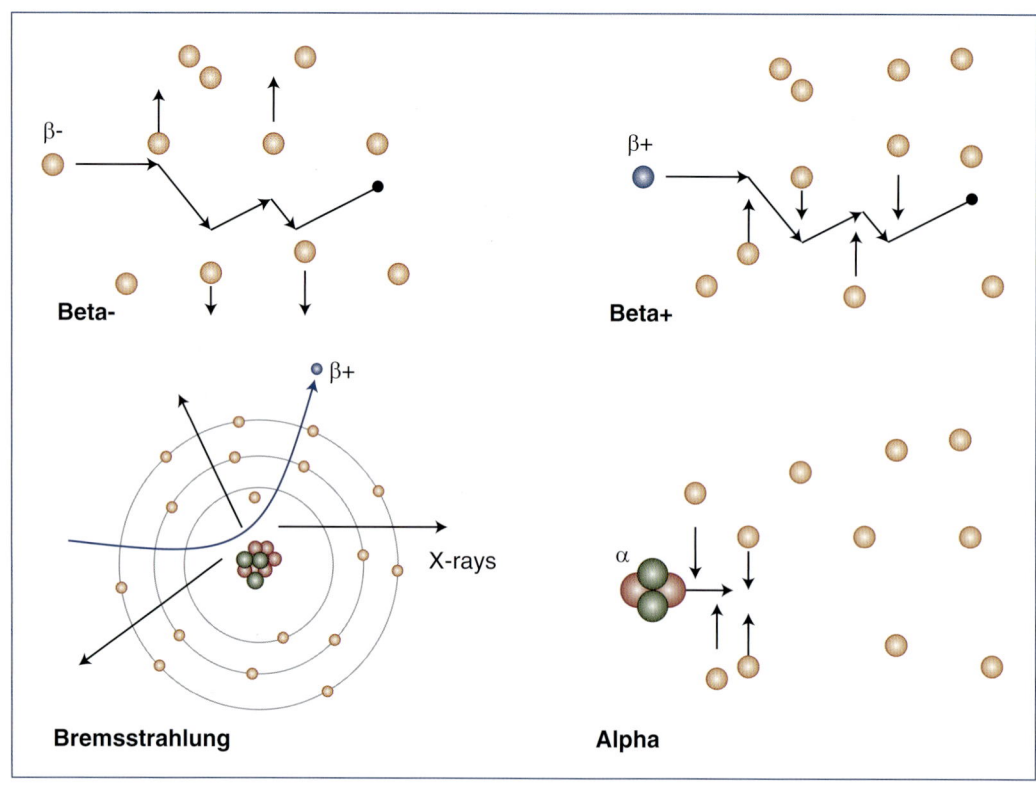

Alpha particles are much more massive than electrons. As collisions occur between alpha particles and electrons, the electrons are excited or swept from orbit, but the encounter has little effect on the direction of the alpha particle. As a result, alpha particles of the same energy all have the same range, with very little straggling. The range is also very small, so that alpha particles present very little danger as an external radiation source given that they are stopped by a few centimeters of air or a few micrometers of tissue.

Figure 1-11. Positron particle range. The table shows the relationship between the maximum energy of the emitted positron and the distance range that these particles travel in air and water. Note that the lower the energy and the denser the medium, the less it travels and thus the higher the resulting spatial resolution. (*Data from Cherry et al.* [5].)

Positron Particle Range

Radionuclide	Maximum energy, MeV	Extrapolated range, cm Air	Extrapolated range, cm Water	Average range, cm Water
Carbon-11	0.961	302	0.39	0.103
Nitrogen-13	1.19	395	0.51	0.132
Oxygen-15	1.723	617	0.80	0.201
Fluorine-18	0.635	176	0.23	0.064
Rubidium-82	3.35	1280	1.65	0.429

6 Atlas of Nuclear Cardiology

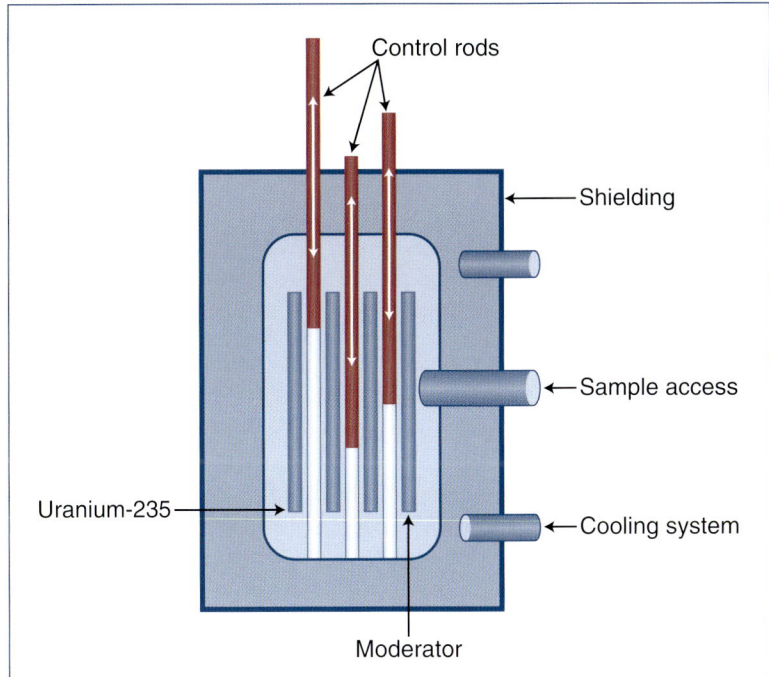

Figure 1-12. Formation of radionuclides: nuclear reactors. The radionuclides used in nuclear cardiology do not occur naturally and must be manufactured. This may be done by extracting them from the spent fuel of a nuclear reactor, bombarding a target nuclide with high-energy neutrons to make a nuclide that is neutron rich (too many neutrons to be stable), or bombarding a target with high-energy positively charged particles, such as protons, using a cyclotron or other particle accelerator to make proton-rich nuclides. Generators are devices that allow separation of a daughter radionuclide from the parent in a shielded container that may be transported long distances from the manufacturing site (reactor or accelerator).

Nuclear reactors are an important source of radionuclides for nuclear medicine, including iodine-131 and xenon-133. Most importantly, molybdenum-99 (^{99}Mo), the parent of technetium-99m, is produced in a nuclear reactor. The heart of a nuclear reactor is a core of fissionable material (usually uranium-235 [^{235}U] and ^{238}U). Fission splits the uranium nucleus into two lighter nuclei and produces two or three fission neutrons. Some of these neutrons strike other uranium nuclei, converting them to ^{236}U. ^{236}U quickly undergoes fission and produces many more fission neutrons, which stimulate even more fission events. The uranium in the core is surrounded by a moderator ("heavy water" and graphite) that slows down the fission neutrons to an energy that is more likely to produce further reactions. The ensuing nuclear chain reaction is regulated by control rods that absorb neutrons made of boron or cadmium. Fission products usually have an excess of neutrons and decay further with emission. More than 100 nuclides are created in the fission process. These fragments can be extracted by chemical means from material removed from the core. Another way to use a nuclear reactor to produce radionuclides, neutron activation, is to place a target into the high-neutron flux of the core while keeping it isolated from the core itself. ^{99}Mo can be produced by either process, but most is extracted as a fission fragment.

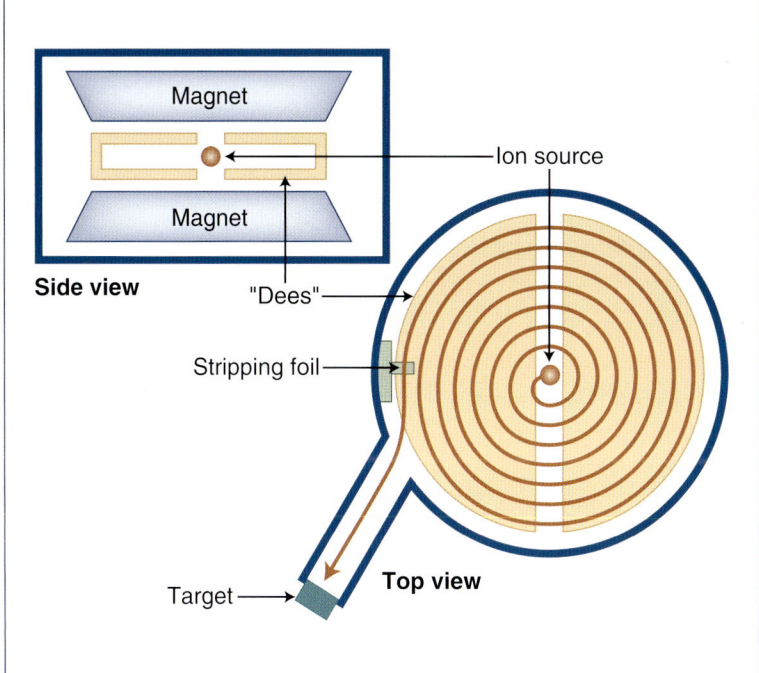

Figure 1-13. Formation of radionuclides: cyclotrons. Cyclotrons are charged particle accelerators that are used to produce radionuclides by bombarding a target with particles or ions that have been accelerated to high rates of speed. The two basic components of a cyclotron are a large electromagnet and semicircular, hollow electrodes called "dees" because of their shape. Ions are injected into the center of the device between the dees. An alternating current applied to the dees causes the ions to be attracted to one side. Once inside the dee, the ion will travel in a curve because any charged particle moving in a magnetic field (supplied by the electromagnet) moves in a circular path. Although there is no electric field inside the dee, the current is carefully timed so that the polarization of the dees changes as the particles emerge from one side. This accelerates the ions, and their arc of travel becomes larger as they move faster and faster, picking up speed each time they cross the gap between the dees. At the maximum radius, the ions are deflected out of the cyclotron and strike a target, creating new nuclides. An example of this is the use of a cyclotron to bombard an oxygen-18 target with protons, resulting in conversion of the nucleus to fluorine-18 (after emission of a neutron). Several cyclotron-produced radionuclides used in nuclear cardiology are listed in Figure 1-14.

Positive-ion cyclotrons accelerate alpha particles or protons and use an electrostatic deflector to direct the ion beam to the target. Negative ion cyclotrons, as shown in the figure, accelerate negative hydrogen (H-) ions, a proton with two electrons. A stripping foil, made of carbon, strips off the two electrons from the ion, leaving a proton. The positive charge of the proton causes it to arch in the opposite direction, causing the beam to exit the cyclotron and strike the target. Most hospital and community-based cyclotrons are negative-ion cyclotrons because they require less shielding and are more compact than positive-ion cyclotrons.

Common SPECT Radionuclides for Use in Nuclear Cardiology

Radionuclide	Production	Decay	Emission, keV	Half-life, h
Iodine-123	Cyclotron	Electron capture	159 (γ-ray)	13.21
Thallium-201	Cyclotron	Electron capture	68–80 (x-ray); 167 (10%; γ-ray)	73
Technetium-99m	Generator	Internal transition	140 (γ-ray)	6

A

Common PET Radionuclides for Use in Nuclear Cardiology

Radionuclide	Production	Positron energy, keV	Half-life, h
Oxygen-15	Cyclotron	735	122 sec
Nitrogen-13	Cyclotron	491	9.96 min
Carbon-11	Cyclotron	385	20.3 min
Fluorine-18	Cyclotron	248	110 min
Rubidium-82	Generator	1523	1.3 min

B

Figure 1-14. Common radionuclides for use in nuclear cardiology. The tables compare the energy of the radiation, half-lives, and modes of production of single-photon emission CT (SPECT) (**A**) versus positron emission tomography (PET) radionuclides (**B**) commonly used in nuclear cardiology procedures. Note that because of the short half-life of most cyclotron-produced PET tracers, a cyclotron must be located nearby. Only fluorine-18 is routinely distributed commercially [6].

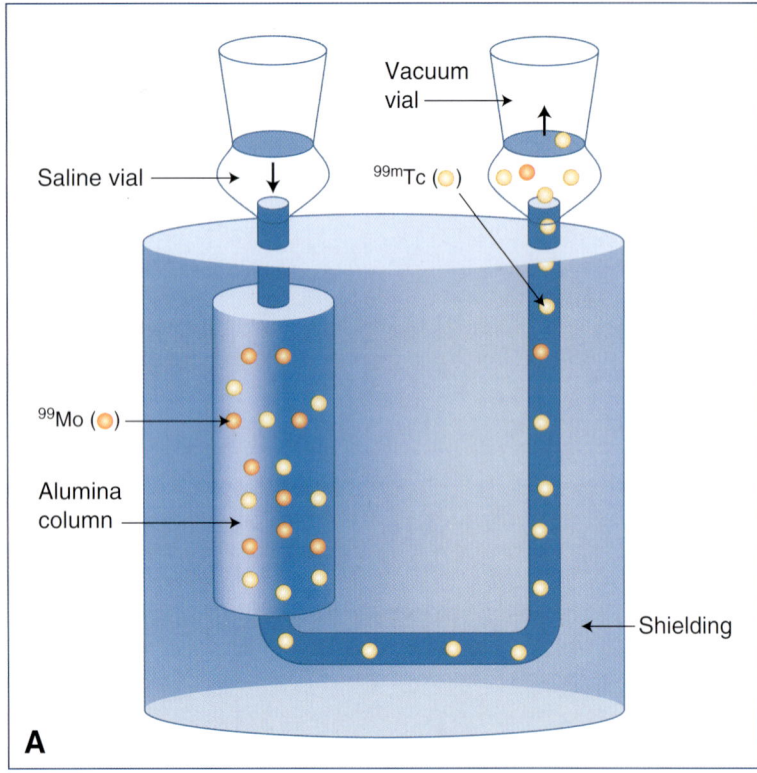

A

Figure 1-15. Formation of radionuclides: molybdenum-99–technetium-99m (^{99}Mo-^{99m}Tc) generator. Generators are devices that allow separation of a radionuclide from a relatively long-lived parent. This allows the production of short-lived radionuclides at a location remote from a reactor or cyclotron (such as a hospital, clinic, or local radiopharmacy). The daughter is continuously replenished by the parent inside the generator, which shields both radionuclides while allowing the daughter to be extracted repeatedly [7].

A, The most common generator used in nuclear medicine is the ^{99}Mo-^{99m}Tc generator, which produces ^{99m}Tc (half-life [t½], 6 hours) from the beta decay of ^{99}Mo (t½, 66 hours). The ^{99}Mo is produced in a nuclear reactor. The heart of the generator is an alumina column impregnated with ^{99}Mo. A vacuum vial is used to pull saline out of a second vial through the porous column. Technetium (both ^{99m}Tc and ^{99}Tc) is washed out of the column by the saline and is collected in a vacuum vial, leaving the ^{99}Mo behind. The generator must be well shielded because ^{99}Mo emits both beta particles and 740 to 780 keV γ-rays. The process of extracting ^{99m}Tc from the generator is called *milking* or *elution*, and the extracted ^{99m}Tc-saline solution is called *eluate*. After milking, the ^{99m}Tc solution must be tested for ^{99}Mo and aluminum. ^{99}Mo is detected using a dose calibrator and a shield that blocks the low-energy photon from ^{99m}Tc. The maximum amount of ^{99}Mo allowed under Nuclear Regulatory Commission regulations is 0.15 Bq ^{99}Mo per kilobecquerel (kBq) ^{99m}Tc (0.15 Ci ^{99}Mo per millicurie [mCi] ^{99m}Tc). Aluminum is detected chemically, with a maximum permissible level of 10 µg/mL of eluate.

Continued on the next page

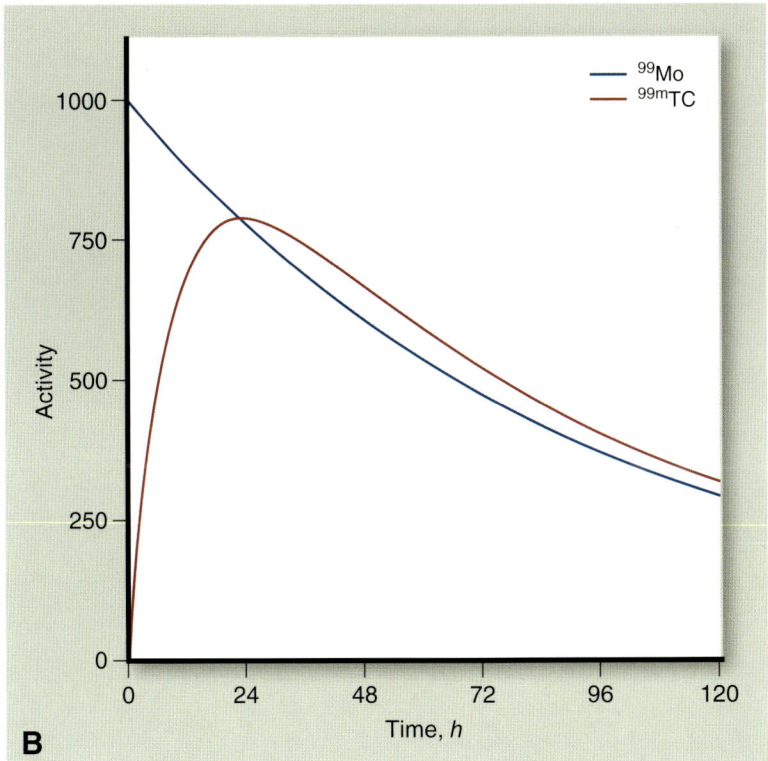

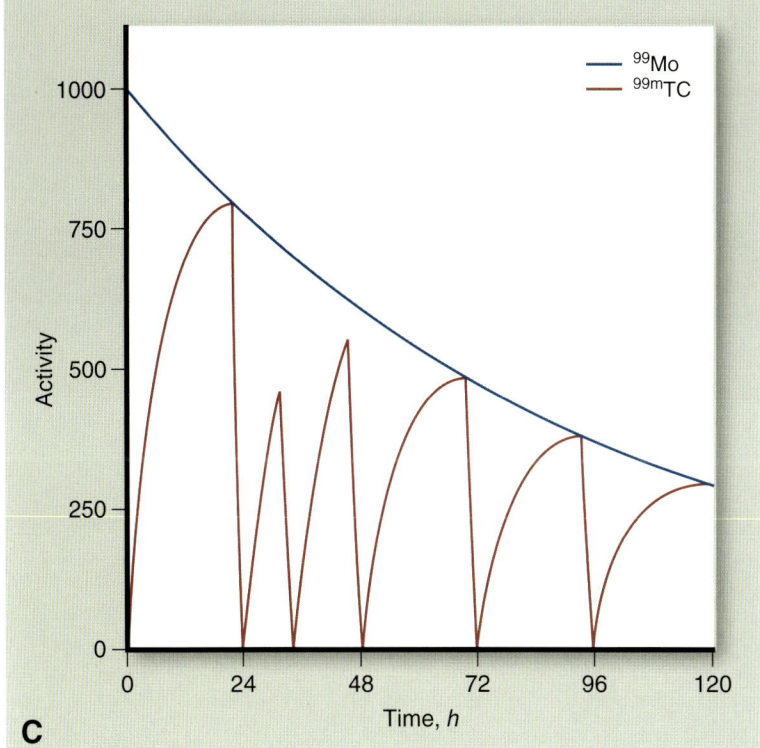

Figure 1-15. *(Continued)* **B,** The ^{99m}Tc produced by beta decay of ^{99}Mo in the alumina column if the generator is undisturbed. This is an example of transient equilibrium in which the parent's half-life is somewhat longer than the daughter's half-life. After a few hours, the daughter activity is almost equal (actually slightly higher) to the parent activity. **C,** Activity in the generator with repeated milkings. Fortunately, the optimal frequency for milking the generator is at intervals slightly less than 24 hours. The dip at 32 hours shows that if the generator is milked, the process of ^{99m}Tc buildup begins again (and in this case results in only slightly less activity at the next regular milking). ^{99}Mo-^{99m}Tc generators are designed to last at least 2 weeks in the nuclear pharmacy.

Another generator of importance to nuclear cardiology is the strontium-82–rubidium-82 (^{82}Sr-^{82}Rb) generator. ^{82}Rb (t½ = 1.3 minutes) is produced by beta decay of ^{82}Sr (t½ = 25 days, manufactured using an accelerator). The daughter activity equals the parent activity very soon after elution and allows elution every hour. This is an example of secular equilibrium in which the parent's half-life is a great deal longer than the daughter's half-life. The short half-life of ^{82}Rb makes it impractical to transport the dose to the patient. The generator is designed to deliver the dose directly into an intravenous line. ^{82}Rb generators are designed to last about a month in the clinic. ^{82}Sr and ^{85}Sr may be low-level contaminants and are found in routine quality control by assaying the eluent after complete decay of the ^{82}Rb.

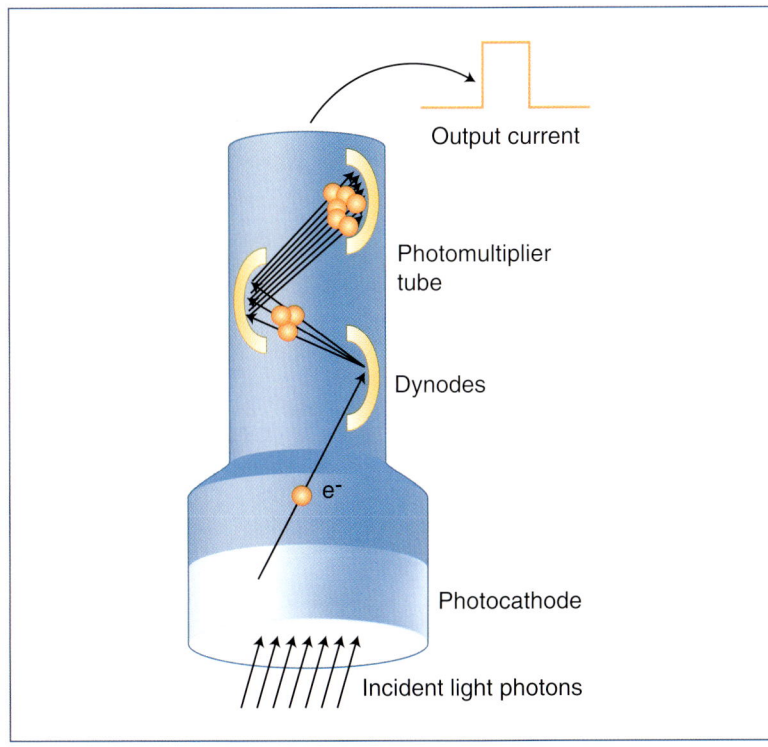

Figure 1-16. Operation of photomultiplier tubes (PMTs). PMTs convert energy from visible light into an electric signal. Light interacting with the material in the photocathode causes it to release electrons, which are accelerated along the tube by a high-voltage differential. As the electrons travel through the tube, they strike metal electrodes called dynodes, at which point even more electrons are ejected. This cascade of multiplication continues until the electrons are output as current at the other end. The voltage (height) of the pulse generated by the PMT is directly proportional to the amount of visible light that strikes the photocathode.

Figure 1-17. Operation of the crystal. The crystal is used to convert γ-rays into visible light. A γ-ray travels through the collimator and interacts with one of the atoms in the crystal, ejecting an electron, called the primary electron, through the photoelectric effect. This ejected electron continues traveling through the crystal, and excites a large number of secondary electrons, which lose their excitation energy by emitting visible light. The glow of the scintillation is converted into electrical signals by the photomultiplier tubes (PMTs). The location of the scintillation event is determined by the positioning circuitry based on the relative signals from the different PMTs. The brightness of the scintillation is proportional to the energy of the photon, measured by the pulse height analyzer.

Note that the γ-ray travels some distance through the crystal before it interacts with a crystal atom. If the crystal is very thin, a γ-ray may travel through the entire width of the crystal with no interaction. Therefore, a thicker crystal results in a higher sensitivity for the detection of γ-rays. Conversely, note that the primary electron travels in an irregular path and may excite atoms far away from its point of origin. The thicker the crystal is, the farther the electron may travel before it exits the crystal. Thus, a thick crystal implies that the scintillation may be more spread out, and this essentially reduces the resolution of the detector. So, just as with collimators, there is a trade-off between sensitivity and resolution with the size and shape of the crystal.

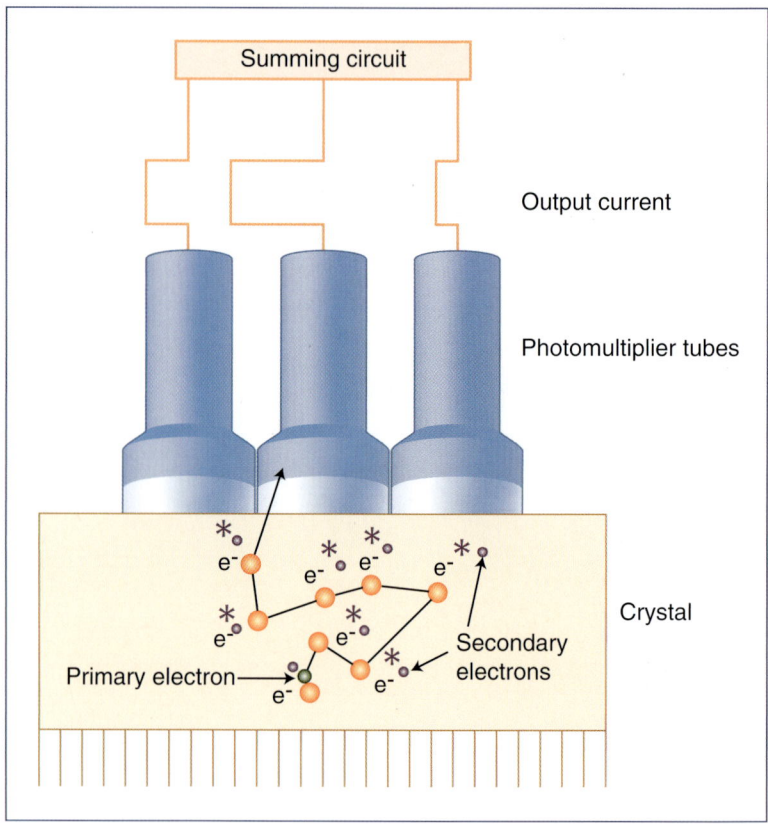

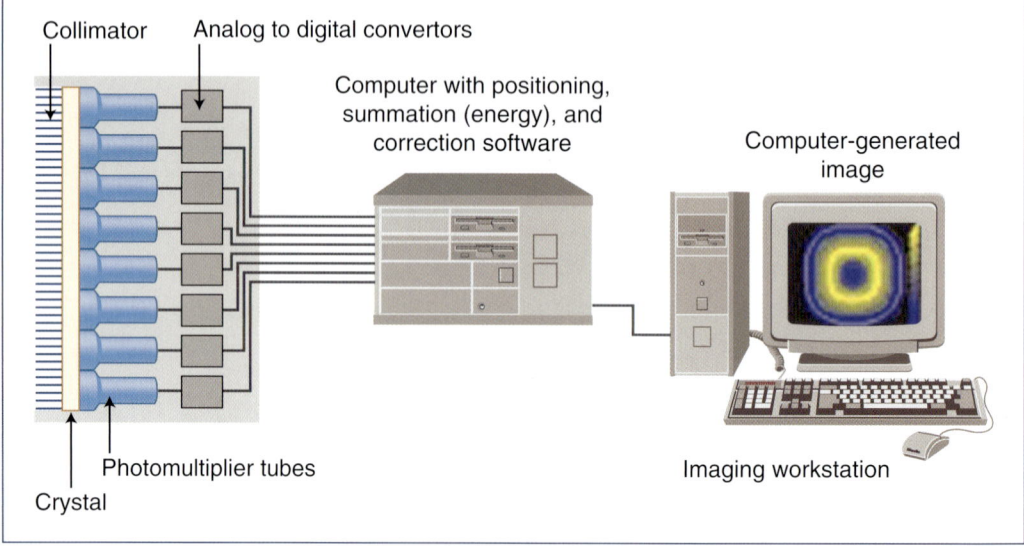

Figure 1-18. Digital scintillation camera. The main components of single-photon emission CT (SPECT) systems are the scintillation camera, the gantry (the frame that supports and moves the heads), and the computer systems (hardware and software). These components work together to acquire and reconstruct the tomographic images.

The basic components of a scintillation camera are a collimator, a sodium iodide crystal, photomultiplier tubes (PMTs), and an analog or digital computer designed to determine the location and energy of a photon striking the crystal. γ-Rays (photons) pass through the collimator and cause a scintillation event (a short burst of visible light) to occur in the crystal. The glow of the scintillation is converted into electrical signals by the PMTs. The location of the scintillation event is determined based on the relative signals from the different PMTs. The brightness of the scintillation is proportional to the energy of the photon. Scintillation cameras were developed in the late 1950s and early 1960s. These cameras used pulse height analyzers and spatial positioning circuitry invented by Hal Anger of the University of California at Berkeley to determine the location and energy of the incident photon [8]. Early cameras were completely analog devices in which the output was sent to an oscilloscope, creating a flash on the screen. A lens focused the screen on a piece of radiographic film that was exposed, one flash at a time. This allowed for planar imaging, but for SPECT, the images must be made available to the computer digitally.

Today, camera systems convert the position and pulse height signals generated from analog circuitry in the camera to digital signals using analog-to-digital converters. The signals may then be further corrected for energy and position through digital processing. Camera designs that convert the output of each PMT to a digital signal, as shown here, have become common. The computer may then perform all of the positioning and pulse height analyses without the need for complicated analog circuitry. This results in greater processing flexibility, greater spatial resolution, and higher count rates.

Another step in the digitization of scintillation cameras is the replacement of PMTs with solid-state detectors called photodiodes. One camera with this design uses individual cesium iodide (CsI) scintillation crystals, each backed with a silicon photodiode. Each CsI crystal is 3 mm^2, giving a resolution similar to that of a conventional camera without the need for positioning circuitry. Elimination of the PMTs greatly reduces the size and weight of the scintillation camera, with some trade-off in cost and energy resolution. These types of cameras are usually known as solid-state cameras.

Figure 1-19. Principle of spatial and contrast resolution. The most common measurements of image quality are spatial resolution and contrast resolution. Spatial resolution refers to how well objects can be separated in space (as opposed to blurring them together), and contrast refers to how well different levels of brightness (representing radionuclide concentration in a scintigram) can be discriminated.

Spatial resolution is the measure of how close two point sources of activity can come together and still be distinguished as separate. Because no medical imaging modality is perfect, a point source never appears as a single bright pixel, but instead as a blurred distribution. Two blurry points eventually smear together into a single spot when they are moved close enough to each other. Resolution is measured by taking a profile (a graph of counts encountered along a line drawn through a region of interest in the image) through a point source and analyzing the resulting curve. A profile through a perfect point source would look like a sharp single spike rising above the flat background. A profile through a real point source appears as a Gaussian-shaped curve; this curve is called the *point spread function*. **A**, When the two Gaussian curves of two point sources get close enough together, they cannot be distinguished as separate. This distance is a measure of image resolution. Two brain tumors are imaged, and a profile is taken through the resulting reconstruction. As the tumors move closer together, the discrete peaks of the profile start to merge into a single peak.

Contrast resolution in nuclear cardiology images can be defined as the measure of counts (or intensity) in the target (the object we are trying to image) compared with the intensity in a background region. High counts in the target increase contrast; high counts in the background region—*eg*, lung uptake—decrease contrast. Low contrast can make the target fade into the background. **B**, Contrast is also easily measured using a profile. The figure shows a count profile taken through a decreased area of a myocardial perfusion image. In this case, the "target" counts are those in the perfusion abnormality and the "background" counts are those in the normal myocardium. The depth of the valley in the profile, compared with the overall height of the rest of the curve, is a measure of contrast.

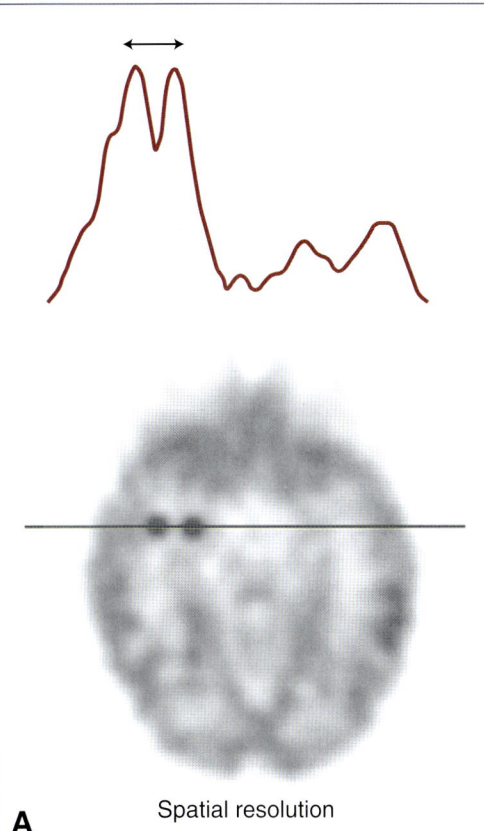
A Spatial resolution

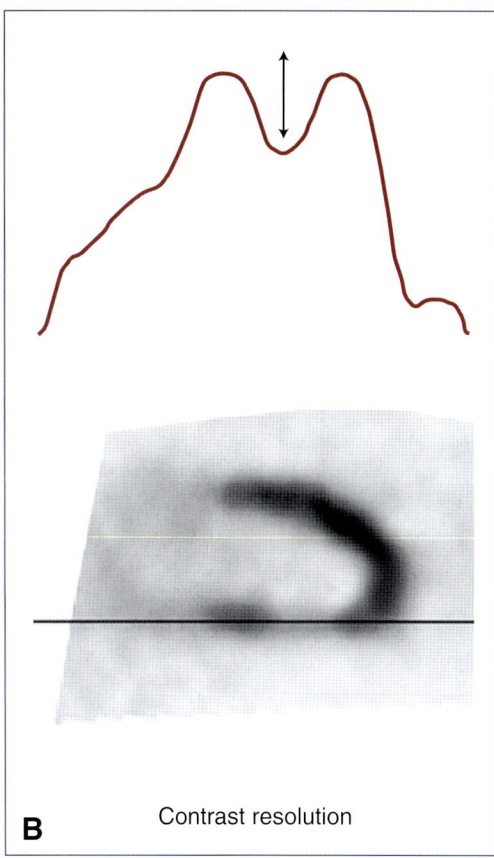
B Contrast resolution

Figure 1-20. Principle of collimation. Because γ-rays are emitted from a source uniformly in all directions, a photon from any area of the body can theoretically strike any area of the detector. Instrumentation is needed to determine the direction of the photon's emission in order to be able to localize the source. This process is called *collimation*. For nuclear cardiology, collimators generally consist of an array of long, narrow (usually) parallel holes that exclude all photons except those that travel parallel to the direction of the hole. Collimators are rated by their sensitivity and resolution. *Resolution* is defined in Figure 1-19; *sensitivity* is the number of photons that travel through the collimator in a certain amount of time (as a fraction of photons emitted from the source), *ie*, counts per second or counts per minute. In this instance, image resolution is affected by collimation because some photons not traveling in exactly a parallel path get through the collimator holes. Thus, a single point source will appear fuzzy on the detector. How much the point "spreads out"—*ie*, the width of its point spread function (PSF)—is related to the spatial resolution and depends on the length and width of the holes. More specifically, spatial resolution is given by the full width of the PSF as half its maximum. Low-energy all-purpose (LEAP) and general-purpose collimators have relatively short, wide holes that accept more photons than do high-resolution collimators with long narrow and/or smaller holes. Increasing the length of the hole increases resolution by decreasing the angle subtended by the hole, and thus, eliminates more γ-rays traveling at angles not parallel to the hole. Thus, a higher resolution is achieved at the cost of sensitivity. In general, the sensitivity and resolution of a collimator are inversely related. A very high-sensitivity collimator will have low resolution, and a very high-resolution collimator will have low sensitivity. Here, the PSFs for different shaped collimators are shown at the *left* of the figure. Note that the width of the PSF curve is broader for LEAP collimators, indicating a lower resolution, but the total area underneath this PSF is higher than that of the high-resolution col-

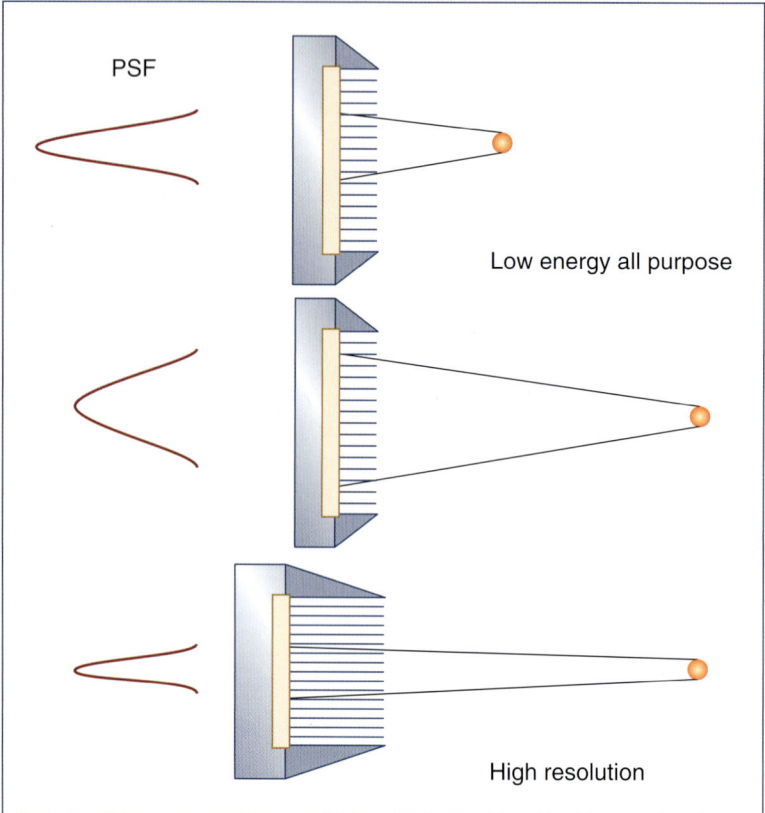

limator, indicating higher sensitivity. The figure also demonstrates that the resolution of the image, as seen by the PSF curves on the *left*, depends on the distance between the source and the collimator. This is discussed in more detail in Figure 1-21.

Figure 1-21. Resolution versus sensitivity. In air, recall that the amount of radiation from a point source falling on a plane decreases as $1/r^2$. However, if a collimator is placed between the source and the detector, this relationship no longer holds. The same number of γ-rays will travel through the collimator, no matter how far the source is from the detector. This is because γ-rays that travel too obliquely from the line of the collimator holes will not pass through any collimator, no matter how close it is to the source. However, a ray that is near enough to parallel to a collimator hole will be able to pass through a collimator, no matter how distant it is to the source. The primary difference between a collimator placed near the source and one placed far away from the source is which collimator hole a γ-ray will pass through.

A γ-ray traveling exactly parallel to the collimator will pass through the hole that is directly "aimed" at the source. If the γ-ray is slightly oblique to the collimator, it may pass through a hole not exactly in line with the source. How far away that hole is from the "correct" hole depends on how far the source is from the collimator. In the figure, notice that when the collimator is close to the source (*A*), most of the γ-rays travel through the collimator holes that are nearly in line with that source, even when those γ-rays are slightly oblique to the holes. However, if the detector is far away from the source (*B*), the same number of γ-rays travel through the collimator but more of the oblique rays travel through holes farther away from the one directly in line with the source. This causes a blurring or loss of resolu-

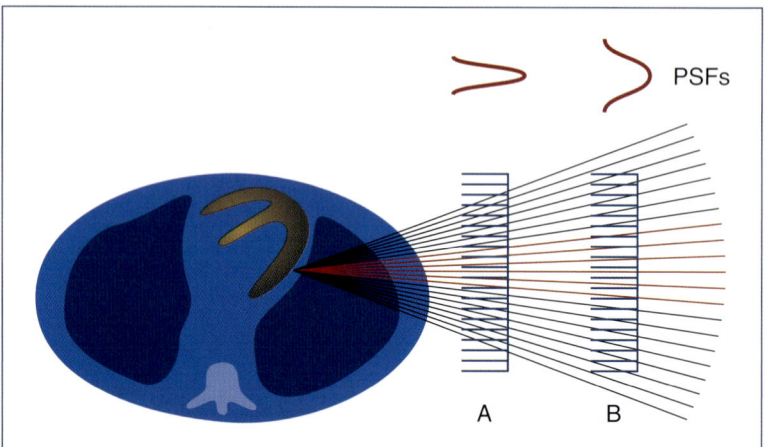

tion, which is seen in the point spread functions (PSFs) shown for each of the collimator positions at the *top* of the figure. Note that the farther away the detector is from the source, the lower and more spread out the PSF; however, the area underneath these curves does not change. Therefore, the number of photons detected stays the same with collimator-source distance, but the image resolution decreases as the distance increases. This resolution decrease with source-to-detector distance is termed *detector response* or *geometric response*.

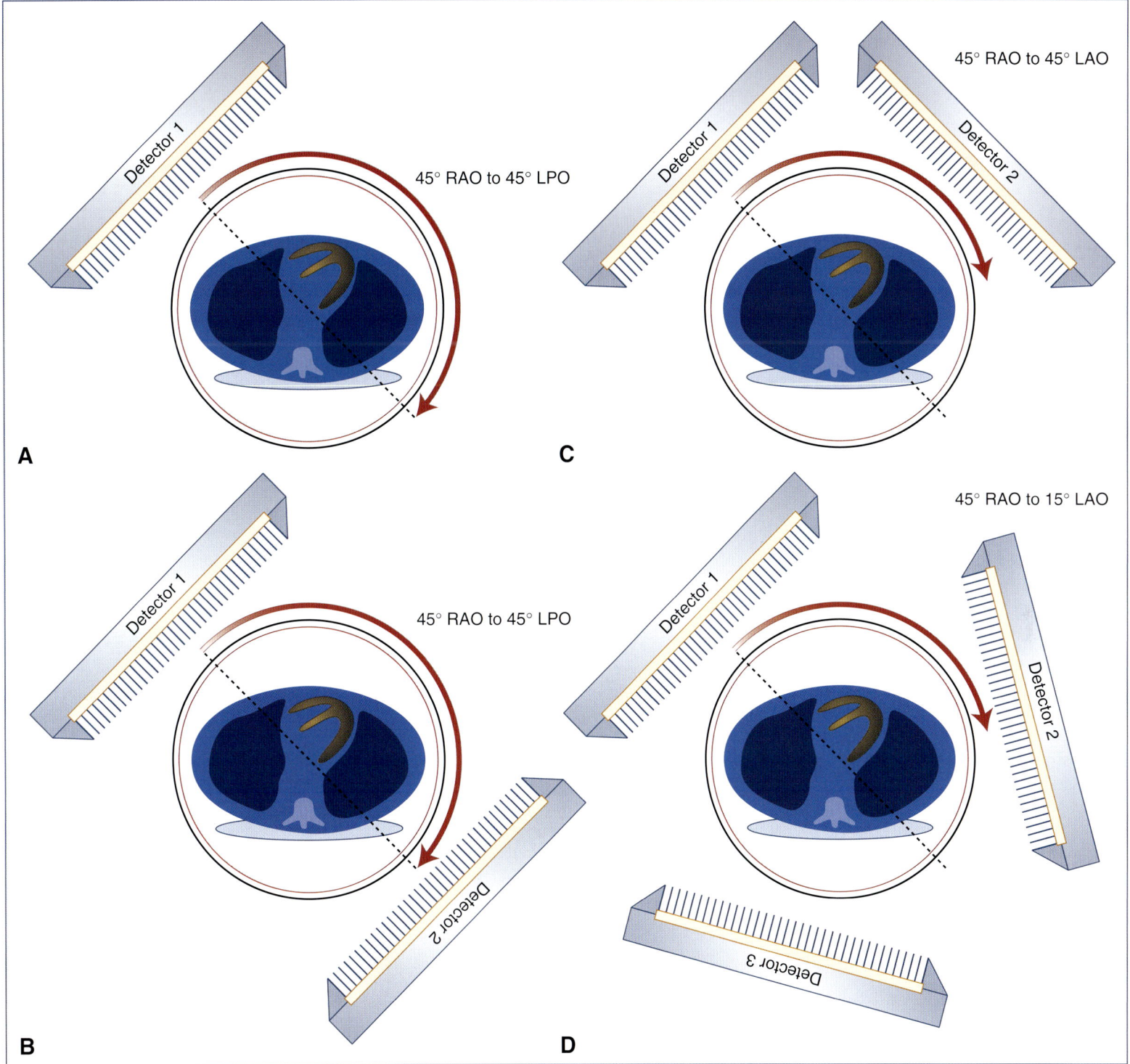

Figure 1-22. Single-photon emission CT (SPECT) cameras: multiheaded cameras. Multidetector SPECT systems have more than one scintillation camera attached to the gantry. **A**, The most obvious benefit of adding more detectors to a scintillation camera system is the increase in sensitivity. Doubling the number of heads doubles the number of photons that may be acquired in the same amount of time. The user may take advantage of the increase in sensitivity by acquiring more counts, adding higher-resolution collimation, or increasing throughput.

B, Two large field-of-view rectangular cameras mounted opposite each other, 180° apart. This configuration may speed 360° SPECT imaging by halving imaging time while collecting the same number of counts, because a full 360° of projections can be acquired by rotating the gantry 180°. **C**, For cardiac SPECT, in which a 180° orbit is recommended, SPECT systems with two detectors mounted next to each other (at 90°) on the gantry allows a full 180° orbit to be acquired while only rotating the gantry through 90°. **D**, Triple detector cameras are usually dedicated to SPECT imaging. The three heads, as discussed for double-headed systems, will result in increased sensitivity that may be used to increase throughput, counts, or resolution. However, if the three detectors are mounted rigidly 120° from one another, the system must rotate through 120° to obtain 180° of data. Thus, these systems also do not have a great impact on cardiac imaging with 180° orbits.

For any multiheaded system, the primary advantage is increase in throughput, because the acquisition will take less time. However, the gain in sensitivity may be traded off to give more precise images by allowing the use of higher-resolution collimators.

Drawbacks of multiple-headed cameras include the increase in quality control required by the addition of the additional heads and some loss of flexibility. Double detector systems do not allow the same flexibility of movement that is enjoyed with many single-headed systems. This may prevent them from being easily used for some types of planar imaging (*eg*, gated blood pool) in which it is often difficult to position the camera correctly. One unique SPECT system acquires planar projections by rotating the patient in an upright position while the camera(s) remain(s) fixed. LAO—left anterior oblique; LPO—left posterior oblique; RAO—right anterior oblique.

Principles of Nuclear Cardiology Imaging 13

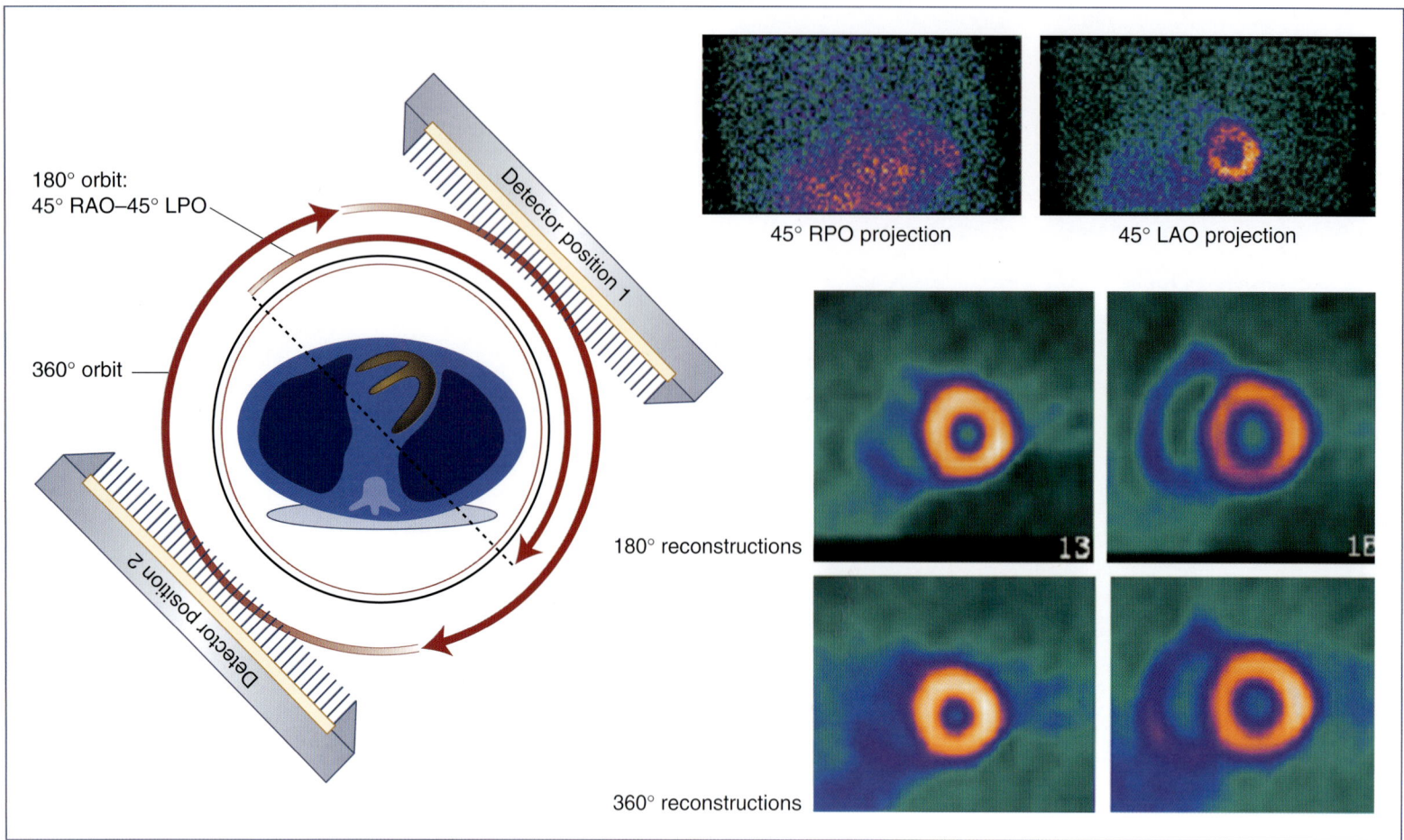

Figure 1-23. Single-photon emission CT (SPECT) cameras: 180° versus 360° data acquisition. Although 360° orbits are generally preferred for body SPECT, 180° orbits may be better for cardiac SPECT. The heart is located forward and to one side of the center of the thorax, resulting in a great deal of attenuation when the camera is behind the patient. The angles chosen for the 180° orbit are those closest to the heart, from 45° right anterior oblique (RAO) to 45° left posterior oblique (LPO). These projections are those that suffer least from attenuation, scatter, and detector response because they are the ones that get the camera head as close as possible to the heart. Projections taken from the posterior aspect of the body are generally noisier and of lower resolution than those taken from the anterior angles. This is easily seen by comparing the 45° left anterior oblique (LAO) projection shown here to the 45° right posterior oblique (RPO) projection. Reconstructions from 180° acquisitions have higher resolution and contrast than those from 360° acquisitions; this is particularly true for thallium-201 images [9–11]. However, because 180° reconstructions are not truly complete—*ie*, new information is available from the other 180° of projections—there are occasional artifacts seen with 180° reconstructions that can be avoided with 360° reconstructions. In particular, 360° reconstructions are generally more uniform than 180° reconstructions. Both of these effects can be seen on the reconstructions on the *bottom right* of the figure.

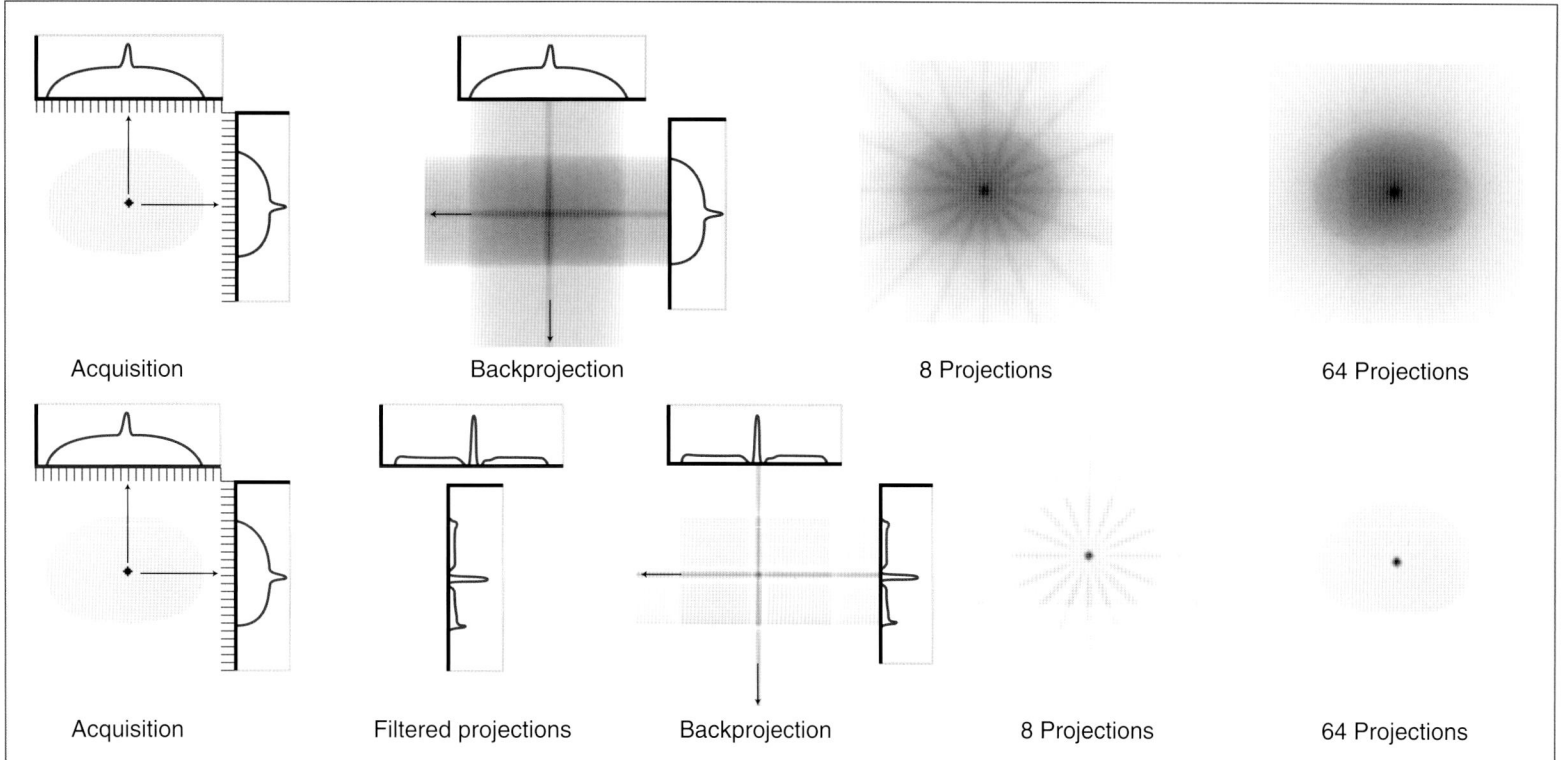

Figure 1-24. Principle of filtered backprojection reconstruction. Filtered backprojection is an analytic method of image reconstruction. Filtered backprojection, as its name implies, is a combination of filtering and backprojection. The principle of backprojection is shown in the *top row*. When a projection image is acquired, each row of the projection contains counts that emanate from the entire transverse plane. When projection images are obtained from many angles about the body, enough information is available in each row of the set of angular projections to reconstruct the original corresponding transverse slice. Backprojection assigns the values in the projection to all points along the line of acquisition through the image plane from which they were acquired. This operation is repeated for all pixels and all angles, adding the new values with the previous, in what is termed a superposition operation. As the number of angles increases, the backprojection improves.

Although simple backprojection is useful for illustrative purposes, it is never used in practice without the step of filtering. Note that the backprojection from the top row is quite blurred compared with the original distribution from which it was created. Also, the reconstructions created from eight projections show instances of the "star artifact," which consists of radial lines near the edges of the object. This artifact is a natural result of backprojection applied without filtering. In clinical practice, the projections are filtered prior to backprojection; filtered backprojection is shown in the *bottom row*. After the projections are acquired, a ramp filter is applied to each of them prior to backprojection. Ramp filters are discussed in more detail in Figure 1-25. The ramp-filtered projections are characterized by enhancement of edge information and the introduction of negative values (or lobes) into the filtered projections. During the backprojection process, these negative values cancel portions of the other angular contributions, and in effect, help to eliminate the star artifact and the blurring seen in the unfiltered backprojection. However, enough projections must be acquired to ensure that proper cancellation is obtained. Radial blurring or streaking toward the periphery of the image often indicates that too few projections were acquired. Finally, a noise-reducing filter such as a Butterworth or Hanning filter is usually applied before, during, or after the backprojection operation. Such filters are discussed in more detail later in the chapter.

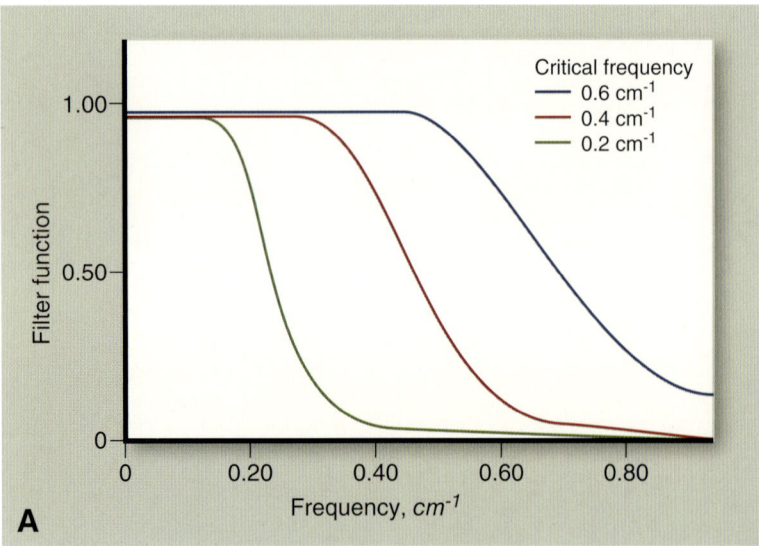
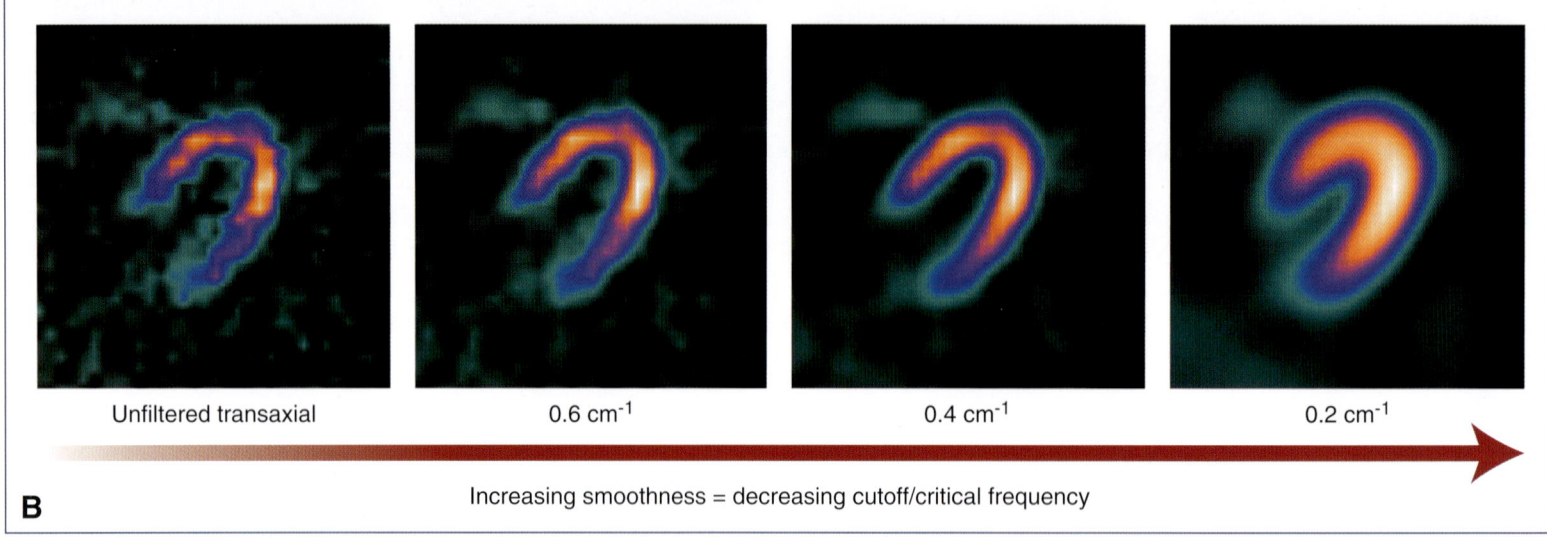

Figure 1-25. Image filtering. Filtering is the process by which images are smoothed, sharpened, reduced in noise, or used in reconstruction, such as the ramp filter in filtered backprojection. Filtering digital images is accomplished by transforming the images from the spatial domain that are used to frequency space [12,13]. This transformation is usually performed using a mathematical process called a Fourier transform. This transform represents images in terms of cycles per centimeter or variations of counts over distance. In this representation, smaller objects, edges of objects that abruptly change in counts, and image noise are all associated with high frequencies. Larger smooth organs are associated with lower frequencies. A filter works by defining a curve that specifies how much of each frequency should be modified. If the filter value is 1 at a specific frequency, then it is not modified; if it is less than 1, it is reduced by that amount; and if it is more than 1, it is enhanced by that amount.

Because the filtered backprojection reconstruction process uses a ramp filter that enhances image noise, smoothing must be applied to the reconstructed images to reduce the image noise. The most common filters used for smoothing cardiac perfusion images are the Hanning and Butterworth filters. Both the Hanning and Butterworth filters are known as low-pass filters because they tend to leave the lower frequencies alone while reducing the higher frequencies. The Butterworth filter is defined by two parameters: the critical frequency and the order of the filter. The critical frequency is used to define when the filter begins to drop to zero (known as the cutoff frequency for a Hanning filter). The order of the filter determines the steepness of the function's downward slope.

A, The *color curves* are three examples of critical frequencies for the Butterworth filter. **B**, The four transaxial cardiac images are examples of that same transaxial image with the various critical frequencies of the Butterworth filter applied. The leftmost transaxial image has had the gray filter applied. Note that the gray filter is 1 for every frequency, and thus no smoothing is performed. This is the original noisy image that results from the filtered backprojection process. The next image has had the purple filter applied with a critical frequency of 0.6 cycles/cm. Note that this image appears slightly smoother than the one with no smoothing. As the other two filters are applied with increasingly lower critical frequencies, the image becomes smoother.

16 Atlas of Nuclear Cardiology

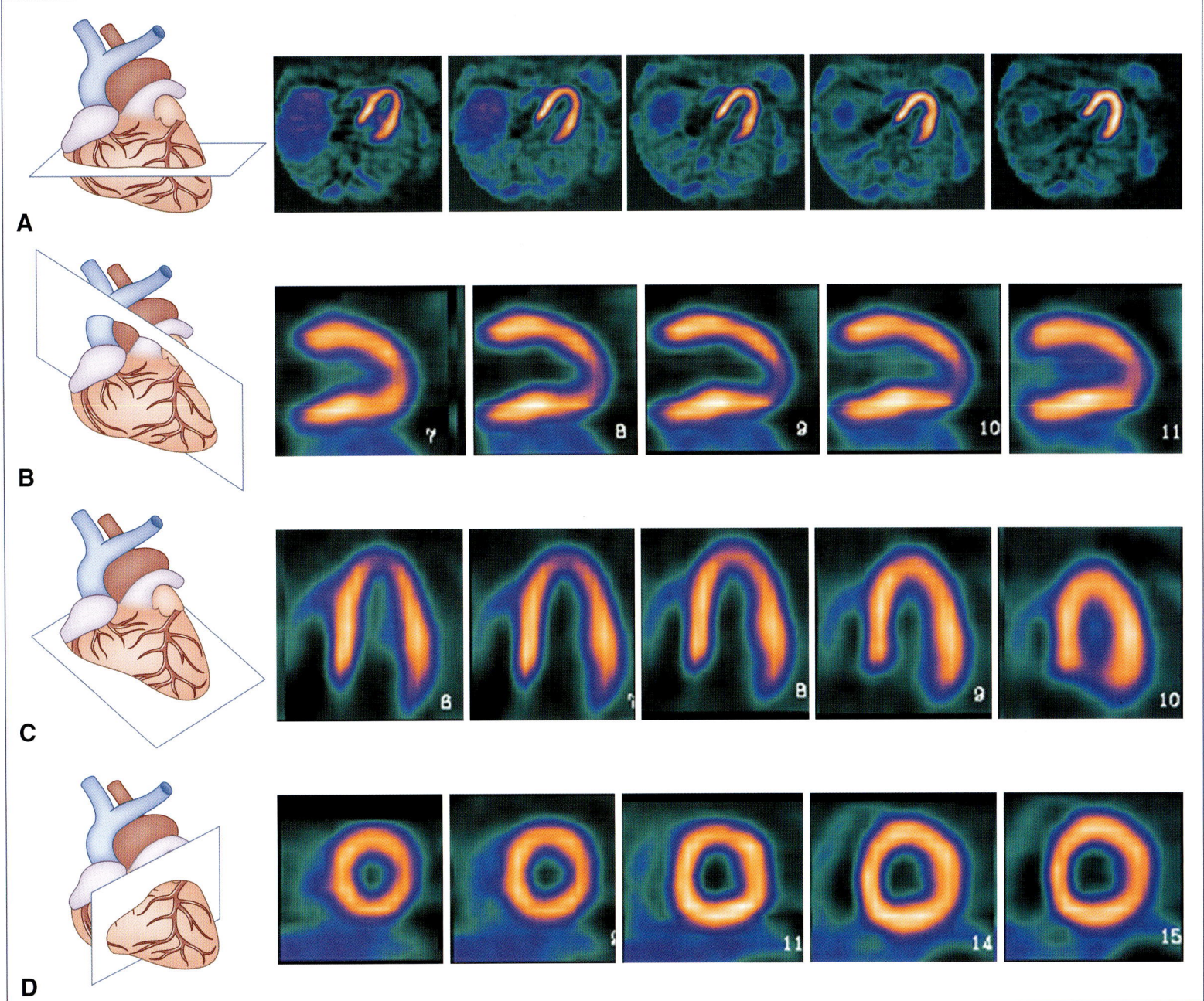

Figure 1-26. Oblique angle reorientation. *Transaxial images:* The natural products of rotational tomography are images that represent cross-sectional slices of the body, perpendicular to the imaging table (or long axis of the body). These images are called transverse or transaxial slices. **A**, An example of transaxial slices.

Oblique images: We are not restricted to the natural x, y, and z directions, however, for the display of images. The computer may be used to extract images at any orientation, and these images are called oblique images. Because of the variation in the heart orientation of different patients, it is important that oblique slices are adjusted to try to match the same anatomy from patient to patient. The important oblique sections used for viewing cardiac images are defined as follows.

Vertical long-axis slices: The three-dimensional set of transaxial sections, some of which are shown in **A**, is resliced parallel to the long axis and perpendicular through the transaxial slices. Each of the resulting oblique images is called a vertical long-axis slice (**B**). They are displayed with the base of the left ventricle toward the left side of the image and the apex toward the right. Serial slices are displayed from medial (septal) to lateral, left to right.

Horizontal long-axis slices: The three-dimensional block of vertical long-axis slices is recut parallel to the denoted long axis and perpendicular to the stack. The resulting oblique cuts are called horizontal long-axis slices (**C**). They contain the left ventricle with its base toward the bottom of the image and its apex toward the top. The right ventricle appears on the left side of the image. Serial horizontal long-axis slices are displayed from inferior to anterior, from left to right.

Short-axis slices: Slices perpendicular to the denoted long axis and perpendicular to the vertical long-axis slices are also cut from the stack. These are termed short-axis slices; they contain the left ventricle with its anterior wall toward the top, its inferior wall toward the bottom, and its septal wall toward the left. **D**, Serial short-axis slices are displayed from apex to base, from left to right.

Principles of Nuclear Cardiology Imaging

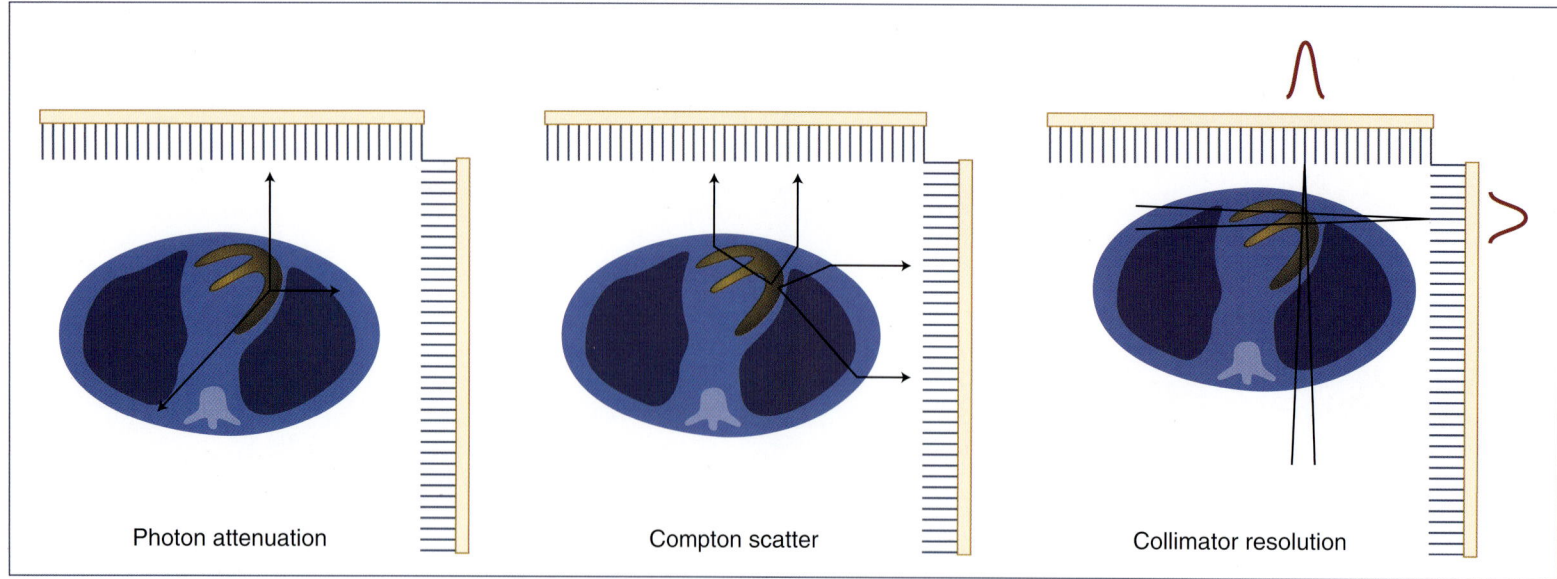

Figure 1-27. Physical factors that may affect single-photon emission CT (SPECT) image formation. Accurate reconstructions of the radionuclide distribution in the body depend on accurate detection of the emitted γ-rays. However, not all of the γ-rays emitted by a radionuclide emerge from the body, and those that do are not all detected in the right place. These complicating factors degrade the resulting image. The three factors that cause degradations in SPECT are attenuation, scatter, and distance-dependent resolution or blur of collimation. Attenuation is the absorption of γ-rays by other materials and includes photons lost because of both the photoelectric effect and Compton scatter. The probability that a γ-ray is absorbed increases with the density of the material through which it must pass, but decreases with increasing energy of the photon.

Other γ-rays may interact with electrons in the material through which they are passing, causing them to change direction and lose energy. These γ-rays may still emerge from the body, but from a direction other than their original path. If these γ-rays are detected by the gamma camera, they appear to be originating from the wrong place. Finally, γ-rays traveling in paths other than parallel to a collimator hole may still travel through that hole and be detected by the camera. This becomes more likely as the source gets farther and farther away from the collimator. The result is a blurring in the final image that depends on the distance between the source and collimator, called the detector response, which is discussed in Figure 1-21.

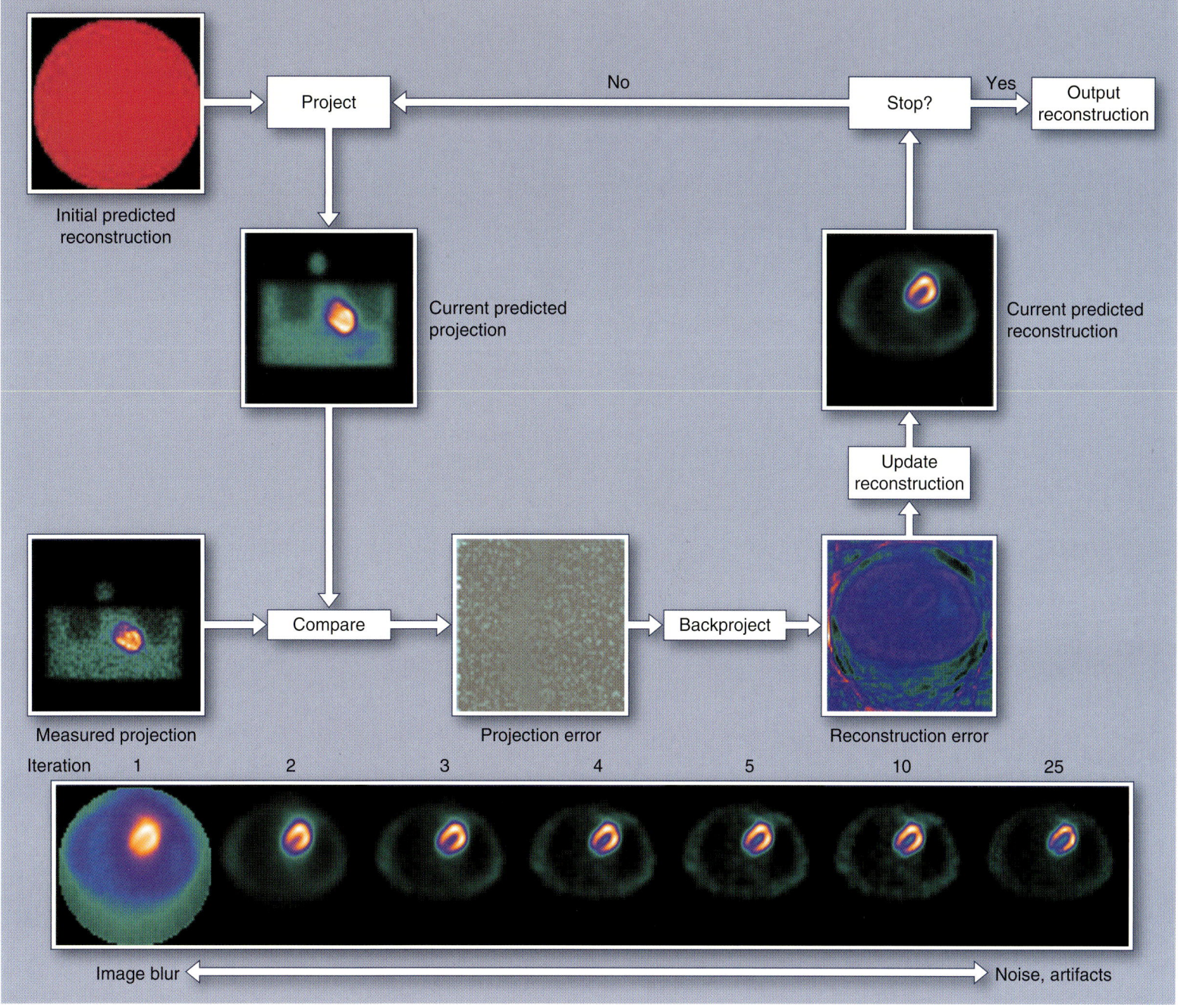

Figure 1-28. Principle of iterative reconstruction. Iterative reconstruction techniques require many more calculations and thus much more computer time to create a transaxial image than does filtered backprojection. However, their great advantage is their ability to incorporate corrections for the factors that degrade single-proton emission CT images into the reconstruction process. Iterative techniques use the original projections and models of the acquisition process to predict a reconstruction. The predicted reconstruction is then used again with the models to recreate new predicted projections. If the predicted projections are different from the actual projections, these differences are used to modify the reconstruction. This process is continued until the reconstruction is such that the predicted projections match the actual projections. The primary differences between various iterative methods are how the predicted reconstructions and projections are created and how they are modified at each step. Practically speaking, the more theoretically accurate the iterative technique, the more time consuming the process. Maximum likelihood methods allow the noise to be modeled, whereas least squares techniques such as the conjugate gradient method generally ignore noise.

The most widely used iterative reconstruction method is maximum-likelihood expectation maximization (MLEM) [14]. The MLEM algorithm attempts to determine the tracer distribution that would "most likely" yield the measured projections given the imaging model and a map of attenuation coefficients, if available. An example of the reconstruction of the myocardium with the MLEM algorithm is shown at the *bottom*. The point of convergence of this algorithm and related number of iterations for clinical use are a source of debate. To date, there is no common rule for stopping the algorithms after an optimal number of iterations on clinical data, and protocols describing the optimal number of iterations are largely empirically based. As can be seen in the reconstructions at the bottom, as iteration number increases, the images generally get less blurry but more noisy.

Another approach to the MLEM algorithm for iterative reconstruction is the ordered-subsets expectation maximization (OSEM) approach [15]. This approach performs an ordering of the projection data into subsets. The subsets are used in the iterative steps of the reconstruction to greatly speed up the reconstruction. The advantage of the OSEM is that an order of magnitude increase in computational speed can be obtained.

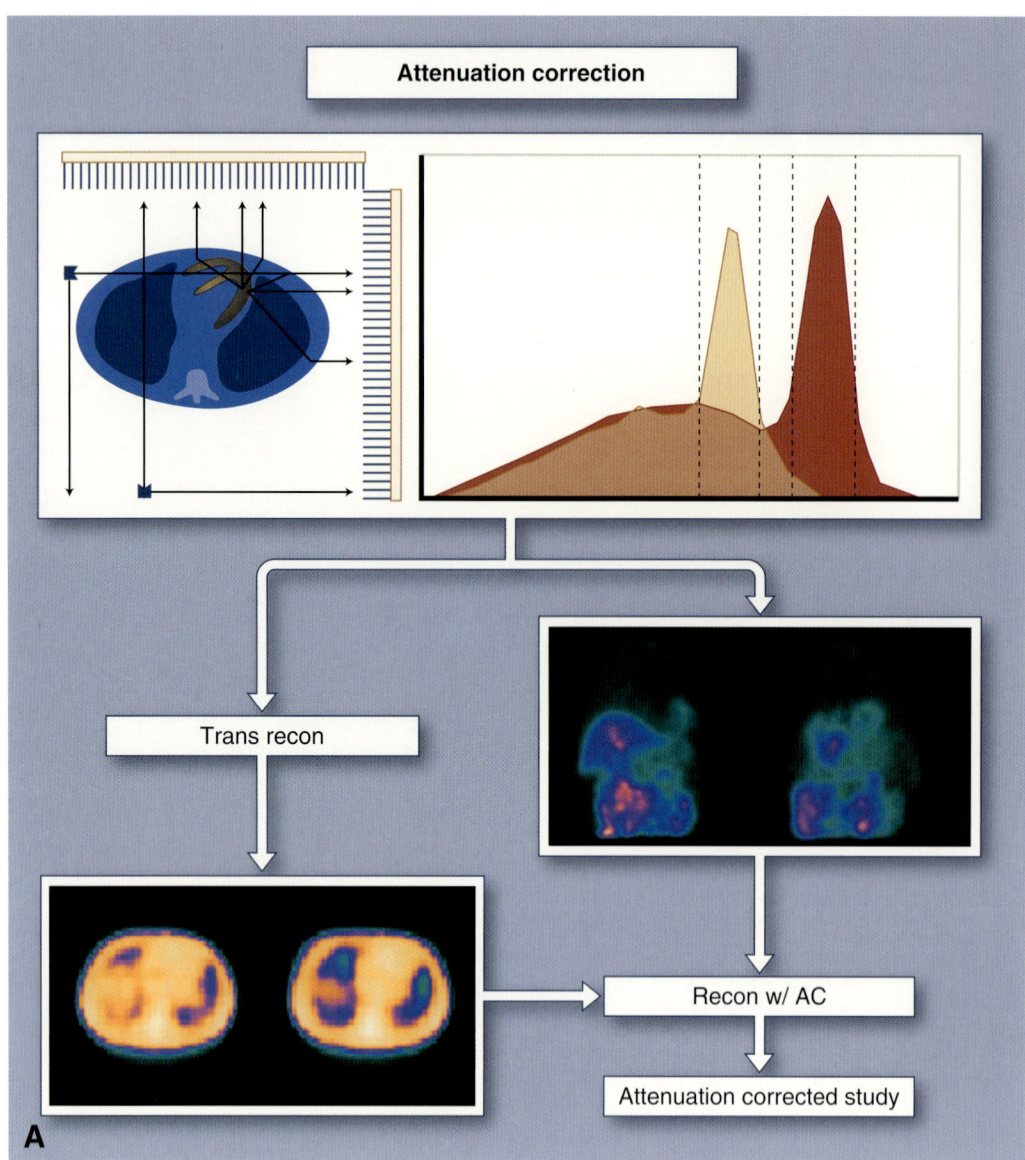

Figure 1-29. Single-photon emission CT (SPECT) attenuation correction (AC) and scatter correction. **A**, SPECT myocardial perfusion imaging uses transmission scan–based AC. Transmission scanning measures the distribution of attenuation coefficients (attenuation map) of the patient, which is used in iterative reconstruction to correct for the decrease in counts resulting from photon attenuation.

Continued on the next page

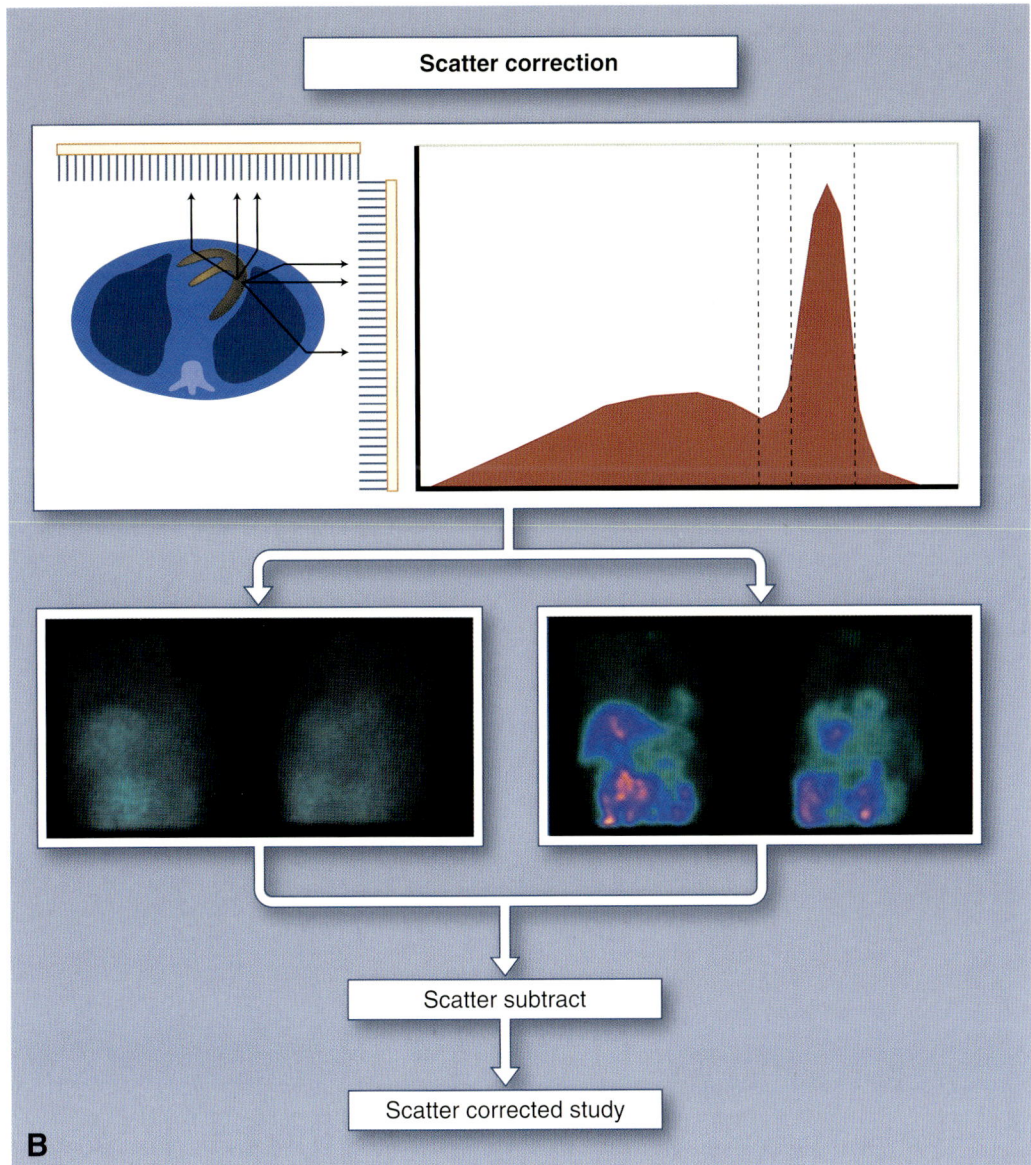

Figure 1-29. *(Continued)* **B,** SPECT scatter correction uses the Compton window subtraction method [16]. In this method, an image that consists of scattered photons is acquired by a second energy window placed below the photopeak window, and this image is multiplied with a scaling factor and then subtracted from the acquired photopeak window image to produce a scatter-corrected image. Another energy window–based approach uses two energy windows, one above and one below the photopeak window, to estimate the portion of scattered photons in the photopeak window [17].

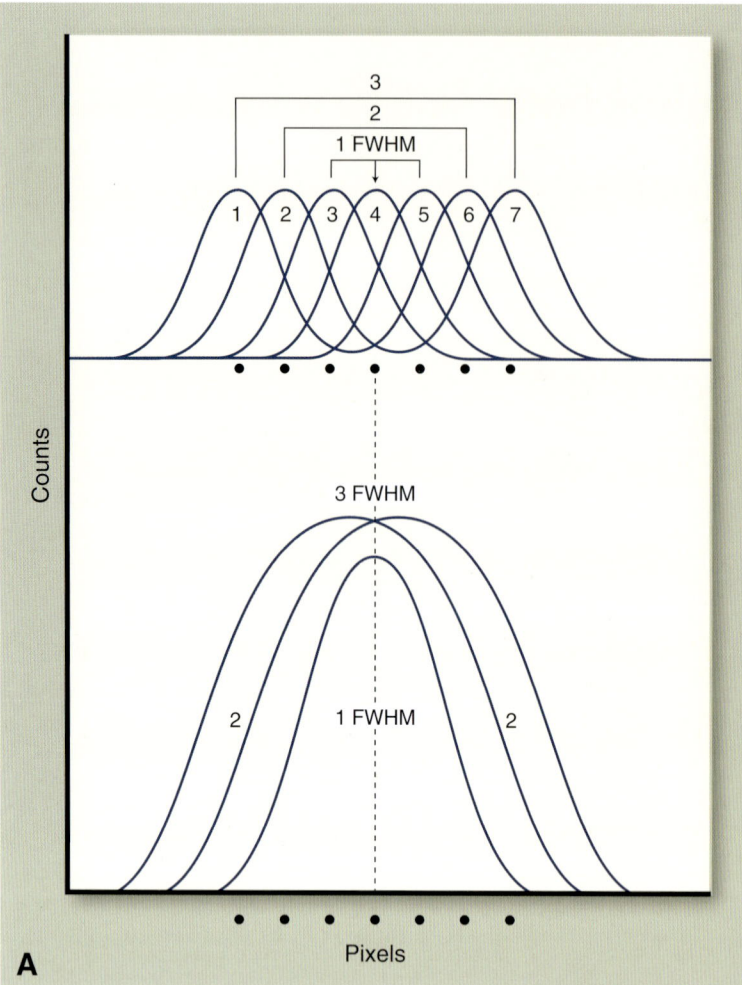
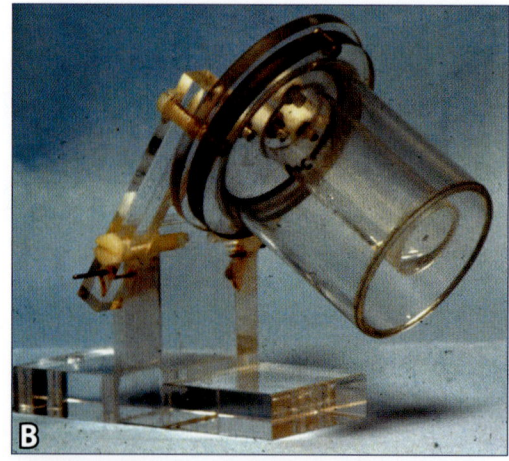
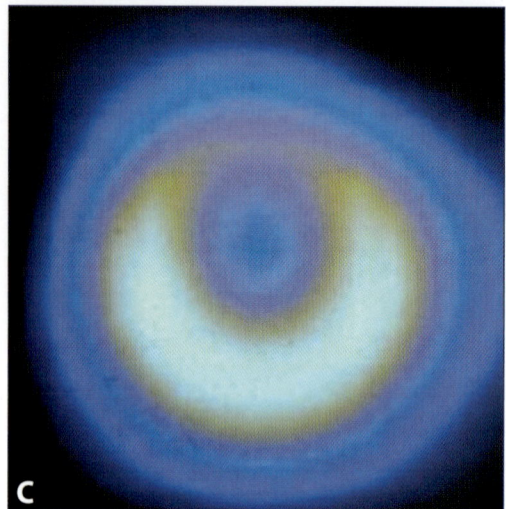

Figure 1-30. A, Partial volume effect. The inherent limitation of the resolution of nuclear imaging systems makes the image of a point source appear as a Gaussian curve. Therefore, the image of an object made up of multiple points appears as overlapping Gaussian curves, which have a value for the center point higher than that for the periphery point, even when the object has uniform distribution of the radiotracer. As a result of this phenomenon, myocardial brightness increases when myocardial thickness increases [18] up to twice the resolution of the system (FWHM), as shown here. If the object is thicker than 2 times FWHM, the resulting count profile will reach a plateau representative of the true expected counts. **B** and **C,** This effect is used quite successfully to assess left ventricular regional myocardial thickness and thickening, but care must be taken when interpreting gated single-photon emission CT images because the myocardium appears brighter in areas where it is thicker and dimmer in areas where it is thinner. The figure shows a study in which a phantom representing an eccentric myocardial chamber is filled with a constant concentration of thallium-201.

Note the thinner anterior wall appears to be hypoperfused in comparison to the inferior wall. This can be a cause of misinterpretation when, for example, the patient has a hypertrophic, thickened septum, making the left ventricular lateral wall with normal thickness and perfusion appear hypoperfused.

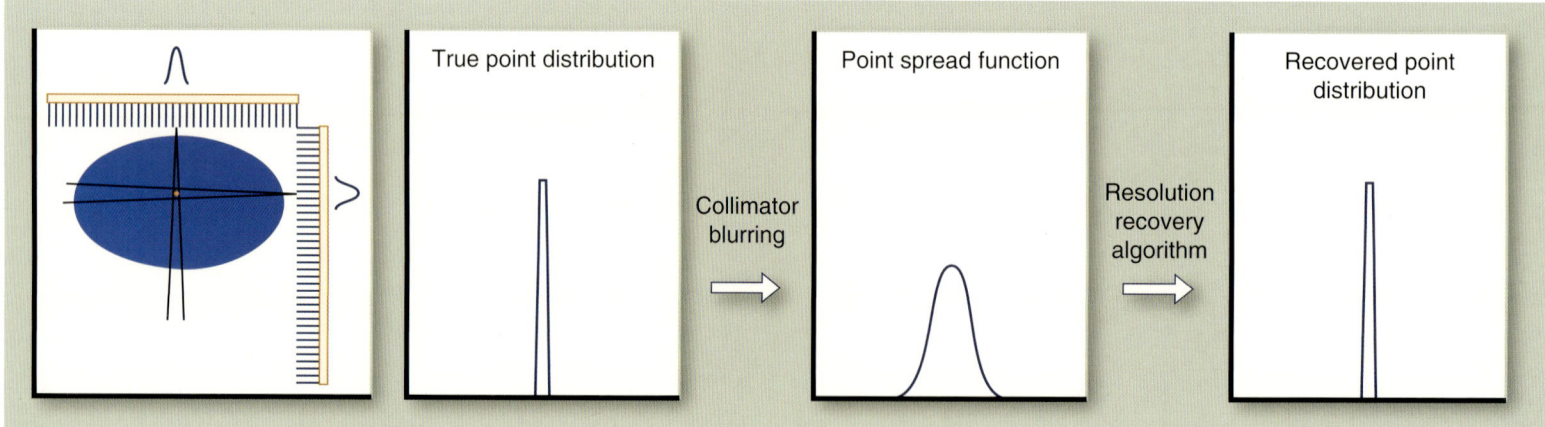

Figure 1-31. Principle of resolution recovery. The limited resolution of nuclear imaging systems makes the image of a point source appear as a Gaussian curve, which is called point spread function (PSF) (*see* Fig. 1-30A). The PSF of a nuclear imaging system increases in width with distance away from the surface of the collimator. Measurement of the PSF of the system at various distances allows the development of a resolution recovery algorithm, which deblurs the image and improves the defect contrast. Two types of resolution recovery algorithms are now commercially available: inverse filtering based on the frequency-distance principle [19] and three-dimensional modeling of the distance-dependent collimator response in iterative reconstruction [20]. As shown in this figure, the main idea of resolution recovery is to apply a mathematical algorithm to transform the blurred image response into a sharp response.

22 Atlas of Nuclear Cardiology

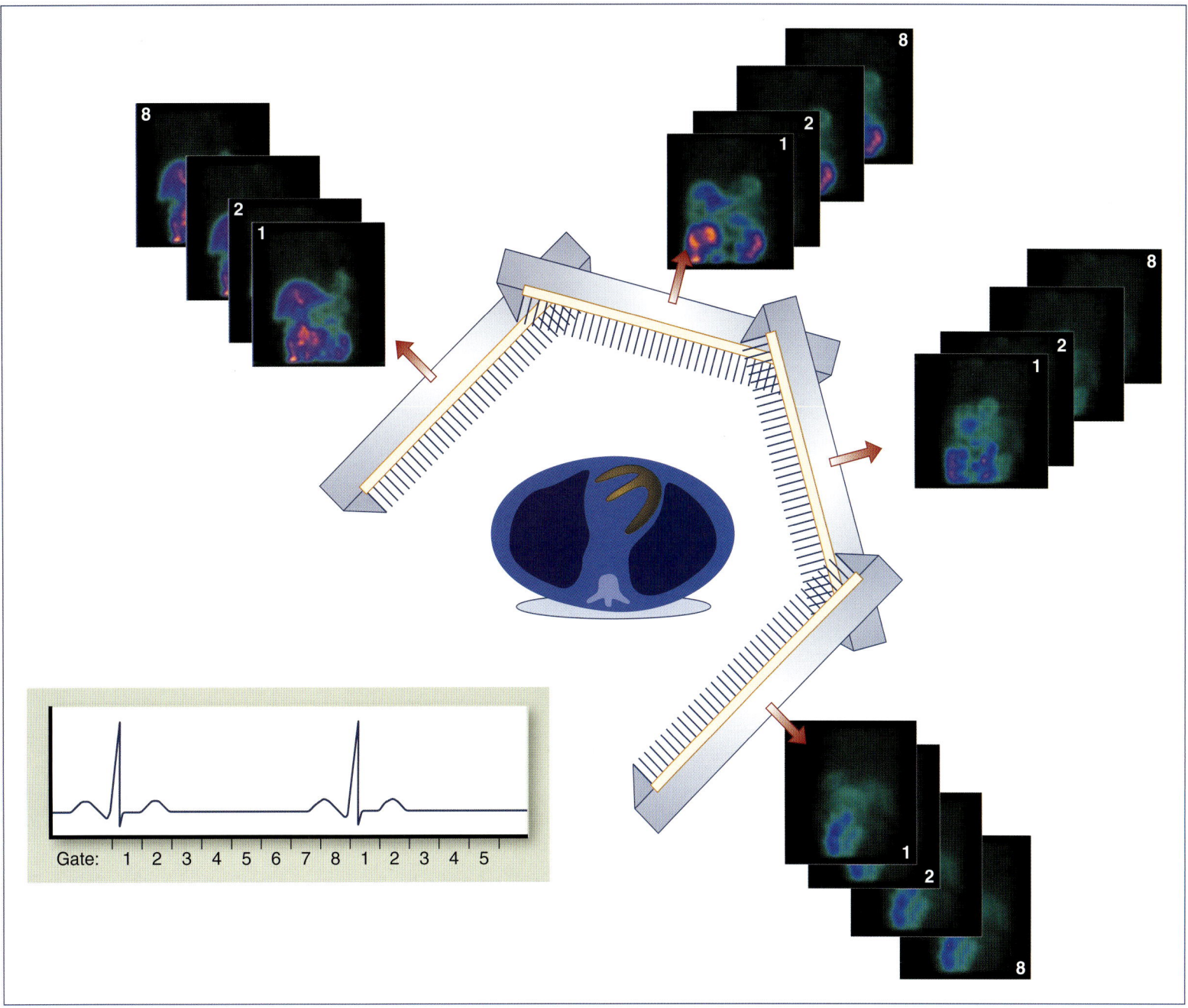

Figure 1-32. Electrocardiogram (ECG)-gated single-photon emission CT (SPECT) myocardial perfusion imaging (MPI) acquisition. Similar to ungated SPECT MPI acquisition, ECG-gated SPECT MPI acquisition collects projection images at equally spaced angles along a 180° or 360° arc during the camera rotation. At each angle, instead of acquiring only one projection in the ungated acquisition mode, the camera acquires several (8, 16, or 32) projection images, each of which corresponds to a specific phase of the cardiac cycle. This is done by synchronizing the computer acquisition to the R wave from the patient's ECG. Here, the cardiac cycle is divided into eight separate frames. If the heart rate is, for example, one beat per second, the computer algorithm assigns each one eighth of a second time interval to each frame. Once the first R wave is detected, all counts are acquired into the first frame; as one eighth of a second elapses, the counts are now acquired into the second frame, and so on until the first second has elapsed or a new R wave is detected, starting the same procedure over again. This technique produces four-dimensional image volumes (three dimensions in space plus time) and allows clinicians to assess not only myocardial perfusion but also myocardial function.

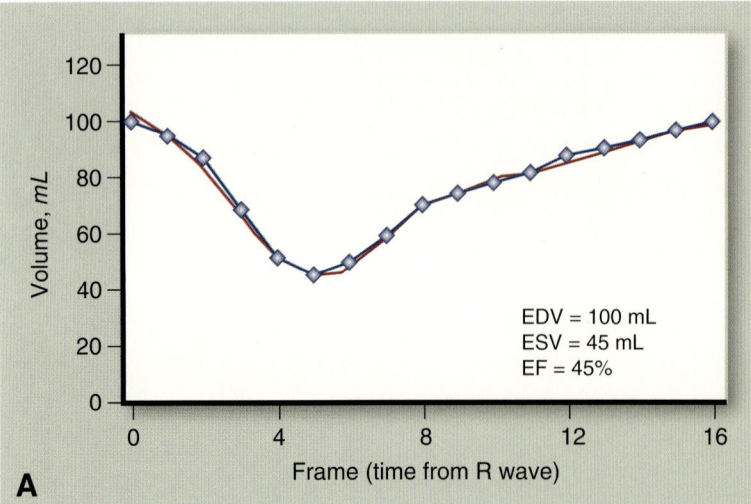
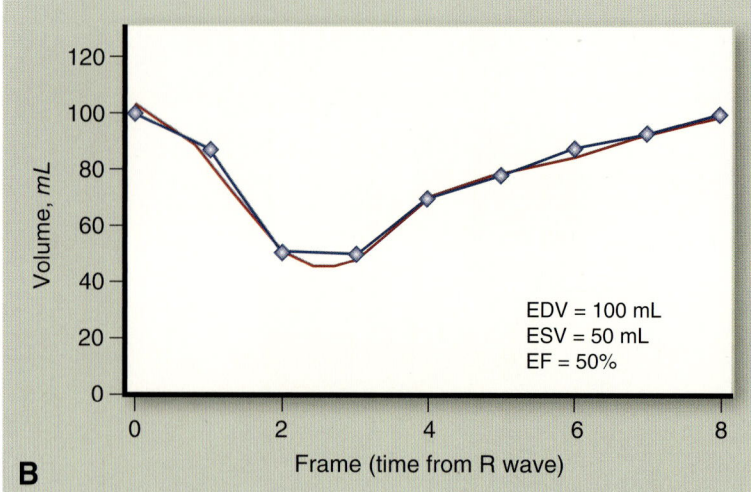

Figure 1-33. **A** and **B**, Principle of temporal resolution. The volume-time curve plots the value of the left ventricular cavity volume as a function of the gated single-photon emission CT (SPECT) time interval. The smaller the time interval (the more the number of frames acquired during a cardiac cycle), the higher the temporal resolution and the closer the volume-time curve is to the "truth" and thus the more accurate the volume and ejection fraction measurements. It is generally agreed that some commonly used eight-frame gated SPECT approaches produce errors in measurement of diastolic function, and it has been suggested that 16-frame imaging is quite effective [21]. There are techniques that use a mathematical algorithm (Fourier transform) to replace the discrete eight samples with a continuous curve on a segment-by-segment basis and thus are less dependent on higher temporal resolution to obtain accurate parameters. EDV—end-diastolic volume; EF—ejection fraction; ESV—end-systolic volume.

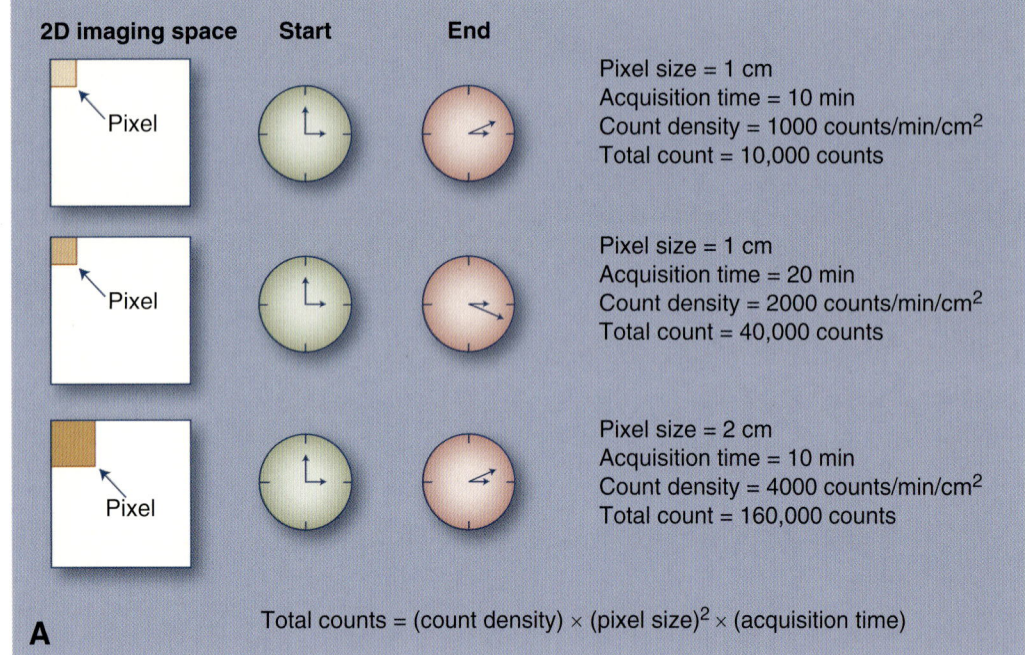

Figure 1-34. Total counts versus count density, preset time of acquisition, and pixel/voxel size. Nuclear imaging acquires photons emitted from the patient and digitizes the data into a matrix (image). Each matrix position corresponds to a pixel, and the pixel value (total counts) corresponds to the number of accepted photons at that position. **A**, The pixel value is proportional to the radiotracer concentration, the length of the acquisition, and the square of the pixel size.

Continued on the next page

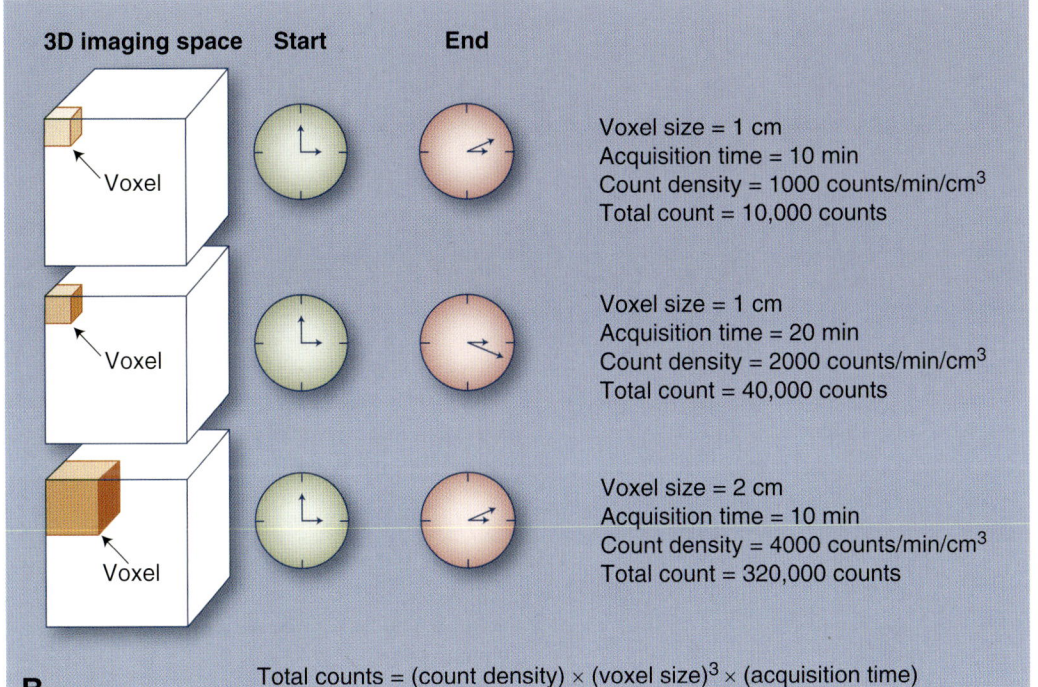

Figure 1-34. *(Continued)* **B,** If the image is three-dimensional (*eg*, reconstructed tomographic image), each element of the image is a cubic instead of a square and is called a "voxel." The voxel value (total counts) is proportional to the radiotracer concentration, the length of the acquisition, and the cubic (not square) of the voxel size. 3D—three-dimensional; 2D—two-dimensional.

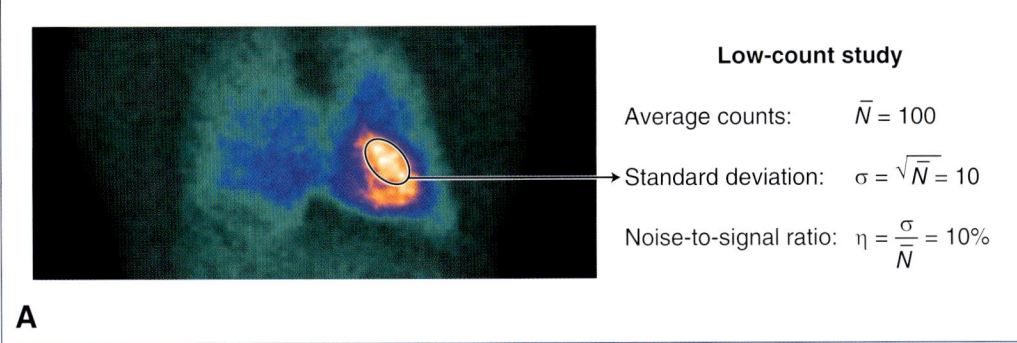

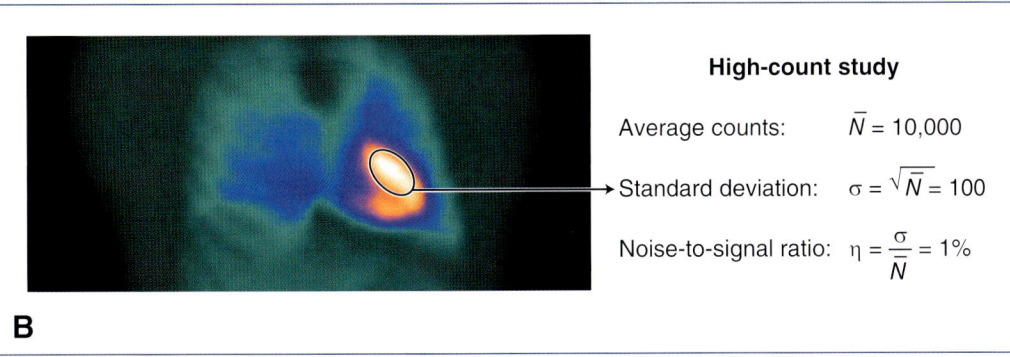

Figure 1-35. Statistics: noise level versus total counts. Nuclear imaging measures radioactive decay, which is a random process and follows the Poisson distribution. The standard deviation of a measured pixel value (counts) from a planar image projection is the square root of the pixel value. A low-count study (**A**) has a bigger standard deviation and a higher noise-to-signal ratio such that the image appears to be noisier than that of a high-count study (**B**). This example shows that if a pixel contains 100 counts, it corresponds to a 10% error, and if another pixel contains 10,000 counts, it corresponds to a 1% error.

Principles of Nuclear Cardiology Imaging 25

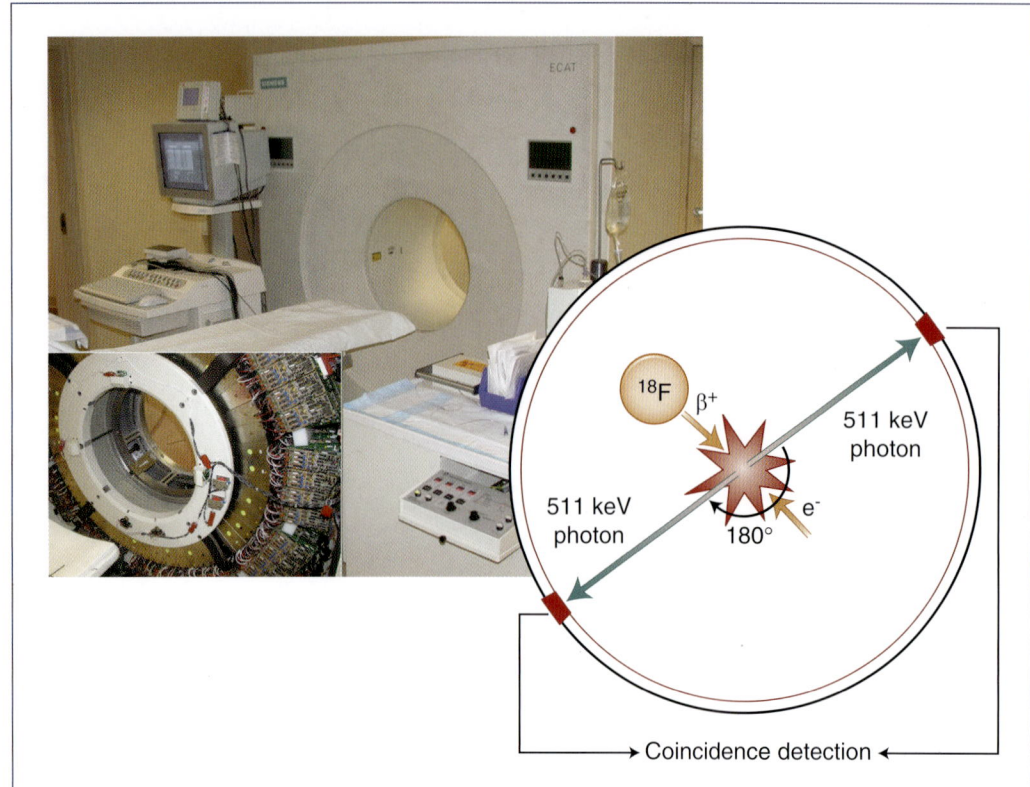

Figure 1-36. Positron emission tomography (PET) scanners; electronic collimation. PET cameras detect paired photons (511 keV of energy each) produced by the positron annihilation effect. The paired 511-keV photons travel in opposite directions at a 180° angle from each other. Thus, positron decay can be localized without collimation with the use of the principle of coincidence detection because if two detectors acquire a count within a short time window, it is assumed that they came from the same pair annihilation and thus the event is positioned by drawing a straight line between the two detectors. Because PET cameras do not require collimators, these systems have a much higher sensitivity than do single-photon emission CT systems. ^{18}F—fluorine-18.

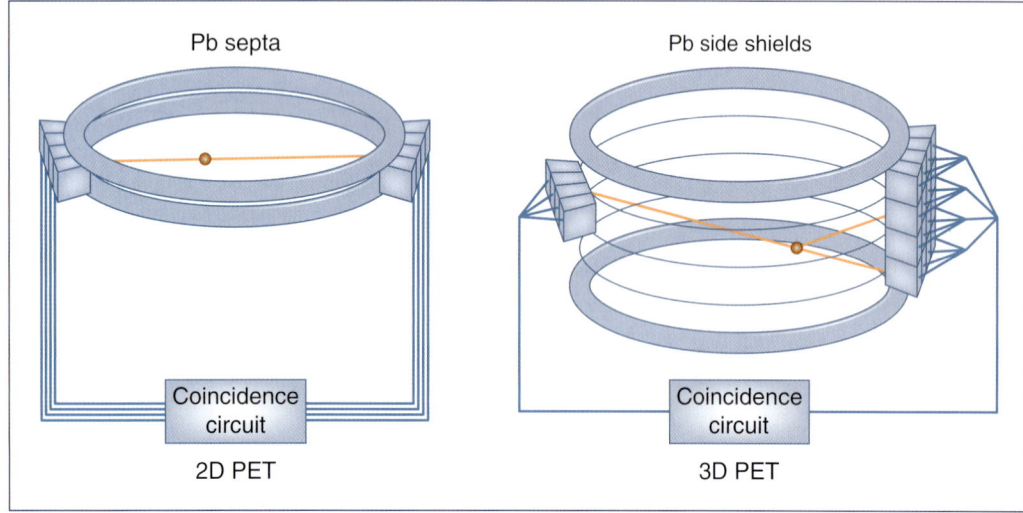

Figure 1-37. Two-dimensional (2D) versus three-dimensional (3D) positron emission tomography (PET) systems. 2D PET systems, equipped with lead (Pb) septa, accept coincidences only from crystals in the same ring of detectors. 3D PET systems, by removing the septa, accept coincidences in any ring and greatly increase count rate and sensitivity. However, the difficulties associated with removing the septa are that it greatly increases scatter, it greatly increases random events, and it greatly increases count rate and so greatly increases dead time [22]. These problems must be effectively compensated for when using 3D PET in cardiac imaging.

Atlas of Nuclear Cardiology

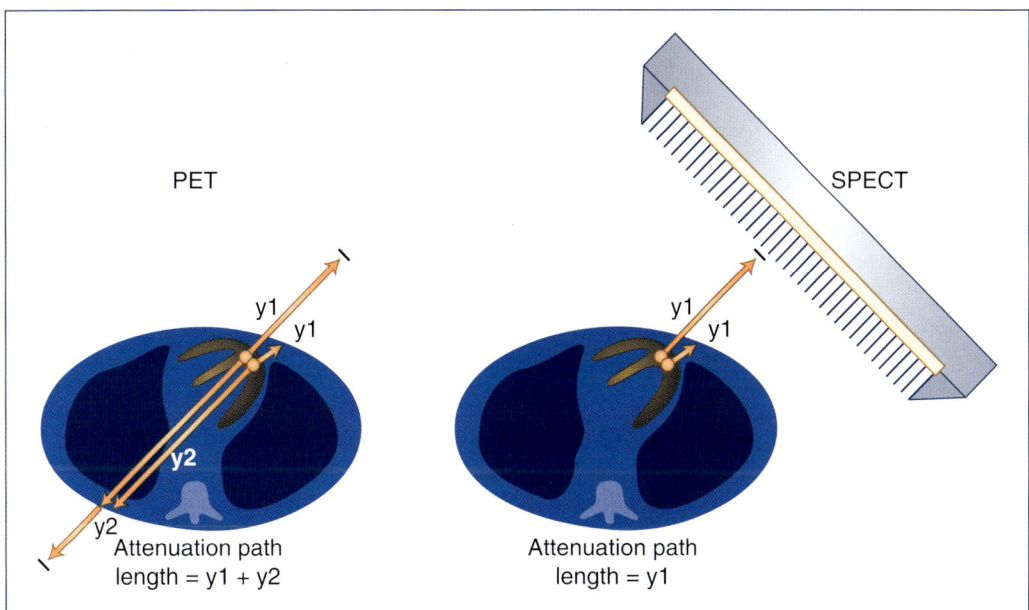

Figure 1-38. Positron emission tomography (PET) versus single-photon emission CT (SPECT) attenuation correction (AC). PET imaging measures 511-keV photons. Because the two photons must be detected to record the event, the entire path length influences the attenuation. In SPECT imaging, even though the energy of the photon is lower, its path length to the detector is much shorter and thus is less affected by attenuation. Thus, the two PET photons undergo higher attenuation when they travel through the body than do the single photons measured in SPECT imaging. Therefore, there is more attenuation in PET studies than in SPECT, making PET more susceptible to attenuation artifacts. Only attenuation-corrected cardiac images should be used in clinical interpretation [23]. Unlike SPECT, PET data can be accurately corrected for attenuation by simply multiplying each projection line by the appropriate AC factor. For both PET and SPECT, measurement of the patient-specific attenuation map is required for accurate AC and can be done either by radionuclide imaging or by radiographic CT.

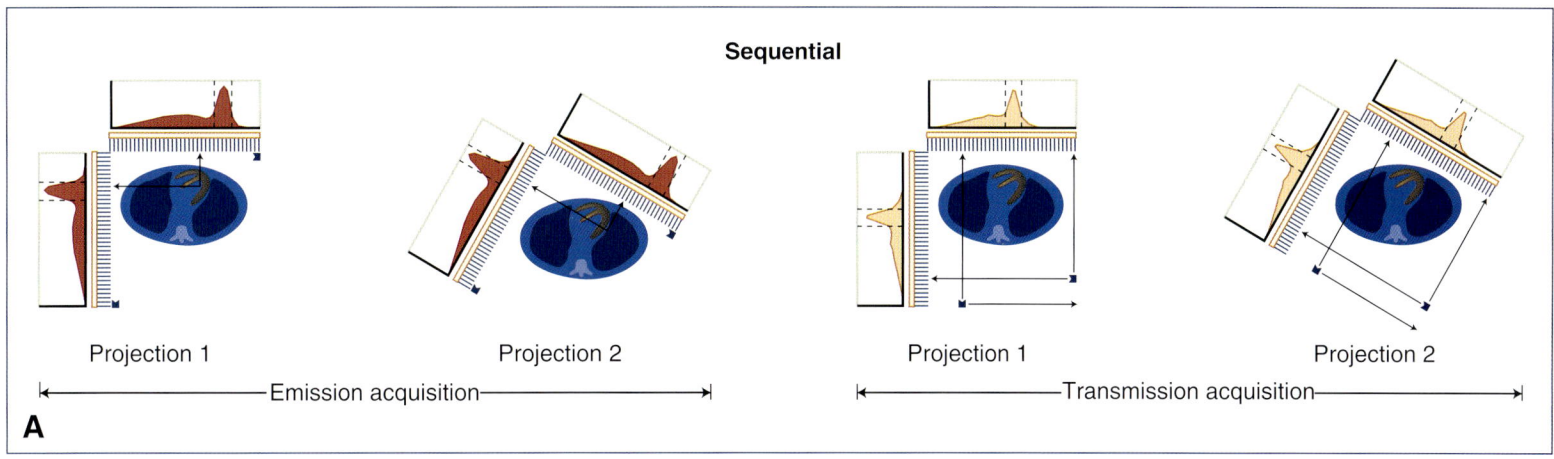

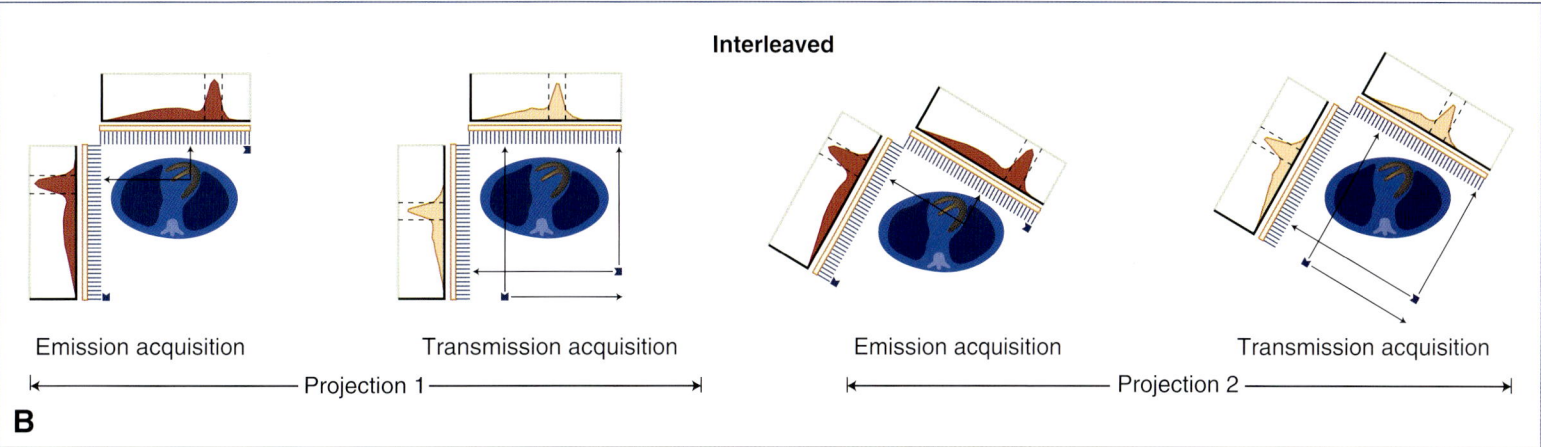

Figure 1-39. Types of attenuation correction (AC): sequential, interleaved, and simultaneous. Accurate AC requires two acquisitions from a single study: emission and transmission. **A,** The two acquisitions can be done sequentially, one following the other; however, registration between the two acquisitions challenges the quality control of this approach in practice. **B,** To reduce the risk of emission/transmission misalignment, the two acquisitions can be done in an interleaved mode, in which the camera acquires emission and transmission projection images sequentially at each stop and rotates around the patient only once in one study.

Continued on the next page

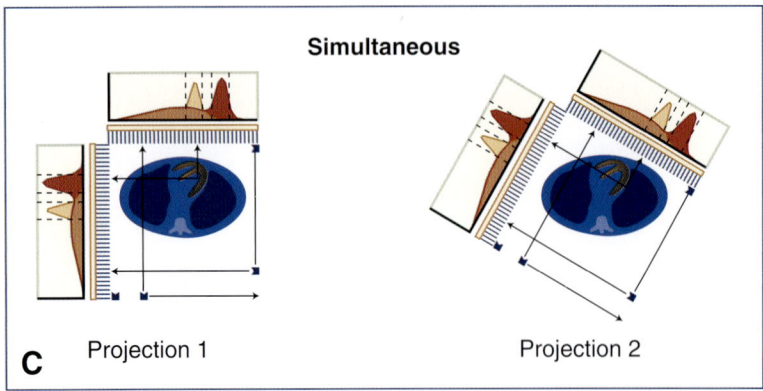

Figure 1-39. *(Continued)* **C**, Simultaneous mode completely solves the problem and reduces the length of the acquisition; however, crosstalk between the emission and transmission photons degrades at least one of the two acquisitions and should be properly compensated for with accurate AC.

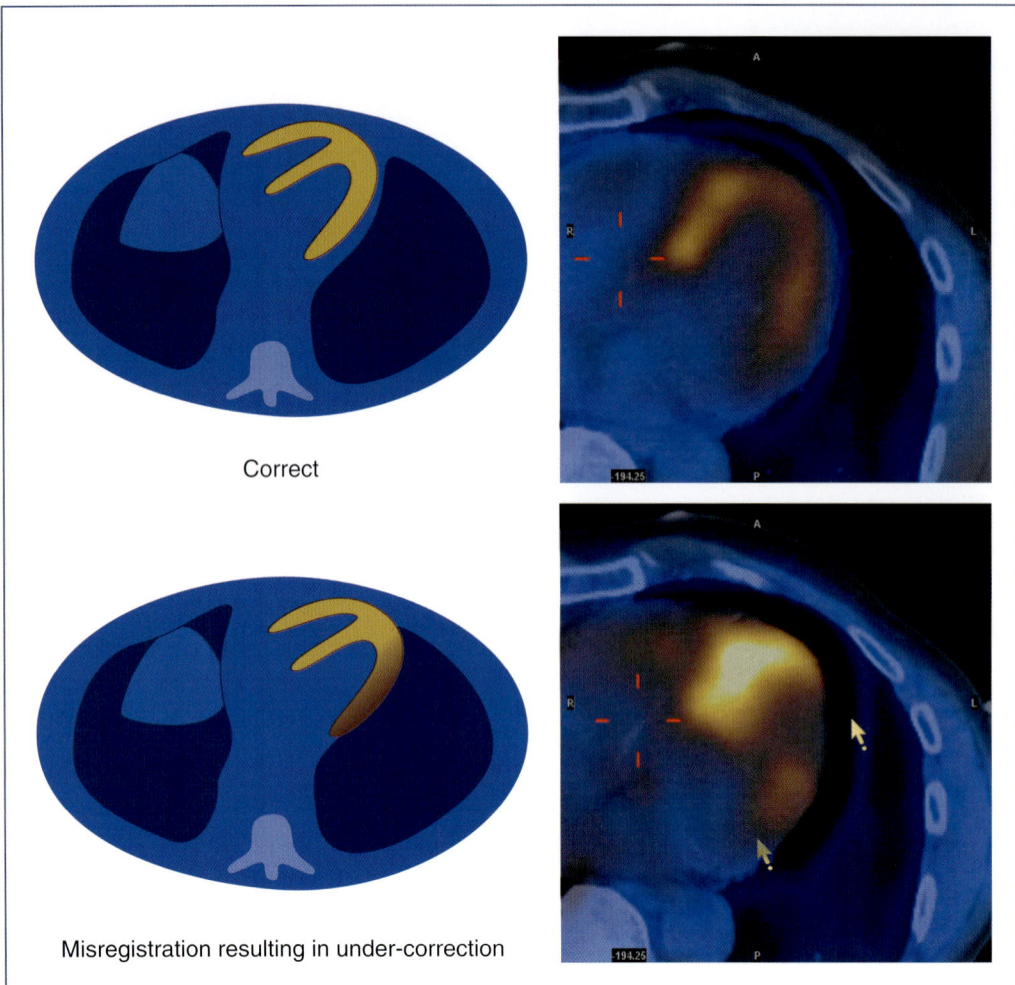

Figure 1-40. Attenuation correction artifact due to misregistration. The figure explains the artifact caused by misregistration between the emission and transmission scans due to patient motion. Attenuation correction requires that the emission scan and the transmission scan that is used to correct for photon attenuation be perfectly registered with each other. Simultaneous acquisitions of both emission and transmission scans ensures that these two are registered. However, when these two acquisitions are performed sequentially and the patient moves between the two acquisitions, artifacts are created.

The *top left panel* shows a diagram of a transaxial emission cardiac image superimposed on the corresponding transaxial transmission image. Note that the entire cardiac silhouette lies in the pericardium, not touching the lung area, represented in *dark blue*. The *top right image* shows an actual attenuation-corrected emission cardiac image when correctly registered with the transmission image. The *bottom left panel* shows a diagram of a transaxial emission cardiac image superimposed on the corresponding transaxial transmission image. Note that the two images are misregistered and that the free left ventricular lateral myocardial wall overlaps a portion of the lung. The *bottom right image* shows an actual attenuation-corrected emission cardiac image that is similarly misregistered in relation to the transmission image. Note that the left ventricular free wall overlaps a portion of the lung. This misregistration causes the lateral wall to be undercorrected, and thus it appears as though it is hypoperfused.

28 Atlas of Nuclear Cardiology

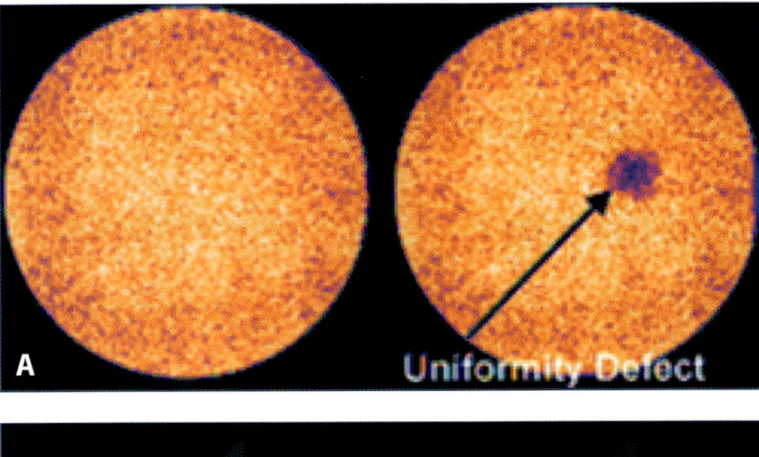

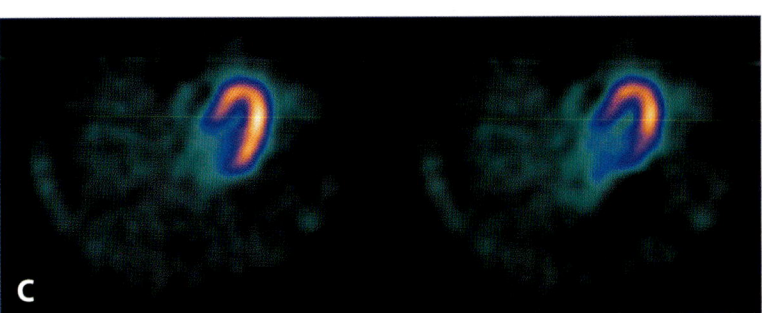

Figure 1-41. Camera uniformity. The Joint Commission on the Accreditation of Healthcare Organizations (JCAHO) requires that a uniformity flood be acquired on each scintillation camera before clinical studies are done for any given day. These 3 million count floods can be used to detect uniformity defects. **A,** Two examples of floods: one using a camera without a uniformity defect (*left*) and one with a uniformity defect that might be caused by a poor photomultiplier tube (*right*). **B,** In the same patient, corresponding thallium planar projections acquired with these cameras. Note that the planar image on the *right* shows decreased counts compared with the one on the *left*. The problem is that even if cine displays of the planar images are viewed, it will be very difficult to detect that the decreased counts in the inferior myocardial wall were caused by a camera uniformity problem as opposed to a true physiologic perfusion abnormality. **C,** Correspondingly, when the transaxial slices are reconstructed, the basolateral wall is decreased in counts. Although a ring artifact is caused by this uniformity problem and can be seen in the transaxial images when imaging a uniform source, in this patient, they are difficult to detect. Therefore, just by looking at the images, it is difficult to detect this uniformity problem if the quality control step is not performed. **D,** The vertical long-axis images make it even harder to detect when a decrease in counts might be the result of a uniformity defect. It is very important that floods be performed on a daily basis to detect uniformity problems before they affect clinical images. Differences in positioning of the patient between rest and stress scans may cause uniformity artifacts to appear in different locations in the two images, possibly mimicking ischemia [12].

Figure 1-42. Quality control (QC) procedures for planar imaging. These are the QC procedures that are necessary to ensure images of diagnostic quality. These procedures are pertinent to guarantee both the quality of studies when performing planar imaging and the quality of the planar projections used in single-photon emission CT imaging.

Energy peaking consists of either manually or automatically placing the correct pulse height analyzer's energy window over the photopeak energy of the radionuclide to be used. This process is usually performed with a radioactive point source imaged a distance away by an uncollimated camera or an extended sheet source on the collimated camera. Either way, the entire field of view should be illuminated by the radioactive source. This process should be performed daily, even in camera systems that perform this function automatically and track the shift of the window. A photograph of the spectrum with the window superimposed is used to record these results [24].

Intrinsic uniformity flood field is another QC procedure that should be performed daily to document the camera uniformity. This procedure is also done using a radioactive point source and without a collimator. This acquisition should be performed using a source of low radioactivity (~ 100 µCi) in a small volume (~ 0.5 mL) to mimic a point source positioned at least five diameters from the camera's crystal, directly over the center of the detector. If this process proves difficult or time consuming, it can be replaced with an extrinsic uniformity flood measurement. Extrinsic uniformity is measured with an extended radioactive sheet source that covers the entire collimated camera face [25].

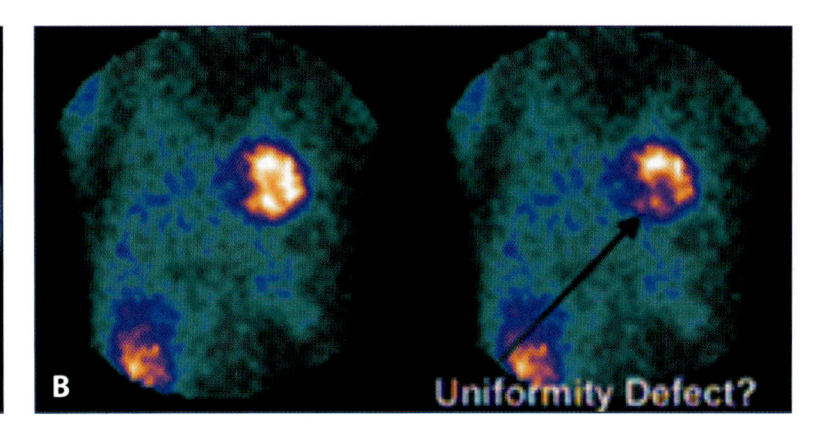

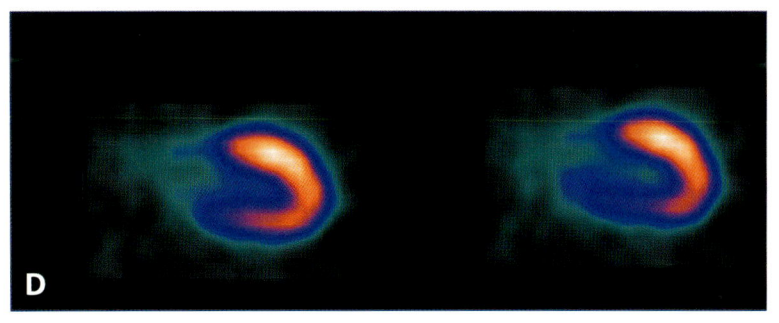

Quality Control Procedures for Planar Imaging

Test	Frequency
Energy peaking	Daily
Intrinsic uniformity	Daily
Intrinsic sensitivity	Daily/weekly
Resolution and linearity	Weekly

Sensitivity QC tests that the device is consistently counting the same radioactive source and should be performed weekly. These tests can be done at the same time the intrinsic (or extrinsic) uniformity tests are done by recording the number of counts acquired for a given time period adjusted to the magnitude of radiation used to create the image.

The resolution and linearity test is performed to document spatial resolution and its change over time as well as how the camera reproduces straight lines. This test consists of imaging an extended radioactive sheet flood source through a spatial resolution test phantom known as a bar phantom. Images of the phantom should be photographed to record the camera's performance and QC procedure. These images are assessed for how straight the bar lines are imaged and for intrinsic spatial resolution. Changes in resolution are assessed by documenting the smallest bars that are discerned [24].

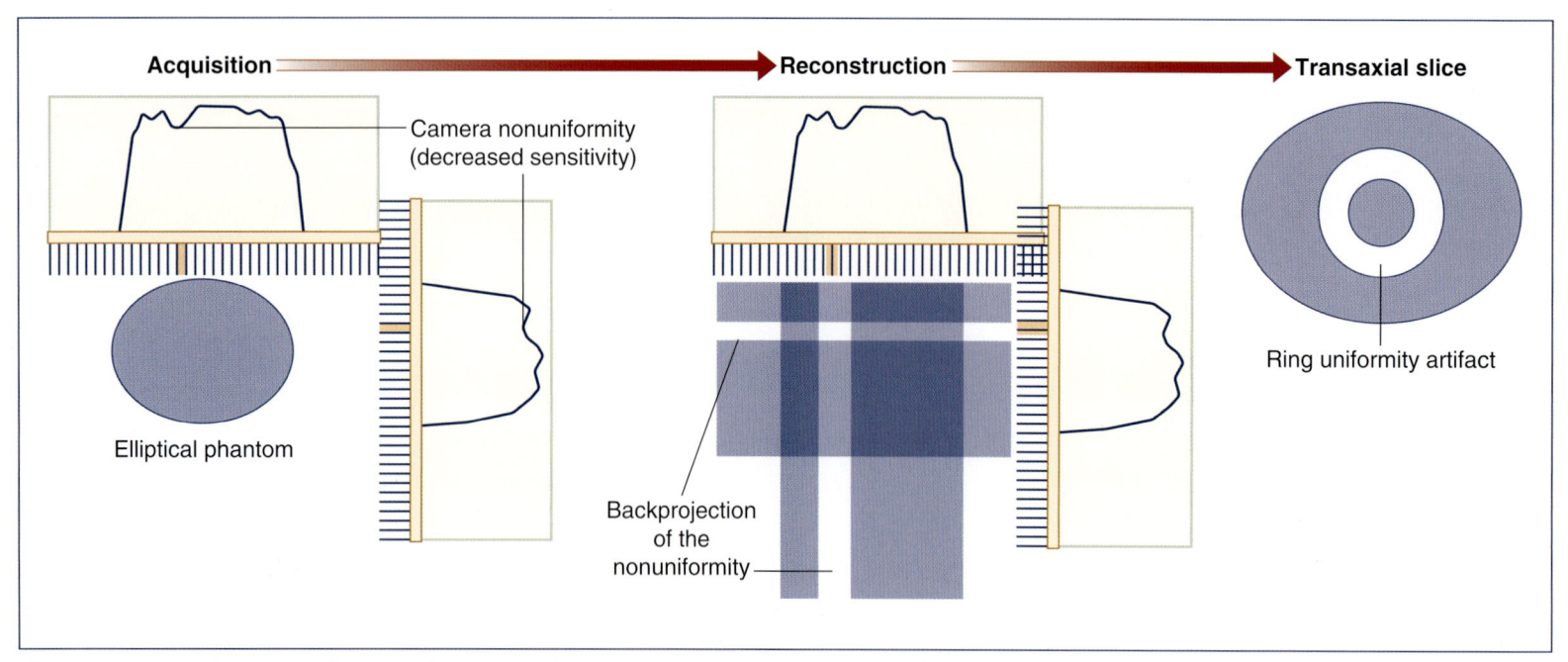

Figure 1-43. Uniformity artifacts. Uniformity artifacts occur when one area of the camera face has decreased sensitivity compared with the other areas. This can occur when a photomultiplier tube begins to work improperly, as in Figure 1-41, or if the collimator is damaged. For example, if an acquisition is performed of an elliptical quality control phantom that was filled with a uniform distribution of technetium, it can generate the two count profiles on the *left side* of the figure. These count profiles should be steep on the sides and fairly flat across the top, depending on the shape of the phantom. In the case of uniformity problems, regions of decreased sensitivity are seen in each of these curves, represented by a small dip at one point. The small dip will correspond to the same location on the camera in all of the projection views. When the images are reconstructed, this small dip is backprojected, as shown in the *middle image*, and with more and more projections, it will scribe out a circle in the transaxial image, as shown on the *right*. This kind of artifact may occur when the collimator is damaged and one or a few of the holes in the lead septa have been closed. To correct for small variations across the face of a collimator, 30 million count floods are used. These high-count floods should be acquired at least once a month and are applied to images acquired with the same collimator being used by the same camera [12].

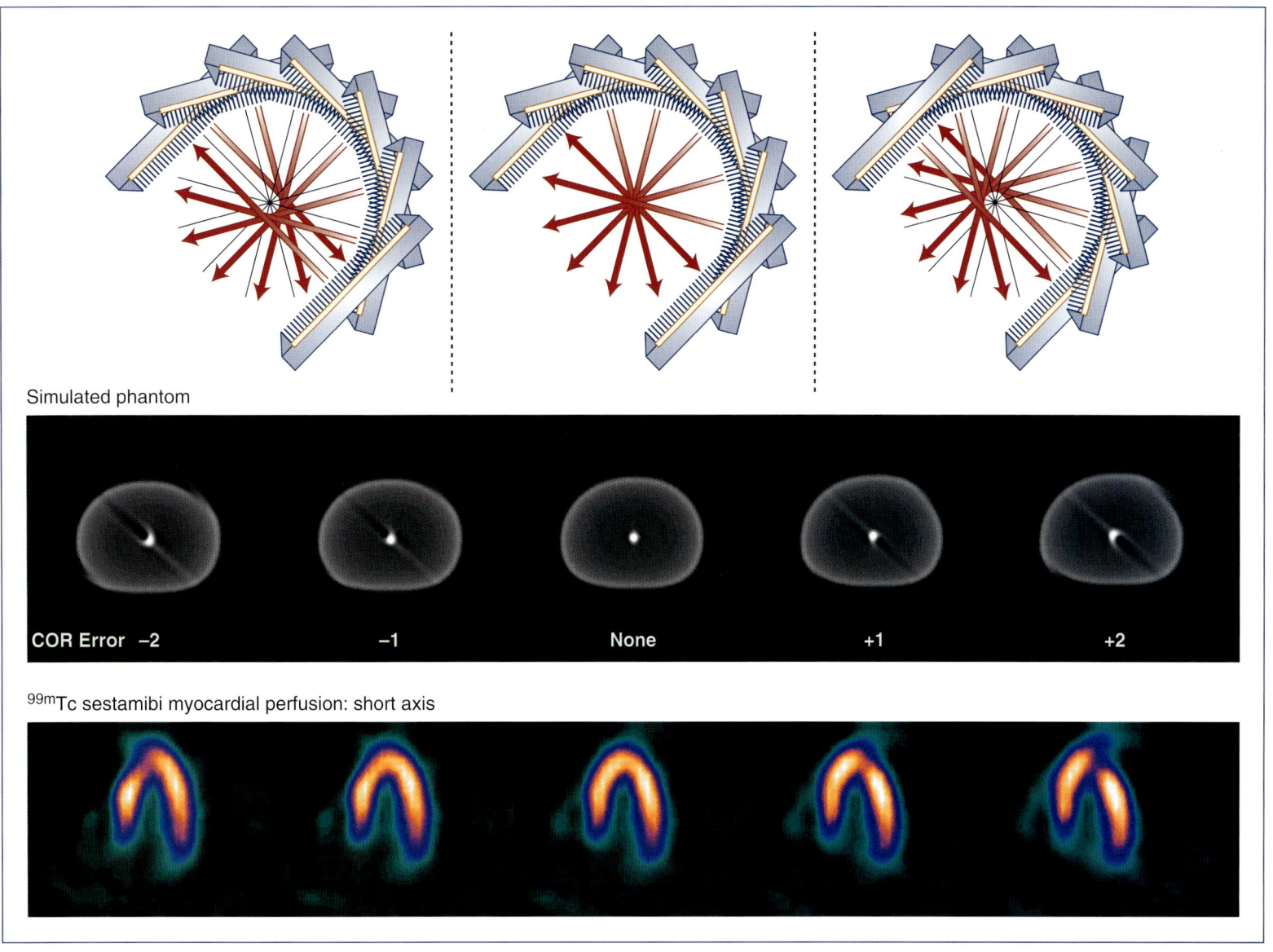

Figure 1-44. Center of rotation (COR). Center of rotation is a calibration performed frequently to ensure that the frame of reference used by the computer in reconstructing images is aligned with the mechanical axis of rotation of the single-photon emission CT (SPECT) camera system. If the center of rotation is properly calibrated, a radioactive point source placed in the center of the camera orbit should project to the center of the computer matrix. These results are seen in the *middle panels*.

For most cardiac SPECT, a 180° orbit is used. When a radioactive point source is used with this orbit, a point source should also be reconstructed as a point in the image. With a center-of-rotation error, however, the reconstruction no longer yields a point. Instead, the point is smeared to make it appear as a tuning fork. This tuning fork artifact is so named because the shape forms two lines in one direction and something that looks like a stem in the opposite direction. If the center-of-rotation calibration errs by a negative amount, the images in the *left panels* are seen. In the *middle left panels*, the smeared radioactive point sources reconstructed with this error are seen. If the error is in the positive direction, the images shown in the *top right* are seen. The camera processes that generated these errors are seen in the *top diagrams*.

Center-of-rotation errors are easy to detect with radioactive point sources. However, these errors may be very difficult to detect with a clinical distribution of activity. In the *bottom panels*, the center-of-rotation errors can be seen that correspond to the images of point sources directly above them. The center-of-rotation error manifests itself in the myocardial perfusion horizontal long-axis images as an area of reduced counts on either side of the myocardium (often surrounding an area of higher counts). It is sometimes difficult to distinguish between the center-of-rotation errors demonstrated here and true clinical defects. This makes it extremely important that the technologists who perform the quality control procedures properly calibrate the center of rotation for the camera [12]. Several excellent reviews on how to detect and account for imaging SPECT artifacts have been published [26,27].

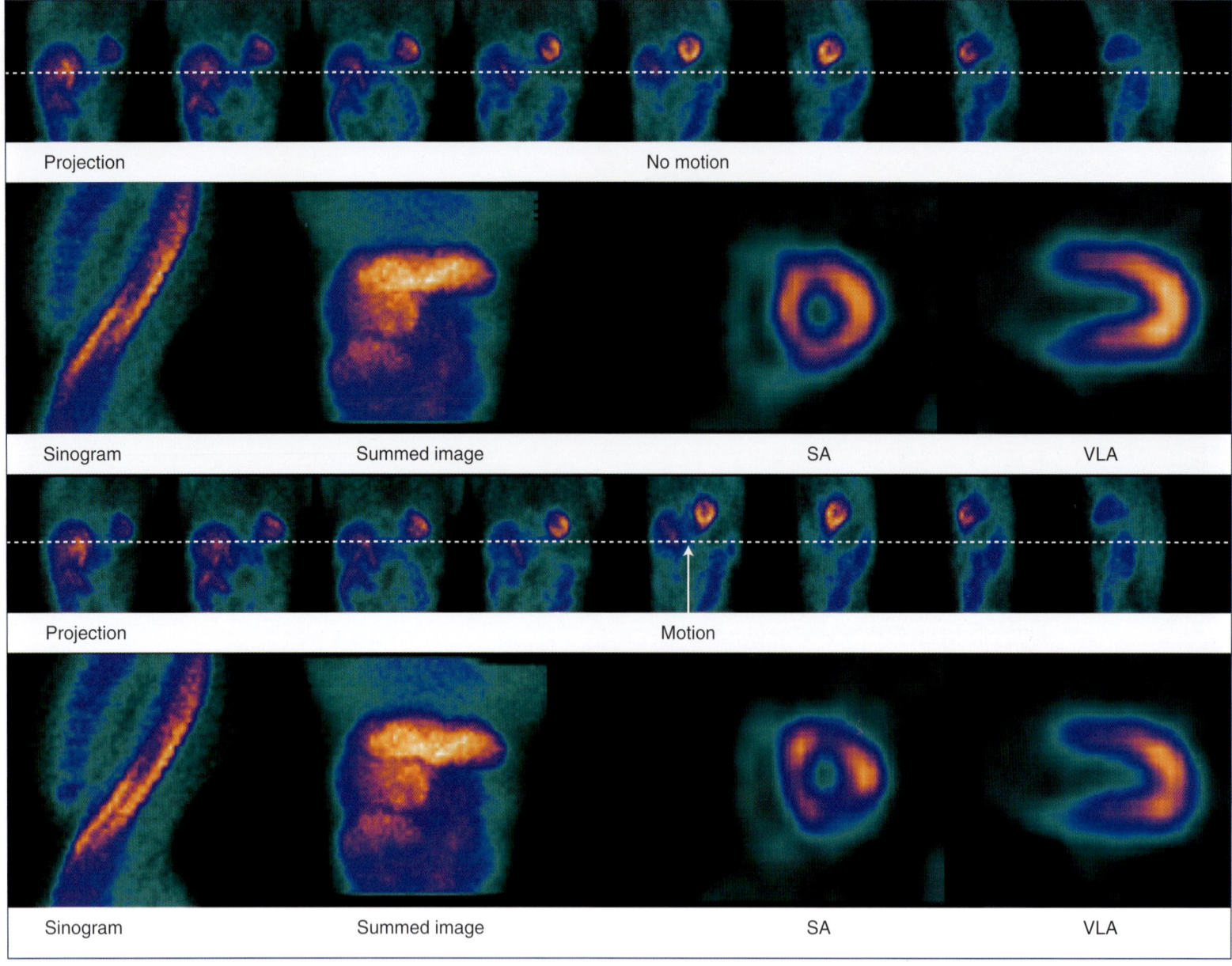

Figure 1-45. Detecting patient motion. Patient motion can be detected by cine displays, sinograms, and summed planar images. Cine displays of the planar projections are perhaps the simplest and best way to detect patient motion. Watching the heart as it moves from right to left in the planar projections can be used to detect all types of motions. The clinician should watch the movie of the planar projections at a fairly rapid cine rate and observe any up-and-down motion of the heart, particularly in relation to a fixed horizontal line just below the heart. The best way to detect and correct motion is for the technologist to observe the patient and repeat the scan if sufficient motion occurs. Immediately repeating the scan might prevent the patient from having to return for a repeated scan as a result of the original acquisition being technically impossible to interpret. The projections at the top of each of the two panels illustrate how patient motion might be detected using a cine display. If the distance between the heart and the horizontal line is compared in each of these planar projections, the *top images* show no variation in the distance between the inferior wall of the left ventricle and the line whereas in the *bottom panel*, the heart is seen to move vertically away from the line starting with the projection to which the arrow points. Note that the short-axis (SA) and vertical long-axis (VLA) images in the *bottom panel* show regions of decreased counts as compared with those in the *upper panel* of the same patient with no motion. Even a slight amount of motion (3 mm) may result in an artifact in the single-photon emission CT (SPECT) images. If this motion is not detected by the clinician before interpretation of the images, a false-positive report may result.

A sinogram is another way to detect patient motion. A sinogram is an image composed of one line of pixels through the planar projections plotted vertically for each of the angular projection views. Thus, the x-axis of the sinogram represents pixels across the camera face, and the y-axis represents different planar projections, with the first planar projection at the top. The heart can be seen as a bright stripe from the top right to the lower left of the sinogram. The clinician looks for a break in this stripe that would represent the patient moving to the left or right. Thus, sinograms are best for detecting horizontal motion across the table. Sinograms may also show vertical motion, but not quite as well as they show the horizontal motion.

Patient motion can also be detected by using summed projections. The summed projection is formed by adding all of the planar projections for the SPECT acquisition. The heart can be traced as a blurry horizontal line across the center of the image. To evaluate patient motion, the clinician should look for a change in the height of the heart that would indicate movement during the acquisition. This is best used for detecting vertical motion, *ie*, motion of the patient along the table.

There are a number of software algorithms, both manual and automatic, for correcting for patient motion [28]. These algorithms work best when the motion is vertical along the table and no twisting motion has occurred. As with any algorithm, although in general they correct for the motion quite well, they may sometimes fail. Sometimes when these algorithms are applied to patients who have not moved during acquisition, the software gets confused and detects and corrects for nonexistent motion. It is advisable to always visually confirm that the motion correction software has performed appropriately.

Quality Control Procedures for SPECT Imaging

Test	Requirement
Center of rotation	Mandatory
Uniformity correction	Mandatory
Motion correction	Optional

Figure 1-46. Quality control (QC) procedures for single-photon emission tomography (SPECT) imaging. The table summarizes the QC procedures necessary to ensure images of diagnostic quality when performing SPECT imaging. These procedures have been described in this chapter. Of course, all the QC procedures required for planar imaging are also required for SPECT imaging.

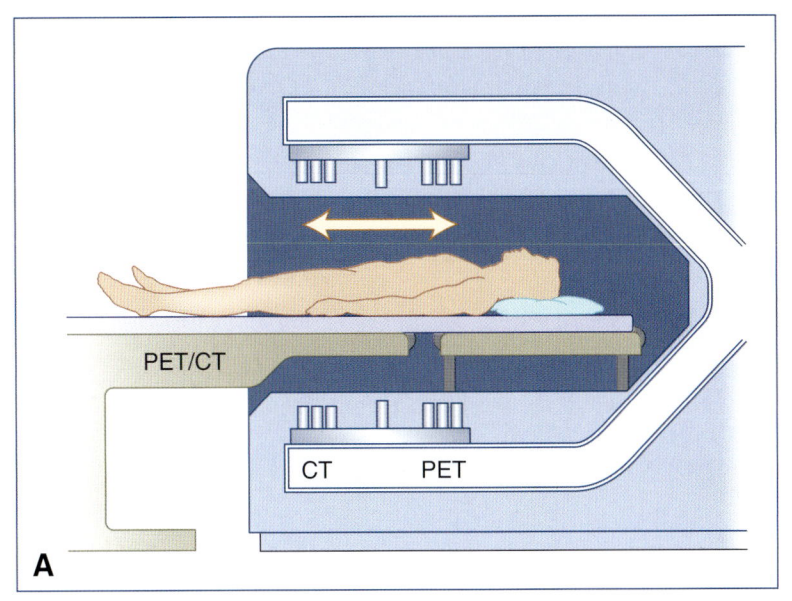

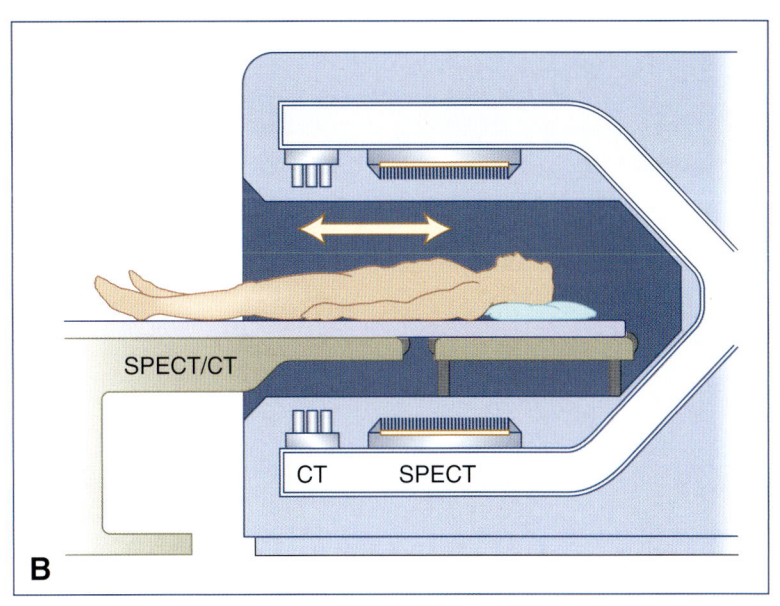

Figure 1-47. Hybrid positron emission tomography (PET)/CT and single-photon emission CT (SPECT)/CT imaging systems. Hybrid systems, which physically couple a CT scanner with a PET (**A**) or a SPECT (**B**) scanner, are now in routine clinical use. The coupled CT scanner, ranging from 1 to 64 slices, is commonly used for attenuation correction, and if supported by the CT scanner, can be used to evaluate coronary calcium and/or perform CT angiographic studies. An advantage of these systems is that they can provide, in one imaging study, comprehensive cardiac evaluation of anatomic information from the CT scan and physiologic information from the PET or SPECT scans [29].

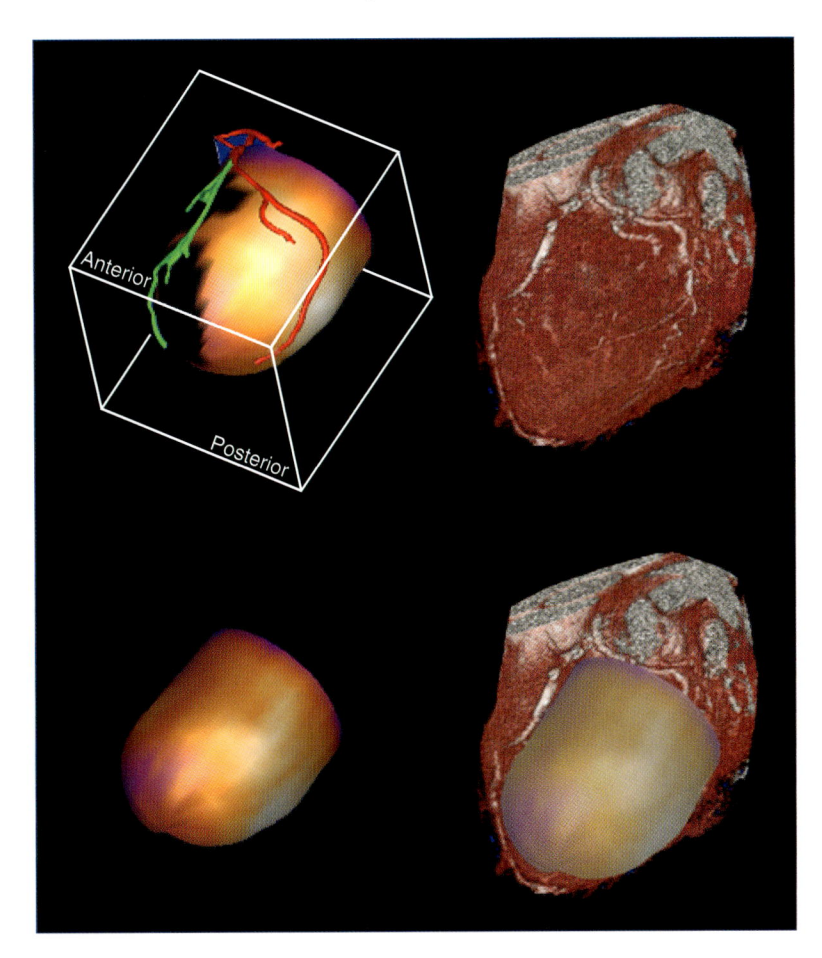

Figure 1-48. Positron emission tomography (PET)/CT and single-photon emission CT (SPECT)/CT image fusion. Software methods are required to fuse the anatomic information from the CT angiographic study and the physiologic information from a nuclear myocardial perfusion PET or SPECT study in three dimensions (3D). Because the emission and transmission studies are not acquired simultaneously, software fusion is needed regardless of whether a hybrid system or two stand-alone systems are used to acquire the information. There are two types of fusion used today: quantitative and qualitative fusion. In quantitative fusion (*top left panel*), the 3D coronary tree is extracted from the CT angiography study and superimposed onto the 3D myocardial perfusion distribution using landmarks and shape operators [30]. In this approach, the quantitatively determined hypoperfused regions are highlighted in *black* and the vessels distal to a coronary stenosis are highlighted in *green*. Compared with the accuracy of CT angiography, this fused information has been shown to provide significantly higher specificity and positive predictive value at no loss of sensitivity or negative predictive value [31]. In the qualitative approach, the 3D surface–rendered CT angiography study (*top right*) is painted with the 3D myocardial perfusion distribution (*bottom left*) angled in the same orientation as the CT angiography study. The fused information (*bottom right*) has also been reported to improve diagnostic accuracy over CT angiography [32].

Principles of Nuclear Cardiology Imaging

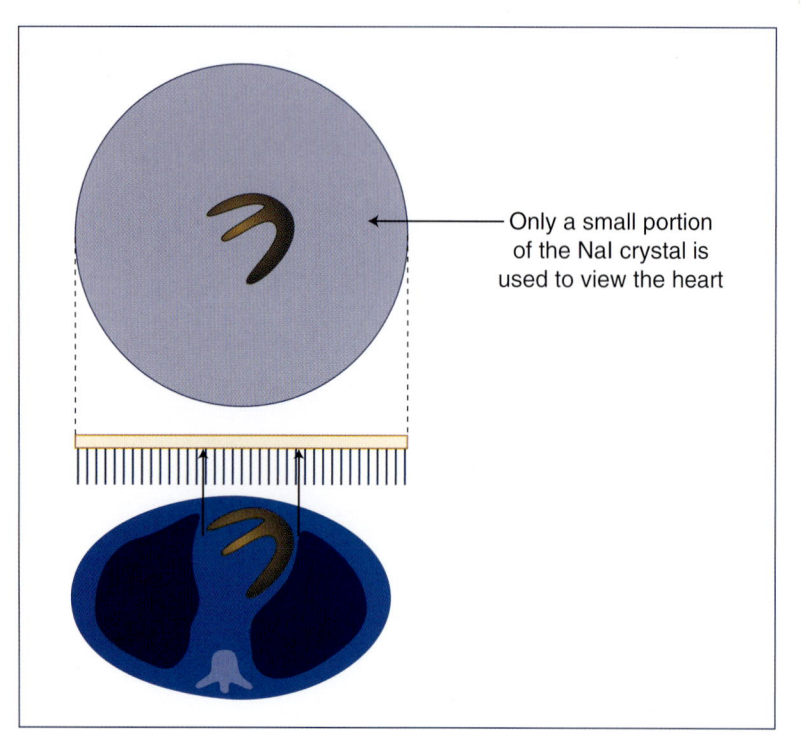

Figure 1-49. Limitations of conventional single-photon emission CT (SPECT) imaging. Myocardial perfusion SPECT imaging has had widespread clinical use because of its well-documented diagnostic accuracy for detecting coronary artery disease. Nevertheless, the basic camera design is more than 50 years old and limited when using standard parallel hole collimators to image the heart, as it uses only a small portion of the available, useful sodium iodide (NaI) crystal detector area.

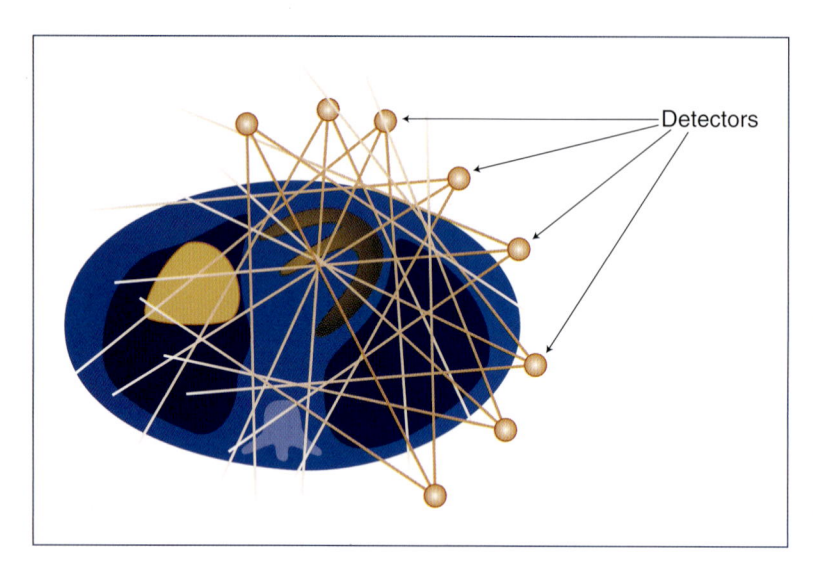

Figure 1-50. Design of new-generation dedicated cardiac ultrafast acquisition scanners. Several manufacturers have begun to break away from the conventional single-photon emission CT imaging approach to create innovative designs of dedicated cardiac scanners. These scanners' designs have in common that all available detectors are constrained to imaging just the cardiac field of view. This diagram shows how eight detectors surrounding the patient are all simultaneously imaging the heart. These new designs vary in the number and type of scanning or stationary detectors, and whether sodium iodide or cadmium zinc telluride solid-state detectors are used. They all have in common the potential for a five- to 10-fold increase in count sensitivity at no loss or even a gain in resolution, resulting in the potential for acquiring a stress myocardial perfusion scan injected with a standard dose in 2 minutes or less [33].

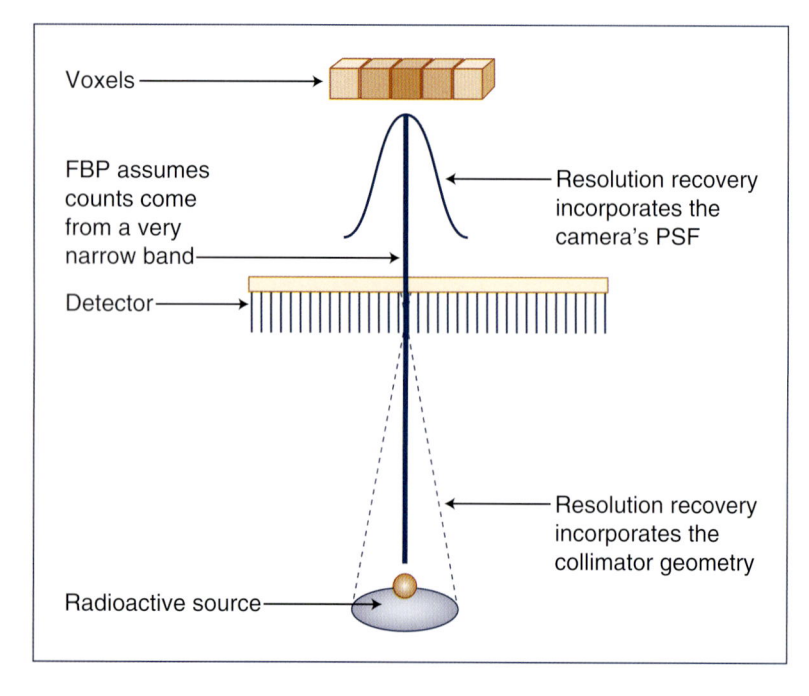

Figure 1-51. Image reconstruction advances allow half-time acquisition. This diagram shows how conventional filtered backprojection (FBP) reconstruction assumes that the photons counted in a voxel over a collimator's parallel hole have emanated in a straight line from a radioactive source perpendicular to the detector surface and aligned with the hole. It assumes that all other photons counted from this source are either image noise or counts from other sources positioned in a very narrow line parallel to and directly in front of the hole. Recent software improvements in image reconstruction take into account the loss of resolution with distance inherent in parallel hole collimators, depicted here by the cone drawn as a dashed line. Using this knowledge in conjunction with the properties of the entire point spread function (PSF) allows for a more accurate resolution recovery. At the same time, noise is suppressed because additional counts are now correctly considered rather than treated as noise. It has been reported that single-photon emission CT (SPECT) myocardial perfusion imaging may be performed with these new resolution recovery algorithms using half the conventional scan time without compromising perfusion imaging results [34]. In another study, it was shown that these new algorithms, applied to half-time electrocardiogram-gated myocardial perfusion imaging SPECT acquisitions, compare favorably with FBP of full-time algorithms in image quality and correlation of functional parameters. However, systematic offset in these parameters were reported due to the increase in contrast of the resolution recovery–gated images over FBP images [35].

34 Atlas of Nuclear Cardiology

References

1. Chandra R: *Introductory Physics of Nuclear Medicine*. Philadelphia: Lea and Febiger; 1992.

2. Christensen EE, Curry TS, Dowdey JE: *An Introduction to the Physics of Diagnostic Radiology*, edn 2. Philadelphia: Lea and Febiger; 1978:159.

3. Powsner RA, Powsner ER: *Essentials of Nuclear Medicine Physics*. Malden MA: Blackwell Science; 1998.

4. Hubble JH, Seltzer SM: Tables of x-ray mass attenuation coefficients, and mass energy-absorption coefficients. Gaithersburg: National Institute of Standards and Technology; 1996. Available at http://physics.nist.gov/PhysRefData/XrayMassCoef/cover.html. Accessed September 15, 2008.

5. Cherry SR, Sorenson JA, Phelps ME: *Physics in Nuclear Medicine*. Philadelphia: WB Saunders; 2003.

6. Beller GA, Bergmann SR: Myocardial perfusion imaging agents: SPECT and PET. *J Nucl Cardiol* 2004, 11:71–86.

7. Saha GB: *Fundamentals of Nuclear Pharmacy*. New York: Springer-Verlag; 2003.

8. Anger HO: Scintillation camera with multichannel collimators. *J Nucl Med* 1964, 5:515–531.

9. Maublant JC, Peycelon P, Kwiatkowski F, et al.: Comparison between 180° and 360° data collection in technetium-99m MIBI SPECT of the myocardium. *J Nucl Med* 1989, 30:295–300.

10. Hoffman EJ: 180° compared to 360° sampling in SPECT. *J Nucl Med* 1982, 23:745–746.

11. Knesaurek K, King MA, Glick SJ, Penney BC: Investigation of causes of geometric distortion in 180° and 360° angular sampling in SPECT. *J Nucl Med* 1989, 30:1666–1675.

12. Garcia EV, Galt JR, Cullom SJ, Faber TL: *Principles of Myocardial Perfusion SPECT Imaging*. North Billerica, MA: DuPont Pharma; 1994:30.

13. Galt JR, Garcia EV, Robbins WL: Effects of myocardial wall thickness on SPECT quantification. *IEEE Trans Med Imaging* 1990, 9:144–150.

14. Shepp LA, Vardi Y: Maximum likelihood reconstruction for emission tomography. *IEEE Trans Med Imaging* 1982, 1:113–122.

15. Hudson HM, Larkin RS: Accelerated image reconstruction using ordered subsets of projection data. *IEEE Trans Med Imaging* 1994, 13:601–609.

16. Jaszczak RJ, Greer KL, Floyd CE Jr, et al.: Improved SPECT quantification using compensation for scattered photons. *J Nucl Med* 1984, 25:893–900.

17. Ogawa K, Ichihara T, Kubo A: Accurate scatter correction in single photon emission CT. *Ann Nucl Med Sci* 1994, 7:145–150.

18. Galt JR, Garcia EV, Robbins WL: Effects of myocardial wall thickness on SPECT quantification. *IEEE Trans Med Imaging* 1990, 9:144–150.

19. Glick SJ, Penney BC, King MA, et al.: Noniterative compensation for the distance-dependent detector response and photon attenuation in SPECT imaging. *IEEE Trans Med Imaging* 1994, 13:363–374.

20. Zeng GL, Gullberg GT, Tsui BM, et al.: Three-dimensional iterative reconstruction algorithms with attenuation and geometric point response correction. *IEEE Trans Med Imaging* 1990, 22:1475–1479.

21. Smith WH, Kastner RJ, Calnon DA, et al.: Quantitative gated single-photon emission computed tomography imaging: a counts-based method for display and measurement of regional and global ventricular systolic function. *J Nucl Cardiol* 1997, 4:451–463.

22. Machac J, Chen H, Almeida OD, et al.: Comparison of 2D and high dose and low dose 3D gated myocardial Rb-82 PET imaging [abstract]. *J Nucl Med* 2002, 43:777.

23. Schelbert HR, Beanlands R, Bengel F, et al.: ASNC PET myocardial glucose metabolism and perfusion imaging guidelines: part II guideline for interpretation and reporting. *J Nucl Cardiol* 2003, 10:557–571.

24. DePuey EG, Garcia EV, eds: Updated imaging guidelines for nuclear cardiology procedures (part 1). *J Nucl Cardiol* 2001, 8:G1–G58.

25. Nichols KJ, Galt JR: Quality control for SPECT imaging. In *Cardiac SPECT Imaging*, edn 2. Edited by DePuey EG, Garcia EV, Berman DS. New York: Lippincott Williams & Wilkins; 2001:17–39.

26. DePuey EG: Artifacts in SPECT myocardial perfusion imaging. In *Cardiac SPECT Imaging*, edn 2. Edited by DePuey EG, Garcia EV, Berman DS. New York: Lippincott Williams & Wilkins; 2001:349.

27. DePuey EG, Garcia EV: Optimal specificity of thallium-201 SPECT through recognition of imaging artifacts. *J Nucl Med* 1989, 30:441–449.

28. Geckle WJ, Frank YL, Links JM, et al.: Correction for patient motion and organ movement in SPECT: application to exercise thallium-201 cardiac imaging. *J Nucl Med* 1988, 29:441–450.

29. Di Carli MF, Hachamovich R: New technology for noninvasive evaluation of coronary artery disease. *Circulation* 2007, 115:1464–1480.

30. Faber TL, Santana CA, Garcia EV, et al.: Three-dimensional fusion of coronary arteries with myocardial perfusion distributions: clinical validation. *J Nucl Med* 2004, 45:745–753.

31. Rispler S, Keidar Z, Ghersin E, et al.: Integrated single-photon emission computed tomography and computed tomography coronary angiography for the assessment of hemodynamically significant coronary artery lesions. *J Am Coll Cardiol* 2007, 49:1059–1067.

32. Gaemperli O, Schepis T, Husman L, et al.: Cardiac image fusion from stand-alone SPECT and CT: clinical experience. *J Nucl Med* 2007, 48:696–703.

33. Patton JA, Slomka PJ, Germano G, Berman DS: Recent technologic advances in nuclear cardiology. *J Nucl Cardiol* 2007, 14:501–513.

34. Borges-Neto S, Pagnanelli RA, Shaw LK, et al.: Clinical results of a novel wide beam reconstruction method for shortening scan time of Tc-99m cardiac SPECT perfusion studies. *J Nucl Cardiol* 2007, 14:555–565.

35. DePuey EG, Gadraju R, Clark J, et al.: Ordered subset expectation maximization and wide beam reconstruction "half-time" gated myocardial perfusion SPECT functional imaging: a comparison to "full-time" filtered backprojection. *J Nucl Cardiol* 2008, 15:547–563.

SPECT and PET Myocardial Perfusion Imaging: Tracers and Techniques

Vasken Dilsizian

The application of radiotracer technique to measure physiologic parameters, such as pulmonary circulation, dates back to 1927. Despite considerable advances in the application of radiotracer technique for interrogating physiologic and pathophysiologic cardiopulmonary conditions in the early 20th century, the spatial resolution of the scintigraphic instruments used to measure tracer concentration in the heart, lungs, and blood was limited. The advent of single photon emission computed tomography (SPECT) in the late 1970s and positron emission tomography (PET) in the 1980s dramatically changed the clinical utility of radiotracer technique for the assessment of myocardial perfusion, viability, and function.

Both SPECT and PET technologies use similar reconstruction processes to obtain tomographic images of the heart. However, they differ in the type of radiopharmaceuticals and the kind of instrumentation used to acquire cardiac images. SPECT allows noninvasive evaluation of myocardial blood flow by extractable tracers such as ^{201}Tl- and ^{99m}Tc-labeled perfusion tracers. PET, on the other hand, allows noninvasive assessment of regional blood flow, function, and metabolism using physiologic substrates prepared with positron-emitting isotopes, such as carbon, oxygen, nitrogen, and fluorine. Radioisotopes commonly used with SPECT emit gamma rays of varying energies and have relatively long physical half-lives. Localization of gamma rays emitted by single photon emitting radiotracers in the heart is accomplished by an Anger scintillation camera (gamma camera), which converts the gamma rays to light photons via sodium iodide scintillation detectors. The gamma camera limits the direction of photons entering the detector by a collimator and then positions each event electronically. Thus, the radioisotopes used for optimal scintigraphic registration with SPECT are limited to those that emit gamma rays with an energy range that is suitable for the gamma camera and related single photon devices, such as ^{201}Tl, ^{99m}Tc, and ^{123}I. The spatial resolution of the SPECT system is in the range of 9 to 12 mm. Although clinically useful, estimates of relative myocardial blood flow by SPECT are significantly affected by attenuation artifacts.

Positron-emitting radioisotopes commonly used with PET emit two gamma rays, 511 keV each, and have relatively short physical half-lives. When the high energy positron is emitted from a nucleus, it travels a short distance and collides with an electron. The result is complete annihilation of both the positron and the electron and conversion of the combined mass to energy in the form of electromagnetic radiation (two gamma rays, 511 keV energy each). Because the gamma rays are perfectly collinear (discharged at 180 degrees to each other) and travel in opposite directions, the PET detectors can be programmed to register only events with temporal coincidence of photons that strike directly at opposing detectors. This results in improved spatial (4–6 mm) and temporal resolution. Moreover, the PET system is more sensitive than a SPECT system (higher count rate) and provides the possibility of attenuation correction. The consequence of these advantages with PET is the possibility for quantitation of tracer concentration in absolute units.

Properties of SPECT Flow Tracers

Tracer	Mechanism of Myocyte Uptake	Usual Dose, mCi
^{201}Tl	Na-K ATPase – sarcolemma	3.0–2.0
^{99m}Tc sestamibi	Negative transmembrane potential – mitochondria	8–40
^{99m}Tc tetrofosmin	Negative transmembrane potential – mitochondria	8–40

A

Properties of PET Flow Tracers

Tracer	Mechanism of Myocyte Uptake	Usual Dose, mCi
^{82}Rb	Na-K ATPase – sarcolemma	30–60
^{13}N ammonia	Trapped as 13N glutamine (mediated by ATP) – cytoplasm	10–20

B

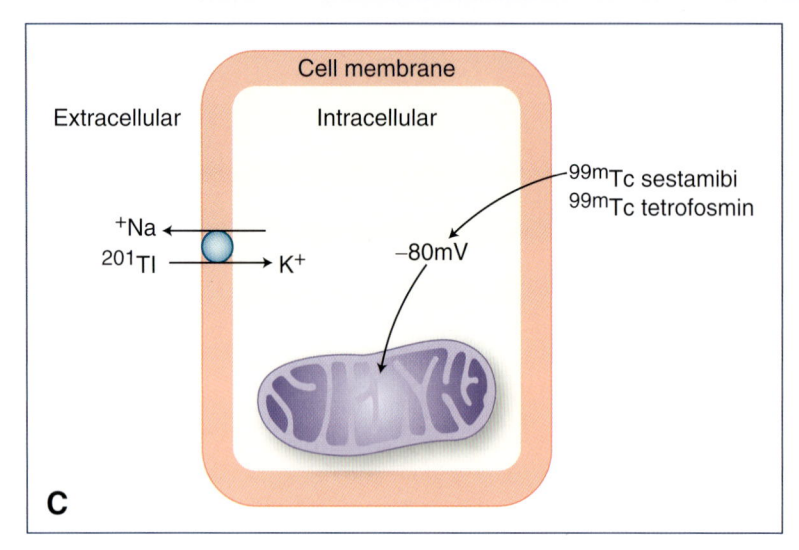

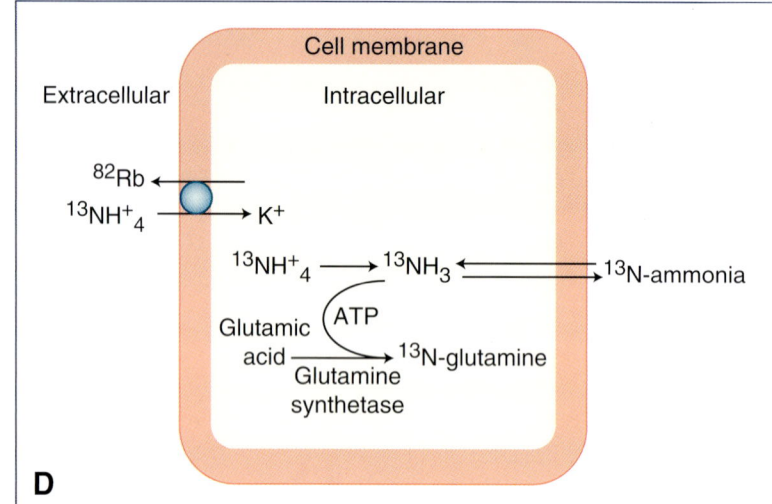

Figure 2-1. **A–D,** Properties of SPECT and PET flow tracers. To reflect regional myocardial perfusion, radiotracers commonly used with SPECT and PET must have high extraction by the heart and rapid clearance from the blood. Clinically available radiopharmaceuticals that meet these criteria are ^{201}Tl and ^{99m}Tc-labeled sestamibi and tetrofosmin with SPECT, and ^{82}Rb and ^{13}N-ammonia with PET. Radiotracers that are not highly extracted (< 50%), or if the residence time in the blood is prolonged (clearance half-time of > 5 minutes), cannot be used to assess regional perfusion.

38 Atlas of Nuclear Cardiology

Myocardial Perfusion, Uptake, and Clearance

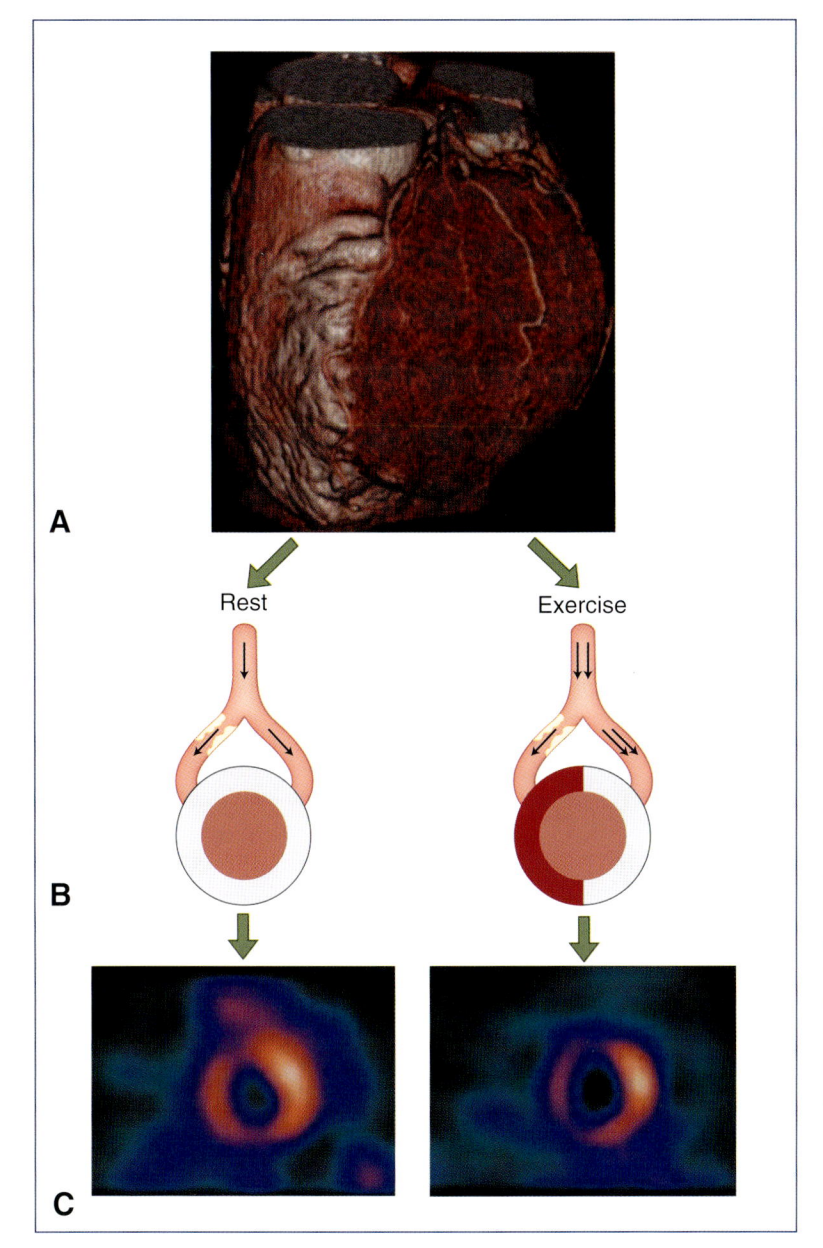

Figure 2-2. Myocardial blood flow and coronary anatomy: disparate yet complementary information. Regional myocardial blood flow is critically dependent on the driving pressure gradient and the resistance of the vascular bed. Advanced degrees of coronary artery disease may exist at rest (**A**) without myocardial ischemia due to compensatory dilatation of the resistance vessels. As illustrated in **B** and **C**, at rest, regional myocardial blood flow is preserved in both patent and stenosed coronary artery branches. Such disparity between myocardial blood flow and coronary anatomy attests to the complementary information that physiologic study such as myocardial perfusion SPECT or PET provides to that of coronary angiography with CT or diagnostic catheterization. In a canine model, over 80% occlusion of the coronary artery was necessary before ischemia was observed under the basal state. Because the pressure drop across a stenosis varies directly with the length of the stenosis and inversely with the fourth power of the radius (Bernoulli's theorem), resistance almost triples as the severity of coronary artery stenosis increases from 80% to 90%. Consequently, during exercise or pharmacologic stress testing, when the resistance to the distal bed and the pressure distending the stenotic coronary artery declines, myocardial ischemia ensues (**B** and **C**).

Coronary blood flow in myocardial regions without coronary artery stenosis may increase about two- to threefold during vigorous aerobic exercise. However, in the setting of moderate-to-severe coronary artery stenosis, the degree of coronary flow increase may be attenuated when compared to myocardial regions without coronary artery stenosis (**B**). The insufficient coronary blood flow increase during stress results in impaired perfusion and myocardial ischemia (**C**). In patients with coronary artery disease, an inverse relationship has been shown between the increase in myocardial blood flow and the percentage of coronary artery stenosis once the lumen is narrowed by approximately 40% to 50%. Thus, when a radiotracer such as thallium is injected at peak exercise, the relative differences in regional myocardial blood flow will be reflected in disproportionate concentrations of regional thallium activity on the stress images. Myocardial perfusion imaging, therefore, identifies subcritical coronary artery stenosis when performed in conjunction with exercise or pharmacologic stress, but not at rest.

Figure 2-3. Schematic illustration of radiotracer uptake in relation to regional myocardial blood flow. The radiotracer that most closely parallels myocardial blood flow would be expected to most accurately identify coronary artery narrowing. There are several classes of radiopharmaceuticals that meet these criteria, such as microspheres, ^{201}Tl, ^{99m}Tc-labeled perfusion tracers, ^{15}O-water, ^{13}N-ammonia, and ^{82}Rb. Differences in the first-pass extraction of these tracers ultimately determine the regional myocardial tracer uptake relative to regional blood flow. The extraction fraction is determined experimentally in a Langendorf preparation and represents first-pass or single-pass extraction of the radiotracer from the blood into the myocardium. An ideal myocardial perfusion tracer would be expected to exhibit a linear relationship to myocardial blood flow over a wide range of flow rates in mL/g/min. ^{15}O-water, a PET myocardial flow tracer, exhibits such a relationship. A linear relationship between tracer uptake and myocardial blood flow would, therefore, differentiate between regions with normal or high blood flow (supplied by normal coronary arteries) and abnormal or low blood flow (supplied by narrowed coronary arteries). However, this is not the case for all other radiotracers commonly used in clinical practice. In an open-chest canine model of regional myocardial ischemia with dipyridamole-induced hyperemia, thallium showed a more ideal linear relationship between tracer uptake and myocardial blood flow assessed by microspheres when compared with ^{99m}Tc-labeled myocardial perfusion agents. While the extraction fraction of ^{201}Tl is high at 85%, the extraction fraction of ^{99m}Tc-sestamibi is only 60%, and that of ^{99m}Tc-tetrofosmin is approximately 54%. Beyond the first-pass extraction, recirculation of the radiotracer in patients allows further extraction of the radiotracers from the blood into the myocardium during that particular physiologic state (rest, exercise, pharmacologic, or mental stress).

At rest, myocardial blood flow is approximately 1 mL/g/min. During physical exercise, myocardial blood flow usually increases two- to three-fold, while with pharmacologic vasodilation (adenosine or dipyridamole) myocardial blood flow exceeds 3 mL/g/min. All clinically available perfusion tracers, SPECT and PET, demonstrate "roll-off" at high coronary blood flow levels (deviation from the line of identity). For SPECT tracers, this "roll-off" phenomenon is particulary marked for ^{99m}Tc-sestamibi and ^{99m}Tc-tetrofosmin, and less so for ^{201}Tl. The implications of this is that at higher flow levels, relative myocardial tracer uptake may underestimate regional myocardial blood flow, and thereby underlying coronary artery disease. Clinical studies have shown that this underestimation of regional blood flow deficits does not affect the detection of significant (> 70%) coronary artery stenosis. However, it is important to point out that coronary artery stenosis between 50% to 70% may go undetected, especially with ^{99m}Tc-sestamibi and ^{99m}Tc-tetrofosmin.

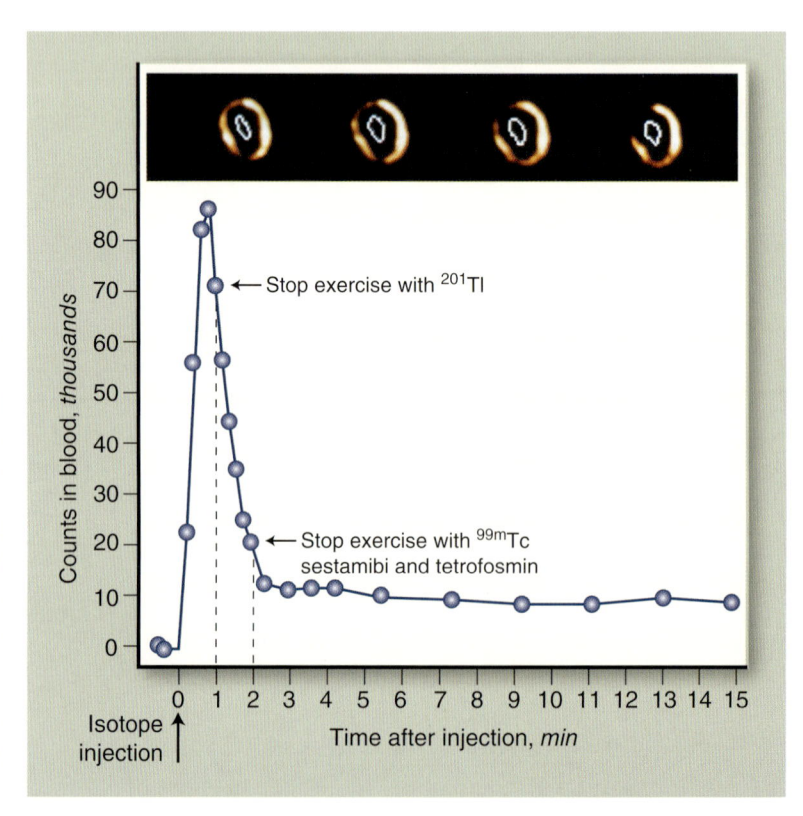

Figure 2-4. Blood clearance of radiotracers. Once a radiotracer is injected intravenously at peak stress, it is extracted rapidly from the blood and accumulated in the myocardium in proportion to regional blood flow. All clinically useful radiotracers have extraction fractions above 50% and are cleared rapidly from the blood in 5 to 7 minutes after injection. Because ^{201}Tl has a higher first-pass extraction fraction and cleared more rapidly from the blood than ^{99m}Tc-sestamibi and ^{99m}Tc-tetrofosmin, patients are encouraged to exercise for an additional 1 minute after injection of ^{201}Tl at peak exercise, and for 2 minutes after injection of ^{99m}Tc-sestamibi or ^{99m}Tc-tetrofosmin at peak exercise. If exercise is stopped too early with the ^{99m}Tc perfusion tracers (that is, 1 minute rather than 2 minutes after injection), residual radiotracer activity in the blood will be taken up at a different physiologic state (under resting condition), thereby underestimating the presence and extent of myocardial ischemia.

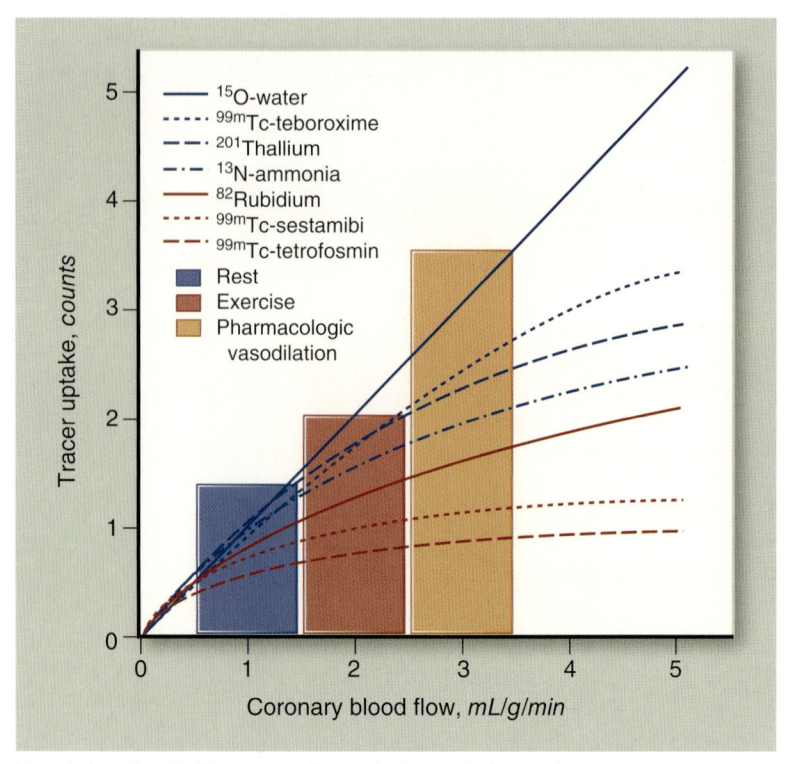

Image Interpretation and Quantitation

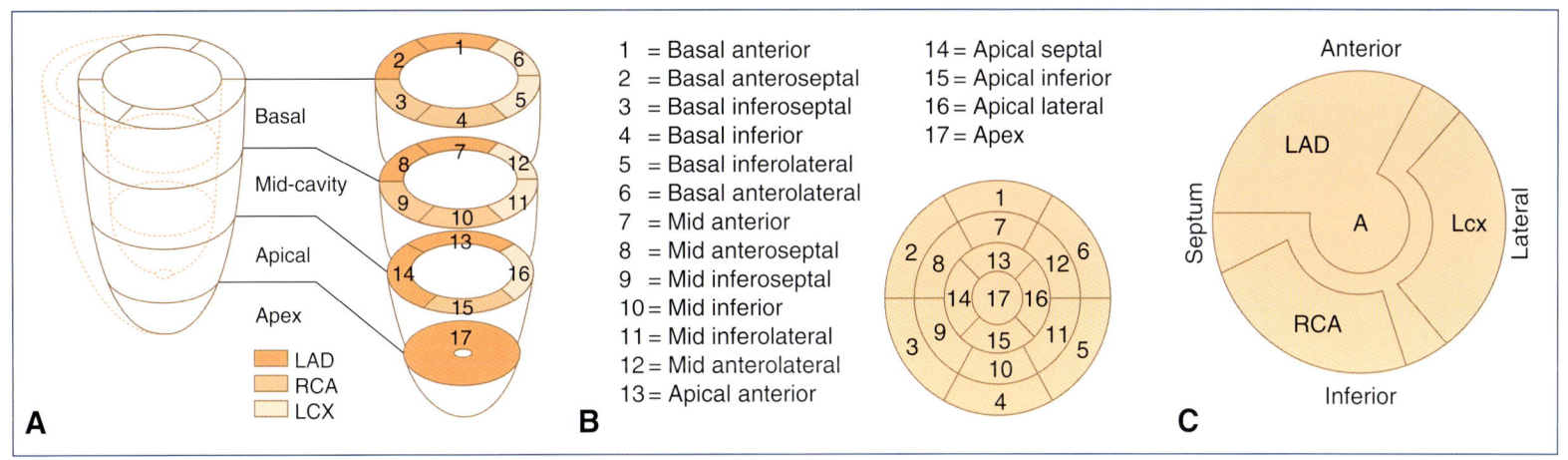

Figure 2-5. Myocardial segmentation, standard nomenclature, and vascular territories. SPECT myocardial perfusion images are interpreted on the basis of the presence, location, extent, and severity of perfusion defects using a standard 17-segment model [1] and visual scoring. **A,** Standard segmentation model divides the left ventricle into three major short-axis slices: apical, mid-cavity, and basal. The apical short-axis slice is divided into four segments, whereas the mid-cavity and basal slices are divided into six segments. The apex is analyzed separately, usually from a vertical long-axis slice. Although the anatomy of coronary arteries may vary in individual patients, the anterior, septal, and apical segments are usually ascribed to the left anterior descending (LAD) coronary artery, the inferior and basal septal segments to the right coronary artery (RCA), and the lateral segments to the left circumflex (LCX) coronary artery. The apex can also be supplied by the RCA and LCX artery. **B,** Data from the individual short-axis tomograms can be combined to create a bull's-eye polar plot representing a two-dimensional compilation of all the three-dimensional short-axis perfusion data. Standard nomenclature for the 17 segments is outlined. **C,** The two-dimensional compilation of perfusion data can then easily be assigned to specific vascular territories.

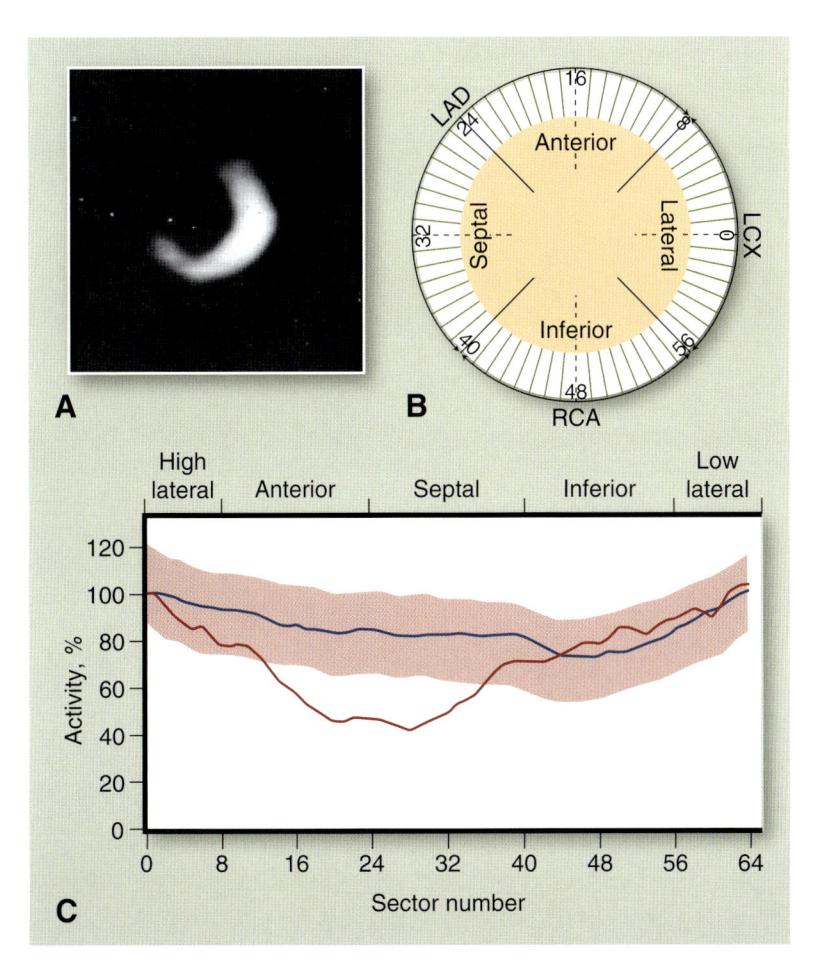

Figure 2-6. Quantitative analysis. Because radionuclide images are intrinsically digital images, true quantification of tracer uptake in myocardial regions is feasible [2]. **A,** The methodology of semiautomatic quantitative cicumferential-profile analysis applied to a short-axis ^{201}Tl tomogram obtained after exercise in a patient with coronary artery disease. **B,** The left ventricular myocardium is divided into 64 sectors, representing four myocardial regions. **C,** The patient's thallium uptake during stress imaging in each section (*red line*) and the normal range (mean ± 2 SD for normal subjects; *shaded area with blue line*). The patient's count profile displays the distribution of counts in the tomogram relative to maximal counts counter-clockwise, starting at 0, representing the high lateral region that is designated the value of 100% (maximal count density). Whenever a region of the circumferential profile falls below the lower limit of normal, that region of the patient's myocardium is considered to have a perfusion defect. In this patient, thallium perfusion defects are apparent in the anterior and septal regions. LAD—left anterior descending; LCX—left circumflex; RCA—right coronary artery.

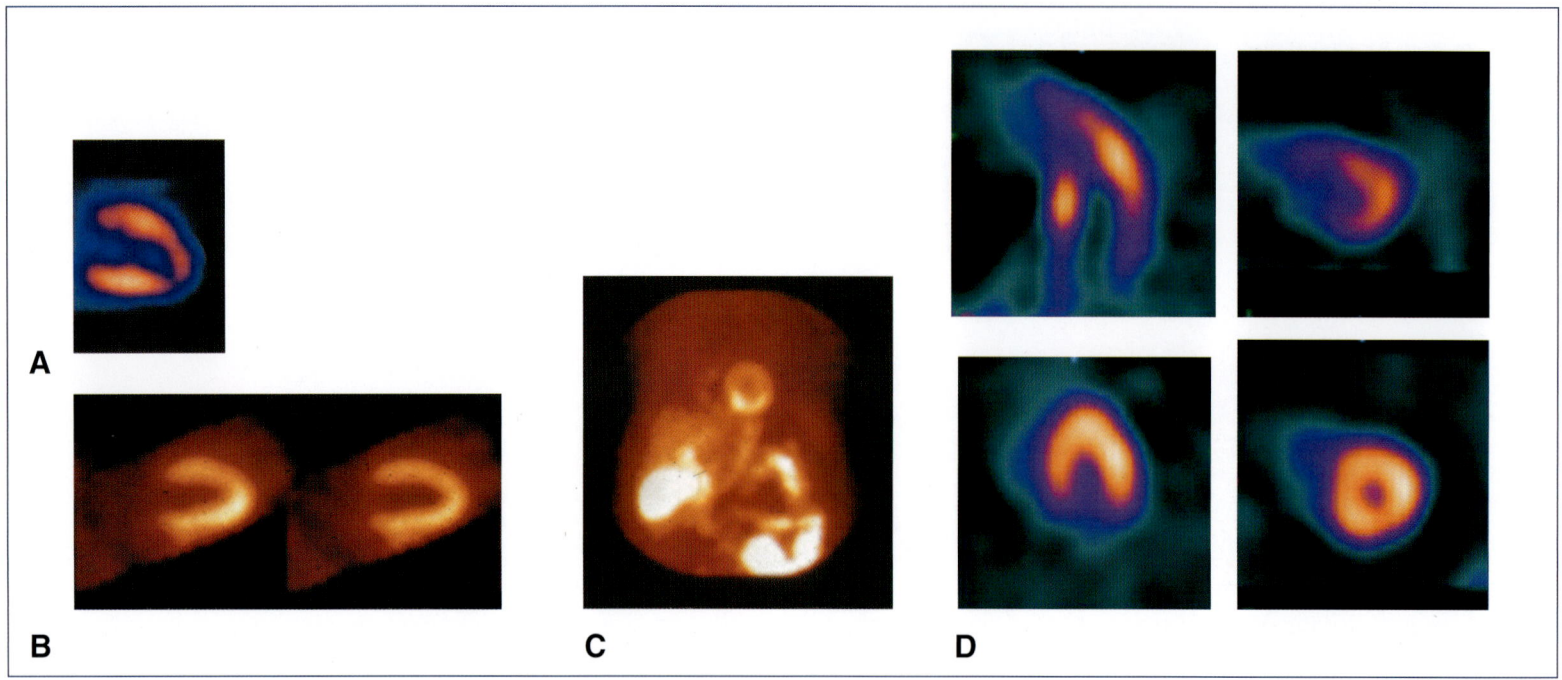

Figure 2-7. Common variations and artifacts of myocardial perfusion SPECT. Although normal myocardial perfusion SPECT images appear to have homogeneous radiotracer uptake, regional inhomogeneities are commonly present that are related to normal structural variation, tissue attenuation, abdominal visceral activity, as well as technical factors associated with image acquisition. On normal SPECT images, the lateral region is usually the area with maximal radiotracer uptake. This should not be interpreted as relative hypoperfusion in all other myocardial regions (which will appear to have slightly less uptake). Rather, during SPECT acquisition, the camera is physically closer to the lateral wall (which is in close proximity to the lateral chest wall) than to the other myocardial regions. Consequently, the lateral region is subject to less soft tissue attenuation and associated with more efficient count capture. Thus, it is often difficult to detect subtle perfusion defects visually within the lateral region because the activity of the radiotracer may remain greater than or similar to other myocardial regions. This would especially be the case in patients with multivessel disease, in whom equivalent reduction in perfusion in several myocardial regions would still result in greater tracer activity in the lateral territory, termed *balanced reduction in flow*. Normal structural variations include the "drop-out" of the upper septum (transition from muscular to membranous septum) and apical thinning (anatomically thinner apex may appear as a perfusion defect). **A,** Example of apical thinning. Soft tissue attenuation can present as breast attenuation (commonly in women with large or dense breasts). **B,** Example of a patient with breast attenuation, which shows mildly decreased uptake in the anterior region. **C,** Breast attenuation can be recognized on the rotating planar projection images as a photopenic shadow over the heart that has the contour of a breast. The demonstration of preserved wall thickening in the anterior region by gated SPECT imaging may be helpful in differentiating attenuation artifact from myocardial infarction. Similarly, inferior wall attenuation can be caused by the diaphragm or by other abdominal visceral structures, such as liver or bowel, either overlapping or near the inferior wall. Adjacent abdominal visceral activity may falsely increase the number of counts that are assigned within the heart (in which case the adjacent myocardium appears "hot") or cause a "ramp filter" or "negative lobe" artifact (in which case the adjacent myocardium appears "cool").

D, An example of a patient motion artifact exhibiting as a "hurricane sign." Images in the *top row* show the consequence of significant patient motion in creating artifactual regional perfusion defects. In the *bottom row*, when the images are reacquired in the same patient, without motion artifact, the distribution of the radiotracer appears homogeneous in all myocardial regions without regional pefusion defects.

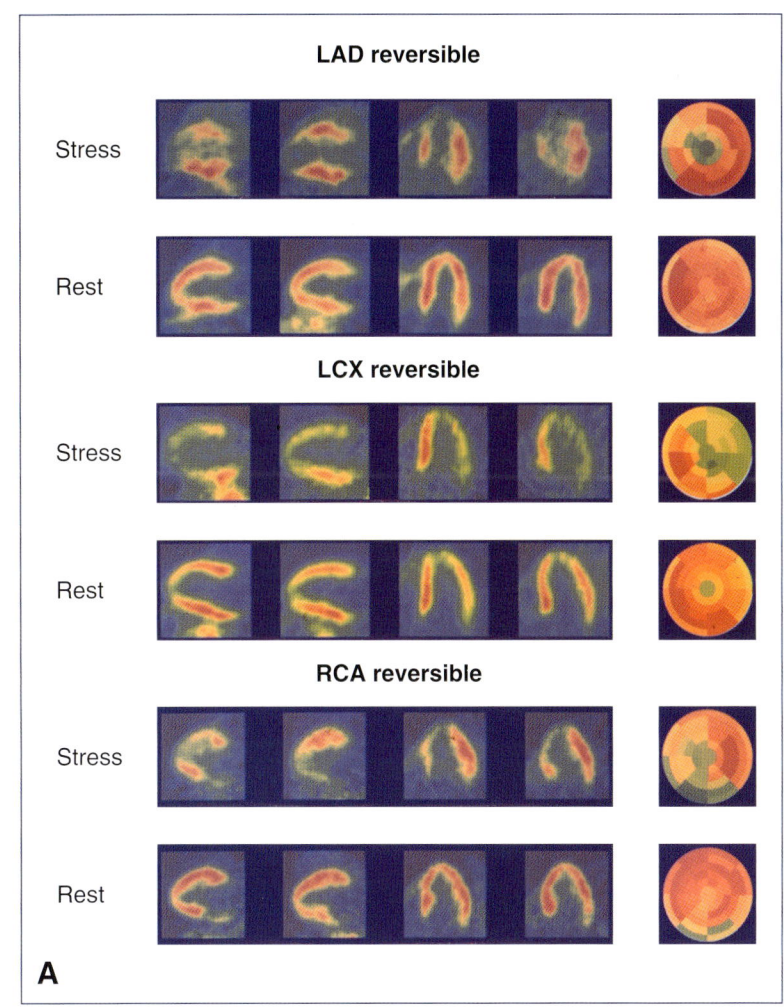

Figure 2-8. Reversible and irreversible perfusion defects: myocardial ischemia and infarction. Imbalance between oxygen supply (usually due to reduced myocardial perfusion) and oxygen demand (determined primarily by the rate and force of myocardial contraction) is termed *ischemic myocardium*. Clinical presentation of such imbalance may be symptomatic (angina pectoris) or asymptomatic (silent ischemia). If the oxygen supply-demand imbalance is transient (*ie*, triggered by exertion) it represents reversible ischemia. The scintigraphic hallmark of reversible ischemia is a reversible perfusion defect. **A**, Examples of patients with reversible perfusion defects in the left anterior descending (LAD), left circumflex (LCX), and right coronary artery (RCA) territories. On the other hand, if regional oxygen supply-demand imbalance is prolonged (*ie*, during myocardial infarction), high-energy phosphates will be depleted, regional contractile function will progressively deteriorate, and cell membrane rupture with cell death will follow (myocardial infarction). The scintigraphic hallmark of myocardial infarction is a fixed or irreversible perfusion defect. **B**, Examples of patients with irreversible (fixed) perfusion defects in the LAD, LCX, and RCA territories.

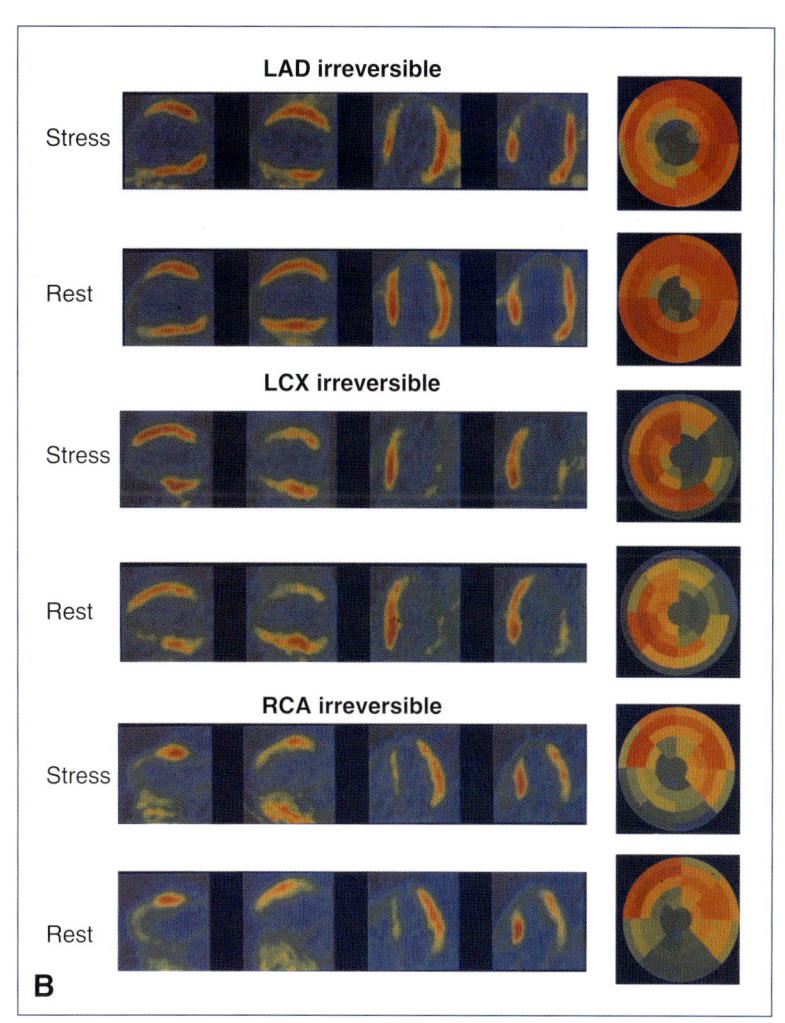

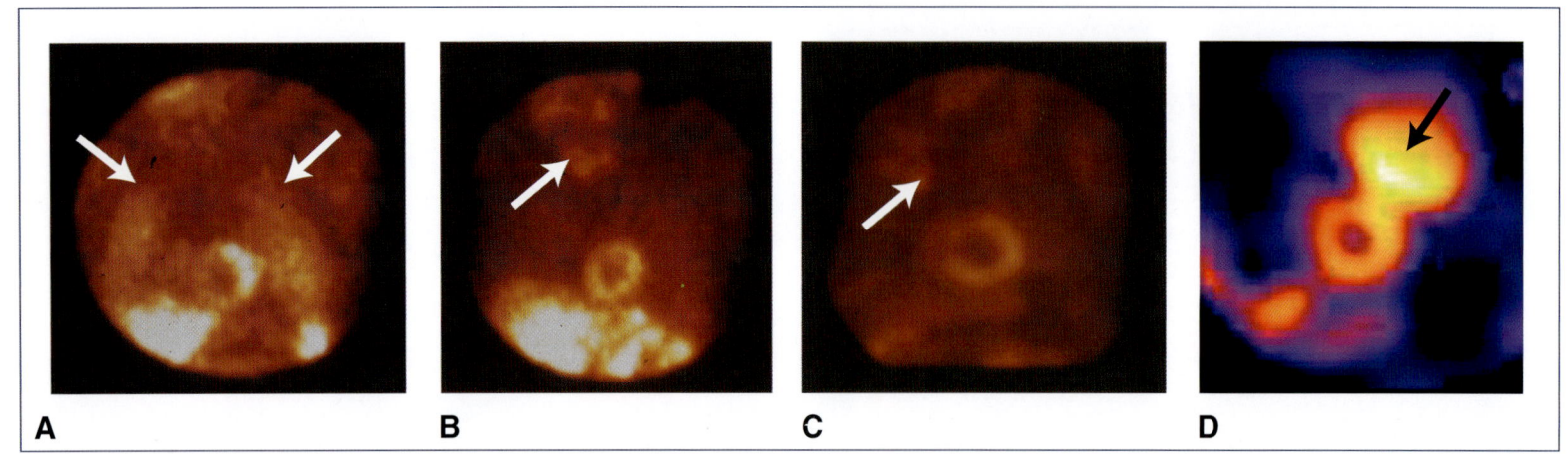

Figure 2-9. Clinically relevant extracardiac activity. Beyond myocardial perfusion, additional important abnormal findings can be present on the rotating planar projection images, such as lung uptake, parathyroid adenoma, or lung cancer, which should be observed and reported. **A**, Increased lung uptake (*arrows*) is associated with extensive coronary artery disease and an adverse prognosis. In patients with extensive myocardial ischemia and/or left ventricular dysfunction, it is likely that increases in left atrial and pulmonary capillary wedge pressures slows the pulmonary transit of the radiotracer, thereby allowing more time for extraction or transudation of the radiotracer into the interstitial spaces of the lung. Lung uptake has been more extensively validated with ^{201}Tl than ^{99m}Tc perfusion tracers. Because of differences in the biodistribution and clearance of ^{201}Tl and ^{99m}Tc perfusion tracers, thallium images are acquired within a few minutes after exercise (minimal splanchnic and background activity) while the ^{99m}Tc-sestamibi and ^{99m}Tc-tetrofosmin are usually acquired 15 to 30 minutes after exercise and 30 to 60 minutes after pharmacologic vasodilation (liver uptake is more prominent than the heart if imaged too early). Thus, lung uptake, even if it had been present early after stress, may be missed with ^{99m}Tc-sestamibi and ^{99m}Tc-tetrofosmin because of more delayed imaging after stress compared with thallium.

The rotating planar projection images allow the visualization of noncardiac structures, such as lung, breast, and the thyroid gland. Abnormal uptake of ^{201}Tl, ^{99m}Tc-sestamibi, and ^{99m}Tc-tetrofosmin in the neck can identify parathyroid adenoma, while in the chest they can identify primary (such as lung or breast cancer) or metastatic lesions. **B**, An example of a patient with findings of a parathyroid adenoma (*arrow*) on a stress ^{99m}Tc-sestamibi myocardial perfusion SPECT. **C**, Similarly, an example of a patient with findings of solitary lung nodule (*arrow*) on a stress ^{99m}Tc-sestamibi myocardial perfusion SPECT. **D**, Intense ^{99m}Tc-sestamibi uptake (*arrow*), superior to the heart, represents an anterior mediastinal mass, compatible with thymoma. While thymomas are the most common neoplasm of the anterior mediastinum, representing 20% of all anterior mediastinal masses in the adult population, their incidence is rather rare, only 0.15 per 100,000 cases. The differentiation of benign from malignant thymoma cannot be made on the basis of size or intensity of ^{99m}Tc-sestamibi uptake. Additional studies are required to further characterize the lesion. (**D**, *courtesy of* Jeffrey R. Folk.)

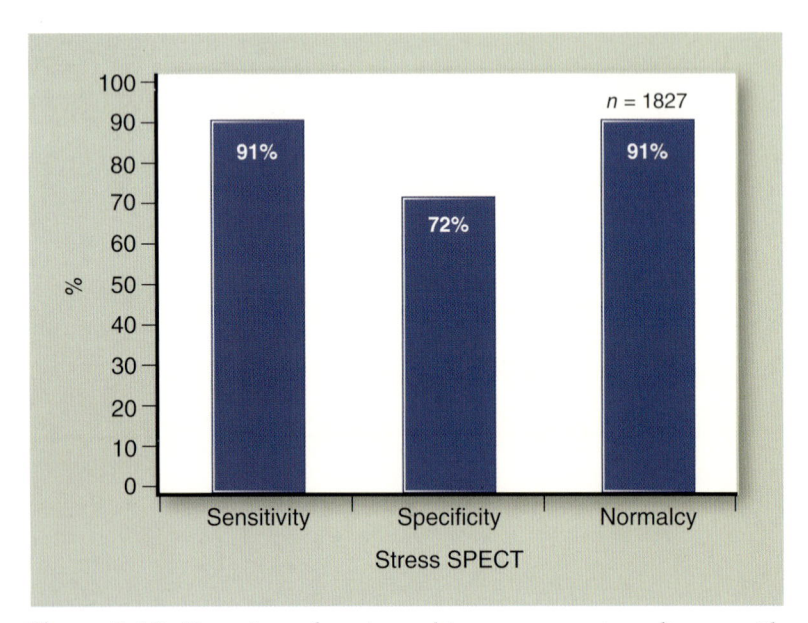

Figure 2-10. Detection of angiographic coronary artery disease with radiotracers. Extensive literature exists on the diagnostic yield of stress SPECT myocardial perfusion imaging [3–14]. Among 1827 patients referred for evaluation of chest discomfort (pooled data from 12 studies performed between 1989 and 1999), the overall sensitivity of myocardial perfusion SPECT for the detection of angiographic coronary artery disease was 91%, the specificity was 72%, and the normalcy rate (in subjects with low likelihood for coronary artery disease who did not undergo coronary angiography) was 91%.

Clinical Indications for Myocardial Perfusion Imaging

Detection of coronary artery disease

Evaluation of known coronary artery disease

Risk stratification

Preoperative evaluation

Differentiation of viable from scarred myocardium

Assessment of acute chest pain in the emergency department

Figure 2-11. Clinical indications for myocardial perfusion imaging. The clinical indications for stress-rest myocardial perfusion SPECT imaging are well established [15]. Most patients are referred because of chest pain symptoms and suspected coronary artery disease (CAD). However, patients with known CAD are referred as well. In these patients, the purpose of testing may be to evaluate the effect of therapy or to determine the cause of changes in symptom patterns. In addition, many patients are referred for risk stratification after acute myocardial infarction. Stress-rest SPECT imaging plays an important role in the preoperative evaluation of patients who are scheduled to undergo major noncardiac surgery. The most important and useful clinical application of SPECT myocardial perfusion imaging is to stratify patients into low- and high-risk categories, and thus contribute to the management of patients.

Figure 2-12. High- and low-risk SPECT images. SPECT images should not be interpreted as either normal or abnormal. The prognosis of a patient is related to the degree of myocardial perfusion abnormality. Quantification or semiquantification provides that important prognostic information. High-risk SPECT images are characterized by large perfusion defects on the stress images that involve multiple coronary artery territories (if two or more coronary territories are involved, the study should be considered high risk). Large stress-induced reversible defects represent extensive myocardial ischemia, which may be associated with increased lung uptake, transient ischemic left ventricular cavity dilation, and transient increased right ventricular myocardial visualization.

One of the strongest features of stress myocardial perfusion SPECT imaging is its ability to identify low-risk patients. Patients with unequivocal normal exercise or pharmacologic stress myocardial perfusion SPECT images exhibit less than a 1% future cardiac event rate, the same as the general population. For those undergoing an exercise study, this presumes that the patient achieved greater than 85% predicted maximum heart rate for a man or woman of their age. Similarly, presuming that adequate exercise was performed, patients with small myocardial perfusion defects on stress and small regions of defect reversibility have low risk for future cardiac events. These patients should be treated aggressively with medical therapy because of the presence of coronary artery disease. It is important to emphasize that stress myocardial perfusion SPECT images should always be interpreted in conjunction with clinical and electrocardiographic data. For example, a rare patient may have a markedly abnormal exercise portion of the test but normal or near-normal SPECT images. It is the responsibility of the nuclear cardiologist to determine the significance of such disparate data.

High- and Low-risk SPECT Images

High Risk
- Large perfusion defect on stress imaging
- Multiple coronary artery territories
- Large reversibility
- Increased lung uptake
- Transient left ventricular dilation

Low Risk
- Normal stress images
- Small stress defect
- Small reversibility

SPECT Techniques: ^{201}Tl

SPECT Techniques: ^{201}Tl

- Monovalent cation with biologic properties similar to potassium
- 60–80 keV mercury x-ray emission, 73-h physical half-life
- High first-pass extraction fraction (~ 85%)
- Transported across myocyte sarcolemmal membrane via the Na-K ATPase transport system and by facilitative diffusion
- Peak myocardial concentration within 5 minutes of intravenous injection
- Rapid clearance from the intravascular compartment
- Redistribution begins 10 to 15 minutes after injection

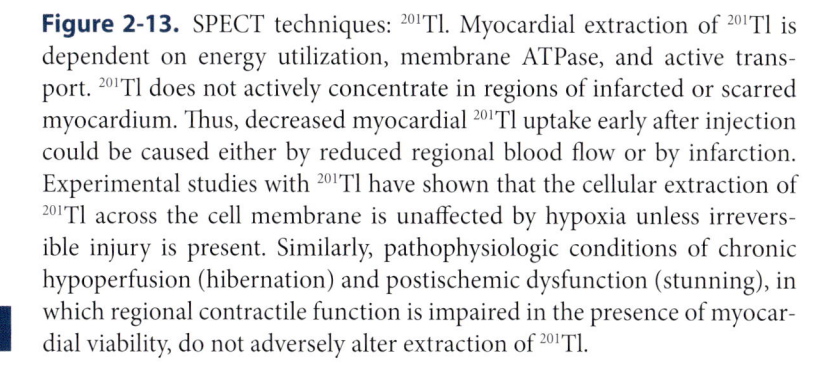

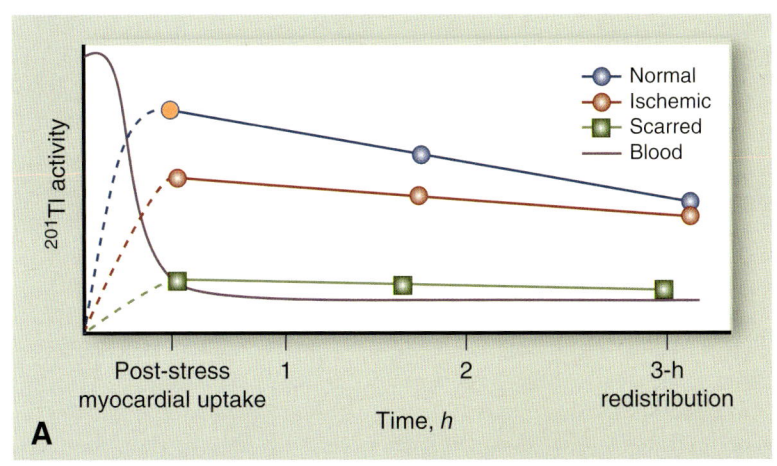

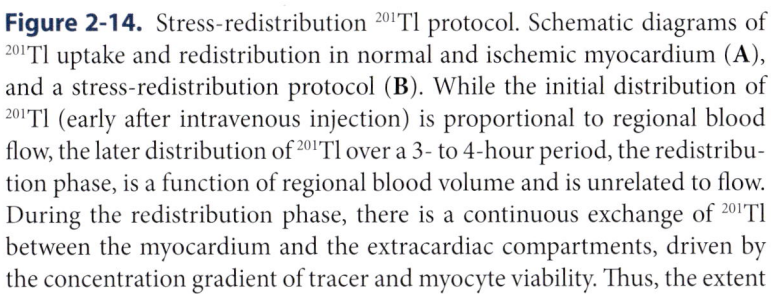

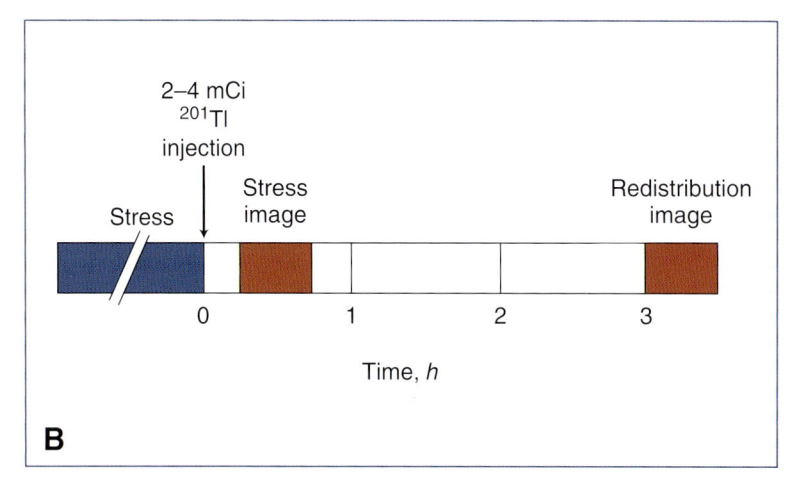

Figure 2-13. SPECT techniques: ^{201}Tl. Myocardial extraction of ^{201}Tl is dependent on energy utilization, membrane ATPase, and active transport. ^{201}Tl does not actively concentrate in regions of infarcted or scarred myocardium. Thus, decreased myocardial ^{201}Tl uptake early after injection could be caused either by reduced regional blood flow or by infarction. Experimental studies with ^{201}Tl have shown that the cellular extraction of ^{201}Tl across the cell membrane is unaffected by hypoxia unless irreversible injury is present. Similarly, pathophysiologic conditions of chronic hypoperfusion (hibernation) and postischemic dysfunction (stunning), in which regional contractile function is impaired in the presence of myocardial viability, do not adversely alter extraction of ^{201}Tl.

Figure 2-14. Stress-redistribution ^{201}Tl protocol. Schematic diagrams of ^{201}Tl uptake and redistribution in normal and ischemic myocardium (**A**), and a stress-redistribution protocol (**B**). While the initial distribution of ^{201}Tl (early after intravenous injection) is proportional to regional blood flow, the later distribution of ^{201}Tl over a 3- to 4-hour period, the redistribution phase, is a function of regional blood volume and is unrelated to flow. During the redistribution phase, there is a continuous exchange of ^{201}Tl between the myocardium and the extracardiac compartments, driven by the concentration gradient of tracer and myocyte viability. Thus, the extent to defect resolution, from the initial to delayed redistribution images over time (a reversible defect), reflects one index of myocardial viability. When only nonviable, scarred myocardium is present, the initial ^{201}Tl defect (an irreversible defect) persists over time without redistribution. When both viable and scarred myocardium are present, ^{201}Tl redistribution is incomplete, giving the appearance of partial reversibility. Thus, the initial phase of ^{201}Tl studies reflect reductions in flow caused by coronary artery narrowing, while the delayed, redistribution phase of ^{201}Tl studies reflect myocardial potassium space, differentiating viable from scarred myocardium.

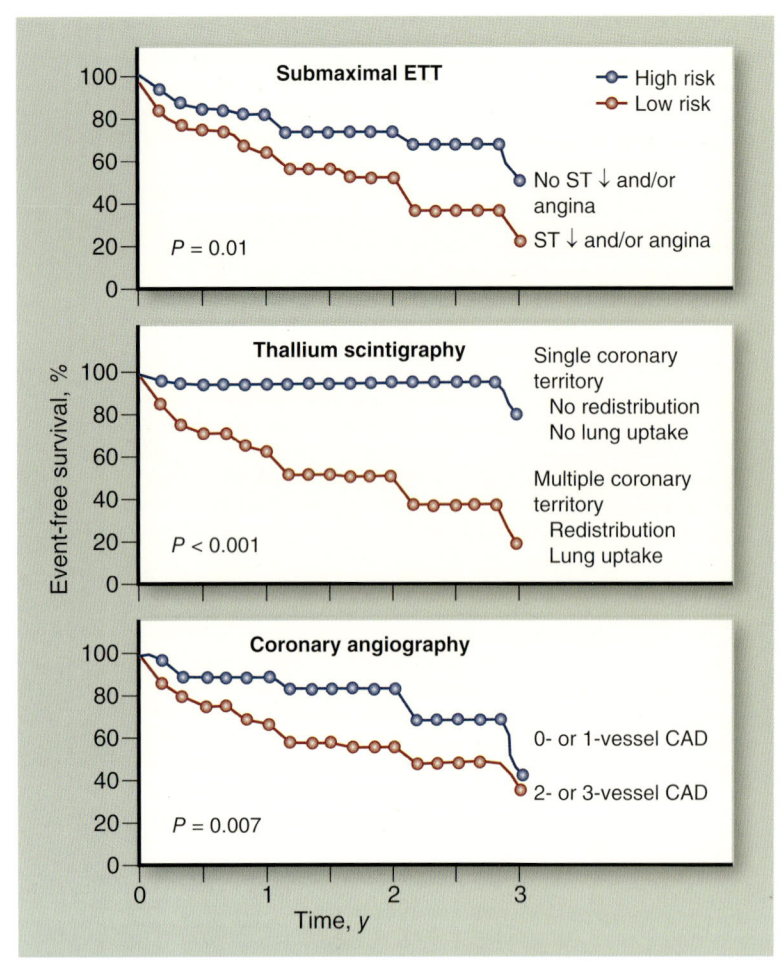

Figure 2-15. Prognostic value of thallium scintigraphy. Beyond its value as a perfusion and viability tracer, the stress-redistribution ^{201}Tl studies provide useful information regarding patient outcome and prognosis. In patients with chronic ischemic heart disease, increased lung-to-heart ratio after stress, transient left ventricular cavity dilatation, and extensive reversible and irreversible ^{201}Tl defects have been shown to be important predictors of adverse outcome. Similarly, the combination of reversible ^{201}Tl defects and increased lung-to-heart ratio has been shown to differentiate between low-risk and high-risk patients after an acute myocardial infarction. Among patients with acute myocardial infarction who underwent a predischarge submaximal exercise treadmill test (ETT), ^{201}Tl scintigraphy, and coronary angiography, ^{201}Tl identified the low-risk subgroup much better than submaximal exercise treadmill testing or coronary angiography. (*Adapted from* Gibson *et al.* [16].)

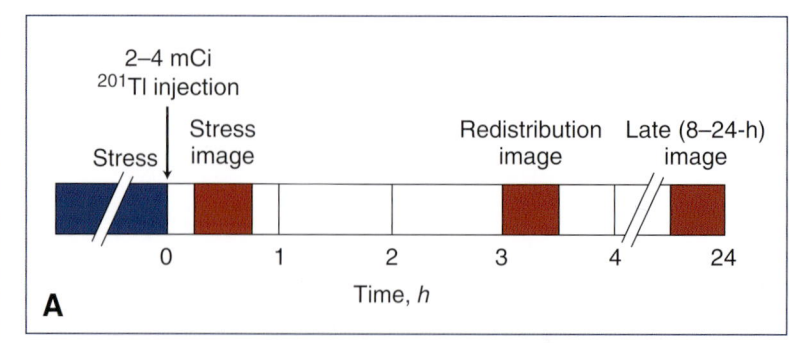

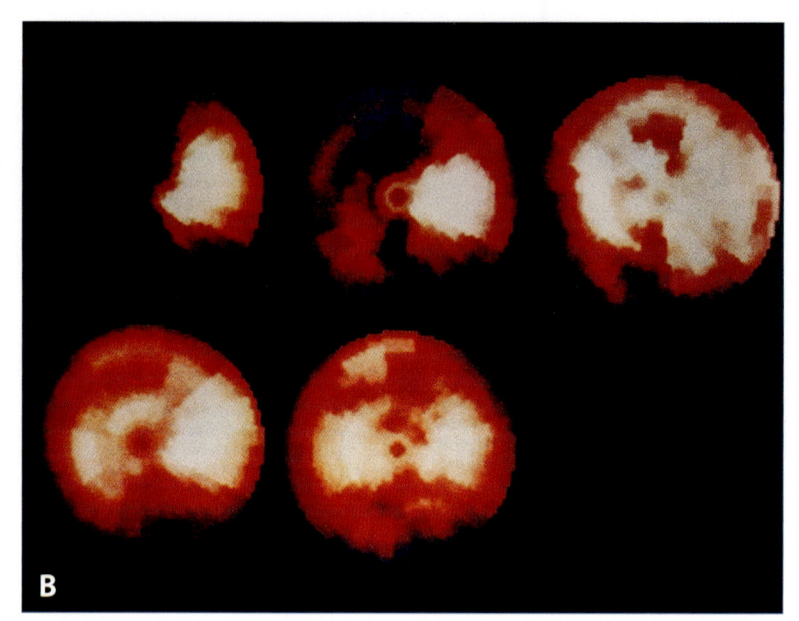

Figure 2-16. Late (24-hour) ^{201}Tl redistribution. **A,** Late redistribution protocol after stress-redistribution ^{201}Tl imaging. In some patients with critically stenosed coronary arteries, the initial uptake of ^{201}Tl in the ischemic region is low and the accumulation of the tracer from the recirculating ^{201}Tl in the blood is slow. Consequently, ischemic but viable myocardium may appear irreversible over the 3- to 4-hour redistribution period and may mimic the appearance of scarred myocardium. However, if more time is allowed for redistribution, a greater number of viable myocardial regions may be differentiated from scarred myocardium.

B, Polar maps demonstrating the effect of late ^{201}Tl redistribution. Bull's-eye image of ^{201}Tl immediately after exercise (*top panel, left*) shows marked decrease in tracer uptake throughout the anterior, septal, apical, and inferoapical regions, with partial redistribution on the 4-hour delayed image (*center*). However, on the late (17-hour) redistribution image (*right*), there is complete reversibility in all myocardial regions, suggestive of extensive myocardial ischemia rather than scar. After successful percutaneous transluminal coronary angioplasty, bull's-eye image of ^{201}Tl immediately after exercise (*bottom panel, left*) shows normal distribution of the tracer throughout all myocardial regions, documenting the accuracy of late redistribution ^{201}Tl and the absence of myocardial scarring. In patients undergoing revascularization, 95% of segments that demonstrated late redistribution showed improved ^{201}Tl uptake after revascularization. However, as with early (3–4 hour) redistribution, the absence of late redistribution underestimates the presence of viable myocardium (*right*). Up to 37% of segments that remained irreversible on both early and late redistribution studies showed improvement in function after revascularization [17]. Moreover, despite implementing longer imaging time, a number of late redistribution studies had suboptimal count statistics at 24 hours. The data suggest that although late ^{201}Tl imaging improves the identification of viable myocardium when compared with early redistribution imaging, it continues to underestimate segmental improvement after revascularization. (**B,** *from* Cloninger *et al.* [18]; with permission.)

46 Atlas of Nuclear Cardiology

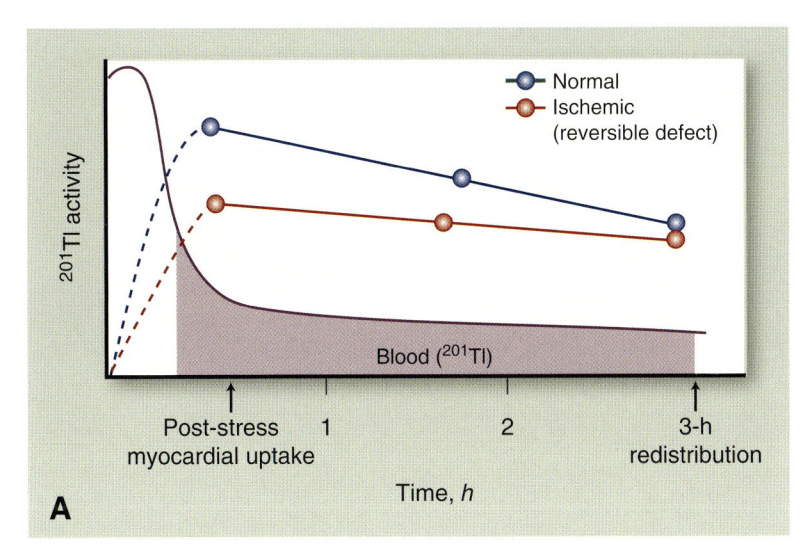

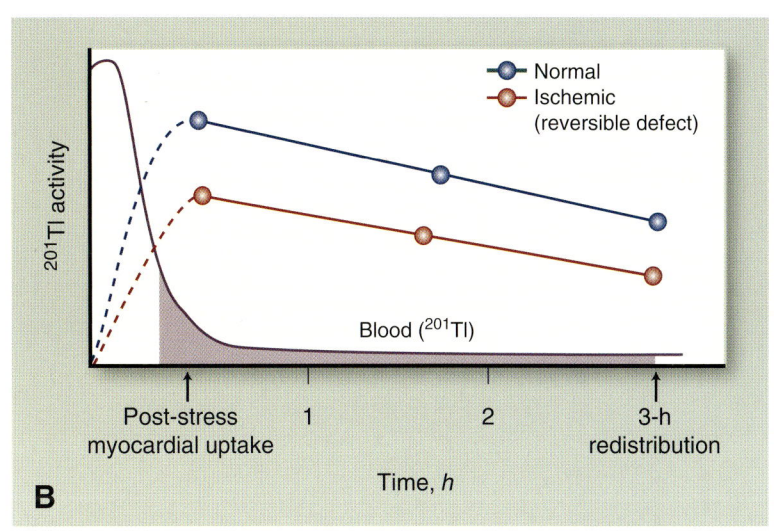

Figure 2-17. Myocardial thallium uptake and clearance in relation to blood activity of thallium. Redistribution of ^{201}Tl is dependent, in part, on blood levels of ^{201}Tl. Redistribution of ^{201}Tl in a given myocardial region depends not only on the severity of the initial defect poststress, but also on the presence of viable myocytes, the concentration of the tracer in the blood, and the rate of decline of ^{201}Tl levels in the blood. During the redistribution phase, there is continuous exchange of ^{201}Tl between the myocardium and the extracardiac compartments, driven by the concentration gradient of the radiotracer across the myocytes and blood and myocyte viability. **A,** If the blood level of ^{201}Tl remains the same (or increases) during the period between stress and redistribution imaging, then a stress-induced defect in a region with viable myocytes that can accumulate ^{201}Tl on the redistribution phase will appear reversible. **B,** If the blood level of ^{201}Tl is low (or decreases) during the imaging interval, the delivery of ^{201}Tl may be insufficient and the stress-induced ^{201}Tl defect may remain irreversible even though the underlying myocardium is viable. Thus, some ischemic but viable regions may show no redistribution on either early (3- to 4-hour) or late (24-hour) imaging, unless blood levels of ^{201}Tl are increased. (*Adapted from* Dilsizian [19].)

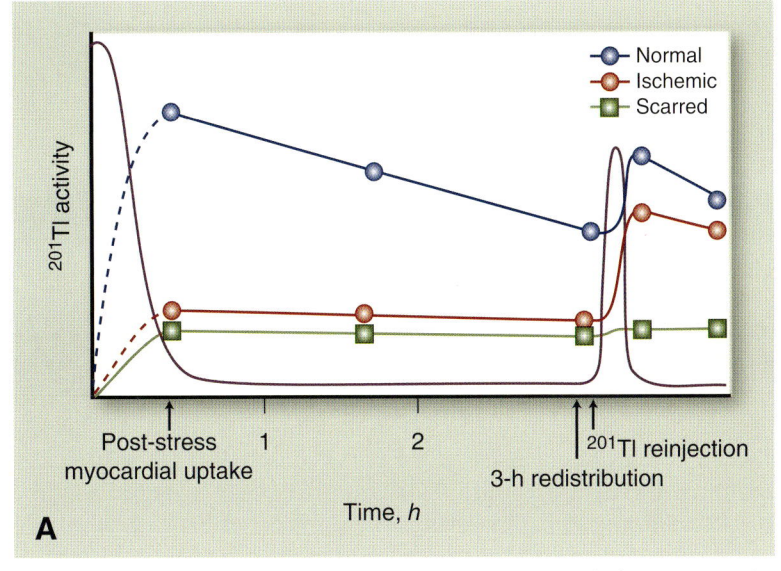

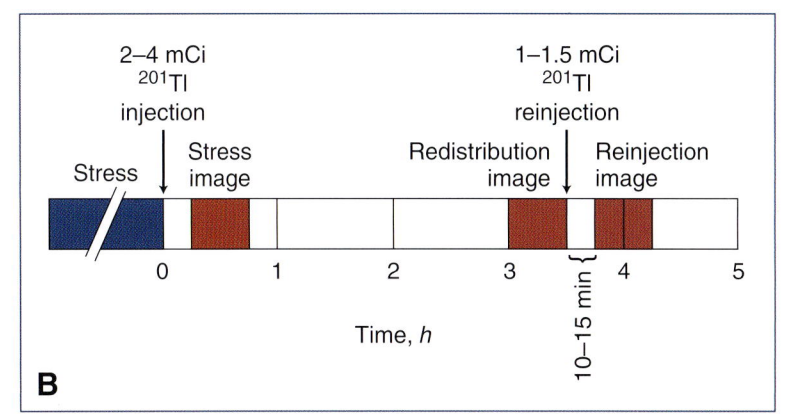

Figure 2-18. Thallium reinjection. **A,** ^{201}Tl reinjection differentiates ischemic but viable myocardium from scarred myocardium by augmenting the blood levels of ^{201}Tl at rest. A viable segment may be asynergic on the basis of repetitive stunning and hibernation. Thus, an asynergic but viable region may have reduced (but not absent) blood flow at rest (hibernation) or transient reduction in blood flow after a period of ischemia (stunning). Although standard stress 3- to 4-hour redistribution ^{201}Tl scintigraphy may underestimate the presence of ischemic but viable myocardium in many patients with coronary artery disease, reinjection of ^{201}Tl at rest after stress 3- to 4-hour redistribution imaging substantially improves the assessment of myocardial ischemia and viability in up to 49% of patients with apparently irreversible defects [2]. The theory that myocardial regions identified by ^{201}Tl uptake following ^{201}Tl reinjection represent viable myocardium is supported by improved regional function after revascularization and preserved metabolic activity by [^{18}F]-fluorodeoxyglucose PET. In addition, a significant inverse correlation between the magnitude of ^{201}Tl activity after reinjection and regional volume fraction of interstitial fibrosis has been demonstrated in comparative clinicopathologic studies [20].

It is possible that the initial myocardial uptake of ^{201}Tl (postinjection) reflects regional blood flow while redistribution of ^{201}Tl in a given defect depends not only on the severity of the initial defect but also on the presence of viable myocytes, the concentration of the tracer in the blood, and the rate of decline of ^{201}Tl levels in the blood. Thus, the heterogeneity of regional blood flow observed on the initial stress-induced ^{201}Tl defects may be independent of the subsequent extent of ^{201}Tl redistribution. If the blood level of ^{201}Tl remains the same (or increases) during the period between stress and 3- to 4-hour redistribution imaging, then an apparent defect in a region with viable myocytes that can retain ^{201}Tl should improve. On the other hand, if the serum ^{201}Tl concentration decreases during the imaging interval, the delivery of ^{201}Tl may be insufficient, and the ^{201}Tl defect may remain irreversible although the underlying myocardium is viable. This suggests that some ischemic but viable regions may never redistribute, even with late (24-hour) imaging, unless serum levels of ^{201}Tl are increased. **B,** This hypothesis is supported by a study where ^{201}Tl reinjection was performed immediately after 24-hour redistribution images were obtained [6]. Improved ^{201}Tl uptake after reinjection occurred in 40% of defects that appeared irreversible on late (24-hour) redistribution images. Thus, reinjection of 1 mCi of ^{201}Tl at rest immediately after either stress 3- to 4-hour redistribution or stress 24-hour redistribution studies, followed by image acquisition 10 to 15 minutes later, significantly improves the assessment of myocardial ischemia and viability. (*Adapted from* Dilsizian [19].)

SPECT and PET Myocardial Perfusion Imaging: Tracers and Techniques

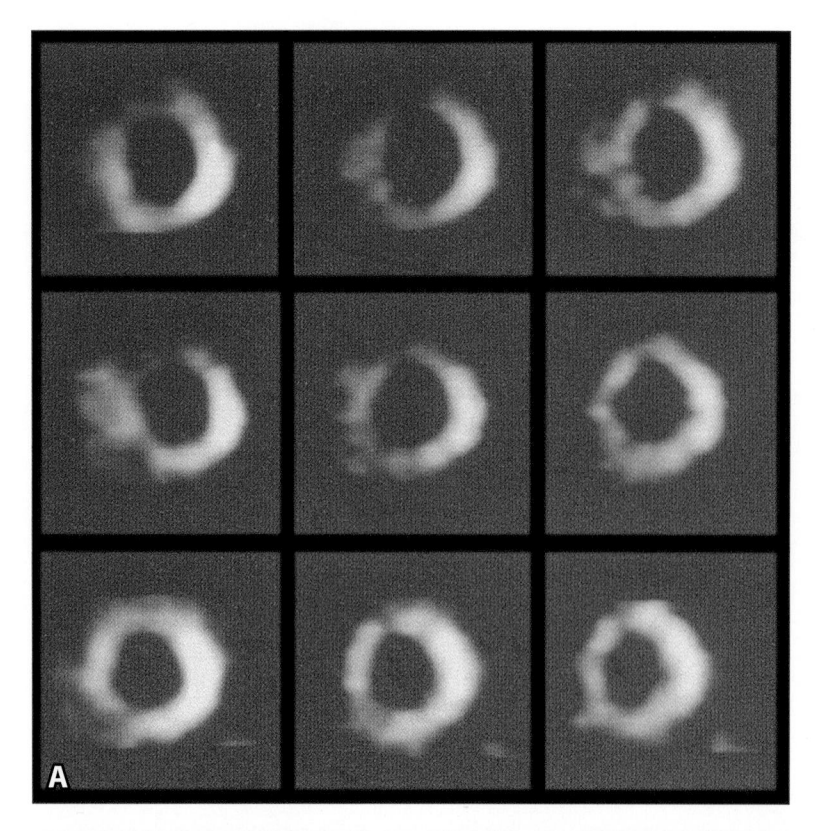

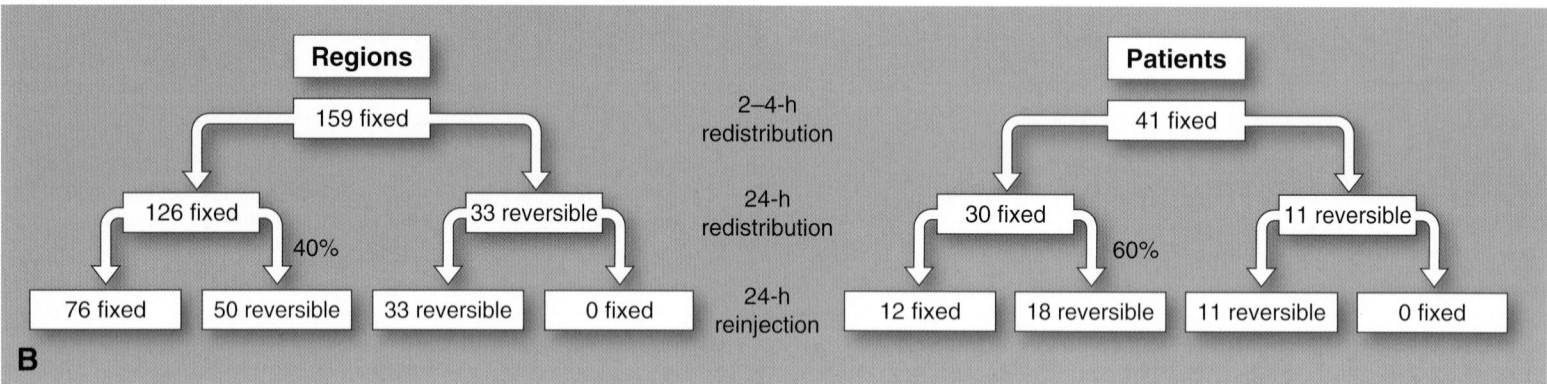

Figure 2-19. The beneficial effect of ^{201}Tl reinjection in the clinical setting. **A,** Short-axis tomograms demonstrate extensive ^{201}Tl defects in the anterior and septal regions on stress images (*top row*) that persist on redistribution images (*center row*) but improve markedly on reinjection images (*bottom row*). Among patients who underwent coronary artery revascularization, 87% of myocardial regions identified as viable by reinjection studies had normal ^{201}Tl uptake and improved regional wall motion after revascularization. In contrast, all regions with irreversible defects on reinjection imaging before revascularization had persistent wall motion abnormality after revascularization [2]. **B,** Similar results were obtained when ^{201}Tl reinjection was performed immediately after late (24-hour) redistribution imaging. Improved ^{201}Tl uptake after reinjection occurred in 40% of regions (involving 60% of patients) that appeared fixed on late redistribution imaging. (**A,** *adapted from* Dilsizian *et al.* [2]; **B,** *adapted from* Kayden *et al.* [21].)

48 Atlas of Nuclear Cardiology

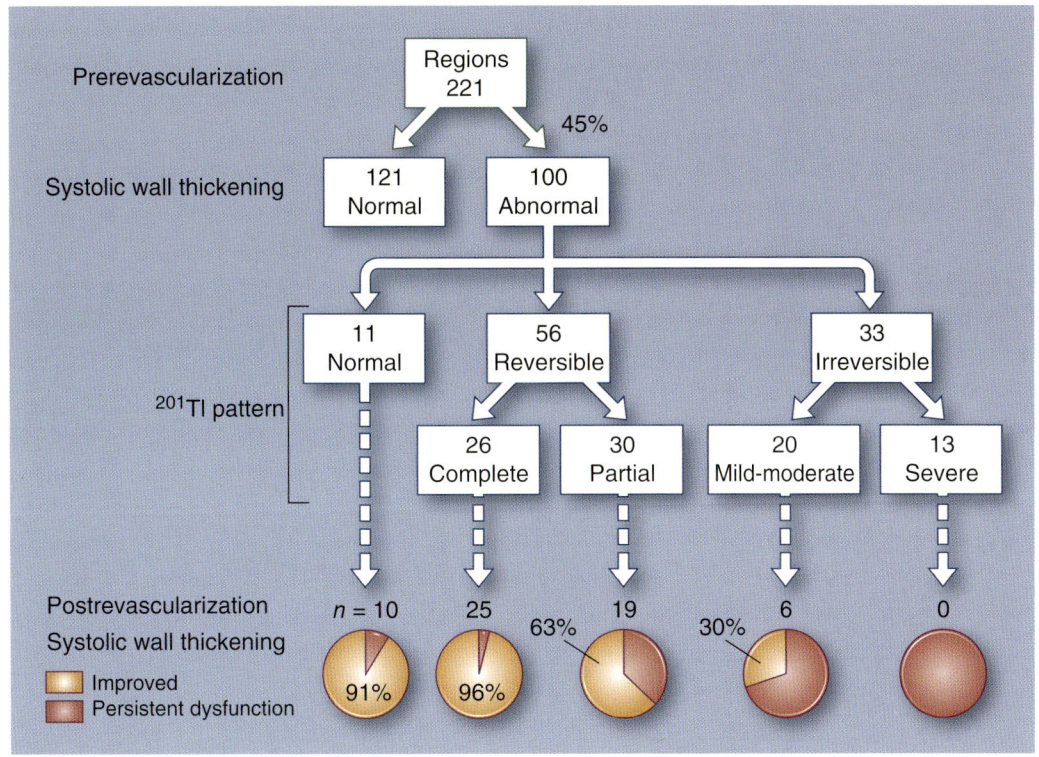

Figure 2-20. Postrevascularization functional outcome of asynergic regions in relation to prerevascularization ^{201}Tl patterns of normal, reversible, partially reversible, mild-to-moderate irreversible, and severe irreversible defects using stress-redistribution-reinjection ^{201}Tl protocol. The probabilities of functional recovery after revascularization were over 90% in normal or completely reversible defects, 63% in partially reversible defects, 30% in mild-to-moderate irreversible defects, and 0% in severe irreversible defects. Asynergic regions with reversible defects (complete or partial) on the prerevascularization ^{201}Tl study were shown more likely to improve function after revascularization when compared with asynergic regions with mild-to-moderate irreversible defects (79% vs 30%, respectively; $P < 0.001$). Even at a similar mass of viable myocardial tissue (as reflected by the final ^{201}Tl content), the presence of inducible ischemia (reversible defect) was associated with an increased likelihood of functional recovery. (Adapted from Kitsiou et al. [22].)

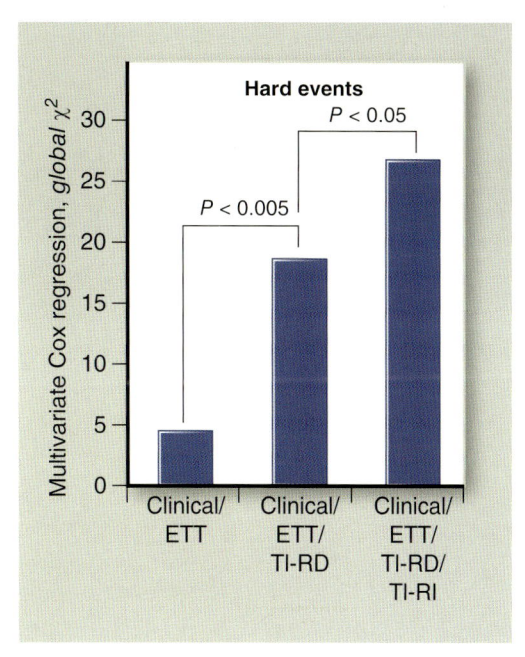

Figure 2-21. Incremental prognostic value of ^{201}Tl reinjection. In patients with prior myocardial infarction and left ventricular dysfunction in whom the assessment of myocardial viability is of clinical relevance, ^{201}Tl reinjection (Tl-RI) imaging provides incremental prognostic information to clinical, exercise tolerance testing (ETT), and ^{201}Tl stress-redistribution (Tl-RD) imaging. Similarly, in patients with chronic coronary artery disease and prior myocardial infarction, the scintigraphic variable that was the strongest predictor of hard events (cardiac death or myocardial infarction) was the presence of more than three irreversible defects that remained irreversible after ^{201}Tl reinjection. (Adapted from Petretta et al. [23].)

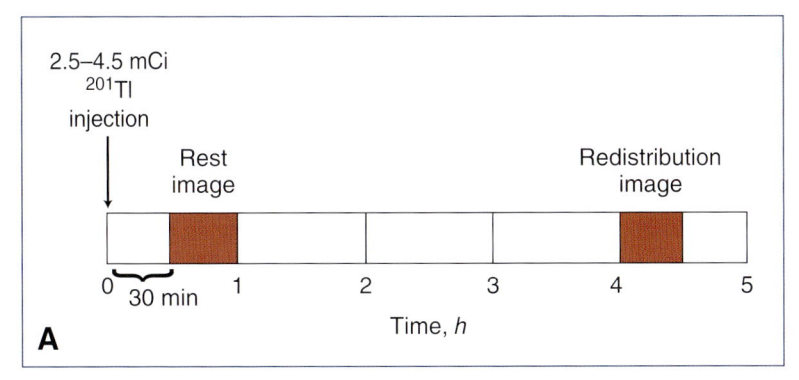

Figure 2-22. Rest-redistribution ^{201}Tl protocol. **A,** The stress-redistribution-reinjection ^{201}Tl protocol provides important diagnostic information regarding both inducible ischemia and myocardial viability. In most cases, the identification of myocardial ischemia is much more important clinically in terms of patient management and risk stratification than knowledge of myocardial viability. However, if the clinical question is one of the presence and extent of viable myocardium within a dysfunctional region and not inducible ischemia, then it is reasonable to perform rest-redistribution ^{201}Tl imaging only.

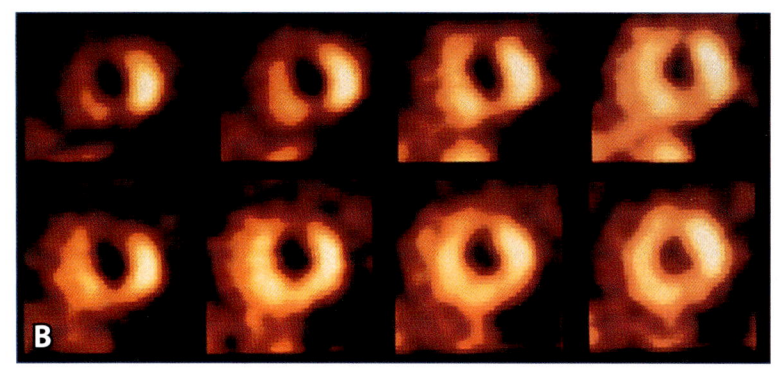

B, Rest-redistribution short-axis ^{201}Tl tomograms are shown from a patient with chronic coronary artery disease. There are extensive ^{201}Tl perfusion defects in the anteroapical, anteroseptal, and inferior regions on the initial rest images (*top row*). On the delayed (3- to 4-hour) redistribution images (*bottom row*), the inferior region remains fixed (scarred myocardium), while the anteroapical and anteroseptal regions show significant reversibility, suggestive of viable myocardium [24].

SPECT and PET Myocardial Perfusion Imaging: Tracers and Techniques

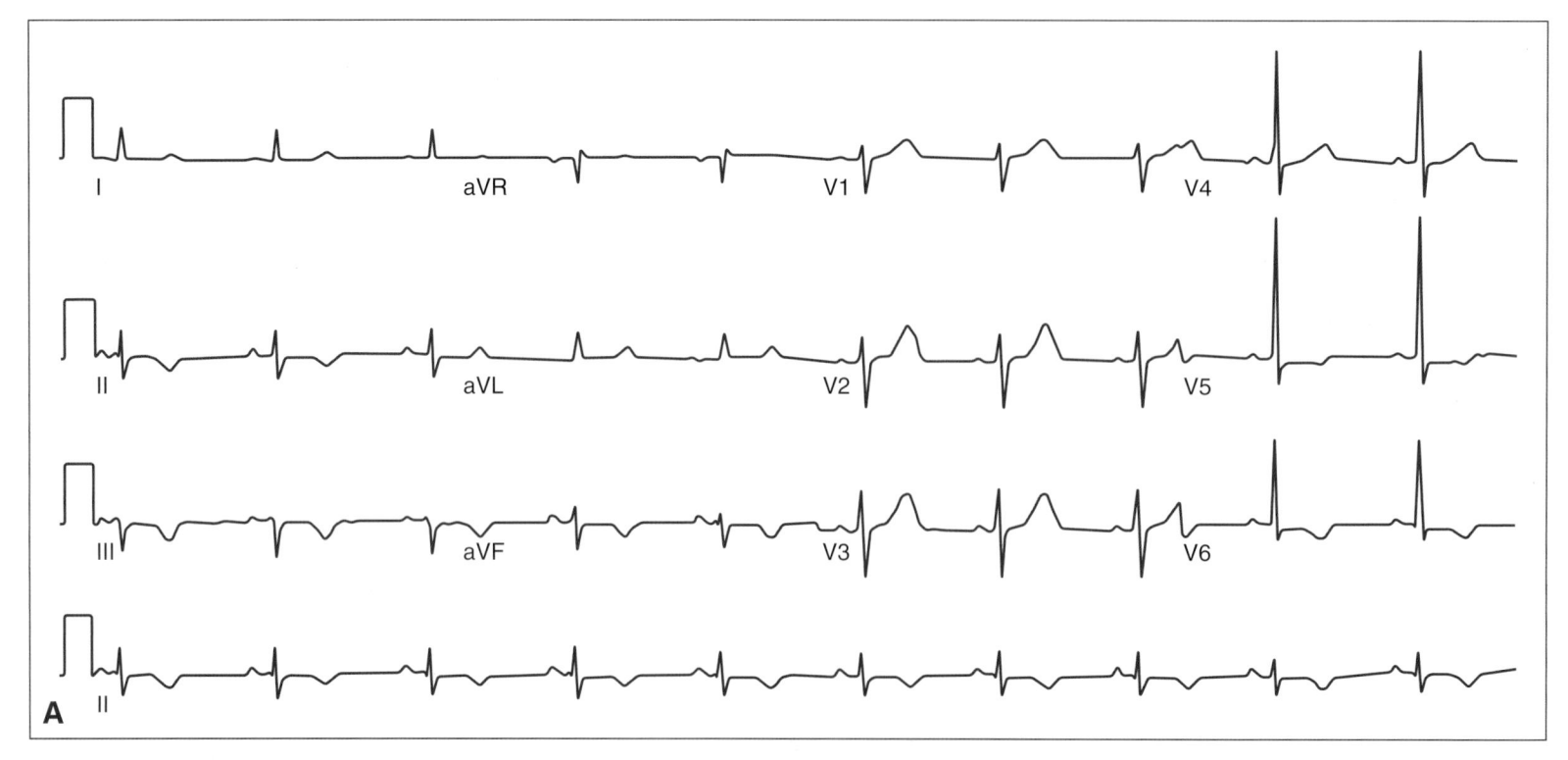

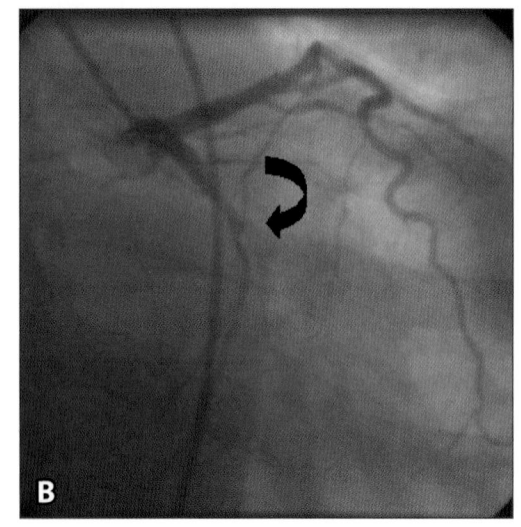

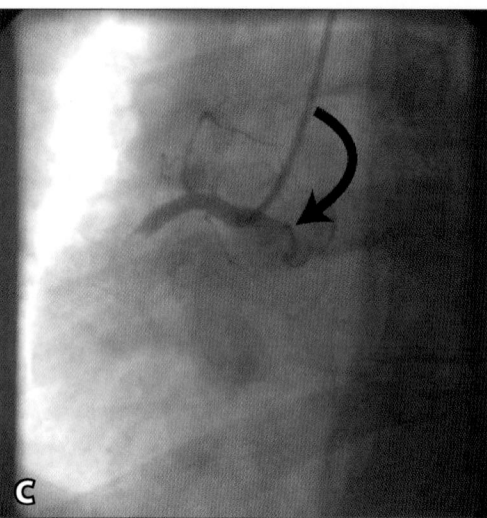

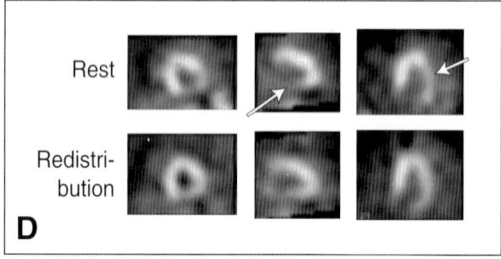

Figure 2-23. Anatomic assessment of the coronary arteries alone does not differentiate viable from scarred myocardium. A patient with prior history of hypertension and hyperlipidemia presents with 2-month history of substernal chest pain. The electrocardiogram shows inverted T waves in the inferolateral leads (**A**) while the coronary angiogram shows total occlusion of the left circumflex (LCX) (**B**) (*arrow*) and the proximal right coronary artery (RCA) (**C**) (*arrow*). There are extensive perfusion defects in the lateral and inferior regions (**D**) on the initial rest images (*top row*) (*arrows*) that become reversible on the delayed (3- to 4-hour) redistribution images (*bottom row*), providing evidence for hypoperfused but viable myocardium in the LCX and RCA vascular territories. The anatomic assessment of the coronary arteries alone is insufficient to determine whether the myocardium subtended by the totally occluded vessels is viable or scarred. Accurate distinction between viable (hibernating or stunned) and scarred myocardium has important clinical implications. Ideally, such information may be used to guide therapeutic decisions for revascularization and risk stratification. The scintigraphic finding of reduced regional blood flow (rest ^{201}Tl images) but preserved cell membrane integrity (redistribution ^{201}Tl images) in dysfunctional myocardial regions provides the most direct evidence of myocardial hibernation. In view of the findings on the rest-redistribution ^{201}Tl study, the patient was referred for coronary artery bypass surgery with an uneventful postoperative course.

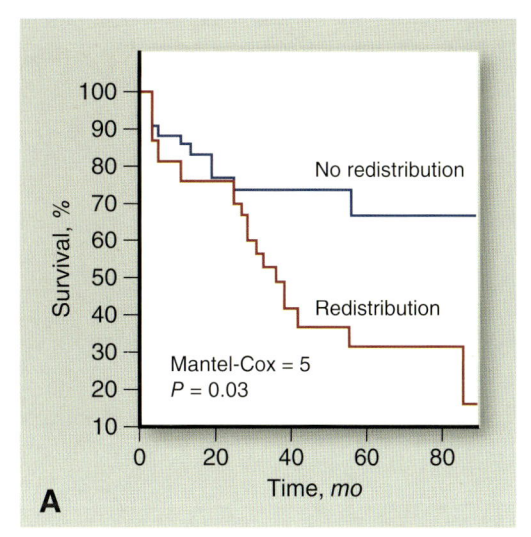

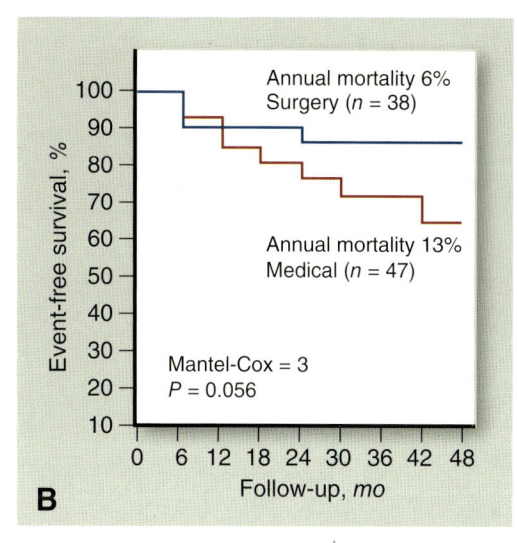

Figure 2-24. Prognostic value of rest-redistribution ^{201}Tl SPECT. In patients with chronic ischemic left ventricular dysfunction, the demonstration of redistribution on rest ^{201}Tl imaging protocols portend a higher mortality rate with medical therapy than do patients with a comparable degree of left ventricular dysfunction without evidence of redistribution. **A**, Actuarial survival curve in 81 medically treated patients is shown; 38 patients (mean left ventricular ejection fraction [LVEF] = 26% ± 7%) showed redistribution on rest ^{201}Tl images and 43 patients (mean LVEF = 27% ± 8%) showed no redistribution. Moreover, in a nonrandomized, retrospective study with rest-redistribution ^{201}Tl, survival and survival without myocardial infarction tended to be significantly higher in patients with chronic ischemic left ventricular dysfunction treated with coronary artery revascularization compared with those treated with medical therapy alone. **B**, Actuarial survival curve in 85 patients with evidence of myocardial viability by rest-redistribution ^{201}Tl is shown; 38 patients underwent coronary artery revascularization and 47 patients were treated medically. (*Adapted from* Gioia et al. [25,26].)

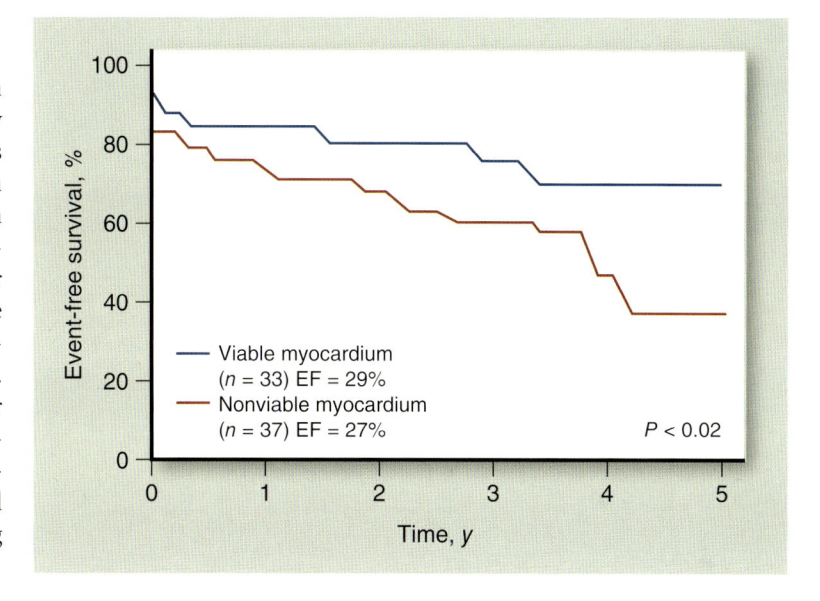

Figure 2-25. Extent of myocardial viability assessed by rest-redistribution ^{201}Tl and patient outcome. Considering the survival advantage of coronary artery revascularization when compared with medical therapy in patients with chronic ischemic left ventricular dysfunction, one might question whether preoperative assessment of myocardial viability is necessary in making revascularization decisions. Should coronary artery revascularization be considered in all patients with chronic ischemic left ventricular dysfunction with or without evidence of myocardial viability? Event-free survival in a retrospective study in patients with preoperative rest-redistribution ^{201}Tl testing undergoing coronary artery bypass surgery is shown. Perioperative and long-term postoperative survival is significantly better in patients with evidence of significant myocardial viability on rest-redistribution ^{201}Tl compared with those patients with less evidence of myocardial viability. The prognostic significance of rest-redistribution ^{201}Tl in large-scale, randomized, prospective studies is the subject of ongoing investigation. EF—ejection fraction. (*Adapted from* Pagley et al. [27].)

SPECT Techniques: ^{99m}Tc-labeled Perfusion Tracers

SPECT Techniques: ^{99m}Tc-labeled Sestamibi and ^{99m}TC-labeled Tetrofosmin

- Lipid-soluble cationic compounds
- 140 keV photopeak energy, 6-h physical half-life
- First-pass extraction fraction ~ 60%
- Uptake is passive across mitochondrial membranes
- At equilibrium, they are retained within the mitochondria because of a large negative transmembrane potential
- Clearance from the intravascular compartment via hepatobiliary excretion
- Minimal redistribution when compared with ^{201}Tl

A

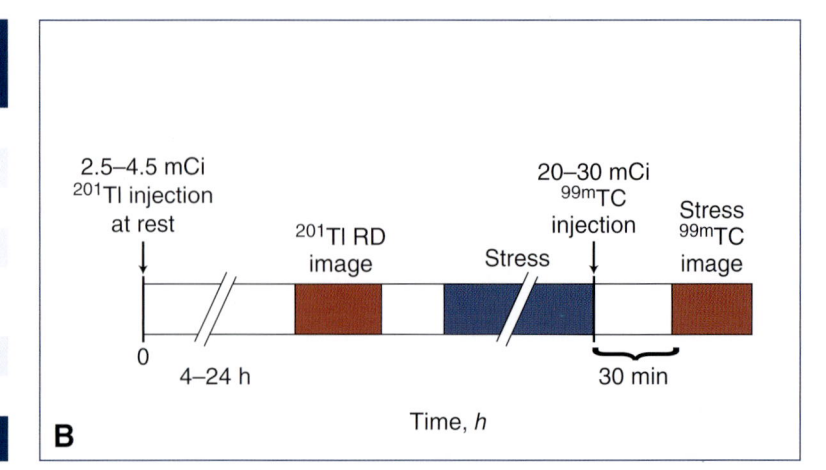

Figure 2-26. SPECT techniques: ^{99m}Tc-labeled sestamibi and ^{99m}TC-labeled-tetrofosmin. **A**, ^{99m}Tc-sestamibi (isonitrile) and ^{99m}Tc-tetrofosmin are both lipophilic cationic complexes with similar myocardial uptake and blood clearance kinetics. However, the clearance of tetrofosmin from the lungs and the liver is faster than ^{99m}Tc-sestamibi, which may improve the resolution of cardiac images and reduce the overall radiation burden. Both ^{99m}Tc-sestamibi and -tetrofosmin are taken up across sarcolemmal and mitochondrial membranes of myocytes by passive distribution, and retained within the mitochondria at equilibrium because of a large negative transmembrane potential. Experimental studies with ^{99m}Tc-sestamibi have shown that myocardial uptake and clearance are related to the mitochondrial transmembrane potential and do not differ from ischemic to nonischemic regions. In addition, experimental studies of myocardial infarction, with and without reperfusion, have fueled optimism in the use of ^{99m}Tc-sestamibi clinically for myocardial viability assessment. In the clinical setting, however, with the exception of a few studies, both ^{99m}Tc-sestamibi and -tetrofosmin appear to underestimate myocardial viability. Compared with ^{201}Tl and PET tracers, factors that may contribute to the impaired ^{99m}Tc-sestamibi or -tetrofosmin accumulation in viable regions at rest include differences in extraction fraction, blood clearance, redistribution (RD), and response to altered metabolic states. Perhaps a likely improvement in viability assessment with ^{99m}Tc-sestamibi and -tetrofosmin could be achieved through nitrate administration before rest ^{99m}Tc-sestamibi injection and quantitation of regional radiotracer uptake. **B**, Alternatively, dual-isotope gated SPECT imaging could be performed, which combines rest-redistribution ^{201}Tl (for viability) with stress ^{99m}Tc-sestamibi or -tetrofosmin (for perfusion), thereby taking advantage of the favorable properties of each of the two tracers.

SPECT Techniques: ^{99m}Tc-Teboroxime

- Neutral, lipophilic compound
- 140 keV photopeak energy, 6-h physical half-life
- High first-pass extraction fraction under hyperemic conditions (~ 91%)
- Extraction by the myocardium remains linear even at high-flow conditions
- Rapid clearance from the myocardium at a rate proportional to regional blood flow
- Uptake and washout are independent of the metabolic status of the myocardial cells

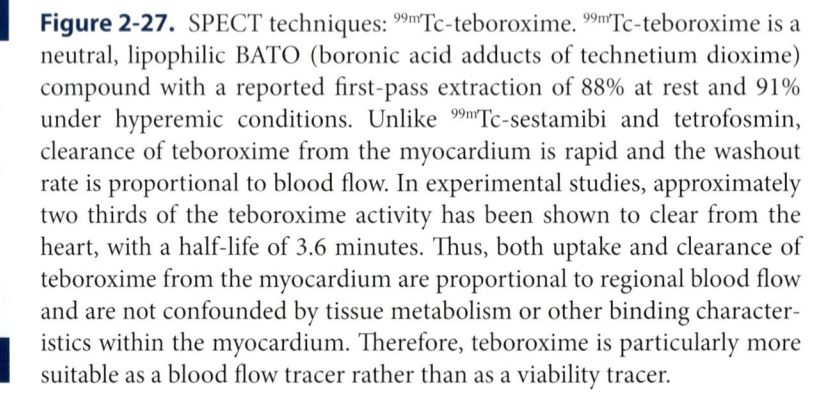

Figure 2-27. SPECT techniques: ^{99m}Tc-teboroxime. ^{99m}Tc-teboroxime is a neutral, lipophilic BATO (boronic acid adducts of technetium dioxime) compound with a reported first-pass extraction of 88% at rest and 91% under hyperemic conditions. Unlike ^{99m}Tc-sestamibi and tetrofosmin, clearance of teboroxime from the myocardium is rapid and the washout rate is proportional to blood flow. In experimental studies, approximately two thirds of the teboroxime activity has been shown to clear from the heart, with a half-life of 3.6 minutes. Thus, both uptake and clearance of teboroxime from the myocardium are proportional to regional blood flow and are not confounded by tissue metabolism or other binding characteristics within the myocardium. Therefore, teboroxime is particularly more suitable as a blood flow tracer rather than as a viability tracer.

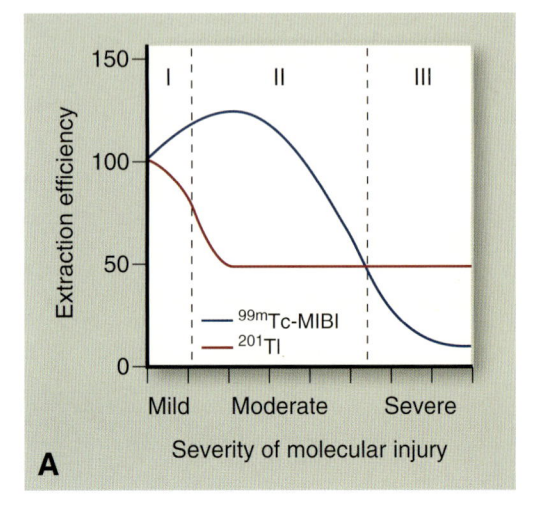

Figure 2-28. Cellular kinetics of ^{201}Tl and ^{99m}Tc-sestamibi (99mTc-MIBI) during metabolic inhibition in cultured chick embryo cardiac myocytes, independent of perfusion. **A**, Oxidative phosphorylation and glycolysis were inhibited simultaneously by rotenone (10 μm) and iodoacetate (1 mmol/L), respectively, producing a decline in myocellular ATP content. Under these conditions, initial extraction efficiency of ^{201}Tl and ^{99m}Tc-sestamibi responded in divergent ways to ATP depletion. Extraction efficiency of ^{201}Tl declined within 20 minutes of metabolic inhibition by 50% to 70%, while extraction efficiency of ^{99m}Tc-sestamibi increased significantly by 10 to 20 minutes and remained elevated for the first 40 to 60 minutes of metabolic inhibition. The observed disparity in initial uptake rates between ^{201}Tl and ^{99m}Tc-sestamibi during mild-to-moderate metabolic injury may explain on a metabolic basis alone the clinical observation that ^{99m}Tc-sestamibi defects are smaller than those assessed by ^{201}Tl.

Continued on the next page

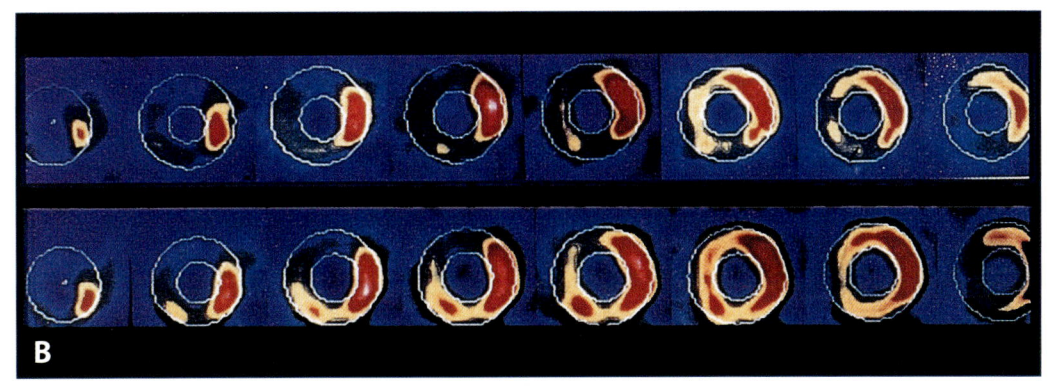

Figure 2-28. *(Continued)* **B**, Images taken with ^{201}Tl 5 to 10 minutes after stress *(top row)* and with ^{99m}Tc-sestamibi 2 hours after stress *(bottom row)* are shown from a patient who performed the same level of exercise with both tracers. Quantitative left ventricular mass algorithm provided similar measures of total mass for ^{201}Tl (197 g) and for ^{99m}Tc-sestamibi (189 g). However, the stress-induced defect mass derived from ^{201}Tl imaging (41 g) is significantly larger than that detected by ^{99m}Tc-sestamibi (30 g). No transmural defects are present on the ^{99m}Tc-sestamibi images. (**A**, *adapted from* Piwnica-Worms *et al.* [28]; **B**, *from* Narahara *et al.* [29]; with permission.)

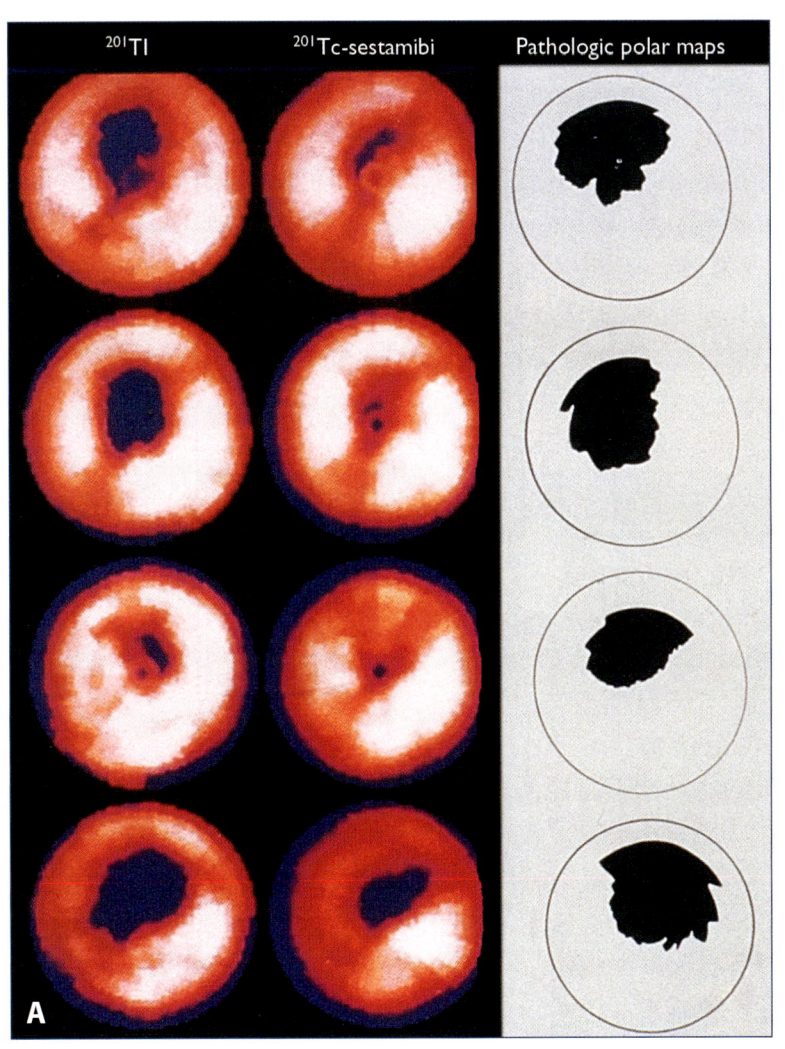

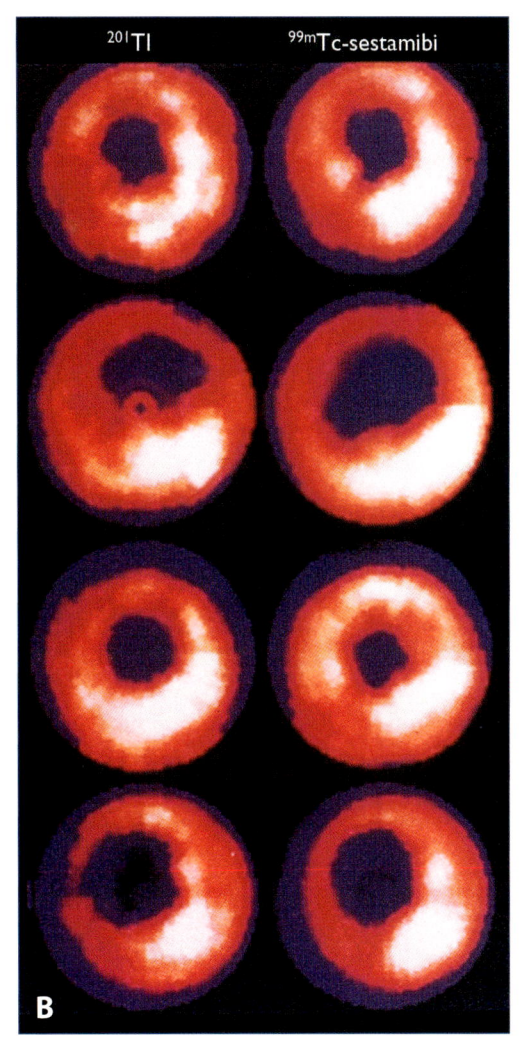

Figure 2-29. Pharmacologic stress. In canine models of moderate (**A**) and severe (**B**) coronary artery occlusion, ^{201}Tl and ^{99m}Tc-sestamibi myocardial perfusion defect size are compared during pharmacologic stimulation and with postmortem staining to define the extent of the hypoperfused region. Bull's-eye displays from four representative experiments of moderate coronary artery stenosis during pharmacologic stimulation for ^{201}Tl and ^{99m}Tc-sestamibi, and corresponding pathologic polar displays from the same four experiments are shown. The extent of ^{201}Tl myocardial perfusion defect size (but not ^{99m}Tc-sestamibi) approaches the hypoperfused area on the corresponding pathologic display. The ^{99m}Tc-sestamibi defect size occupies only 37% of the area of the defect on the ^{201}Tl images of the same dog, and the counts within the defects are 39% higher for ^{99m}Tc-sestamibi compared to ^{201}Tl (**A**). On the other hand, when coronary artery occlusion is near total (severe), ^{201}Tl and ^{99m}Tc-sestamibi show similar defect contrast and areas (**B**). These observations in canines are similar to the experimental observations made in cultured myocytes. (*From* Leon *et al.* [30]; with permission.)

SPECT and PET Myocardial Perfusion Imaging: Tracers and Techniques

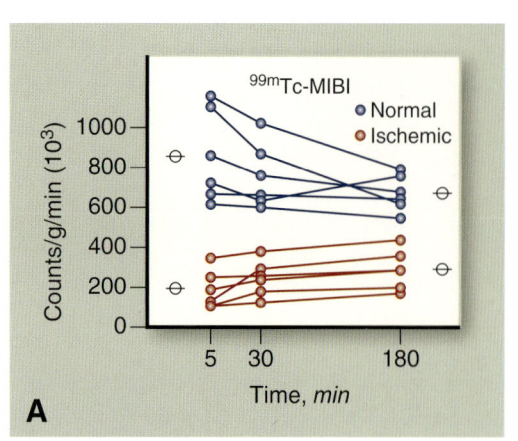

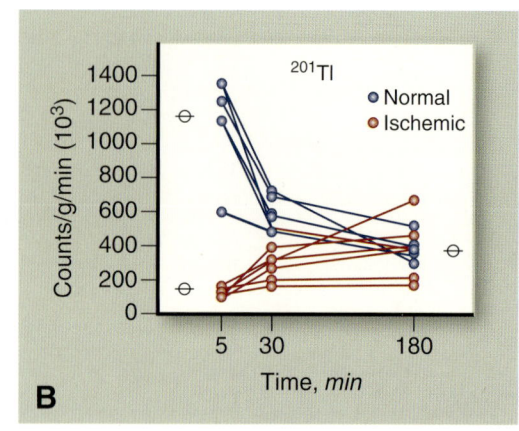

Figure 2-30. ^{99m}Tc-sestamibi and ^{201}Tl activities in myocardial biopsies. Change in defect size of ^{99m}Tc-sestamibi (MIBI) with time (redistribution) has been shown both in animal models and in patients with chronic coronary artery disease [31,32]. Depending on the level of blood activity of ^{99m}Tc-sestamibi after stress, continued uptake by the myocardium after the first pass may reduce the defect severity and area in the hypoperfused region. In the early comparative studies of ^{201}Tl and ^{99m}Tc-sestamibi, ^{201}Tl images were acquired 5 to 10 minutes after injection, while ^{99m}Tc-sestamibi images were acquired 1 to 2 hours after injection. The 1- to 2-hour delay between ^{99m}Tc-sestamibi injection and imaging was based on the best compromise between a high myocardial count rate and low background activity and on the assumption that ^{99m}Tc-sestamibi does not "redistribute" over time.

Following transient ischemia and reperfusion after 5 minutes in a canine model, there was evidence for change in defect size of ^{99m}Tc-sestamibi with time (**A**), albeit more slowly and less completely when compared to ^{201}Tl redistribution (**B**). For both ^{99m}Tc-sestamibi and ^{201}Tl, the consistent fall in normal zone activity and rise in ischemic zone activity over the 3-hour time interval, consistent with redistribution, is noted. It is important to point out, however, that there is no change in ^{99m}Tc-sestamibi defect size between the 5-minute and 30-minute time intervals. In view of these and other similar reports, it is now recommended that ^{99m}Tc-sestamibi images be acquired earlier, approximately 30 minutes after injection of the tracer. (*Adapted from Li et al.* [31].)

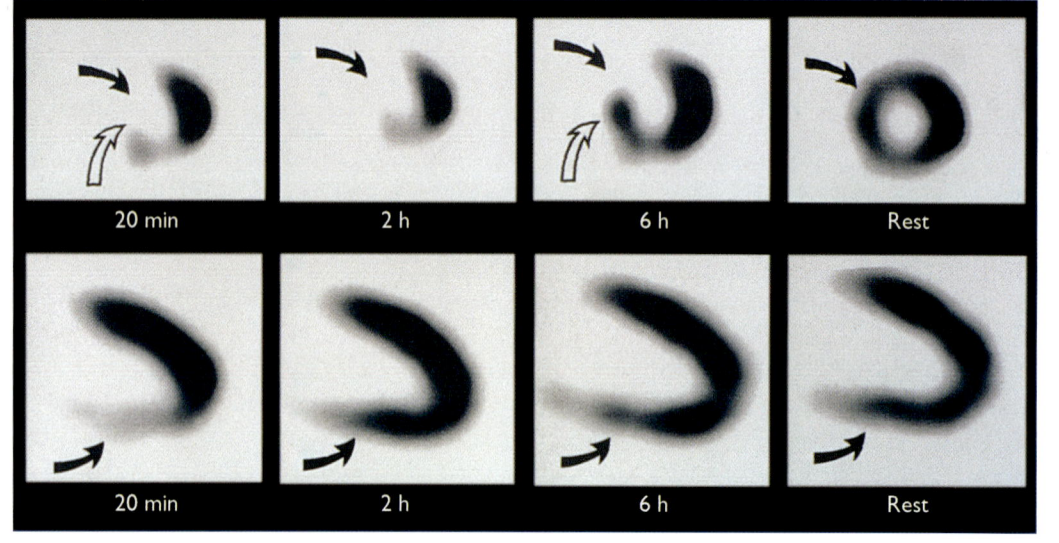

Figure 2-31. Clinically relevant change in defect size of ^{99m}Tc-sestamibi with time (redistribution) in two patients undergoing exercise ^{99m}Tc-sestamibi studies. Myocardial SPECT images obtained from two different patients are presented in the short-axis plane (*top row*) and in the vertical long-axis plane (*bottom row*) after exercise and at rest. In the short-axis plane, there is no change in ^{99m}Tc-sestamibi defect size from 20 minutes to 2 hours after exercise. However, by 6 hours there is significant change in defect size in the inferoseptal region (*open arrow*) but not in the anteroseptal region (*closed arrow*). On the injected image taken at rest, complete normalization of all perfusion defects is seen, which suggests that delayed ^{99m}Tc-sestamibi images alone do not provide accurate information regarding defect reversibility. In the vertical long-axis plane, there is significant change in ^{99m}Tc-sestamibi defect in the inferior region (*closed arrows*) from 20 minutes to 2 hours after exercise (redistribution), without further fill-in at 6 hours or on rest-injected ^{99m}Tc-sestamibi images. Although interpretation of ^{99m}Tc-sestamibi data should be viewed cautiously when imaging is delayed by 2 hours or more after stress (underestimation of defect size and extent of myocardial ischemia), the same concept does not apply for rest-injected ^{99m}Tc-sestamibi studies. On the contrary, delaying ^{99m}Tc-sestamibi images by 2 hours or more after rest injection may improve myocardial viability assessment. (*From Franceschi et al.* [33]; with permission.)

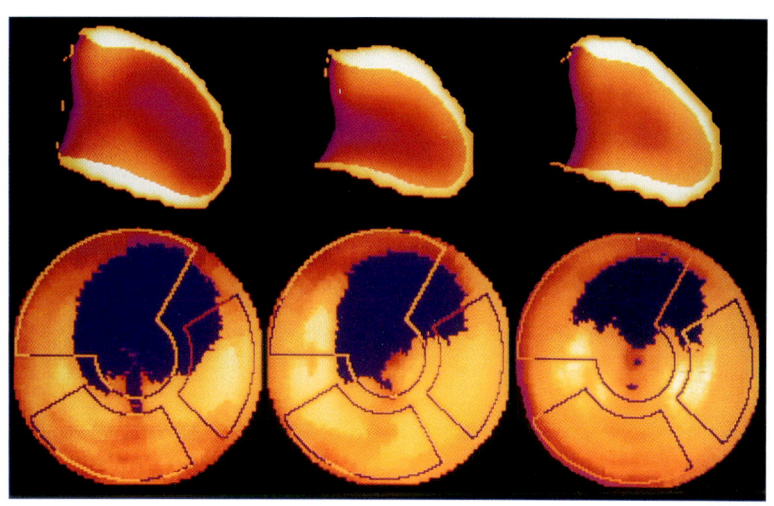

Figure 2-32. Nitrate administration before rest ^{99m}Tc-sestamibi or ^{99m}Tc-tetrofosmin injection. Considering the kinetics of ^{99m}Tc-sestamibi and ^{99m}Tc-tetrofosmin, uptake of these radiotracers in myocardial regions with reduced perfusion and partially impaired viability appear to be influenced by regional perfusion rather than myocyte viability. In view of the limitations in the clinical setting of rest-injected ^{99m}Tc-sestamibi and ^{99m}Tc-tetrofosmin for assessing myocardial viability, some investigators have proposed injection of the radiotracers during nitrate infusion. In addition to lowering preload and afterload, nitrates may cause vasodilatation of the flow, limiting epicardial coronary arteries as well as collateral vessels. The injection of ^{99m}Tc-sestamibi during nitrate infusion (10 mg of isosorbide dinitrate in 100 mL solution of isotonic saline solution infused over 20 minutes) is shown to improve the accuracy of ^{99m}Tc-sestamibi for predicting recovery of regional and global left ventricular function after revascularization. In this patient example with anterior myocardial infarction and single vessel left anterior descending (LAD) coronary artery disease, prerevascularization baseline images (*left*) show anteroapical akinesis and global left ventricular ejection fraction (LVEF) of 38% on first-pass radionuclide angiography associated with a large anterior and apical ^{99m}Tc-sestamibi perfusion defect (63% of the LAD vascular territory in the bull's-eye image at rest). ^{99m}Tc-sestamibi images acquired after nitrate infusion (*center*) show improvement in the anteroapical wall motion associated with an increase in global LVEF to 42% and a decrease in the extent of ^{99m}Tc-sestamibi perfusion defect size to 42% of the LAD vascular territory. After revascularization of the LAD (*right*), there is improvement in the anteroapical wall motion at rest, increase in global LVEF to 45%, and decrease in the extent of ^{99m}Tc-sestamibi perfusion defect to 38% of the LAD vascular territory [34]. (*Courtesy of* Roberto Sciagra.)

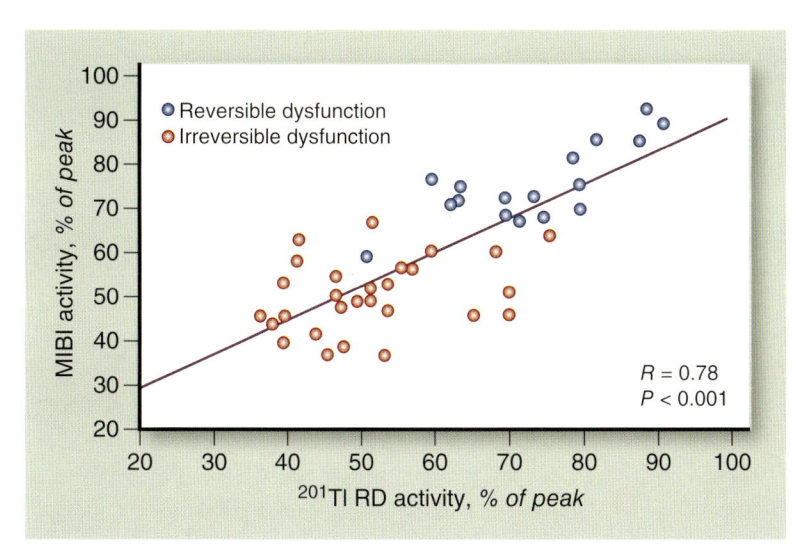

Figure 2-33. Quantitation of severity of reduction in myocardial perfusion at rest. Unlike ^{201}Tl studies, there are a growing number of studies in the literature to suggest that ^{99m}Tc-sestamibi and -tetrofosmin studies underestimate defect reversibility and myocardial viability in patients with chronic coronary artery disease. One approach that may overcome, in part, the limitations of ^{99m}Tc-sestamibi and -tetrofosmin in assessing myocardial viability is to quantify the severity of regional tracer activity, *ie*, severity of myocardial perfusion at rest. Among 18 patients with coronary artery disease undergoing revascularization, good correlation between quantitative regional activities of ^{201}Tl (on redistribution imaging after rest injection) and ^{99m}Tc-sestamibi (at rest) is shown. Moreover, the scatterplot shows that at 60% threshold level for both radiotracers, dysfunctional myocardial regions that improve function after revascularization (*blue circles*) can be differentiated from dysfunctional myocardial regions that do not improve function after revascularization (*red circles*). The positive and negative predictive accuracies attained when the severity of radiotracer defects were quantitated are 80% and 96%, respectively. Considering the kinetics of ^{99m}Tc-sestamibi, in myocardial regions with decreased blood flow and partially impaired viability, uptake of ^{99m}Tc-sestamibi appears to be influenced by regional perfusion rather than myocyte viability [35]. (*Adapted from* Udelson et al. [36].)

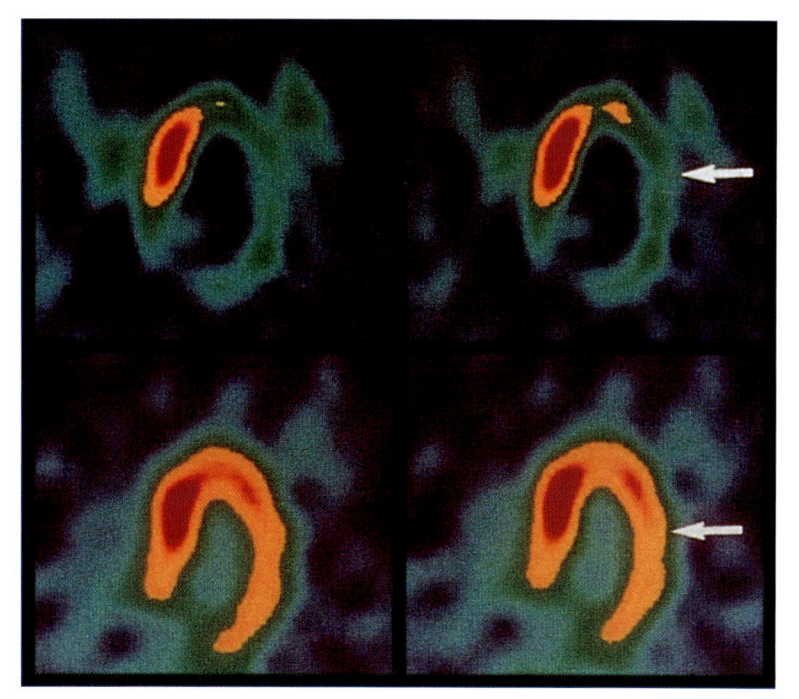

Figure 2-34. Underestimation of myocardial viability by rest ^{99m}Tc-sestamibi SPECT. Using dual-isotope injection at rest (same physiologic state) and simultaneous acquisition using SPECT (accurate anatomical alignment), these images show mismatch between rest cardiac perfusion assessed by ^{99m}Tc-sestamibi and metabolism assessed by [^{18}F]-fluorodeoxyglucose (FDG). After oral glucose loading, the patient was injected with 10 mCi of FDG and 25 mCi of ^{99m}Tc-sestamibi at rest. Dual-isotope single acquisition SPECT was performed approximately 60 minutes later by positioning two 20% pulse-height analyzer windows symmetrically around the 140 keV photopeak of ^{99m}Tc and the 511 keV photopeak of FDG. The digital electronics of the camera permitted frame-by-frame decay correction for short-lived FDG. Thus, two separate sets of slices mapping the ^{99m}Tc-sestamibi and FDG distribution were simultaneously obtained, resulting in one-to-one correspondence in spatial registration. Rest ^{99m}Tc-sestamibi images in the horizontal long-axis plane (*top row*) show reduced perfusion in the apical and lateral regions (*arrow*). Corresponding FDG images (*bottom row*) show preserved metabolism in the apical and lateral regions suggestive of viable myocardium (*arrow*). (*From* Delbeke et al. [37]; with permission.)

SPECT and PET Myocardial Perfusion Imaging: Tracers and Techniques

PET Tracers and Techniques

PET Techniques: ^{82}Rb

Positron-emitting cation with biologic properties similar to potassium
Emits two gamma rays, 511 keV each, with a short physical half-life of 75 s
Transported across the sarcolemmal membrane via the Na-K ATPase system
Initial uptake reflects myocardial blood flow
Kinetics of washout phase may be used as an index of viability

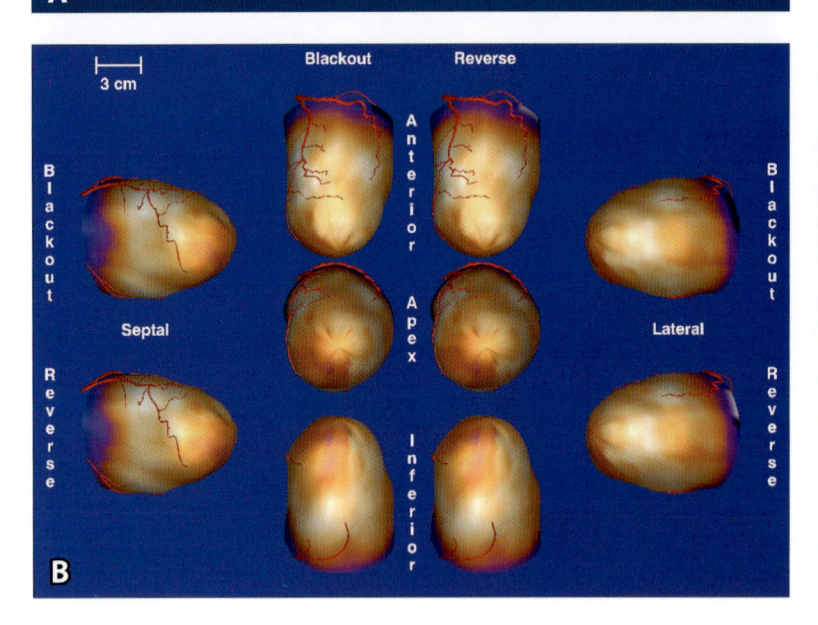

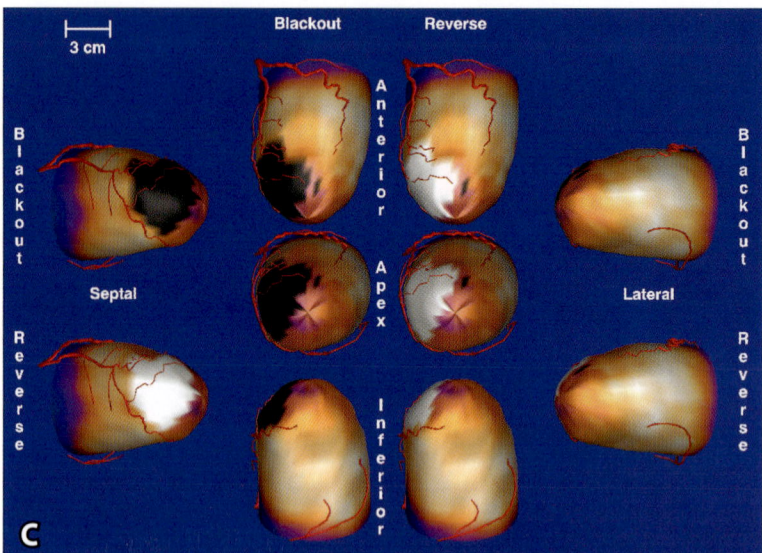

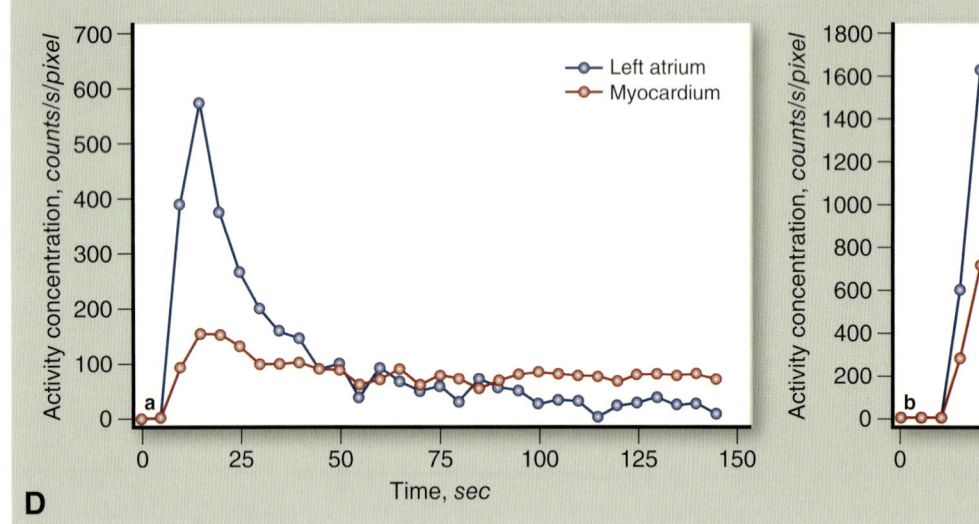

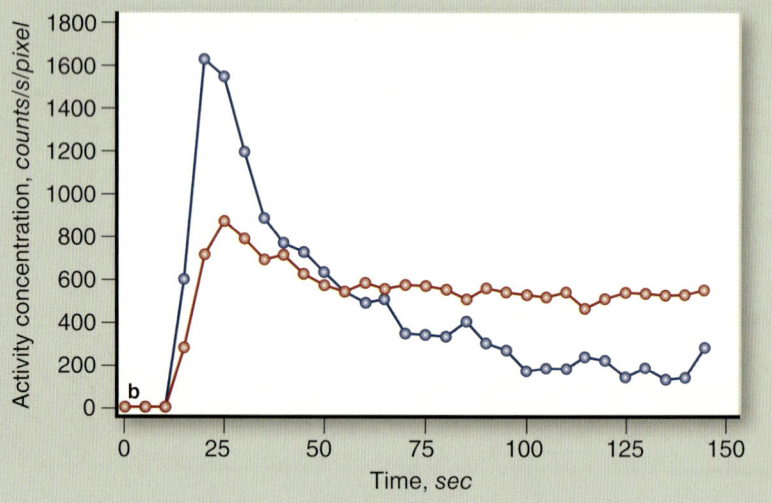

Figure 2-35. PET techniques: ^{82}Rb. **A**, ^{82}Rb is a generator-produced, short-lived, positron-emitting cation with biologic properties that are similar to potassium and ^{201}Tl. As with potassium and ^{201}Tl, intracellular uptake of ^{82}Rb across the sarcolemmal membrane reflects active cation transport via the Na-K ATPase transport system. In patients with chronic coronary artery disease, myocardial uptake of ^{82}Rb is preserved in viable regions and severely reduced in scarred regions. In the setting of acute myocardial injury and reperfusion, initial uptake of ^{82}Rb reflects blood flow.

Examples of three-dimensional surface-rendered models of normal (**B**) and abnormal (**C**) ^{82}Rb PET myocardial perfusion images are shown with the potential for overlaying coronary anatomic information from hybrid PET/CT angiography.

D, Although the first few minutes after the infusion of ^{82}Rb are not usually included in clinical acquisition protocols, it is precisely this period that is of interest if myocardial perfusion is to be quantified. Dynamic imaging of the heart during this time allows analysis of the ^{82}Rb concentration in both arterial blood and myocardial tissue as a function of time. ^{82}Rb time-activity curves at rest (*a*) and after adenosine stress (*b*). *Blue circles* represent the activity concentration in the left atrium and the *red circles* represent the activity concentration in myocardial tissue.

Continued on the next page

56 Atlas of Nuclear Cardiology

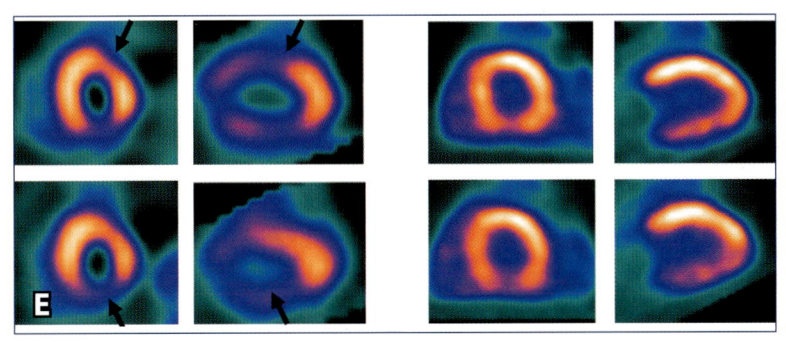

Figure 2-35. *(Continued)* **E,** Disparity between myocardial perfusion SPECT and ^{82}Rb-PET studies is shown. Clinically indicated adenosine dual-isotope gated SPECT images (*left panel*) without attenuation correction show regional ^{99m}Tc sestamibi perfusion defect in the anterior and inferior regions (*arrows*). On the rest ^{201}Tl images, the anterior defect became reversible while the inferior defect persisted. Corresponding ^{82}Rb PET myocardial perfusion tomograms performed in the same patient are shown on the *right panel*. PET images acquired on a PET/CT scanner after an infusion of adenosine and 30 mCi of ^{82}Rb (*top*) and at rest following another 30 mCi infusion of ^{82}Rb (*bottom*). ^{82}Rb PET images show normal distribution of the radiotracer in all myocardial regions, without evidence for reversible or fixed defect to suggest myocardial ischemia or infarction. Although the high energy positrons of ^{82}Rb degrade spatial resolution and the short half-life increases statistical noise, high-quality images free from attenuation artifacts can be produced with ^{82}Rb PET with only 30 mCi injected dose.

F, Three-dimensional display of gated ^{82}Rb PET images acquired during pharmacologic stress with adenosine. While gated myocardial perfusion SPECT images are acquired poststress, reflecting regional and global left ventricular function in the resting state, gated ^{82}Rb PET images are acquired during pharmacologic stress as well as at rest. As such, gated ^{82}Rb PET images provide an indirect evaluation of abnormal myocardial perfusion as reflected in regional wall motion abnormalities during stress as opposed to poststress with SPECT. In this patient example, surface rendering of end-diastolic and end-systolic images from gated adenosine ^{82}Rb PET are shown along with the time activity curve. The left ventricular ejection fraction is calculated to be 36% during adenosine ^{82}Rb PET and 28% at rest. Postexercise gated SPECT left ventricular ejection fraction acquired in the same patient was calculated to be 32% [38].

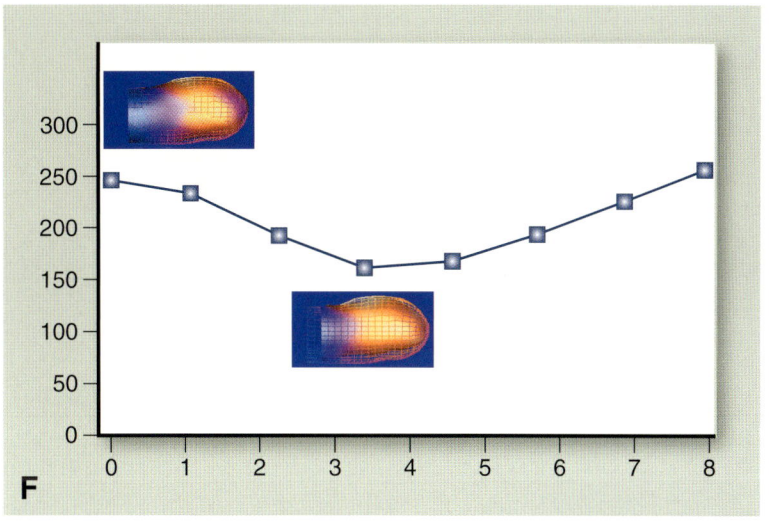

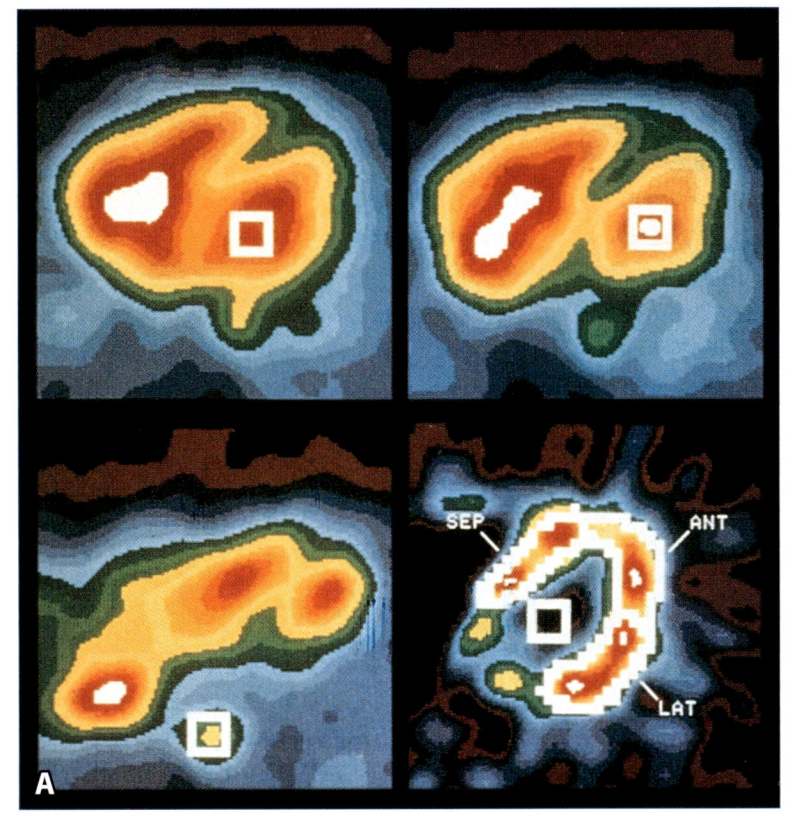

Figure 2-36. PET techniques: ^{15}O-water. ^{15}O-water is a freely diffusable tracer that correlates closely with perfusion as assessed by microspheres with a first-pass extraction fraction approaching unity. Because ^{15}O-water is both in the vascular space and myocardium, visualization of myocardial activity requires correction for activity in the vascular compartment. **A,** Correction for activity in the left atrium (*top left*), left ventricle (*top right*), and thoracic aorta (*bottom left*) is shown in a healthy patient after inhalation of 30 to 40 mCi of ^{15}O-carbon monoxide, which labels erythrocytes in vivo. The distribution of ^{15}O-water is shown in the left ventricular myocardium (*bottom right*) after correction for vascular space.

Continued on the next page

Figure 2-36. *(Continued)* **B,** The ability of ^{15}O-water to assess myocardial viability through modification of the blood flow information is shown. This method, termed *water perfusable tissue index* (PTI), is based on measurement of perfusable tissue fraction (PTF) as a method to correct for the partial volume effects in ^{15}O-water studies [39]. PTF is defined as the fractional volume of a given region of interest occupied by myocardium that is capable of exchanging water rapidly. Using transmission and ^{15}O-blood pool images, the anatomic tissue fraction (ATF), a quantitative estimate of extravascular tissue density, is derived. The ratio of PTF to ATF thus represents the proportion of the extravascular tissue that is perfusable by ^{15}O-water. Because water can freely exchange across all normal tissue cells, the PTF should approach unity in normal myocardium and be reduced in scarred myocardium.

A myocardial region of interest containing a mixture of ^{15}O-water perfusable and nonperfusable tissue is diagrammed. The volume of the region of interest is shown (*A*). ATF for the region of interest is produced by subtraction of the blood pool (^{15}O-carbon monoxide) from the transmission images after normalization of the latter to tissue density (1.04 g/mL). Total ATF (*B*) represents the total extravascular tissue and contains both perfusable and nonperfusable tissue components. ^{15}O-water PTF for the region of interest calculated from the ^{15}O-water data set identifies the mass of tissue within the region of interest that is capable of rapid trans-sarcolemmal exchange of water. Note that the nonperfusable or necrotic region is excluded from this parameter. The ^{15}O-water PTI is calculated by dividing ^{15}O-water PTF (*C*) by the total ATF (*B*), and represents the fraction of the total anatomic tissue that is perfusable by water. ANT—anterior; LAT—lateral; SEP—septal. (**A**, from Bergmann *et al.* [40]; with permission; **B**, adapted from Yamamoto *et al.* [41].)

Figure 2-37. PET techniques: ^{13}N-ammonia. ^{13}N-ammonia is the extractable perfusion tracer most commonly used with PET. At physiologic pH, ammonia is in its cationic form with a physical half-life of 10 minutes. Myocardial distribution of ammonia is related inversely and nonlinearly to blood flow. Although the exact mechanism of ^{13}N-ammonia transport across the myocardial membrane has not been conclusively established, it has been suggested that ^{13}N-ammonia may cross cell membranes by passive diffusion or as ammonium ion (^{13}NH$^+_4$) by the active sodium-potassium transport mechanism influenced by the concentration gradient across the cell membrane. Once in the myocyte, myocardial retention of ^{13}N-ammonia involves predominantly the conversion of ^{13}N-ammonia and glutamic acid to ^{13}N-labeled glutamine mediated by ATP and glutamine synthetase. Hence, absolute quantification requires two- and three-compartment kinetic models that incorporate both extraction and retention rate constants. Quantification of ammonia is further complicated by the rapid degradation of ammonia, which occurs within 5 minutes after administration, producing metabolic intermediates such as urea and glutamine that are also extracted by the heart. Experimental studies suggest that myocardial uptake of ammonia reflects absolute blood flows up to 2 to 2.5 mL/g/min and plateaus at flows in the hyperemic range. In the clinical setting, 10 to 20 mCi of ^{13}N-ammonia is administered intravenously.

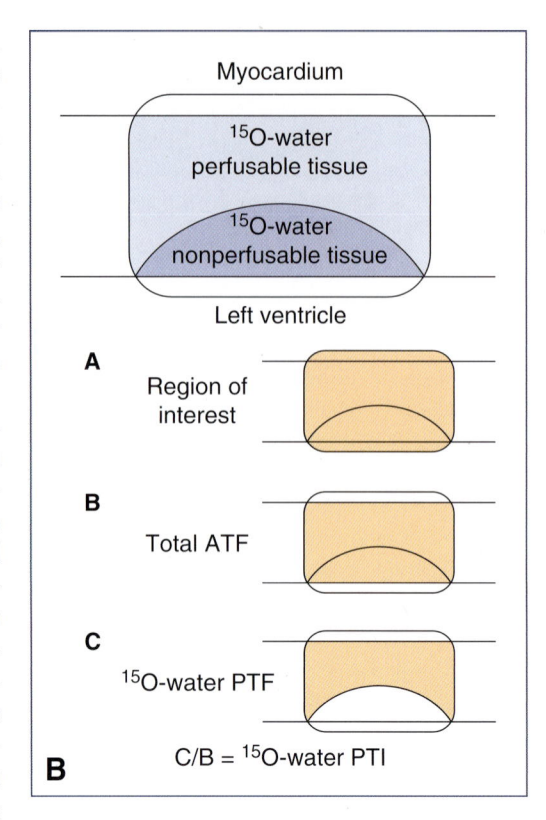

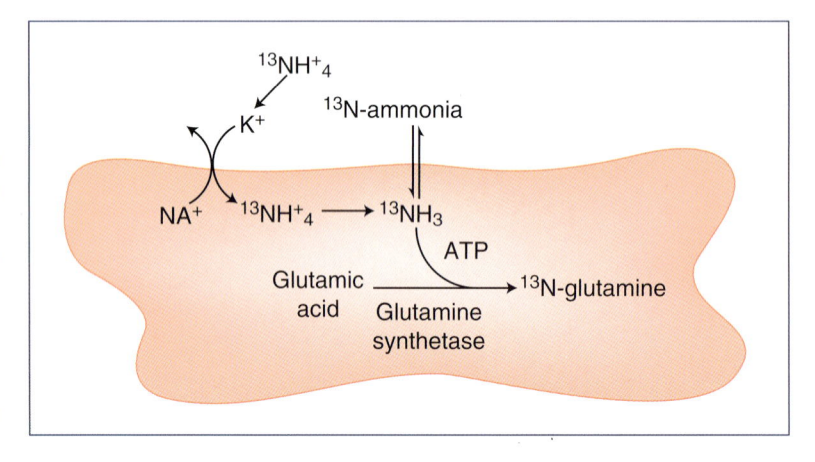

58 Atlas of Nuclear Cardiology

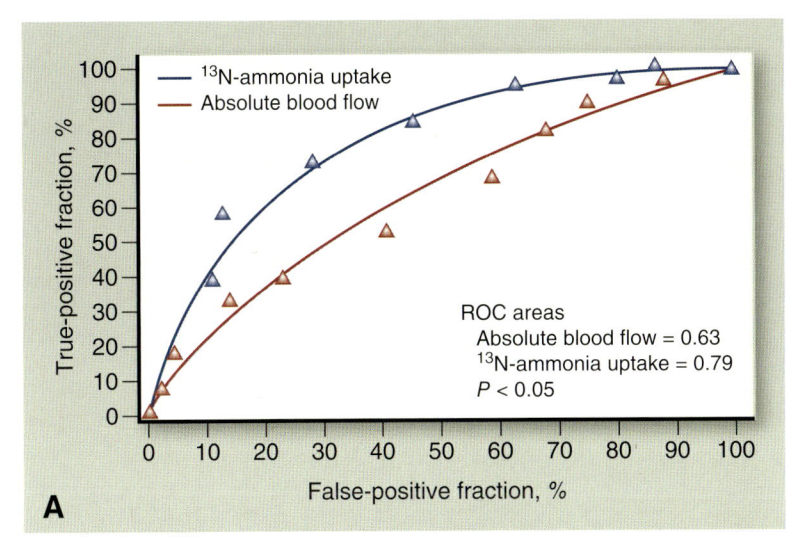

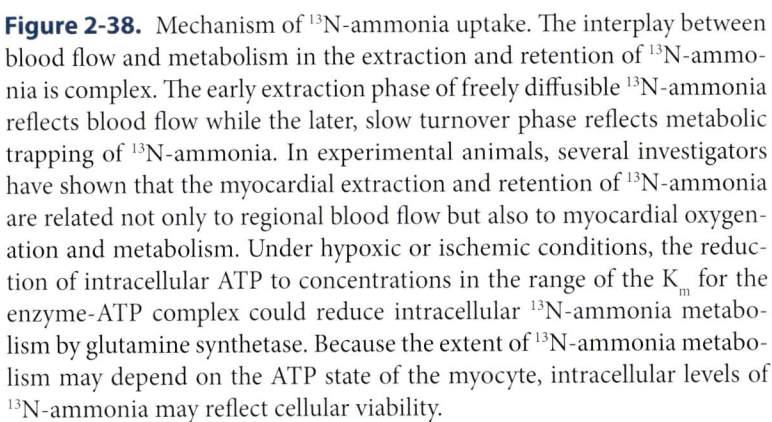

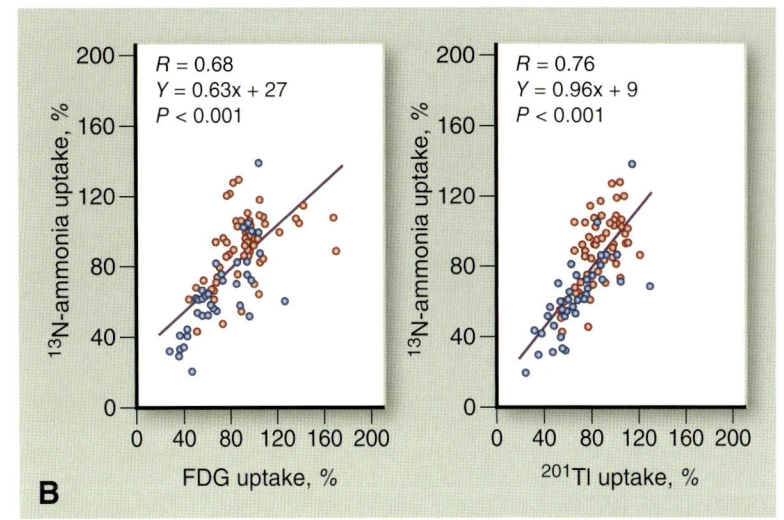

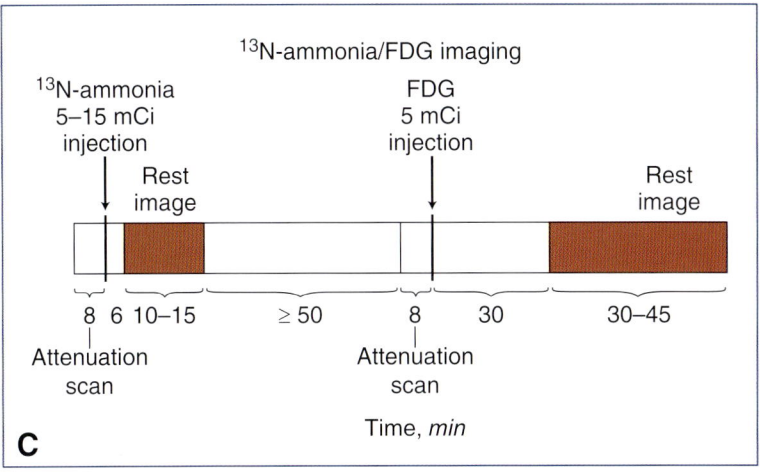

Figure 2-38. Mechanism of ^{13}N-ammonia uptake. The interplay between blood flow and metabolism in the extraction and retention of ^{13}N-ammonia is complex. The early extraction phase of freely diffusible ^{13}N-ammonia reflects blood flow while the later, slow turnover phase reflects metabolic trapping of ^{13}N-ammonia. In experimental animals, several investigators have shown that the myocardial extraction and retention of ^{13}N-ammonia are related not only to regional blood flow but also to myocardial oxygenation and metabolism. Under hypoxic or ischemic conditions, the reduction of intracellular ATP to concentrations in the range of the K_m for the enzyme-ATP complex could reduce intracellular ^{13}N-ammonia metabolism by glutamine synthetase. Because the extent of ^{13}N-ammonia metabolism may depend on the ATP state of the myocyte, intracellular levels of ^{13}N-ammonia may reflect cellular viability.

A, In patients with chronic coronary artery disease and left ventricular dysfunction, receiver-operating characteristic (ROC) curves were used to compare the abilities of late ammonia uptake (final 10 to 15 minutes of image acquisition) and absolute blood flow (early extraction phase, approximately 3 minutes after injection) to predict functional improvement of asynergic regions after revascularization. The results show that late ammonia uptake (metabolic trapping) is a significantly better predictor of functional improvement after revascularization when compared to absolute blood flow. **B,** There is a linear relationship between percent late ammonia uptake and [^{18}F]-fluorodeoxyglucose (FDG) uptake (*left*), and ^{201}Tl uptake on redistribution imaging (*right*) in reversible (*red circles*) and irreversible (*blue circles*) asynergic regions after revascularization. **C,** Sequence and timing of ^{13}N-ammonia and FDG PET imaging for assessment of myocardial viability. Thus, beyond ammonia's value as a perfusion tracer, late ammonia images provide important insight regarding cell membrane integrity and myocardial viability. (*Adapted from* Kitsiou *et al.* [42].)

References

1. Cerqueira MD, Weissman NJ, Dilsizian V, *et al.*: Standardized myocardial segmentation and nomenclature for tomographic imaging of the heart. AHA Writing Group on Myocardial Segmentation and Registration for Cardiac Imaging. *Circulation* 2002, 105:539–542.

2. Dilsizian V, Rocco TP, Freedman NM, *et al.*: Enhanced detection of ischemic but viable myocardium by the reinjection of thallium after stress-redistribution imaging. *N Engl J Med* 1990, 323:141–146.

3. Maddahi J, Van Train K, Prigent F, *et al.*: Quantitative single photon emission computed thallium-201 tomography for detection and localization of coronary artery disease: optimization and prospective validation of a new technique. *J Am Coll Cardiol* 1989, 14:1689–1995.

4. Fintel DJ, Links JM, Brinker JA, *et al.*: Improved diagnostic performance of exercise thallium-201 single photon emission computed tomography over planar imaging in the diagnosis of coronary artery disease: a receiver operating characteristic analysis. *J Am Coll Cardiol* 1989, 13:600–608.

5. Iskandrian AS, Heo J, Kong B, *et al.*: Effect of exercise level on the ability of thallium-201 tomographic imaging in detecting coronary artery disease: analysis of 461 patients. *J Am Coll Cardiol* 1989, 14:1477–1482.

6. Go RT, Marwick TH, MacIntyre WJ, *et al.*: A prospective comparison of rubidium-82 PET and thallium-201 SPECT myocardial perfusion imaging utilizing a single dipyridamole stress in the diagnosis of coronary artery disease. *J Nucl Med* 1990, 31:1899–1905.

7. Mahmarian JJ, Boyce, Goldberg RK, *et al.*: Quantitative exercise thallium-201 single photo emission computed tomography for the enhanced diagnosis of ischemic heart disease. *J Am Coll Cardiol* 1990, 15:318–323.

8. Van Train KF, Maddahi J, Berman DS, *et al.*: Quantitative analysis of tomographic stress thallium-201 myocardial scintigrams: A multicenter trial. *J Nucl Med* 1990, 31:1168–1177.

9. Kiat H, Maddahi J, Roy L, *et al.*: Comparison of technetium 99m methoxy isobutyl isonitrile and thallium-201 for evaluation of coronary artery disease by planar and tomographic methods. *Am Heart J* 1989, 117:111–117.

10. Iskandrian AS, Heo J, Long B, *et al.*: Use of technetium-99m isonitrile (RP-30A) in assessing left ventricular perfusion and function at rest and during exercise in coronary artery disease, and comparison with coronary arteriography and exercise thallium-201 SPECT imaging. *Am J Cardiol* 1989, 64:270–278.

11. Kahn JK, McGhie I, Akers MS, *et al.*: Quantitative rotational tomography 201Tl and 99mTc 2-methoxly-isobutyl-isonitrile. *Circulation* 1989, 79:1282–1289.

12. Solot G, Hermans J, Merlo P, *et al.*: Correlation of 99Tcm-sestamibi SPECT with coronary angiography in general hospital practice. *Nucl Med Commun* 1993, 14:23–28.

13. Van Train KF, Garcia EV, Maddahi J, *et al.*: Multicenter trial validation for quantitative analysis of same-day rest-stress technetium-99m-sestamibi myocardial tomograms. *J Nucl Med* 1994, 35:609–615.

14. Azzarelli S, Galassi AR, Foti R, *et al.*: Accuracy of 99m-tetrofosmin myocardial tomography in the evaluation of coronary artery disease. *J Nucl Cardiol* 1999, 6:183–191.

15. Ritchie JL, Bateman TM, Bonow RO, *et al.*: Guidelines for the clinical use of cardiac radionuclide imaging: a report of the ACC/AHA Task Force on assessment of diagnostic and therapeutic procedures. *J Am Coll Cardiol* 1995, 25:521–547.

16. Gibson RS, Watson DD, Craddock GB, *et al.*: Predication of cardiac events after uncomplicated myocardial infarction: A prospective study comparing predischarge exercise thallium-201 scintigraphy and coronary angiography. *Circulation* 1983, 68:321–336.

17. Kiat H, Berman DS, Maddahi J, *et al.*: Late reversibility of tomographic myocardial thallium-201 defects: An accurate marker of myocardial viability. *J Am Coll Cardiol* 1988, 12:1456–1463.

18. Cloninger KG, DePuey EG, Garcia EV, *et al.*: Incomplete redistribution in delayed thallium-201 single photon emission computed tomographic (SPECT) images: An overestimation of myocardial scarring. *J Am Coll Cardiol* 1988, 12:955–963.

19. Dilsizian V: Thallium-201 scintigraphy: experience of two decades. In *Myocardial Viability: A Clinical and Scientific Treatise*. Edited by Dilsizian V. Armonk, New York: Futura; 2000:265–313.

20. Zimmermann R, Mall G, Rauch B, *et al.*: Residual Tl-201 activity in irreversible defects as a marker of myocardial viability: clinicopathological study. *Circulation* 1995, 91:1016–1021.

21. Kayden DS, Sigal S, Soufer R, *et al.*: Thallium-201 for assessment of myocardial viability: Quantitative comparison of 24-hour redistribution imaging with imaging after reinjection at rest. *J Am Coll Cardiol* 1991, 18:1480–1486.

22. Kitsiou AN, Srinivasan G, Quyyumi AA, *et al.*: Stress-induced reversible and mild-to-moderate irreversible thallium defects: are they equally accurate for predicting recovery of regional left ventricular function after revascularization? *Circulation* 1998, 98:501–508.

23. Petretta M, Cuocolo A, Bonaduce D, *et al.*: Prognostic value of thallium reinjection after stress-redistribution imaging in patients with previous myocardial infarction and left ventricular dysfunction. *J Nucl Med* 1997, 38:195–200.

24. Arrighi JA, Dilsizian V: Identification of viable, nonfunctioning myocardium. In *Cardiac Intensive Care*. Edited by Brown DL. Philadelphia: WB Saunders; 1998:307–327.

25. Gioia G, Milan E, Giubbini R, *et al.*: Prognostic value of tomographic rest-redistribution thallium-201 imaging in medically treated patients with coronary artery disease and left ventricular dysfunction. *J Nucl Cardiol* 1996, 3:150–156.

26. Gioia G, Powers J, Heo J, Iskandrian AS: Prognostic value of rest-redistribution tomographic thallium-201 imaging in ischemic cardiomyopathy. *Am J Cardiol* 1995, 75:759–762.

27. Pagley PR, Beller GA, Watson DD, *et al.*: Improved outcome after coronary artery bypass surgery in patients with ischemic cardiomyopathy and residual myocardial viability. *Circulation* 1997, 95:793–800.

28. Piwnica-Worms D, Chiu ML, Kronauge JF, *et al.*: Divergent kinetics of 201Tl and 99mTc-SESTAMIBI in cultured chick ventricular myocytes during ATP depletion. *Circulation* 1992, 85:1531–1541.

29. Narahara KA, Vilaneuva-Meyer J, Thompson CJ, *et al.*: Comparison of thallium-201 and technetium-99m hexakis 2-methoxyisobutyl isonitrile single-photon emission computed tomography for estimating the extent of myocardial ischemia and infarction in coronary artery disease. *Am J Cardiol* 1990, 66:1438–1444.

30. Leon AR, Eisner RL, Martin SE, *et al.*: Comparison of single-photon emission computed tomographic (SPECT) myocardial perfusion imaging with thallium-201 and technetium-99m sestamibi in dogs. *J Am Coll Cardiol* 1992, 20:1612–1625.

31. Li QS, Solot G, Frank TL, *et al.*: Myocardial redistribution of technetium-99m-methoxyisobutyl isonitrile (sestamibi). *J Nucl Med* 1990, 31:1069–1076.

32. Dilsizian V, Arrighi JA, Diodati JG, *et al.*: Myocardial viability in patients with chronic coronary artery disease: comparison of 99mTc-sestamibi with thallium reinjection and 18F-fluorodeoxyglucose. *Circulation* 1994, 89:578–587.

33. Franceschi M, Guimond J, Zimmerman RE, *et al.*: Myocardial clearance of Tc-99m hexakis-2-methoxy-2-methylpropyl isonitrile (MIBI) in patients with coronary artery disease. *Clin Nucl Med* 1990, 15:307–312.

34. Bisi G, Sciagra R, Santoro GM, *et al.*: Technetium-99m-sestamibi imaging with nitrate infusion to detect viable hibernating myocardium and predict postrevascularization recovery. *J Nucl Med* 1995, 36:1994–2000.

35. Mehry Y, Latour JG, Arsenault A, Rousseau G: Effect of coronary reperfusion on technetium-99m methoxyisobutylisonitrile uptake by viable and necrotic myocardium in the dog. *Eur J Nucl Med* 1992, 19:503–510.

36. Udelson JE, Coleman PS, Metherall JA, *et al.*: Predicting recovery of severe regional ventricular dysfunction: comparison of resting scintigraphy with 201Tl and 99mTc-sestamibi. *Circulation* 1994, 89:2552–2561.

37. Delbeke D, Videlefsky S, Patton JA, *et al.*: Rest myocardial perfusion/metabolism imaging using simultaneous dual-isotope acquisition SPECT with technetium-99m-MIBI/fluorine-18-FDG. *J Nucl Med* 1995, 36:2110–2119.

38. Lodge MA, Braess H, Mahmood F, *et al.*: Developments in nuclear cardiology: transition from SPECT to PET/CT. *J Inv Cardiol* 2005, 17:491–496.

39. Iida H, Rhodes CG, de Silva R, *et al.*: Myocardial tissue fraction: Correction of partial volume effects and measure of tissue viability. *J Nucl Med* 1991, 32:2169–2175.

40. Bergmann SR, Herrero P, Markham J, *et al.*: Noninvasive quantitation of myocardial blood flow in human subjects with oxygen-15-labeled water and positron emission tomography. *J Am Coll Cardiol* 1989, 14:639–652.

41. Yamamoto Y, de Silva R, Rhodes CG, *et al.*: A new strategy for the assessment of viable myocardium and regional myocardial blood flow using 15O-water and dynamic positron emission tomography. *Circulation* 1992, 86:167–178.

42. Kitsiou AN, Bacharach SL, Bartlett ML, *et al.*: 13N-ammonia myocardial blood flow and uptake: Relation to functional outcome of asynergic regions after revascularization. *J Am Coll Cardiol* 1999, 33:678–686.

Pharmacologic Stressors in Coronary Artery Disease

D. Douglas Miller

Given the phenomena of population aging and obesity, both in the United States and globally [1], the current pattern of stress imaging and the expected future trend indicates that pharmacologic stress imaging will grow in clinical importance [2]. Clinical demand for this service has driven significant evolution in pharmacologic stress protocols, new drug development, and indications for testing. Published evidence, expert guidelines, and clinical practice all reflect, to varying degrees, this growth and evolution. The results of pharmacologic stress imaging studies, whether positive or negative for myocardial ischemia, continue to influence patient management decisions in the diverse population of patients with known or suspected coronary artery disease (CAD).

The target populations who benefit most from the incremental diagnostic and prognostic value of drug stress imaging are those at higher risk of severe CAD and related serious cardiac events due to their comorbid conditions (ie, generalized vascular disease) and/or poor functional capacity, which renders them unable to perform the preferred stress modality, maximal dynamic exercise stress.

Triaging patients for further cardiac evaluation based on clinical risk predictors and the type of surgical procedure is now recommended and widely practiced. Pharmacologic stress myocardial perfusion imaging is an excellent adjunctive method for identifying high- and low-risk patients from within an intermediate clinical risk pool. The stress imaging results with each of the available pharmacologic stressors are qualitatively similar for discriminating low- and high-risk groups for postoperative cardiac events, although the reported clinical experience to date with adenosine and dobutamine is somewhat limited. With the routine use of electrocardiograph-gated SPECT imaging, the left ventricular ejection fraction can also be obtained, adding further prognostic value to the perfusion data. Patients with more extensive stress-induced myocardial hypoperfusion or ischemia are at highest risk, and are best evaluated with coronary angiography with the goal of preoperative revascularization based on the current published guidelines. Although the American College of Cardiology/American Heart Association Task Force guidelines have not been prospectively validated, several small studies support these expert, evidence-based recommendations.

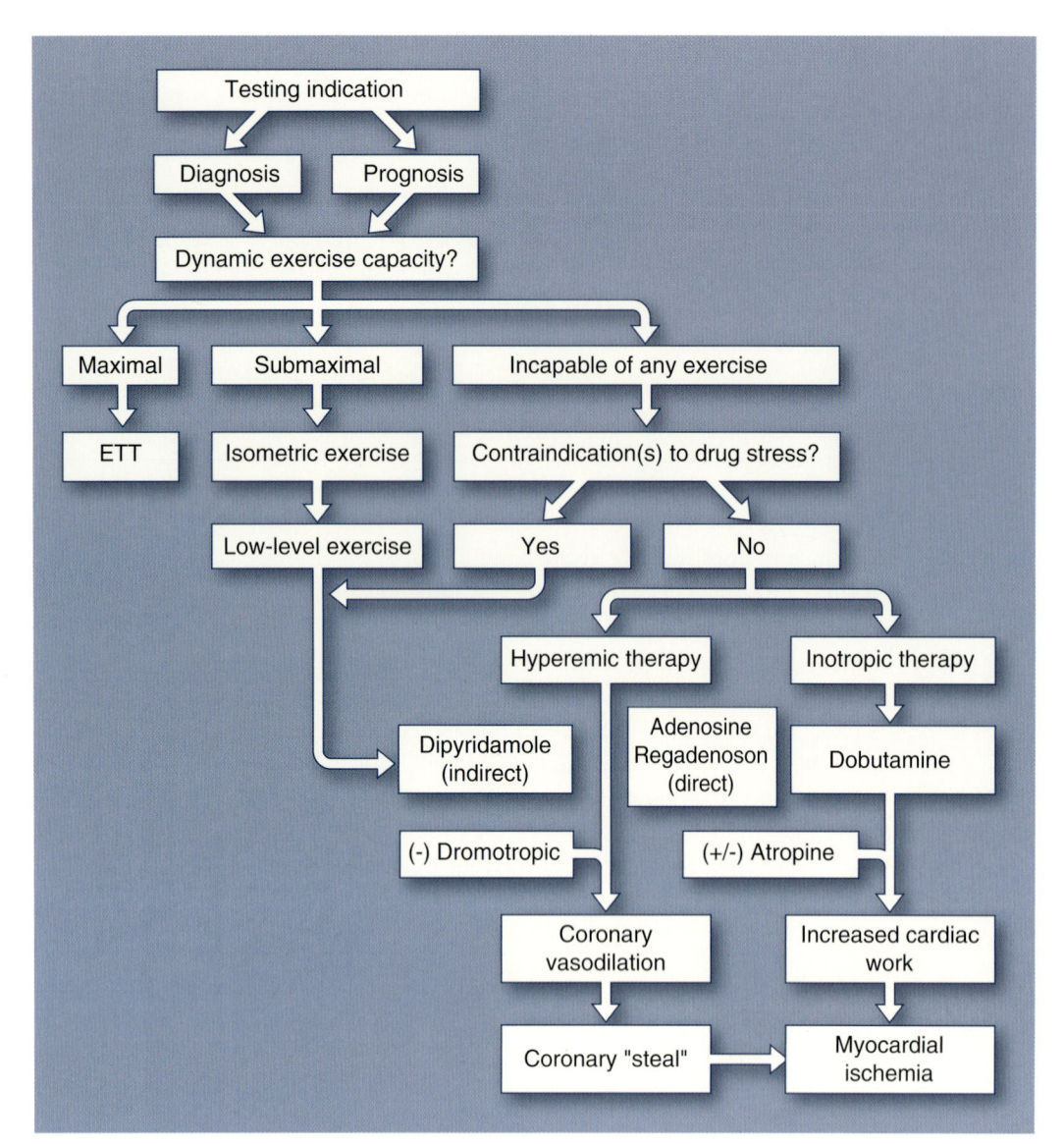

Figure 3-1. Patient protocol selection algorithm. The decision analysis for pharmacologic stress imaging illustrates the clinical issues that should be addressed: whether the patient can perform dynamic exercise, whether there are contraindications for drug stress, the type of drug stress (*ie*, hyperemic or inotropic), and the resulting physiologic and pathophysiologic endpoints. ETT—exercise treadmill testing.

Indications for Pharmacologic Imaging

Inability to exercise
  Physical limitations (amputations, etc.)
  Recent operation
  Comorbidity
Limited exercise capacity
  Deconditioning
  Limiting physical conditions (COPD, claudication)
  Medications (ß-blockers)
  Poor motivation
Contraindications to exercise
  Early post–myocardial infarction
  Unstable angina
  Aortic aneurysm (coexisting medical conditions)
  LBBB

Figure 3-2. Indications for pharmacologic stress imaging. These indications include inability to exercise, limited exercise capacity, and relative or absolute contraindications to exercise. While exercise remains the preferred modality of stress testing in the majority of cases, a significant number of patients cannot complete a maximum stress test. Some patient populations are well suited for vasodilator stress imaging, such as patients with aortic stenosis, where excellent diagnostic accuracy and safety have been shown [3]. Patients with electrocardiographic left bundle branch block (LBBB) have a high false-positive rate with exercise or dobutamine stress testing due to abnormal patterns of septal perfusion and contraction [4,5]. The diagnostic accuracy in patients with LBBB is 86% to 90% with adenosine or dipyridamole, compared with 50% or less with exercise perfusion imaging. Supplemental exercise is not advised for patients with LBBB. COPD–chronic obstructive pulmonary disease.

Options for Nonexercise Stress Testing

- Cold pressor test
- Atrial pacing
  - Transthoracic
  - Intravenous
  - Transesophageal
- Pharmacologic stress
  - Vasodilator stress
    - Dipyridamole
    - Adenosine
    - Regadenoson
  - Inotropic/chronotropic
    - Dobutamine

Figure 3-3. Options for nonexercise stress testing. These options include less frequently used techniques such as cold pressor testing and atrial pacing, and more commonly used pharmacologic stress with vasodilators or inotropic agents. General contraindications for pharmacologic stress testing include hypersensitivity to the particular stress agent or its antidote, testing within 24 hours of an acute coronary syndrome, and uncompensated congestive heart failure. Dipyridamole, adenosine, and regadenoson are contraindicated for patients with hypotension, bronchospasm, and advanced atrioventricular block; dobutamine is contraindicated for patients with hypertension, high-grade ventricular ectopy, uncontrolled atrial fibrillation/flutter, left ventricular outflow tract obstruction, and expanding aortic aneurysm. Published data support the safety of adenosine or dipyridamole in patients with lung disease in the absence of wheezing, and if peak flow rates on spirometry are normal before testing [6,7]. Regadenoson safety has been established in a small series of patients with mild-to-moderate asthma [8] and chronic obstructive pulmonary disease [9].

Characteristics of Methods of Stress Testing

	Exercise	Dobutamine	Dipyridamole	Adenosine	Regadenoson
CBF increase	2–3 times	2 times	3–4 times	3–5 times	2–3 times
Ischemia provocation	Frequent	Common	Rare	Uncommon	Uncommon
Onset of effect	3–5 min	2–4 min	4–6 min	1–2 min	1–4 min
Duration after stopping	2–5 min	4–6 min	10–30 min	0.5–1 min	15–30 min
AV block occurrence	No	No	Rare	Common (transient)	Uncommon (transient)
Ventricular ectopy	Uncommon	Common	Rare	Rare	Rare

Figure 3-4. Characteristics of stress testing with regard to responses from exercise, dobutamine, and clinically available vasodilators dipyridamole, adenosine, and regadenoson. AV—atrioventricular; CBF—coronary blood flow.

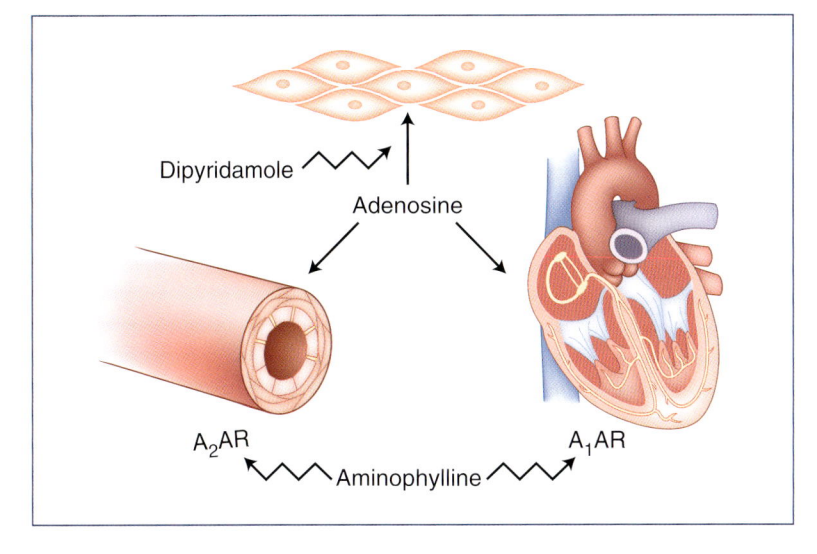

Figure 3-5. The direct and indirect action of adenosine and dipyridamole on vascular smooth muscle cells (A_2 receptors [$A_{2A}R$]) and on cardiac conduction cells (A_1 receptors [$A_{1A}R$]).

Adenosine is a small, heterocyclic, endogenous compound produced by the endothelial cell. It activates A_2 receptors, causing vasodilatation via the production of adenyl cyclase and the subsequent local increase in cylic AMP. Theophylline and other methylxanthines, including caffeine, are competitive antagonists of adenosine, blocking their effects at the A_2 receptor. Adenosine enters endothelial and red blood cells by a facilitated transport mechanism. Intracellular adenosine is then deaminated or converted to other inactive metabolites.

The "antidote" that reverses the effects of dipyridamole or adenosine is aminophylline. Patient preparation for pharmacologic stress testing is similar to that for 12 to 24 hours for exercise stress, although all methylxanthines must be withheld before adenosine or dipyridamole testing [10]. β-Blockers should be withheld for 24 hours before dobutamine stress testing. With vasodilator SPECT imaging, the increased splanchnic activity mandates a delay in image acquisition for 30 to 60 minutes following the injection of a ^{99m}Tc agent [11,12].

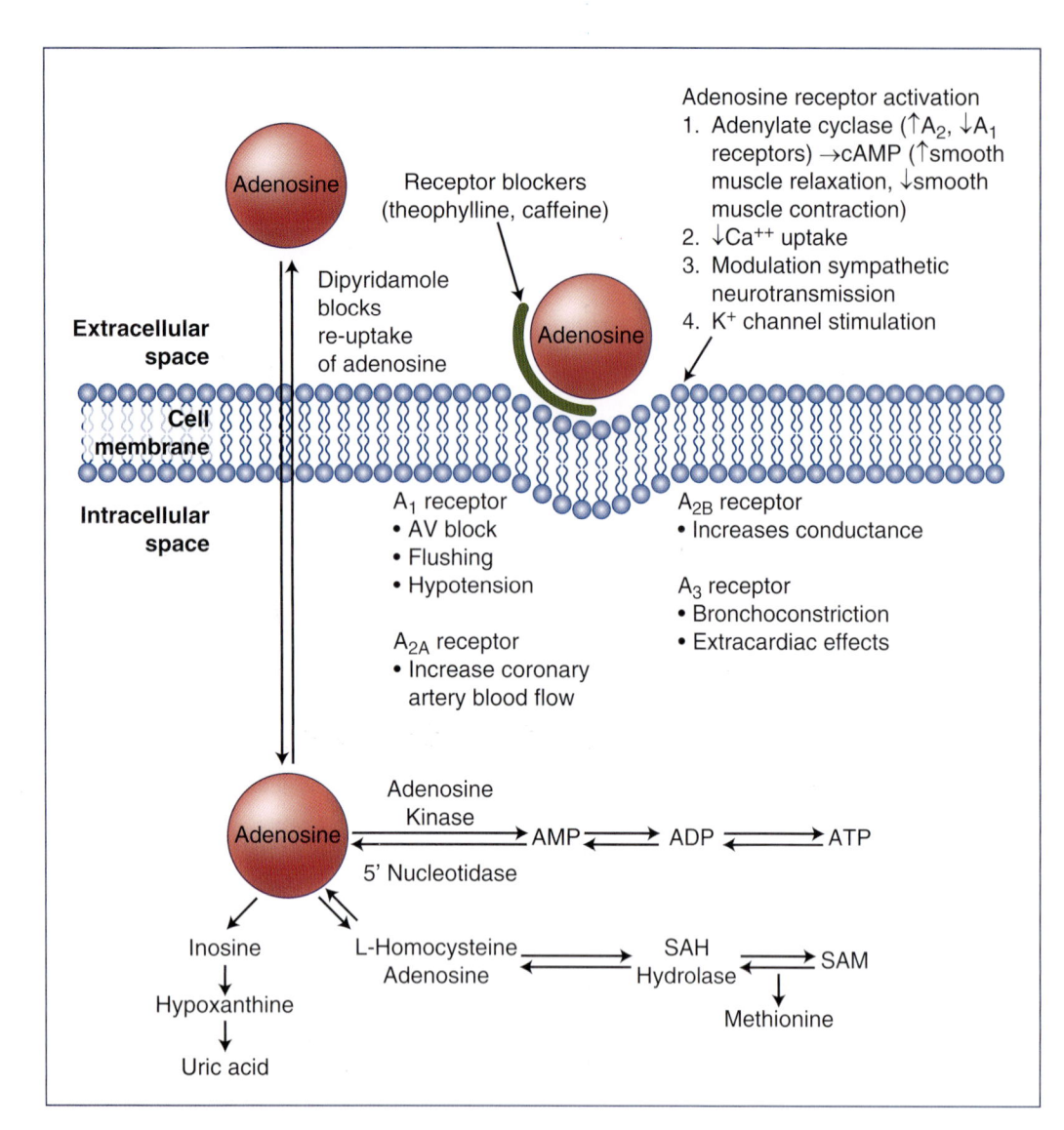

Figure 3-6. Adenosine receptor subtypes and mechanisms of action. The clinical utility of pharmacologic vasodilators is in their ability to produce hyperemic coronary flow by stimulating A_{2A} adenosine receptors on arteriolar vascular smooth muscle cells. However, both adenosine and dipyridamole activate other adenosine receptor subtypes, A_1, A_{2B}, and A_3, nonselectively, which explains many common and undesirable side effects that patients experience, such as bronchospasm and high-grade atrioventricular block. A pharmacologic vasodilator that is A_{2A} subtype receptor specific would in theory result in reduction of these undesirable side effects while targeting coronary artery vasodilation. There are three selective A_{2A} adenosine receptor agonists that have been studied in clinical trials: regadenoson, binodenoson, and apadenoson. Current US Food and Drug Administration–approved and Centers for Medicare & Medicaid Services–reimbursable selective A_{2A} adenosine receptor agonists are limited to regadenoson. SAH—S-adenosyl homocysteine; SAM—S-adenosyl methionine.

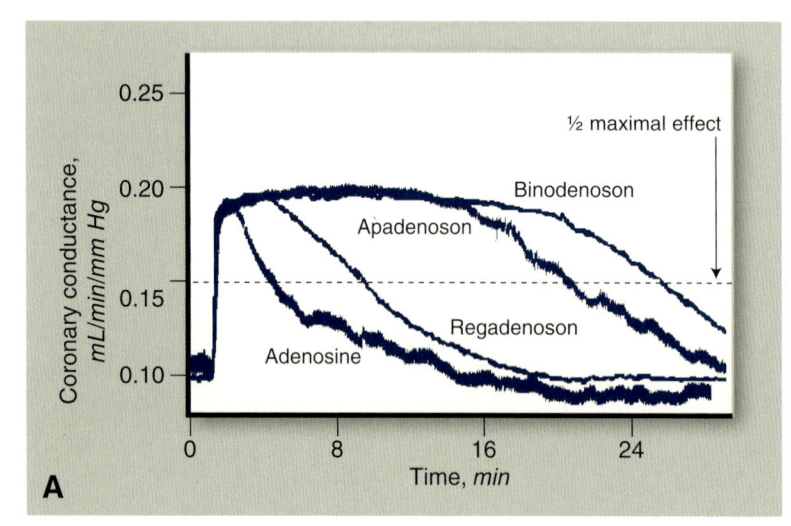

Figure 3-7. A, Time course of changes in coronary conductance caused by adenosine, regadenoson, binodenoson, and apadenoson. All of the A_{2A} agonists tested achieved comparable maximal increases in coronary vasodilation to that of adenosine. However, there were differences in the duration of the coronary conductance, which is likely explained by the inverse relationship between affinity for the A_{2A} receptor and duration of action. Low-affinity agonists, such as adenosine and regadenoson, can cause maximal coronary vasodilation that is rapid in both onset and termination. On the other hand, high-affinity agonists, such as binodenoson and apadenoson, achieve rapid maximal coronary vasodilation but exhibit much longer termination phase, with longer duration of coronary vasodilation [13].

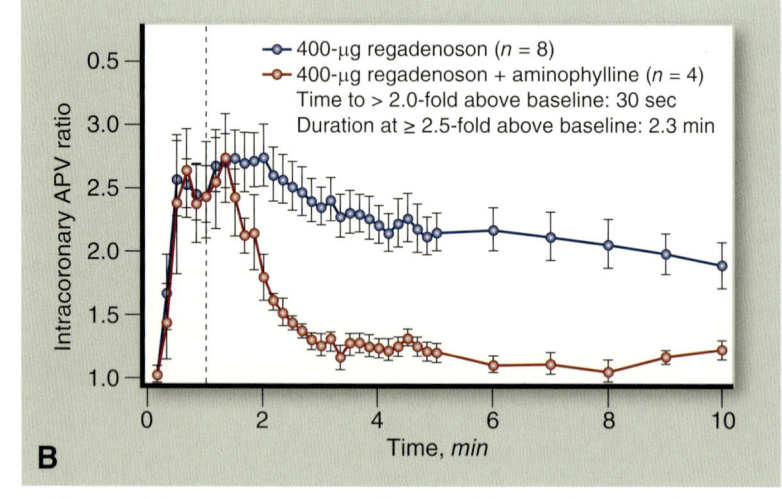

B, The effect of regadenoson on intracoronary blood flow. A rapid increase (to ≥ 2.5-fold over baseline) is sustained for approximately 2.3 minutes and decreases to less than twice the baseline level within 10 minutes. Flow velocity is evaluated by pulsed-wave ultrasonography in patients undergoing coronary catheterization [14]. When regadenoson is followed by aminophylline (100 mg slow intravenous bolus) 1 minute later, there is prompt and rapid decrease of coronary vasodilation. Thus, aminophylline can be use as an "antidote" to reverse the effects of regadenoson. APV—average peak velocity.

64 Atlas of Nuclear Cardiology

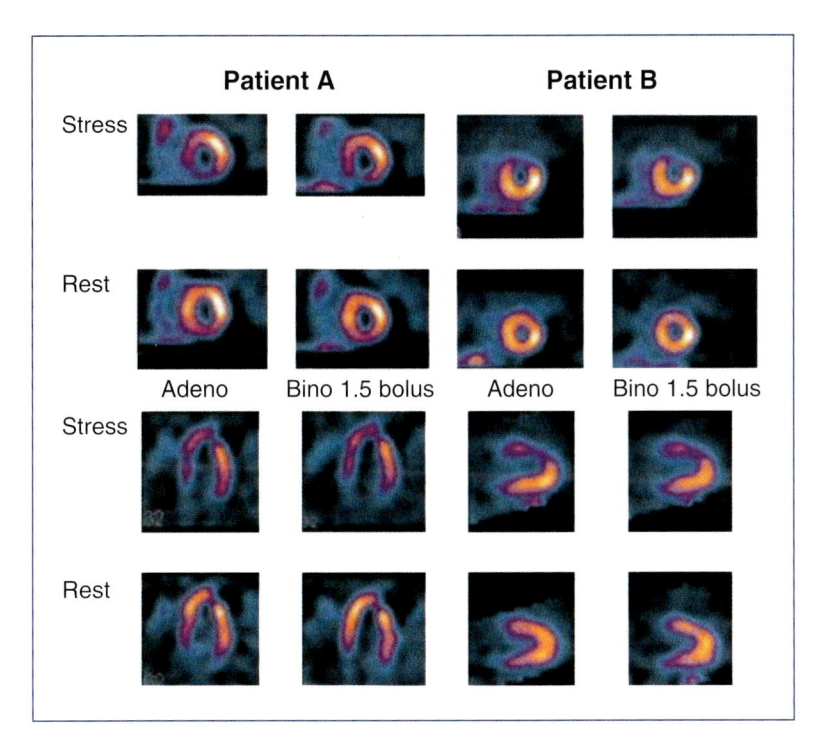

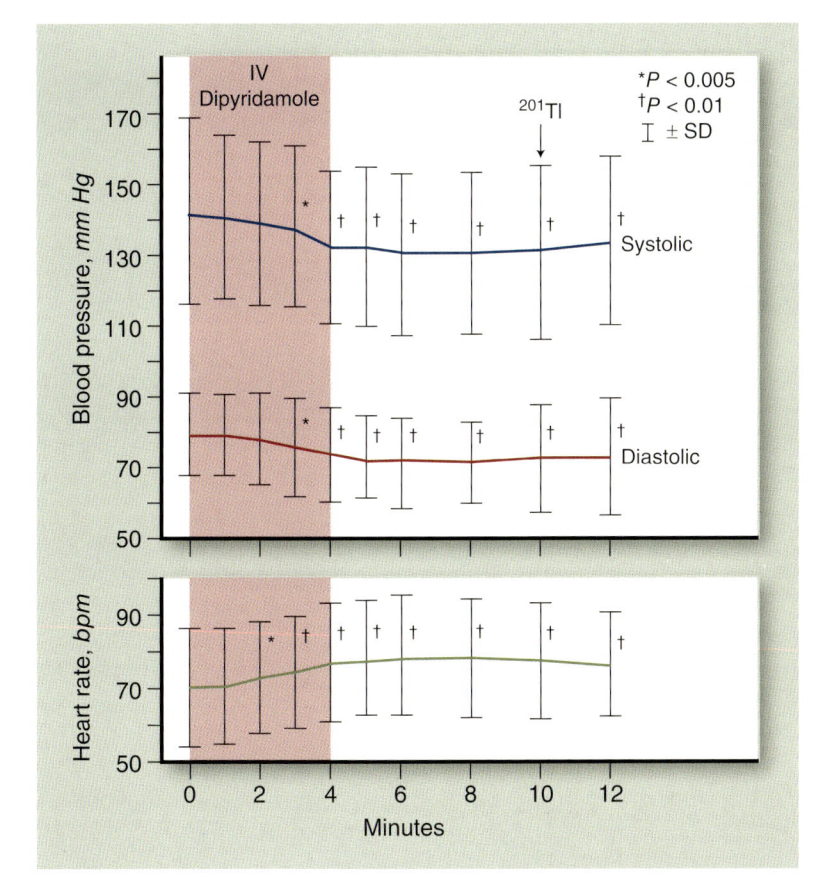

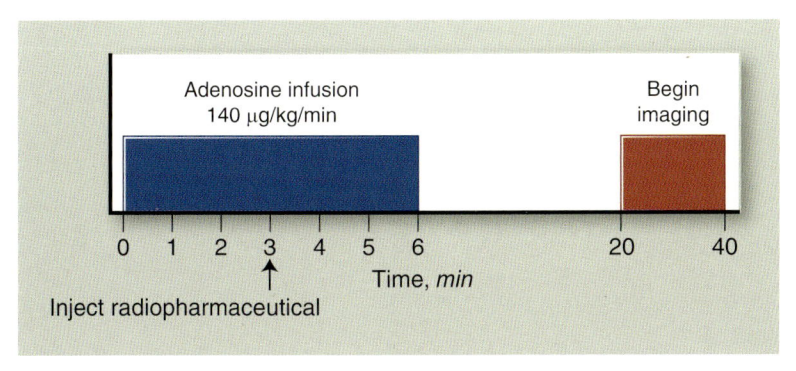

Figure 3-8. The desirable arteriolar vasodilator effect on the coronary adenosine A_{2A} receptor is the basis for the differential effects of pharmacologic stress agents on coronary flow reserve in stenotic versus unobstructed vascular beds. The undesirable nonselective activation of the adenosine A_1, A_{2B}, and A_3 receptors contributes to the side-effect profile of these drugs, including atrioventricular heart block and bronchospasm.

Selective adenosine A_{2A} receptor agonists have been tested in several clinical trials to take advantage of greater drug receptor specificity during pharmacologic stress myocardial perfusion imaging. Dose-ranging studies have identified the optimal doses to maximize coronary A_{2A}-mediated vasodilation while reducing concomitant side effects due to nonspecific stimulation of lower affinity receptor sites. Utilizing the agent binodenoson in doses ranging from 0.5 to 1.5 µg/kg as a 30-second intravenous (IV) bolus or 1.5 µg/kg IV infusion for 3 minutes demonstrated good-to-excellent image concordance with adenosine SPECT [12].

The figure illustrates two examples of the concordance of SPECT image results between adenosine (Adeno) and binodenoson at 1.5 µg/kg bolus dose (Bino 1.5 bolus). The short axis (*top left*) and horizontal long axis (*bottom left*) SPECT images in patient A demonstrate septal and apical reversible defects similar in extent and severity after pharmacologic stress with the two agents and a fixed inferior defect. In patient B, short axis (*top right*) and vertical long axis (*bottom right*) adenosine and binodenoson SPECT images show a concordantly severe reversible anterior defect.

Figure 3-9. Hemodynamic responses to intravenous (IV) dipyridamole. The response usually entails a slight (10%–15%) decrease in blood pressure with compensatory (reflex) tachycardia. (*Adapted from* Homma et al. [15].)

Figure 3-10. Adenosine infusion protocol. This timeline indicates that optimal injection of the radiopharmaceutical should occur at approximately 3 to 4 minutes after the onset of continuous pump infusion. The peak hyperemic effect is established by 3 minutes. ^{99m}Tc-agent imaging is started 20 to 40 minutes thereafter. Adenosine is administered in a dose of 140 µg/kg/min over 6 minutes, although protocols using infusion times of 3 to 4 minutes have been successful. Adenosine is administered by an infusion pump through a small caliber tube to avoid sudden bolus administration.

Pharmacologic Stressors in Coronary Artery Disease 65

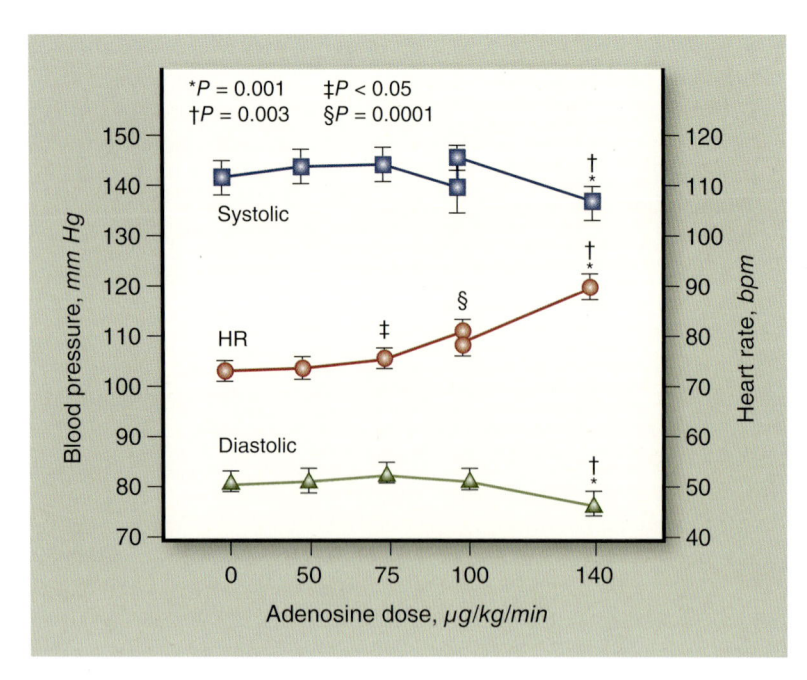

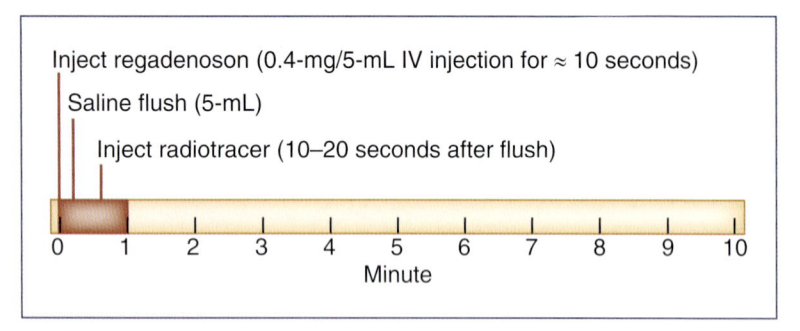

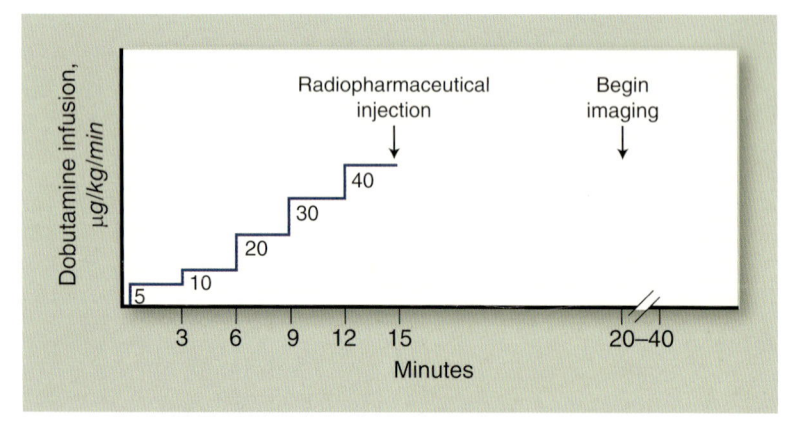

Figure 3-11. Peripheral hemodynamic responses to adenosine. Blood pressure decreases by 10% to 15% in a dose-dependent fashion during infusion, with compensatory (reflex) tachycardia. BPM—beats per minute; HR—heart rate. (*Adapted from* Verani et al. [16].)

Figure 3-12. Regadenoson infusion protocol. Regadenoson is administered as a single 400-μg peripheral intravenous (IV) bolus (< 10 seconds) followed immediately by a 5-mL solution of saline flush. The radiotracer is then injected 10 to 20 seconds after the saline flush. The subsequent image acquisition protocol is dependent on the extraction and clearance properties of the injected radiotracer.

Figure 3-13. Intravenous (IV) dobutamine infusion protocol. Incremental doses of dobutamine are given at 3-minute intervals to a maximum of 50 μg/kg/min over 15 to 20 minutes. Radiopharmaceutical injection is performed at the peak of drug effect (measured by cardiac double product), with imaging initiated 20 to 40 minutes thereafter. Dobutamine, a synthetic catecholamine, produces a predominantly β-adrenergic effect, causing increased inotropy and relatively small changes in blood pressure. Atropine can be safely added to increase heart rate and to help reach the target heart rate in most patients. Side effects include frequent supraventricular and ventricular ectopy; ventricular tachycardia occurs in only 4% of patients [17]. These arrhythmias are successfully treated with termination of the infusion and the occasional use of an IV β-blocker (esmolol or metoprolol). Radiopharmaceutical (IV) injection should occur at the peak heart rate that should be maintained for at least one additional minute [18]. No deaths or myocardial infarctions attributable to dobutamine have occurred.

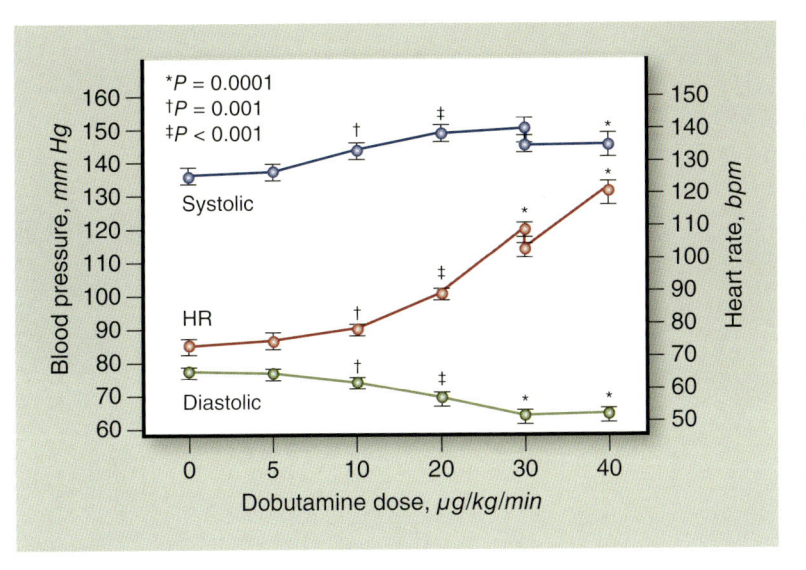

Figure 3-14. Peripheral hemodynamic responses to dobutamine. The responses entail a predictable increase in systolic blood pressure, widening of the pulse pressure, and a chronotropic impact on heart rate (HR), which may be augmented by atropine (0.4–0.6 mg intravenous bolus). ST segment alterations are predictive of significant coronary disease with exercise, but there is controversy regarding the diagnostic value of ST depression with pharmacologic stress testing [19]. ST depression is predictive of both scintigraphic evidence of myocardial ischemia and more severe coronary artery disease. Electrocardiographic changes are more common with dobutamine than with vasodilators, perhaps due to the increased cardiac workload (demand) [10]. With adenosine and dipyridamole, ST depression reflects coronary "steal," as collateral vessels are usually associated with adenosine- or dipyridamole-induced ST depression [20]. BPM—beats per minute. (*Adapted from* Hays *et al.* [18].)

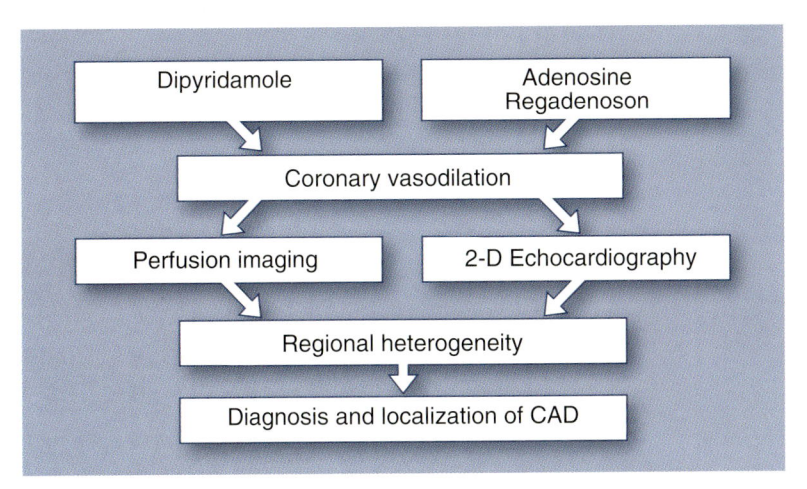

Figure 3-15. The effects of hyperemic stress with dipyridamole, adenosine, or regadenoson on coronary vasodilation, establishing flow heterogeneity (usually in the absence of ischemia), leading to the diagnosis and localization of coronary artery disease (CAD). Adenosine, regadenoson, and dipyridamole reduce coronary vascular resistance and increase blood flow two- to fivefold, to near maximal levels. Myocardial ischemia is not a prerequisite for the detection of obstructive CAD, because poststenotic flow disparities may be imaged in the setting of critical stenoses. In a direct comparison, dipyridamole and adenosine had similar diagnostic accuracy, with a myocardial segmental concordance of 87% [21].

Combined Vasodilator Plus Exercise Stress Imaging

Study	Patients, n	Vasodilator Protocol	Exercise Protocol	Tracer	Vasodilator + Exercise Benefits
Samady *et al.* [22]	41	Adenosine (6′)	Modified Bruce (stage 2)	MIBI	ST changes improved, scan quality improved, heart:liver improved
Vitola *et al.* [23]	90	Dipyridamole (4′)	Bruce (stages 1–2)	MIBI	ST changes improved, no hypotension, heart:liver improved
Thomas *et al.* [24]	507	Adenosine (6′)	Treadmill (METS = 2.2)	MIBI or TI	Adverse reactions decreased (hypotension, arrhythmias), heart:liver improved
Elliott *et al.* [25]	19	Adenosine (4′)	Modified Bruce (stage 0–1/2)	MIBI	Adverse reactions decreased (severity, duration), heart:liver improved
Jamil *et al.* [26]	32	Adenosine (6′)	Modified Bruce (stage 0–1)	MIBI	Scan ischemia improved, sensitivity improved, NPV improved
Candell-Riera *et al.* [27]	72	Dipyridamole (4′)	Bicycle (METS ≥ 4)	MIBI	Scan ischemia improved, sensitivity improved, NPV improved
Pennell *et al.* [28]	173	Adenosine (6′)	Bicycle (25–150 W)	TI	Noncardiac side effects decreased, major arrhythmia decreased, heart:liver improved, defect reversibility improved
Thomas *et al.* [29]	60	Regadenoson (10 sec)	Treadmill (1.7 mph, 4 min)	MIBI	Adverse reactions decreased (cardiac flushing, second degree AV block); liver:heart improved vs adenosine

Figure 3-16. Combined vasodilator plus exercise stress imaging. The feasibility of combining low-level treadmill or bicycle exercise with adenosine or dipyridamole is well established. Consistently demonstrated benefits include 1) improved target-to-background activity by virtue of reduced liver and/or gut tracer uptake; 2) reduced frequency, duration, and severity of cardiac and noncardiac adverse effects; and 3) greater provocation of electorcardiogram and scan evidence of myocardial ischemia (excluding patients with left bundle branch block) compared with vasodilator stress without combined exercise.

Potential mechanisms for these benefits include 1) shunting of splanchnic blood flow to the skeletal musculature, 2) increased sympathetic nervous system activity, and 3) increased cardiac work with associated "demand" type myocardial ischemia. AV—atrioventricular; METS—metabolic equivalents; MIBI—^{99m}Tc-sestamibi; NPV—negative predictive value; TI—thalium 201.

Pharmacologic Stressors in Coronary Artery Disease

Reported Side Effects of FDA-Approved Intravenous Vasodilator Drug Stress Imaging

	Adenosine, %	Dipyridamole, %	Regadenoson, %
Noncardiac			
Flushing	36.5	3.4	16
Dyspnea	35.2	2.6	28
Chest pain	34.6	19.7	13
Gastrointestinal distress	14.6	5.6	5
Headache	14.2	12.2	26
Dizziness	8.5	11.8	8
Cardiorespiratory			
Second degree AV block	1	0	0.1
ST-T wave changes	5.7	7.5	12
Arrhythmia	3.3	5.2*	20‡
Hypotension	1.8	4.6	7
Bronchospasm	0.1	0.15	N/A
Myocardial infarction	0.000	0.05	N/A
Death	0†	0.05	0

*Ventricular arrhythmias.
†One subsequent death reported.
‡PACs, PVCs, atrial fibrillation, wandering atrial pacemaker, asystole.

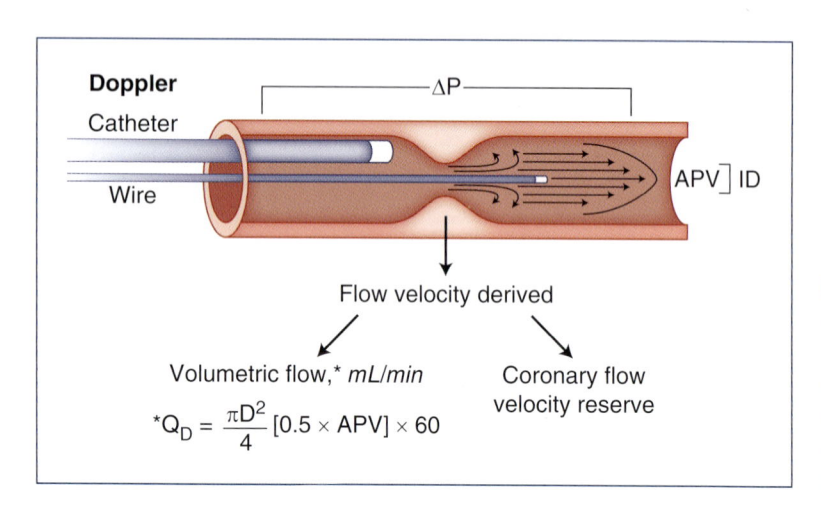

Figure 3-17. Side effect comparison between intravenous adenosine, dipyridamole [30,31], and regadenoson [32,33] imaging in multicenter studies for both noncardiac and cardiorespiratory events. Chest pain is not necessarily associated with the presence of coronary artery disease, because these agents also stimulate the nociceptors. Caution is advised in patients with severe asthma or chronic obstructive pulmonary disease due to the direct bronchoconstrictive effects of A_{2B} and A_3 receptor agonists; A_{2A} receptor agonists also have the potential to cause or worsen bronchospasms in asthmatics [9] and patients with chronic obstructive pulmonary disease [10]. Second degree heart block occurs in up to 1% of patients, but is generally well tolerated and brief [34]. AV—atrioventricular; FDA—US Food and Drug Administration; N/A—not applicable; PACs—premature atrial contractions; PVCs—premature ventricular contractions.

$$Q_D = \frac{\pi D^2}{4}[0.5 \times APV] \times 60$$

Figure 3-18. Schematic illustration of a Doppler flow wire crossing a coronary stenosis for measurement of average peak velocity (or pressure drop using a pressure wire). Flow velocity can be used to derive volumometric flow or coronary flow velocity reserve, which normally increases twofold or greater under the effects of hyperemic drug stress. This physiologic catheterization laboratory technique has been correlated with SPECT and PET imaging. APV—average peak velocity; ΔP—pressure drop.

Clinical Predictors of Perioperative Events

Major

Unstable coronary syndromes

  Recent MI* with evidence of important ischemic risks by clinical symptoms or noninvasive study

  Unstable or severe† angina (Canadian class III or IV)

Decompensated congestive heart failure

Significant arrhythmias

  High-grade AV block

  Symptomatic ventricular arrhythmias in the presence of underlying heart disease

  Supraventricular arrhythmias with uncontrolled ventricular rate

Severe valvular disease

Intermediate

Mild angina pectoris (Canadian class I or II)

Prior MI by history of pathologic Q waves

Compensated or prior congestive heart failure

Diabetes mellitus

Minor

Advanced age

Abnormal ECG (LV hypertrophy, LBBB, ST-T abnormalities)

Rhythm other than sinus (*eg*, atrial fibrillation)

Low functional capacity
  (*eg*, inability to climb one flight of stairs with a bag of groceries)

History of stroke

Uncontrolled systemic hypertension

*Recent is defined as more than 7 days but less than or equal to 30 days.
†May include stable angina in unusually sedentary patients.

Figure 3-24. Clinical predictors of perioperative events. The American College of Cardiology/American Heart Association Task Force has published and updated practice guidelines for perioperative cardiovascular evaluation prior to noncardiac surgery [67]. These recommendations embody expert and evidence-based considerations, and identify specific clinical markers, patient functional capacity, and the type of surgery to be performed as crucial factors for deciding which patients need more intensive preoperative evaluation.

The major, intermediate, and minor clinical predictors of increased perioperative cardiovascular risk are summarized. A medical history and physical examination can elicit clinical risk predictors including angina, prior myocardial infarction (MI), congestive heart failure, arrhythmias, diabetes, peripheral vascular disease, and prior coronary revascularization procedures. Asymptomatic patients with known coronary artery disease who have had coronary revascularization within the past 5 years require no further evaluation. Surgery can also proceed in patients with coronary artery disease when the results of a recent cardiac catheterization or stress test reflect clinical stability.

In patients who have any of the recognized major clinical predictors of risk, a full cardiac work-up is warranted prior to surgery. The appropriate assessment would include coronary angiography, echocardiography to assess left ventricular (LV) ejection function and valvular abnormalities, or noninvasive stress imaging to detect myocardial ischemia. In the intermediate-risk category, the functional capacity of the patient and the type of surgical procedure determine whether further testing is indicated. Cardiac testing is necessary in intermediate-risk patients with a functional capacity of fewer than 4 metabolic equivalents and those with moderate or excellent functional capacity who are undergoing a high-risk surgical procedure.

Patients with good functional capacity who are undergoing an intermediate- or low-risk surgical procedure do not generally require preoperative cardiac testing. In patients with minor or no clinical risk predictors, surgery can be performed without further evaluation unless patients have poor functional capacity or surgery is high risk.

Although functional capacity is an important determinant of risk, exercise stress testing (with or without imaging) is not possible in many patients who require further preoperative evaluation. Elderly or obese patients; those with prior MI, congestive heart failure, or pulmonary disease; and patients referred for peripheral vascular, orthopedic, and neurologic procedures may not be able to exercise adequately. In this setting, pharmacologic stress myocardial perfusion imaging is the preferred method of preoperative screening. AV—atrioventricular; ECG—electrocardiogram; LBBB—left bundle branch block. (*Adapted from* Eagle *et al.* [67].)

Dipyridamole–^{201}Tl Imaging for Preoperative Assessment of Cardiac Risk

Study[†]	n	Patients with Ischemia by ^{201}Tl–RD, n (%)	MI/Death, n (%)	Perioperative Events* RD Scan Positive Predictive Value, % (n/n)	Normal Scan Negative Predictive Value, % (n/n)
Vascular Surgery		16 (33)	3 (6)	19 (3/160)	100 (32/32)
Boucher et al. [47]	48	54 (47)	11 (10)	20 (11/54)	100 (60/60)
Cutler and Leppo [61]	116	15 (22)	3 (4)	20 (3/15)	100 (56/56)
Fletcher et al. [68]	67	14 (31)	2 (4)	14 (2/14)	100 (24/24)
Sachs et al. [77]	46	82 (41)	15 (8)	16 (13/82)	98 (61/62)
Eagle et al. [49]	200	34 (36)	7 (7)	9 (3/34)	96 (44/46)
McEnroe et al. [64]	95	40 (36)	8 (7)	15 (6/40)	100 (51/51)
Younis et al. [69]	111	22 (37)	3 (5)	5 (1/22)	95 (19/20)
Mangano et al. [62]	60	NA	4 (6)	NA	100 (21/21)
Strawn and Guernsey [70]	68	15 (58)	3 (12)	20 (3/15)	100 (11/11)
Watters et al. [66]	26	167 (51)	28 (9)	14 (23/167)	99 (97/98)
Hendel et al. [52]	327	161 (45)	30 (8)	17 (28/161)	99 (160/162)
Lette et al. [57]	355	45 (69)	5 (8)	11 (5/45)	100 (20/20)
Madsen et al. [51]	65	77 (33)	12 (5)	13 (10/77)	99 (120/121)
Brown and Rowen [38]	231	67 (39)	5 (3)	4 (3/67)	98 (64/65)
Kresowik et al. [54]	170	160 (35)	22 (5)	4 (7/160)	96 (195/203)[‡]
Baron et al. [63]	457	110 (46)	17 (7)	11 (12/110)	100 (97/97)
Bry et al. [59]	237	107 (41)	178 (6.6)	12 (33/1079)	99 (1132/1149)
Total	2679				
Nonvascular Surgery		9 (23)		67 (6/9)	
Camp et al. [45]	40	11 (41)	6 (15)	27 (3/11)	100 (23/23)
Iqbal et al. [46]	31	36 (36)	3 (11)	8 (3/36)	100 (20/20)
Coley et al. [60]	100	28 (47)	4 (4)	21 (6/28)	98 (63/64)
Shaw et al. [75]	60	15 (28)	6 (10)	27 (4/15)	100 (19/19)
Takase et al. [65]	53	50 (31)	6 (11)	18 (9/50)	100 (32/32)
Younis et al. [71]	161	149 (33)	15 (9)	21 (31/149)	98 (87/89)
Total	445		40 (9)		99 (244/247)

*Patients with fixed defects were omitted from calculation of positive and negative predictive value.
[†]All studies except those by Coley et al. [60] acquired patient information prospectively. Only in reports by Mangano et al. [62] and Baron et al. [63] were scan results blinded from attending physicians.
[‡]Nonfatal MI only.

Figure 3-25. Dipyridamole–^{201}Tl imaging for preoperative assessment of cardiac risk. Dipyridamole–^{201}Tl myocardial scintigraphy has been used extensively as a noninvasive approach to assess perioperative cardiac risk in patients prior to vascular and nonvascular surgery [66,68–72]. Dipyridamole–^{99m}Tc-sestamibi scintigraphy for preoperative risk stratification has also been evaluated [73,74]. Patients with a normal ^{201}Tl or sestamibi myocardial perfusion study are at very low likelihood for peri- or postoperative cardiac events. Events (including death and nonfatal myocardial infarction [MI]) occur in approximately 20% of patients with scintigraphic evidence of ischemia. Patients with fixed perfusion defects are at lower risk for perioperative cardiac events, but their long-term prognosis is similar to that in patients with chronic coronary artery disease with myocardial ischemia. Although drug-induced myocardial hypoperfusion or ischemia predicts a high risk for cardiac events, approximately 80% of patients survive the surgical procedure without complications (ie, low positive predictive value). Risk stratification may be improved by identifying not only the presence but also the extent of myocardial ischemia. Patients with multiple ischemic defects in several vascular beds are at higher risk than those with a single ischemic segment. Quantitative SPECT imaging permits the determination of the percent and location of ischemic myocardium. Of 231 patients undergoing noncardiac surgery who had dipyridamole studies with 1 month of operation [38], the number of segments with ^{201}Tl redistribution (RD) was the best predictor of perioperative cardiac death or nonfatal MI ($P = 0.0001$), although a history of diabetes mellitus was also predictive in this study ($P = 0.006$). When dipyridamole perfusion scintigraphy was performed in 66 consecutive patients undergoing predominantly vascular surgeries, only 9% of patients with a "small" ischemic defect had a cardiac event compared with 80% of patients with more extensive ischemia. Levinson et al. [58] reported a significantly higher cardiac event rate in patients with ^{201}Tl redistribution in four or more segments (38%) compared with those with less extensive ischemia (12%).

The optimal approach for identifying risk in surgical candidates should integrate clinical and imaging variables. In 200 patients undergoing major vascular surgery [48], clinical and imaging parameters were evaluated to optimize risk stratification in patient subsets. Logistic regression analysis identified five clinical predictors of cardiac event risk: electrocardiographic Q waves; ventricular ectopic activity; diabetes; age over 70 years; and a history of angina. The presence of ^{201}Tl redistribution was also found to be a significant risk predictor. In the 64 patients who had no clinical predictors, only 3.1% had ischemic events, with no deaths.

Continued on the next page

Figure 3-25. *(Continued)* Most of these patients also had no scintigraphic evidence of ischemia, and therefore would have been classified as low risk by imaging. Conversely, 50% of patients with more than three clinical risk factors had cardiac events, and scintigraphic ischemia involving multiple vascular territories was frequent in this subgroup. The majority of patients had one or two clinical variables (68%); of these, 15.5% had a postoperative event, defining a large group at intermediate clinical risk. Without dipyridamole–^{201}Tl redistribution, 3.2% had a subsequent cardiac event compared with 30% with defect redistribution. Among younger patients without a prior cardiovascular history, clinical criteria can effectively define a low-risk group, and stress imaging is generally not warranted [67]. In patients with multiple cardiac risk factors, imaging is useful as a guide to coronary revascularization prior to surgery. In heterogeneous clinical populations with variable risk, drug stress perfusion imaging is valuable for defining patients most likely to have cardiac events based on the presence and extent of myocardial ischemia.

Despite the increased use of adenosine and dobutamine as pharmacologic stressors [39,40,53,72,75,76], less data are available for these agents in preoperative risk stratification than for dipyridamole. When adenosine–^{201}Tl tomography was used as a preoperative screening test in patients referred for vascular orthopedic or general surgery, patients with defect redistribution had a 25% event rate, whereas no events occurred in patients without myocardial ischemia [75].

Adenosine–^{201}Tl tomography, when performed in 106 patients undergoing vascular surgery, was abnormal in 54% of patients, of whom 82% demonstrated defect ischemia [53]. Eleven percent of the patients with scintigraphic ischemia had an event, but none of the patients without ischemia had an event. By quantitative analysis, the size of the total and reversible perfusion defect was larger in patients with events compared with those without events.

In 126 patients awaiting vascular surgery, dobutamine was administered in doses up to 20 μg/kg/min, with atropine given to 47 patients to further increase heart rate [72]. Sixty-seven percent had either a normal ^{201}Tl SPECT or only a fixed defect, with cardiac event rates of 1.8% and 11%, respectively. In the 42 patients who demonstrated ^{201}Tl defect redistribution, 15 operations were canceled, nine underwent coronary revascularization, and 18 proceeded with their vascular procedures. Nine of the 18 patients who did not undergo revascularization with scintigraphic ischemia (50%) had a postoperative cardiac event.

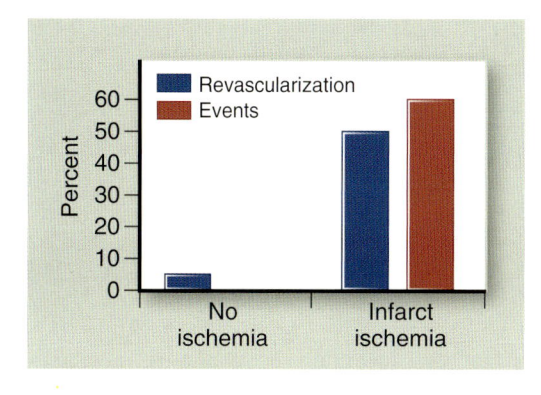

Figure 3-26. Predictive accuracy of early post–myocardial infarction (MI) imaging with dipyridamole–^{201}Tl. The presence of infarct zone ischemia is predictive of a higher rate of coronary revascularization and other cardiac events. In the absence of ischemia, revascularization and cardiac events are very low. Imaging in this multicenter study was safely performed 2 to 4 days following uncomplicated MI. Pharmacologic testing is useful for identifying both early and late risk for cardiac events. For example, data demonstrate that early (2–4 days) dipyridamole sestamibi perfusion imaging after an uncomplicated MI is a safe and powerful predictor of future cardiac death and recurrent MI [39], and offers incremental prognostic value to that of submaximal exercise testing. *(Adapted from* Brown et al. [78].*)*

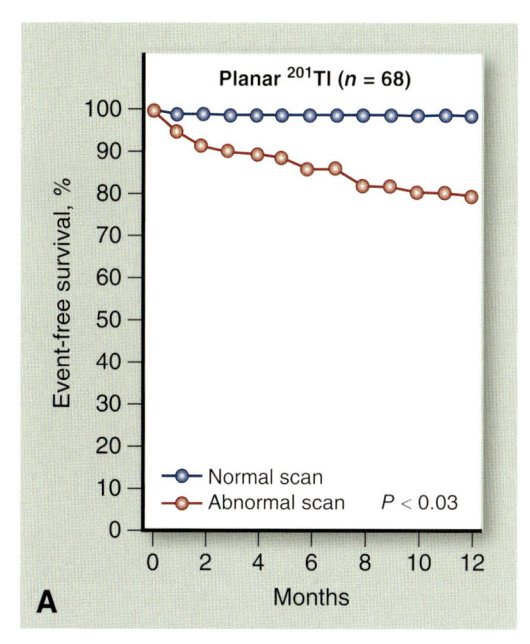

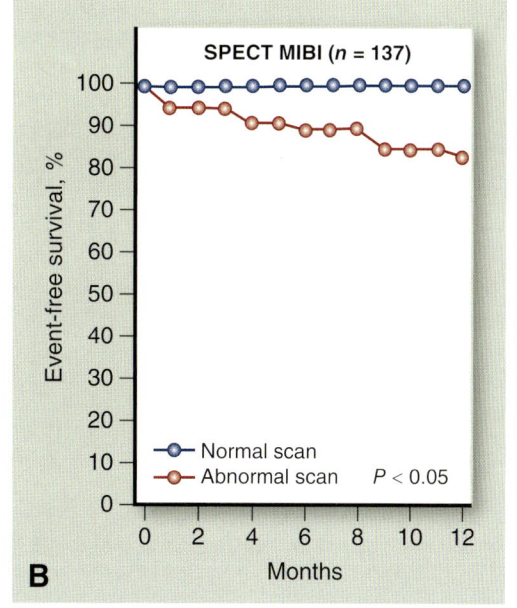

Figure 3-27. Prognostic value of predischarge dipyridamole stress myocardial imaging for predicting cardiac death or myocardial infarction (MI) in combination with planar ^{201}Tl (n = 68) (**A**) or SPECT sestamibi (MIBI) (n = 137) (**B**) in patients with a medically stabilized recent ischemic event (MI or unstable angina). Both techniques identify a low-risk subset with a normal scan and few cardiac events over 1 year following the acute ischemic event. The event rate in patients with an abnormal scan is significantly higher, regardless of the imaging technique. In patients with unstable angina, the very low mortality rate associated with a normal scan supports a conservative medical management approach [43,64]. (**A**, *adapted from* Younis et al. [79]; **B**, *adapted from* Miller et al. [44].)

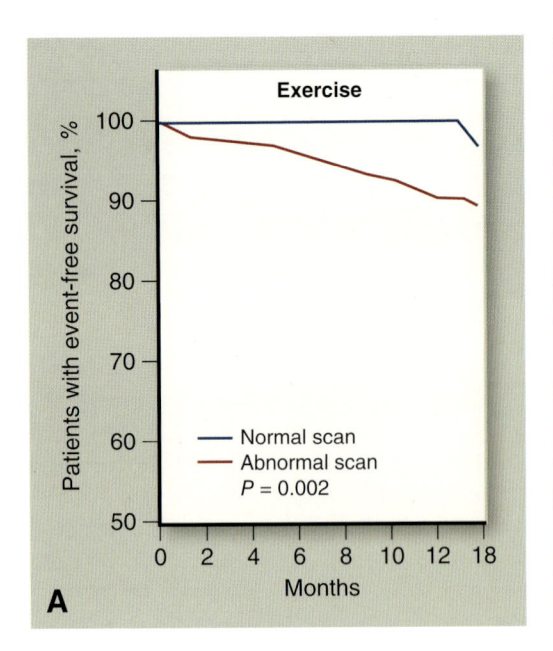

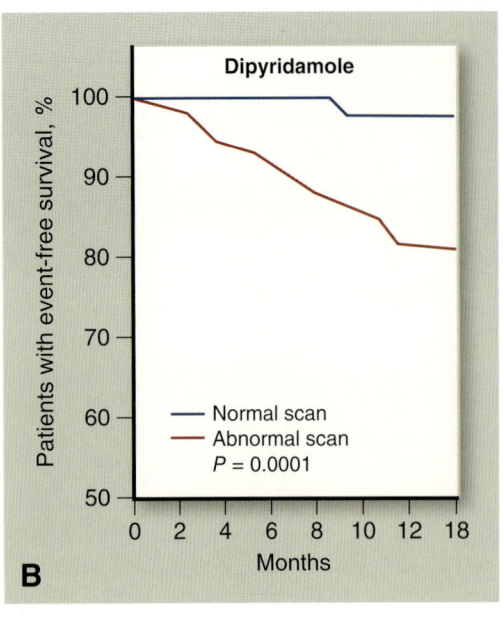

Figure 3-28. Prognostic value of ^{99m}Tc-sestamibi imaging in patients with stable chest pain, comparing exercise testing (**A**) with dipyridamole testing (**B**) in similar populations. A normal scan is associated with a low 18-month cardiac event rate and good cardiac event-free survival, regardless of the stress approach utilized. Significantly higher cardiac event rates and poorer cardiac event-free survival occur in the presence of an abnormal dipyridamole scan in stable chest pain patients [80,81]. (**A**, *adapted from* Stratmann *et al.* [80]; **B**, *adapted from* Stratmann *et al.* [82].)

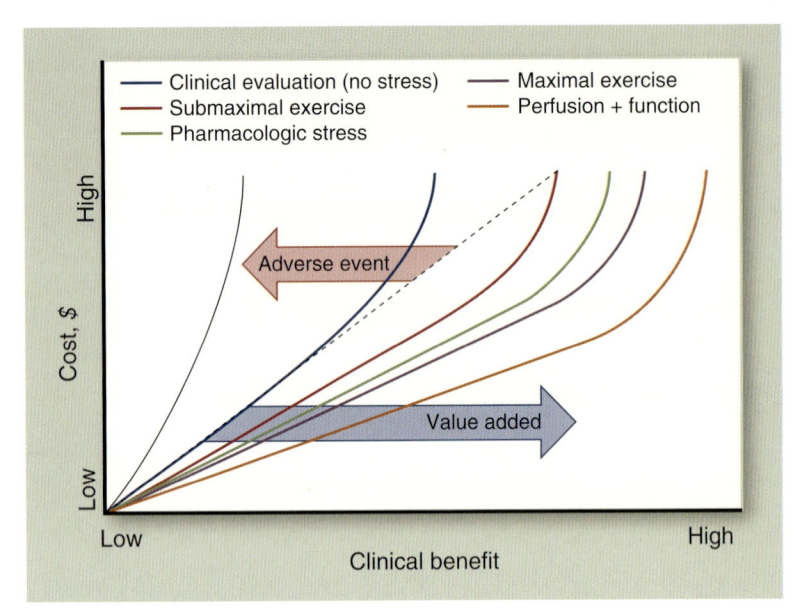

Figure 3-29. Relationship between cost and clinical benefit (incremental diagnostic or prognostic data derived) for various stress imaging techniques to evaluate coronary artery disease. Value is added to a baseline level of clinical benefit (incremental value in proportion to incremental cost) when submaximal exercise, pharmacologic stress, maximal exercise, and perfusion plus function imaging are utilized. An adverse event during testing can reduce the clinical benefit and significantly accelerate the incremental cost of patient care [83].

74 Atlas of Nuclear Cardiology

Figure 3-30. American College of Cardiology/American Heart Association/American Society of Nuclear Cardiology (ACC/AHA/ASNC) guidelines for clinical use of pharmacologic stress in cardiac radionuclide imaging. In 2003, the scientific organizations responsible for the development of practice guidelines published their updated recommendations on radionuclide imaging, including specific comments on the use of pharmacologic stress imaging in patients with known or suspected coronary artery disease (CAD) [84]. After performing an extensive literature search, including the key words adenosine and dipyridamole, the committee concluded that both agents are "very useful for risk stratifying patients after an acute myocardial infarction." The principal advantage cited was the capacity to use pharmacologic stress earlier after infarction than exercise (between 2 and 5 days), with "a very good safety record." A large prospective randomized trial, the Adenosine Sestamibi SPECT Post-infarction Evaluation (INSPIRE) trial, was designed to determine the value of sequential perfusion imaging to assess postinfarction myocardium at risk and changes following medical and revascularization therapy [85]. The ACC/AHA 2002 guideline update for management of patients with unstable angina (UA) and non-ST elevation myocardial infarction (NSTEMI) [84] also recommended the use of dipyridamole imaging in selected patients with UA on the basis of multiple observational studies.

ACC/AHA/ASNC Guidelines for Clinical Use of Pharmacologic Stress in Cardiac Radionuclide Imaging (2003)

Indication	Test	Class	Evidence Level*
Diagnosis of CAD in low-risk ACS patients with negative serum marker, nondiagnostic ECG	Same day rest-stress MPI	I	B
Risk assessment/prognosis in patients with NSTEMI and UA	Stress MPI with ECG gating	I	A or B
Patients with intermediate CAD likelihood and/or risk stratifying patients with high-intermediate risk unable to exercise to 85% MPHR	Stress MPI		
Extent, severity, and location of ischemia		I	B
Functional significance of intermediate stenosis		I	B
Re-assess risk of cardiac event with change in symptoms		I	C
At 3–5 years after PCI or CABG		IIa	B
In patients with > 20% 10-year risk of cardiac events		IIa	B
For risk assessing patients with equivocal SPECT MPI studies	PET	I	B
Extent, severity, and location of ischemia	PET	I	B
Before noncardiac surgery	Stress MPI or PET	I	B
Patient able to exercise but with			
LBBB on resting ECG	Stress MPI or PET	I	B
Electronic pacemaker			

*Evidence applies to pharmacologic stress with either adenosine or dipyridamole.

Another conclusion rendered by the experts [84] was that over the period from 1990 to 2000, multiple studies evaluating the specificity and sensitivity of tracers used with coronary hyperemic stress demonstrated its ability to identify CAD in individual arteries and to assess the overall extent of disease. The three most commonly utilized drugs, dipyridamole, adenosine, and dobutamine, create physiologic changes that are conducive to the detection of coronary stenosis in the definition of future cardiac risk. The limited experience with dobutamine stress perfusion imaging did not permit the guideline writers to confirm its diagnostic or prognostic accuracy as an alternative to dipyridamole or adenosine stress in all situations. Two studies [86,87] using adenosine stress sestamibi imaging confirmed a less than 5% to 10% likelihood of CAD in patients with a normal scan. Other studies have demonstrated that lung uptake of ^{201}Tl or ^{99m}Tc-sestamibi following pharmacologic stress is an indicator of global left ventricular dysfunction and possible multivessel disease. Transient ischemic dilation may be seen in patients with severe and/or extensive CAD with either exercise or vasodilator stress.

The guidelines recommended the use of pharmacologic stress imaging for patients with a normal resting electrocardiogram (ECG) who are unable to exercise, and among patients with left bundle branch block (LBBB) or electronic pacemaker devices. Pharmacologic stress was considered to be preferable to exercise stress for imaging purposes in both the diagnosis and risk stratification of patients with these conditions. In patients with LBBB, a reversible or fixed septal defect may be observed during exercise stress, but is "often absent during pharmacologic stress" [84]. As such, a patient with LBBB on a resting ECG would "be most appropriately tested using pharmacologic stress imaging." Pharmacologic stress agents have also been evaluated for risk stratification in LBBB patients, and have demonstrated the capacity to prognosticate in several studies.

Final recommendations of the 2003 ACC/AHA/ASNC guidelines [84] rendered pharmacologic stress imaging a Class I indication for diagnosing patients at intermediate likelihood of CAD, or for risk stratification of patients with intermediate-to-high likelihood of CAD who are unable to exercise, or who demonstrate LBBB on the resting ECG or an electronically paced rhythm (strength of evidence level B). Either adenosine or dipyridamole SPECT was recommended to identify the extent, severity, and location of myocardial ischemia; the functional significance of intermediate coronary lesions; and/or the definition of future cardiac event risk as a Class I indication (strength of evidence level B or C). Class IIa guideline indications for adenosine or dipyridamole SPECT included high-risk asymptomatic subjects 3 to 5 years after coronary revascularization with percutaneous coronary intervention (PCI) or coronary artery bypass graft (CABG), and high risk patients (*ie*, diabetics) with a more than 20% 10-year risk of CAD events based on Framingham study criteria [88]. Dobutamine may be used as an alternative among patients with a medical contraindication to adenosine or dipyridamole (level of evidence C). Finally, the guidelines considered pharmacologic stress imaging as a Class I indication among patients undergoing risk stratification in combination with PET imaging, and prior to noncardiac surgery in selected populations such as those with LBBB and those unable to perform diagnostic levels of exercise stress (strength of evidence level B or C).

While concluding that maximal exercise stress imaging is "preferable to pharmacologic stress," the guidelines reiterated that pharmacologic stress is preferable among patients unable to exercise and those with LBBB and electronically paced rhythms. For this reason, the guidelines note that "pharmacologic stress testing now comprises more than 30% of the myocardial perfusion studies performed in the United States."

References

1. Miller DD: Medical globalization: "A Fin de Siecle Phenomenon." *Multinat Business Rev* 2003, 11:113–142.

2. Miller DD: Cost efficiency of nuclear cardiology services in the modern health care environment. *Curr Cardiol Rep* 2004, 6:41–52.

3. Samuels B, Kiat H, Friedman JD, Berman DS: Adenosine pharmacologic stress myocardial perfusion tomographic imaging in patients with significant aortic stenosis. Diagnostic efficacy and comparison of clinical, hemodynamic and electrocardiographic variables with 100 age-matched control subjects. *J Am Coll Cardiol* 1995, 25:99–106.

4. O'Keefe JH Jr, Bateman TM, Barnhart CS: Adenosine thallium-201 is superior to exercise thallium-201 for detecting coronary artery disease in patients with left bundle branch block. *J Am Coll Cardiol* 1993, 21:1332–1338.

5. Wagdy HM, Hodge D, Christian TF, et al.: Prognostic value of vasodilator perfusion imaging in patients with left bundle-branch block. *Circulation* 1998, 97:1563–1570.

6. Shaffer J, Simbartl L, Render ML, et al.: Patients with stable chronic obstructive pulmonary disease can safely undergo intravenous dipyridamole thallium-201 imaging. *Am Heart J* 1998, 36:307–313.

7. Miller DD, Labovitz AJ: Dipyridamole and adenosine vasodilator stress for myocardial imaging: vive la difference! *J Am Coll Cardiol* 1994, 23:390–392.

8. Leaker BR, O'Connor B, Hansel TT, et al.: Safety of regadenoson, an adenosine A_{2A} receptor agonist for myocardial perfusion imaging, in mild asthma and moderate asthma patients: a randomized, double-blind, placebo-controlled trial. *J Nucl Cardiol* 2008, 15:329–336.

9. Thomas GS, Tammelin BR, Schiffman GL, et al.: Safety of regadenoson, a selective adenosine A_{2A} agonist, in patients with chronic obstructive pulmonary disease: a randomized, double-blind, placebo-controlled trial (RegCOPD trial). *J Nucl Cardiol* 2008, 15:319–328.

10. Pennell DJ, Ell PJ: Whole-body imaging of thallium-201 after six different stress regimens. *J Nucl Med* 1994, 35:425–428.

11. Wu JC, Yuyn JJ, Heller EN, et al.: Limitations of dobutamine for enhancing flow heterogeneity in the presence of single coronary artery stenosis: implications for technetium-99m-sestamibi imaging. *J Nucl Med* 1998, 39:417–425.

12. Udelson JE, Heller GV, Wackers Frans JT, et al.: Randomized, controlled dose-ranging study of the selective adenosine a2a receptor agonist binodenoson for pharmacological stress as an adjunct to myocardial perfusion imaging. *Circulation* 2003, 104:457-464.

13. Gao Z, Otero DH, Zablock JA, et al.: Time course of changes in coronary conductance caused by regadenoson, binodenoson, CGS21680, and adenosine. Pharmacological characterization of novel A_{2A} adenosine receptor (A_{2A}AdoR) agonists. *Drug Dev Res* 2000, 50:92.

14. Lieu HD, Shryock JC, von Mering GO, et al. Regadenoson, a selective A_{2A} adenosine receptor agonist, causes dose-dependent increases in coronary blood flow velocity in humans. *J Nucl Cardiol* 2007, 14:514–520.

15. Homma S, Gilliland Y, Guiney TE, et al.: Safety of intravenous dipyridamole for stress testing with thallium imaging. *Am J Cardiol* 1987, 59:152–154.

16. Verani MS, Mahmarian JJ, Hixson JB, et al.: Diagnosis of coronary artery disease by controlled coronary vasodilation with adenosine and thallium-201 scintigraphy in patients unable to exercise. *Circulation* 1990, 82:80–87.

17. Elhendy A, Valkema R, van Domburg RT, et al.: Safety of dobutamine-atropine stress myocardial perfusion scintigraphy. *J Nucl Med* 1998, 39:1662–1669.

18. Hays JT, Mahmarian JJ, Cochran AJ, Verani MS: Dobutamine thallium-201 tomography for evaluating patients with suspected coronary artery disease unable to undergo exercise or vasodilatory pharmacologic stress testing. *J Am Coll Cardiol* 1993, 21:1583–1590.

19. Marshall ES, Raichlen JS, Tighe DA, et al.: ST-segment depression during adenosine infusion as a predictor of myocardial ischemia. *Am Heart J* 1994, 127:305–311.

20. Nishimura S, Mahmarian JJ, Boyce TM, Verani MS: Equivalence between adenosine and exercise thallium-201 myocardial tomography: a multicenter, prospective, crossover trial. *J Am Coll Cardiol* 1992, 20:265–275.

21. Taillefer R, Amyot R, Turpin S, et al.: Comparison between dipyridamole and adenosine as pharmacologic coronary vasodilators in detection of coronary artery disease with thallium 201 imaging. *J Nucl Cardiol* 1996, 3:204–211.

22. Samady H, Wackers FJ, Joska TM, et al.: Pharmacologic stress perfusion imaging with adenosine: role of simultaneous low-level treadmill exercise. *J Am Coll Cardiol* 2002, 9:188–196.

23. Vitola JV, Brambatti JC, Caligaris F, et al.: Exercise supplementation to dipyridamole prevents hypotension, improves electrocardiogram sensitivity, and increases heart-to-liver activity ratio on Tc-99m sestamibi imaging. *J Nucl Cardiol* 2001, 8:652–659.

24. Thomas GS, Prill NV, Majmundar H, et al.: Treadmill exercise during adenosine infusion is safe, results in fewer adverse reactions, and improves myocardial perfusion image quality. *J Nucl Cardiol* 2000, 7:439–446.

25. Elliott MD, Holly TA, Leonard SM, et al.: Impact of an abbreviated adenosine protocol incorporating adjunctive treadmill exercise on adverse effects and image quality in patients undergoing stress myocardial perfusion imaging. *J Nucl Cardiol* 2000, 7:584–589.

26. Jamil G, Ahlberg A, Elliott MD, et al.: Impact of limited treadmill exercise on adenosine Tc-99m sestamibi single-photon emission computed tomographic myocardial perfusion imaging in coronary artery disease. *Am J Cardiol* 1999, 84:400–403.

27. Candell-Riera J, Santana-Boado C, Castell-Conesa J, et al.: Simultaneous dipyridamole/maximal subjective exercise with 99mTc-MIBI SPECT: improved diagnostic yield in coronary artery disease. *J Am Coll Cardiol* 1997, 29:531–536.

28. Pennell DJ, Mavrogeni SI, Forbat SM, et al.: Adenosine combined with dynamic exercise for myocardial perfusion imaging. *J Am Coll Cardiol* 1995, 25:1300–1309.

29. Thomas GS, Thompson RC, Miyamoto MI, et al.: The RegEx trial: a randomized, double-blind, placebo- and active-controlled pilot study combining regadenoson, a selective A_{2A} adenosine agonist, with low-level exercise, in patients undergoing myocardial perfusion imaging. *J Nucl Cardiol* 2009, 16: 63–72.

30. Lette J, Waters D, Bernier H, et al.: Preoperative and long-term cardiac risk assessment: predictive value of 23 clinical descriptors, 7 multivariate scoring systems, and quantitative dipyridamole imaging in 360 patients. *Ann Surg* 1992, 216:192–204.

31. Ranhosky A, Kempthorne-Rawson J: The safety of intravenous dipyridamole thallium myocardial perfusion imaging. Intravenous Dipyridamole Thallium Imaging Study Group. *Circulation* 1990, 81:1205–1209.

32. Iskandrian AE, Bateman TM, Belardinelli L, et al.: Adenosine versus regadenoson comparative evaluation in myocardial perfusion imaging: results of the ADVANCE phase 3 multicenter international trial. *J Nucl Cardiol* 2007, 14:645–658.

33. Cerqueira MD, Nguyen P, Staehr P, et al.: Effects of age, gender, obesity and diabetes on the efficacy and safety of the selective A_{2A} agonist regadenoson versus adenosine: integrated ADVANCE-MPI Trial results. *J Am Coll Cardiol: Cardiovasc Imaging* 2008, 1:307–316.

34. Henzlova M, Cerqueira MD, Hansen CL, et al. : Stress protocols and tracers. *J Nucl Cardiol* 2009 [Epub ahead of print], http://www.asnc.org/imageuploads/ImagingGuidelinesStressProtocols021109.pdf.

35. Miller DD, Donohue TJ, Younis LT, et al.: Correlation of pharmacological 99mTc-sestamibi myocardial perfusion imaging with poststenotic coronary flow reserve in patients with angiographically intermediate coronary artery stenoses. *Circulation* 1994, 89:2150–2160.

36. Joye JD, Schulman DS, Lasorda D, et al.: Intracoronary Doppler guide wire versus stress single-photon emission computed tomographic thallium-201 imaging in assessment of intermediate coronary stenoses. *J Am Coll Cardiol* 1994, 24:940–947.

37. Heller LI, Popma J, Cates C, et al.: Functional assessment of stenosis in the cath lab: a comparison of Doppler and Tl-201 imaging. *J Interv Cardiol* 1995, 7:23A.

38. Brown KA, Rowen M: Extent of jeopardized viable myocardium determined by myocardial perfusion imaging best predicts perioperative cardiac events in patients undergoing noncardiac surgery. *J Am Coll Cardiol* 1993, 21:325–330.

39. Hachamovitch R, Berman DS, Kiat H, et al.: Incremental prognostic value of adenosine stress myocardial perfusion single-photon emission computed tomography and impact on subsequent management in patients with or suspect of having myocardial ischemia. *Am J Cardiol* 1997, 80:426–433.

40. Shaw LJ, Eagle KA, Gersh BJ, Miller DD: Meta-analysis of intravenous dipyridamole-thallium-201 imaging (1985 to 1994) and dobutamine echocardiography (1991 to 1994) for risk stratification before vascular surgery. *J Am Coll Cardiol* 1996, 27:787–798.

41. Stratmann HG, Tamesis BR, Younis LT, *et al*.: Prognostic value of predischarge dipyridamole technetium 99m sestamibi myocardial tomography in medically treated patients with unstable angina. *Am Heart J* 1995, 130:734–740.

42. Brown KA, Heller GV, Landin RS, *et al*.: Early dipyridamole Tc-99m sestamibi single photon emission computed tomographic imaging 2 to 4 days after acute myocardial infarction predicts in-hospital and postdischarge cardiac events: comparison with submaximal exercise. *Circulation* 1999, 100:2060–2066.

43. Mahmarian JJ, Mahmarian AC, Marks GF, *et al*.: Role of adenosine thallium-201 tomography for defining long-term risk in patients after acute myocardial infarction. *J Am Coll Cardiol* 1995, 25:1333–1340.

44. Miller DD, Stratmann HG, Shaw LJ, *et al*.: Dipyridamole technetium 99m sestamibi myocardial tomography as an independent predictor of cardiac event-free survival after acute ischemic events. *J Nucl Cardiol* 1994, 1:72–82.

45. Camp AD, Garvin PJ, Hoff J, *et al*.: Prognostic value of intravenous dipyridamole thallium imaging in patients with diabetes mellitus considered for renal transplantation. *Am J Cardiol* 1990, 65:1459–1463.

46. Iqbal A, Gibbons RJ, McGoon MD, *et al*.: Noninvasive assessment of cardiac risk in insulin-dependent diabetic patients being evaluated for pancreatic transplantation using thallium-201 myocardial perfusion scintigraphy. *Transplant Proc* 1991, 23(pt 2):1690–1691.

47. Boucher CA, Brewster DC, Darling RC, *et al*.: Determination of cardiac risk by dipyridamole-thallium imaging before peripheral vascular surgery. *N Engl J Med* 1985, 312:389–394.

48. Eagle KA, Singer DE, Brewster DC, *et al*.: Dipyridamole-thallium scanning in patients undergoing vascular surgery: optimizing preoperative evaluation of cardiac risk. *JAMA* 1987, 257:2185–2189.

49. Eagle KA, Coley CM, Newell JB, *et al*.: Combining clinical and thallium data optimizes preoperative assessment of cardiac risk before major vascular surgery. *Ann Intern Med* 1989, 110:859–866.

50. Lette J, Waters D, Bernier H, *et al*.: Preoperative and long-term cardiac risk assessment: predictive value of 23 clinical descriptors, 7 multivariate scoring systems, and quantitative dipyridamole imaging in 360 patients. *Ann Surg* 1992, 216:192–204.

51. Madsen PV, Vissing M, Munck O, Kelbaek H: A comparison of dipyridamole thallium 201 scintigraphy and clinical examination in the determination of cardiac risk before arterial reconstruction. *Angiology* 1992, 43:306–311.

52. Hendel RC, Whitfield SS, Villegas BJ, *et al*.: Prediction of late cardiac events by dipyridamole thallium imaging in patients undergoing elective vascular surgery. *Am J Cardiol* 1992, 70:1243–1249.

53. Koutelou MG, Asimacopoulos PJ, Mahmarian JJ, *et al*.: Preoperative risk stratification by adenosine thallium-201 single-photon emission computed tomography in patients undergoing vascular surgery. *J Nucl Cardiol* 1995, 2:389–394.

54. Kresowik TF, Bower TR, Garner SA, *et al*.: Dipyridamole thallium imaging in patients being considered for vascular procedures. *Arch Surg* 1993, 128:299–302.

55. Lane SE, Lewis SM, Pippin JJ, *et al*.: Predictive value of quantitative dipyridamole-thallium scintigraphy in assessing cardiovascular risk after vascular surgery in diabetes mellitus. *Am J Cardiol* 1989, 64:1275–1279.

56. Leppo JA, Plaja J, Gionet M, *et al*.: Noninvasive evaluation of cardiac risk before elective vascular surgery. *J Am Coll Cardiol* 1987, 9:269–276.

57. Lette J, Walters D, Cerino M, *et al*.: Preoperative coronary artery disease risk stratification based on dipyridamole imaging and a simple three-step, three-segment model for patients undergoing noncardiac vascular surgery or major general surgery. *Am J Cardiol* 1992, 69:1553–1558.

58. Levinson JR, Boucher CA, Coley CM, *et al*.: Usefulness of semiquantitative analysis of dipyridamole-thallium-201 redistribution for improving risk stratification before vascular surgery. *Am J Cardiol* 1990, 66:406–410.

59. Bry JD, Belkin M, OÕDonnell TF Jr, *et al*.: An assessment of the positive predictive value and cost-effectiveness of dipyridamole myocardial scintigraphy in patients undergoing vascular surgery. *J Vasc Surg* 1994, 19:112–121.

60. Coley CM, Field TS, Abraham SA, *et al*.: Usefulness of dipyridamole-thallium scanning for preoperative evaluation of cardiac risk for nonvascular surgery. *Am J Cardiol* 1992, 69:1280–1285.

61. Cutler BS, Leppo JA: Dipyridamole thallium-201 scintigraphy to detect coronary artery disease before abdominal aortic surgery. *J Vasc Surg* 1987, 5:91–100.

62. Mangano DT, London MJ, Tubau JF, *et al*.: Dipyridamole thallium-201 scintigraphy as a preoperative screening test: a reexamination of its predictive potential. Study of Perioperative Ischemia Research Group. *Circulation* 1991, 84:493–502.

63. Baron JF, Mundler O, Bertrand M, *et al*.: Dipyridamole-thallium scintigraphy and gated radionuclide angiography to assess cardiac risk before abdominal aortic surgery. *N Engl J Med* 1994, 330:663–669.

64. McEnroe CS, O'Donnell RF Jr, Yeager A, *et al*.: Comparison of ejection fraction and Goldman risk factor analysis of dipyridamole-thallium-201 studies in the evaluation of cardiac morbidity after aortic aneurysm surgery. *J Vasc Surg* 1990, 11:497–504.

65. Takase B, Younis LT, Byers SL, *et al*.: Comparative prognostic value of clinical risk indexes, resting two-dimensional echocardiography, and dipyridamole stress thallium-201 myocardial imaging for perioperative cardiac events in major nonvascular surgery patients. *Am Heart J* 1993, 126:1099–1106.

66. Watters TA, Botvinick EH, Dae MW, *et al*.: Comparison of the findings on preoperative dipyridamole perfusion scintigraphy and intraoperative transesophageal echocardiography: implications regarding the identification of myocardium at ischemic risk. *J Am Coll Cardiol* 1991, 18:93–100.

67. Eagle KA, Brundage BH, Chaitman BR, *et al*.: Report of the American College of Cardiology/American Heart Association Task Force on Practice Guidelines (Committee on Perioperative Cardiovascular Evaluation for Noncardiac Surgery). *J Am Coll Cardiol* 1996, 27:910–948.

68. Fletcher JP, Antico JF, Gruenewald S, *et al*.: Dipyridamole-thallium scan for screening of coronary artery disease prior to vascular surgery. *J Cardiovasc Surg (Torino)* 1988, 29:666–669.

69. Younis LT, Aguirre F, Byers SL, *et al*.: Perioperative and long-term prognostic value of intravenous dipyridamole thallium scintigraphy in patients with peripheral vascular disease. *Am Heart J* 1990, 119:1287–1292.

70. Strawn DJ, Guernsey JM: Dipyridamole thallium scanning in the evaluation of coronary artery disease in elective abdominal aortic surgery. *Arch Surg* 1991, 126:880–884.

71. Younis LT, Stratmann HG, Takase B, *et al*.: Preoperative clinical assessment and dipyridamole thallium-201 scintigraphy for prediction and prevention of cardiac events in patients having major noncardiovascular surgery and known or suspected coronary artery disease. *Am J Cardiol* 1994, 74:311–317.

72. Elliott BM, Robison JG, Zellner JL, *et al*.: Dobutamine-thallium-201 imaging: Assessing cardiac risks associated with vascular surgery. *Circulation* 1991, 84(suppl III):III54–III60.

73. Stratmann HG, Younis LT, Wittry MD, *et al*.: Dipyridamole technetium-99m sestamibi myocardial tomography for preoperative cardiac risk stratification before major or minor nonvascular surgery. *Am Heart J* 1996, 132:536–541.

74. Amanullah AM, Berman DS, Erel J, *et al*.: Incremental prognostic value of adenosine myocardial perfusion single-photon emission computed tomography in women with suspected coronary artery disease. *Am J Cardiol* 1998, 15:725–730.

75. Shaw LJ, Miller DD, Kong BA, *et al*.: Determination of perioperative cardiac risk by adenosine thallium-201 myocardial imaging. *Am J Heart J* 1992, 124:861–869.

76. Stratmann HG, Younis LT, Wittry MD, *et al*.: Dipyridamole technetium-99m sestamibi myocardial tomography in patients evaluated for elective vascular surgery: Prognostic value for perioperative and late cardiac events. *Am Heart J* 1996, 131:923–929.

77. Sachs RN, Tellier P, Larmignat P, *et al*.: Assessment by dipyridamole-thallium-201 myocardial scintigraphy of coronary risk before peripheral vascular surgery. *Surgery* 1988, 103:584–587.

78. Brown KA, O'Meara J, Chambers CE, Plante DA: Ability of dipyridamole-thallium-201 imaging one to four days after acute myocardial infarction to predict in-hospital and late recurrent myocardial ischemic events. *Am J Cardiol* 1990, 65:160–167.

79. Younis LT, Byers S, Shaw L, *et al*.: Prognostic value of intravenous dipyridamole thallium scintigraphy after an acute myocardial ischemic event. *Am J Cardiol* 1989, 64:161–166.

80. Stratmann HG, Williams GA, Wittry MD, *et al*.: Exercise technetium-99m sestamibi tomography for cardiac risk stratification of patients with stable chest pain. *Circulation* 1994, 89:615–622.

81. Younis LT, Stratmann H, Takase BR, *et al.*: Preoperative clinical assessment and dipyridamole thallium-201 scintigraphy for the prediction of prevention of cardiac events in major nonÐcardiovascular surgery patients. *Am J Cardiol* 1994, 74:311–317.

82. Stratmann HG, Tamesis BR, Younis LT, *et al.*: Prognostic value of dipyridamole technetium-99m sestamibi myocardial tomography in patients with stable chest pain who are unable to exercise. *Am J Cardiol* 1994, 73:647–652.

83. Miller DD: Cost efficacy of diagnostic and management strategies. *2nd International Conference of Nuclear Cardiology*; April 25, 1995; Cannes, France.

84. ACC/AHA practice guidelines –full text. ACC/AHA/ASNC guidelines for the clinical use of cardiac radionuclide imaging. 2003:1–69. Available at www.acc.org., www.americanheart.org, www.asnc.org.

85. Mahmarian JJ, Shaw LJ, Olszewski GH, *et al.*: Adenosine sestamibi SPECT post-infarction evaluation (INSPIRE) trial: a randomized, prospective multicenter trial evaluating the role of adenosine Tc-99m sestamibi spect for assessing risk and therapeutic outcomes in survivors of acute myocardial infarction. *J Nucl Cardiol* 2004,11:458–469.

86. Amanullah AM, Lindvall K: Prevalence and significance of transient-predominately asymptomatic-myocardial ischemia on Holter monitoring in unstable angina pectoris, and correlation with exercise test and thallium-201 myocardial perfusion imaging. *Am J Cardiol* 1993, 72:144–148.

87. Nicolai E, Cuocolo A, Pace L, *et al.*: Adenosine coronary vasodilation quantitative technetium 99m methoxy isobutyl isonitrile myocardial tomography in the identification and localization of coronary artery disease. *J Nucl Cardiol* 1996, 3:9–17.

88. Wilson WF, D'Agostino RB, Levy D, *et al.*: Prediction of coronary heart disease using risk factor categories. *Circulation* 1998, 97:1837–1847.

PET Perfusion Tracers: Quantitation of Myocardial Blood Flow

Thomas H. Schindler and Heinrich R. Schelbert

Conventional scintigraphic myocardial perfusion imaging with SPECT and, more recently, with PET, has emerged as the primary diagnostic modality for the identification and therapy decision-making process of coronary artery disease (CAD). By assessing the relative myocardial distribution of the myocardial blood flow (MBF) during treadmill exercise or pharmacologic stress—for example with dobutamine stimulation or pharmacologic vasodilation—and during rest, the presence of flow-limiting epicardial coronary artery lesions can be determined. Stress-induced relative reductions in regional MBF, as denoted by diminished regional radiotracer uptake during stress, identify myocardial regions that are subtended to advanced stages of epicardial artery lesions. In contrast, myocardial regions with the highest radiotracer uptake are commonly considered to be supplied by normal epicardial arteries or subclinical stages of the coronary artery process. Further, a homogenous distribution of left ventricular radiotracer uptake during both stress and rest commonly denotes the absence of flow-limiting epicardial coronary artery lesions.

Although the imaging of only the relative distributions of MBF at rest and during stress has yielded a high diagnostic and predicative accuracy in assessing flow-limiting epicardial artery lesions, there are limitations worthy of some considerations. First, myocardial regions with the highest radiotracer uptake are deemed as "normal" when in fact such regions may also be subtended by diseased coronary vessels, though less severely than the coronary vessels associated with downstream reductions in myocardial tracer uptake. Second, evaluation of only the relative distributions of MBF may fail to detect "balanced" CAD in which the relative distribution of MBF may be uniformly depressed rather than lead to regional reductions in myocardial tracer uptake. In both instances, images of the relative distribution of MBF would fail to detect even significant obstructive or flow-limiting CAD. Thirdly, and importantly, qualitative perfusion images are unlikely to identify early stages of coronary atherosclerosis. Such stages are associated with only mild and fluid-dynamically nonsignificant coronary lesions with only mild luminal irregularities as angiographic evidence of early structural changes or, further, with only functional alterations of the endothelial and/or vascular smooth muscle cells. Apart from these considerations, it must be kept in mind that the majority of acute coronary events originate in coronary vessels without flow-limiting epicardial artery lesions [1]. In addition, vasomotor abnormalities of the coronary circulation, even in the absence of structural substrates in the arterial wall and mostly related to the endothelium, have been recognized to be an independent predictor for the initiation and/or progression of the coronary atherosclerotic process and future coronary events [2–7].

The limitations inherent to qualitative myocardial perfusion imaging or imaging of the relative distributions of the myocardial radiotracer uptake underscores the necessity and, at the same time, potential benefits of quantitative approaches that measure MBF and its changes in response to interventions in absolute units. PET in concert with tracer kinetic modeling [8–10] and combined with pharmacologic or physical stimuli affords measurements of regional MBF in milliliters per gram per minute (mL/g/min) and, thereby, offers the opportunity to characterize coronary circulatory function and to identify its disturbances noninvasively [11–17]. By assessing alterations of MBF in milliliters per gram per minute in response to various stress stimuli, the functional consequences of structural and functional alterations in the coronary arterial wall may be identified before angiographic–morphologic changes may manifest. Thus, the concurrent ability of PET to assess regional MBF in quantitative estimates (mL/g/min) expands the diagnostic scope of conventional SPECT perfusion imaging in the identification of flow-limiting epicardial lesions, based on the stress-induced heterogeneity of relative myocardial perfusion, to early functional disturbances of the coronary circulation in the absence of clinically manifest CAD. Notably, the noninvasive identification and characterization of coronary circulatory dysfunction by PET entails not only diagnostic but potentially also important prognostic information [6,7,18] and allows monitoring of responses to medical therapy and risk factor modification [12,19–24].

As initial investigations demonstrate, PET quantification of regional MBF at rest and during hyperemic flow increases may indeed lead to an improvement in the detection of multivessel CAD and in characterizing the fluid-dynamic consequences of coronary artery stenosis [25–30].

Other investigations in asymptomatic individuals but with coronary risk factors, as described below, indicate the possibility of exploring the effects of coronary risk factors on coronary vasomotor function as well as of responses to risk factor modification and to therapeutic interventions. Other studies again suggest the predictive value of indices of coronary vasomotor function in early stages of developing CAD for future cardiac events. Whether therapeutic improvements or restoration of coronary circulatory function do indeed translate into an improved clinical outcome remains to be explored. Moreover, recent investigations [19,20,22] have shown that the noninvasive characterization of the normal coronary circulatory function as well as of its disturbances by PET can provide insight into the complex nature of underlying disease mechanisms. As such, these noninvasive approaches may aid in unmasking pathophysiology of early, developing coronary atherosclerosis [31–34]. These insights to pathophysiologic processes of developing atherosclerosis as made with PET can further contribute to design and testing of therapeutic strategies for primary and secondary prevention of CAD.

The following section of this atlas illustrates technical and methodologic aspects of PET-based measurements of MBF, describes approaches for the characterization of the coronary vasomotor function in the human heart, reviews findings in patients with cardiovascular disease or at risk of CAD, and examines the possibility of monitoring responses to risk-modifying treatments.

The Coronary Circulation

Figure 4-1. Schematic representation of the functional compartments of the coronary circulation. The coronary circulation can be viewed as a two-compartment system that consists of the large epicardial conductance and the small resistance vessels. In the normal coronary circulation, the intraluminal pressure in the conductance vessels equals that in the aortic root (coronary driving pressure). There is little resistance to flow along the conductance vessels so that the intracoronary pressure remains relatively constant throughout the epicardial vessels but steeply declines within the resistance vessels to values that are moderately higher than those in the right atrium. This maintains a pressure gradient between the coronary circulation and the right atrium. Changes in resistance—mostly at the level of the pre-arterioles but also arterioles affected by vascular smooth muscle relaxation and constriction—and extravascular factors regulate coronary blood flow and adjust it to metabolic needs. Changes in coronary blood flow are further modulated in close concert with the endothelium and endothelium-derived vasoactive substances. Increases in coronary blood flow velocity, for example, lead to shear stress–mediated increases in the synthesis and release of nitric oxide from the endothelium, which in the normal coronary circulation results in about a 15% to 25% increase in conductance vessel diameter [35,36]. This flow-dependent dilation offsets and thus adjusts for the flow velocity–related increase in resistance so that resistance to high flow rates remains low in the coronary conductance vessels. F—blood flow.

Figure 4-2. Autoregulation of coronary blood flow. The coronary circulation underlies an active autoregulation [37] that keeps coronary blood flow relatively constant despite changes in coronary driving pressure. Autoregulation of coronary blood flow depends on myocardial oxygen requirements [38], so that coronary flow changes in proportion to changes in oxygen demand and consumption. Mechanisms responsible for the active changes in coronary vascular resistance relate to both myogenic control and local metabolic needs. Myogenic control implies that pressure distension of the vessel due to increases in coronary perfusion pressure lead to active vasoconstriction that increases vascular resistance and maintains flow relatively constant. In contrast, local metabolic feedback control entails intrinsic local mechanisms that adjust coronary blood flow to changes in oxygen consumption. An increase in oxygen consumption (*eg*, due to increases in contractile state or heart rate and thus in myocardial work) is associated with a decrease in myocardial oxygen tension. This leads to release or activation of local vasodilator substances such as adenosine, K^+-adenosine triphosphate channels, and/or nitric oxide, which in turn increase coronary blood flow and oxygen supply.

The vasodilator capacity represents the increase in flow from rest to hyperemia either during exercise or, more correctly, the pharmacologically stimulated maximum vasodilation. However, the autoregulation is lost at coronary driving pressures less than 60 mm Hg. Further, during maximum vasodilation, as induced by vascular smooth muscle–relaxing agents, coronary flow becomes dependent on coronary driving pressure.

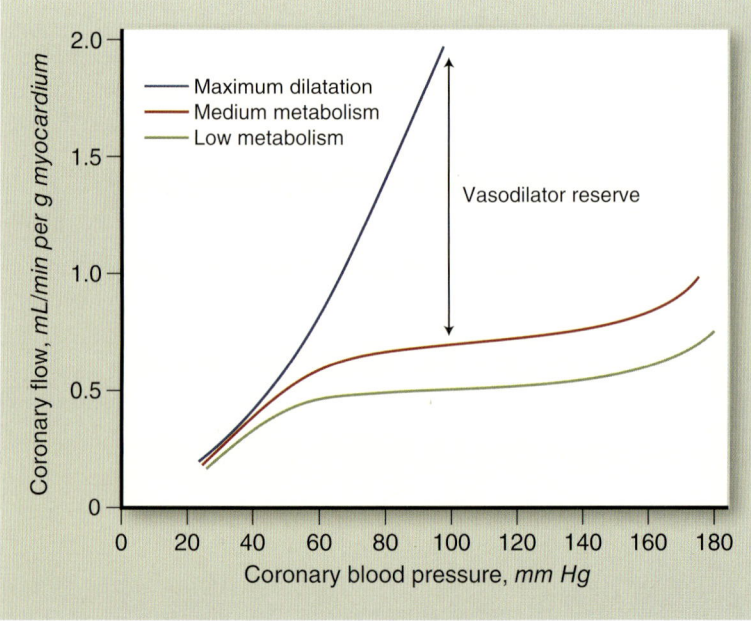

Technical and Methodologic Aspects of PET Measurements of Myocardial Blood Flow

Components essential to the noninvasive measurement of myocardial blood flow (MBF) include the high spatial and temporal resolution PET imaging system and the use of appropriate positron-emitting tracers of MBF and of an appropriate tracer kinetic model.

Several positron-emitting tracers of MBF are available. Their ultra-short physical half-time allows serial measurements at time intervals ranging from 8 to 50 minutes. Retention of these positron-emitting flow tracers follows MBF generally in a curvilinear fashion. In the low-flow range, myocardial tracer concentrations rise steeply with increases in MBF, whereas flow increases in the hyperemic flow range are associated with progressively smaller increments in flow tracer concentrations. The exception is ^{15}O water, which rapidly exchanges between blood and tissue, so that its initial uptake into myocardium increases linearly with MBFs. Tracer compartment models describe the kinetics of the radiotracer in blood and in tissue relative to MBF and correct for the flow-dependent, nonlinear radiotracer uptake in the myocardium. Measurements of MBF are performed through intravenous administration of the flow tracer; acquisition of serial images or dynamic imaging of the tracer transit through the central circulation and accumulation of the tracer in the myocardium; determination of the arterial tracer input function and the myocardial tissue response from regions of interest assigned to the left ventricular blood pool and myocardium; and, finally, fitting of the resulting time activity curves with the tracer compartment model.

Positron-Emitting Tracers of Myocardial Blood Flow

Tracer	Abbreviation	Physical half-life
Oxygen-15 water	$H_2{}^{15}O$	2.4 minutes
Nitrogen-13 ammonia	$^{13}NH_3^+$	9.8 minutes
Rubidium-82 chloride	$^{82}Rb^+$	78 seconds

Figure 4-3. Positron-emitting tracers of myocardial blood flow.

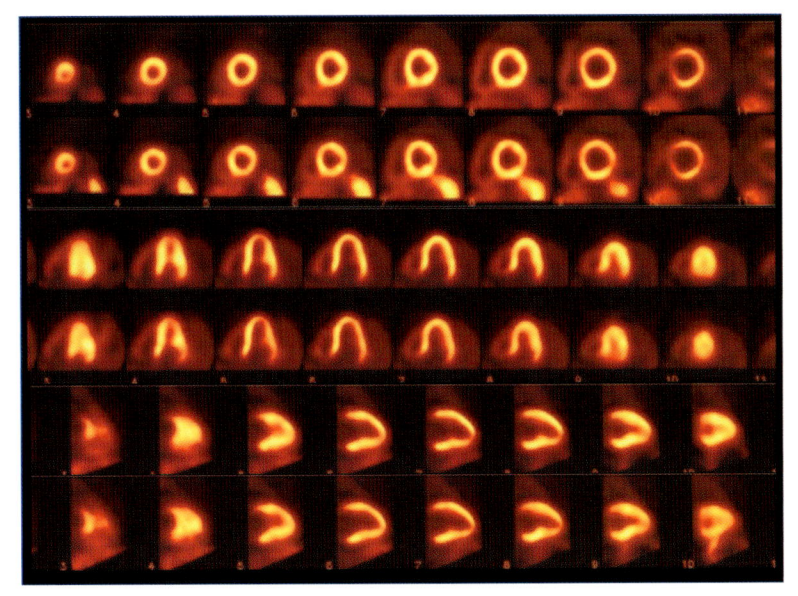

Figure 4-4. Images of the relative distribution of myocardial blood flow in the normal human heart. Distribution of the flow tracer ^{13}N-ammonia in the normal human myocardium during dipyridamole-induced hyperemic coronary flow increases and during rest as depicted on reoriented, short-axis and horizontal and vertical long-axis images. The activity is distributed homogenously throughout the left and, although less intensely, right ventricular myocardium (seen best in the horizontal long-axis views).

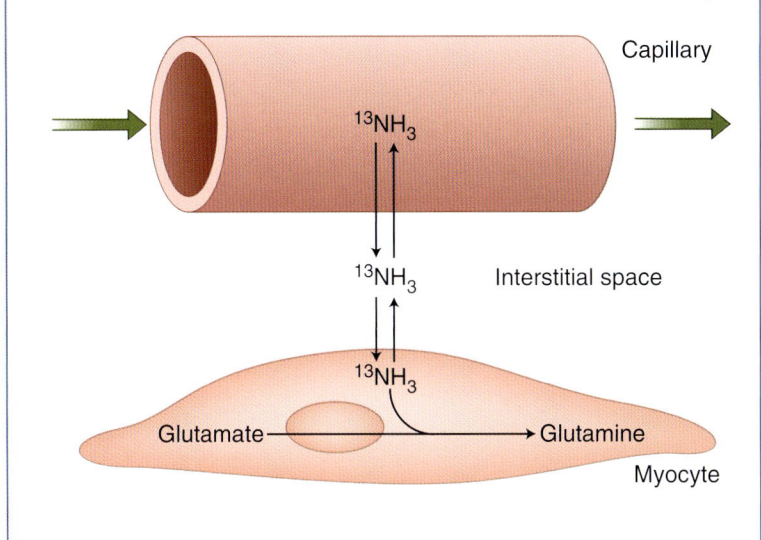

Figure 4-5. Myocardial tissue kinetics of the flow tracer ^{13}N-ammonia ($^{13}NH_3$). Injected intravenously in minute, true tracer quantities, ^{13}N-ammonia exchanges across the capillary wall and transits through the interstitial spaces and reaches the myocardial cell. A fraction of tracer then diffuses back from tissue into blood while another fraction becomes metabolically trapped and retained in the myocardium through the α-ketoglutarate-to-glutamate and the glutamate-to-glutamine reactions [9]. Over the 10- to 20-minute time interval of serial image acquisition required for flow measurements, myocardial ^{13}N-ammonia concentrations remain constant without loss of the ^{13}N-labeled glutamine from the myocardium.

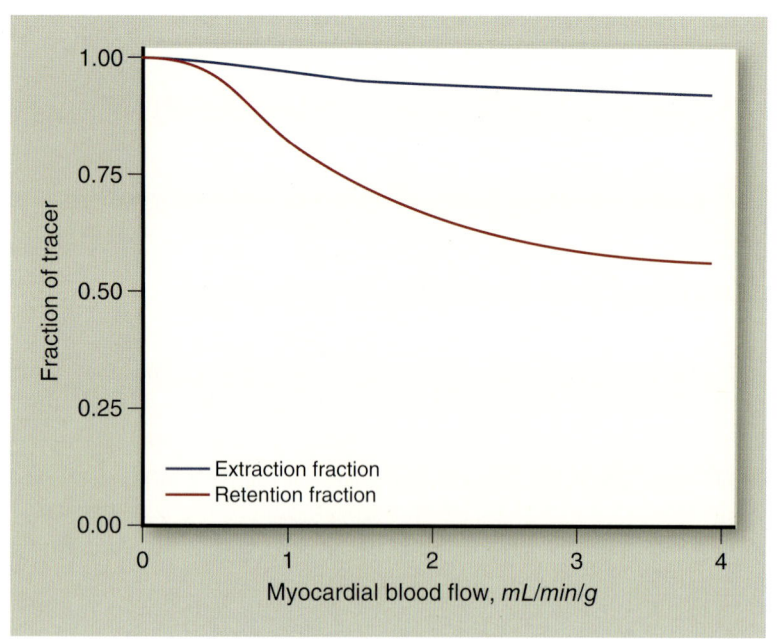

Figure 4-6. First-pass extraction and retention fractions of flow tracers. The tracer first-pass extraction fraction is defined as the fraction of tracer that crosses the capillary membrane during the first transit through the coronary circulation that approaches unity for ^{13}N-ammonia, for example, and does not significantly decline with higher-flow velocities [9]. However, back diffusion of tracer from tissue to blood increases with higher flows, so that an increasingly smaller fraction becomes available for metabolic trapping and the first-pass retention fraction progressively declines with higher coronary flows.

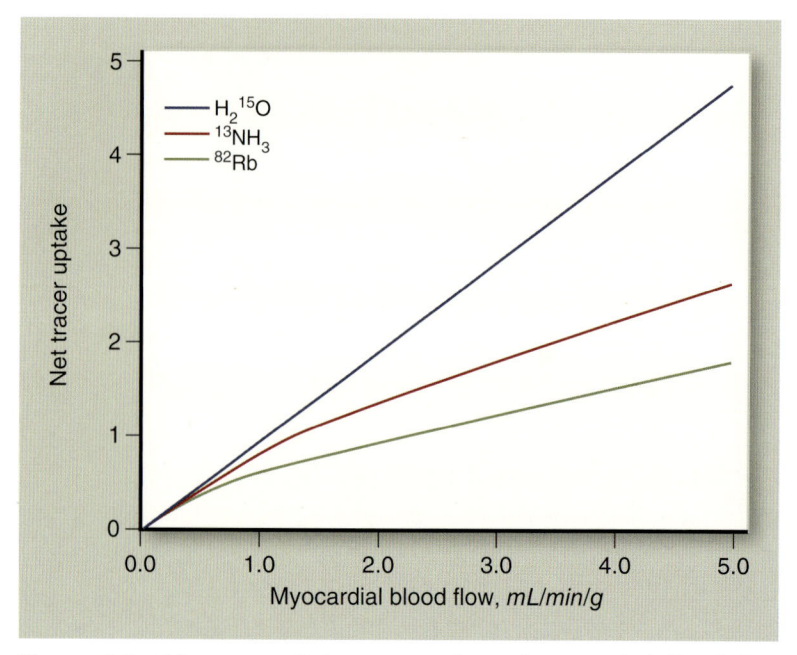

Figure 4-7. Net myocardial tracer uptake and myocardial blood flow (MBF). The net myocardial uptake of a tracer is the product of the first-pass retention fraction of the tracer and of MBF (eg, the amount of tracer delivered to the myocardium). Because the first-pass extraction fraction for ^{15}O water (H$_2$^{15}O) approaches 1 and is independent of blood flow, its net uptake increases linearly with MBF. In contrast, the net uptake of ^{13}N-ammonia (^{13}NH$_3$) and rubidium-82 (^{82}Rb) increases nonlinearly with higher flows. For the same flow, the net uptake of ^{13}NH$_3$ is higher than that of ^{82}Rb because of its higher first-pass extraction fraction.

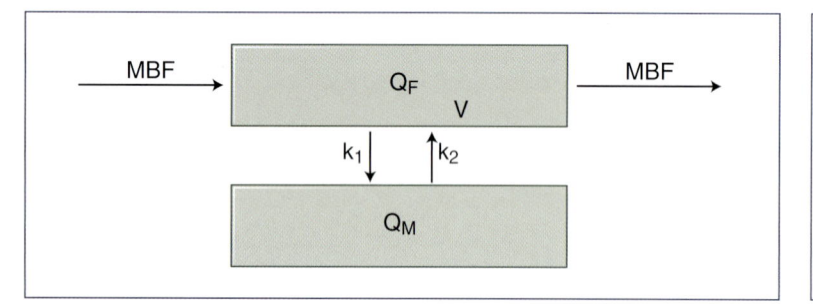

Figure 4-8. Compartment models for tracers of myocardial blood flow (MBF). Tracer compartment models are fundamental for establishing operational equations that permit estimates of MBF. The tracer kinetic model, shown here for the flow tracer ^{13}N-ammonia, describes quantitatively the exchange of tracer between blood and tissue and within tissue in terms of functional compartments of different sizes or volumes of distribution (V) of that tracer [8,39]. For example, in this model, compartment 1 describes the amount of radiotracer Q$_F$ present at any time after tracer injection in freely diffusible form. Because the first-pass extraction fraction of ^{13}N-ammonia approaches unity, freely diffusible tracer present in blood, in the interstitium, and in the cell is "lumped" into a single functional compartment. The metabolically trapped tracer activity (Q$_M$) is described by compartment 2. Forward and reverse (back diffusion) tracer exchange between the two functional compartments is described by first-order rate constants or k$_1$ and k$_2$. For example, the product of the forward rate constant k$_1$ and the concentration (or mass) of ^{13}N-ammonia then describes the mass flux of ^{13}N-ammonia from blood into tissue (K$_1$).

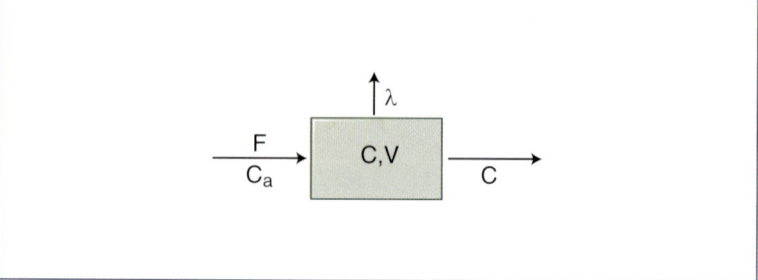

Figure 4-9. One-compartment tracer kinetic model for ^{15}O water. Because the capillary and sarcolemmal membranes do not exert a barrier effect to the exchange of water, the activity of ^{15}O-labeled water observed in a region of interest assigned to the myocardium on the serially acquired images can be described by a one-compartment tracer kinetic model. λ—physical decay constant of ^{15}O; C$_a$—tracer concentrations in arterial blood; F—blood flow; V—volume of distribution in tissue [10].

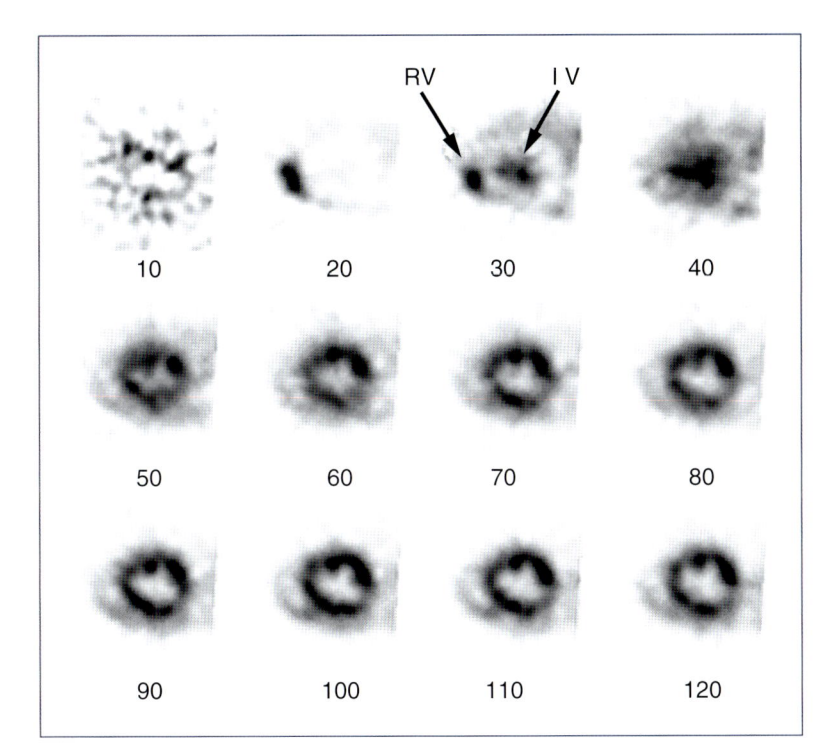

Figure 4-10. Serially acquired images of a bolus transit of ^{13}N-ammonia through the central circulation. The serially acquired 10-second short-axis images illustrate the transit of the intravenously administered radiotracer bolus through the central circulation (from left to right and top to bottom). The initial images depict the tracer activity mostly in the right heart, followed by dispersion of the tracer bolus into both lungs, return into the left ventricular cavity, and subsequent clearance of tracer activity from arterial blood into the myocardium. The late, static image depicts the tracer activity retained in the left ventricular myocardium after the radiotracer has largely disappeared from the blood. LV—left ventricle; RV—right ventricle.

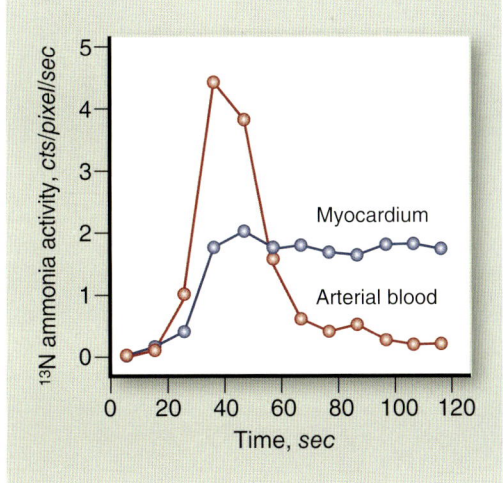

Figure 4-11. Arterial radiotracer input function and myocardial tissue response. From regions of interest assigned to the left ventricular blood pool and the left ventricular myocardium on the serially acquired images, time activity curves are derived that describe the changes in radiotracer activity in arterial blood (counts/pixel/sec) and in myocardium (counts/pixel/sec) as a function of time. Through fitting of the time activity curves with the operational equation formulated from the tracer kinetic model, estimates of myocardial blood flow in units of milliliters of blood per minute per gram of myocardium are obtained.

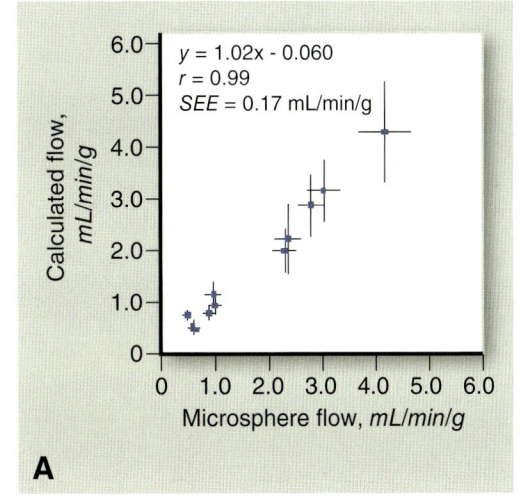

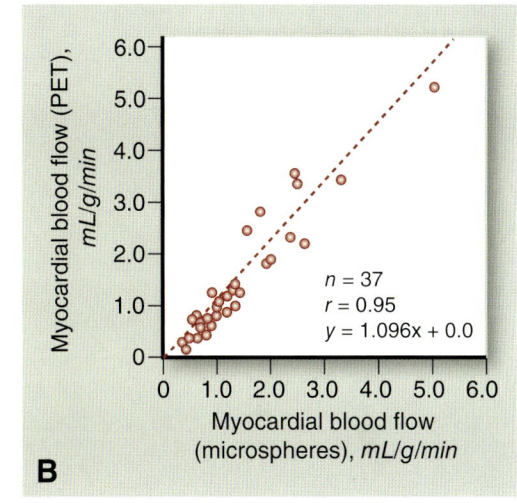

Figure 4-12. Animal experimental validation of PET-based measurements of myocardial blood flow (MBF). Comparison of MBFs measured simultaneously with ^{13}N-ammonia and PET (**A**) and with ^{15}O water and PET (**B**) and radiolabeled microspheres injected into the left ventricular cavity and postmortem tissue counting in dog experiments [8,10]. The error bars in **A** indicate the standard deviations of the segmental about the mean left ventricular MBF. SEE—standard error of the estimate.

PET Perfusion Tracers: Quantitation of Myocardial Blood Flow

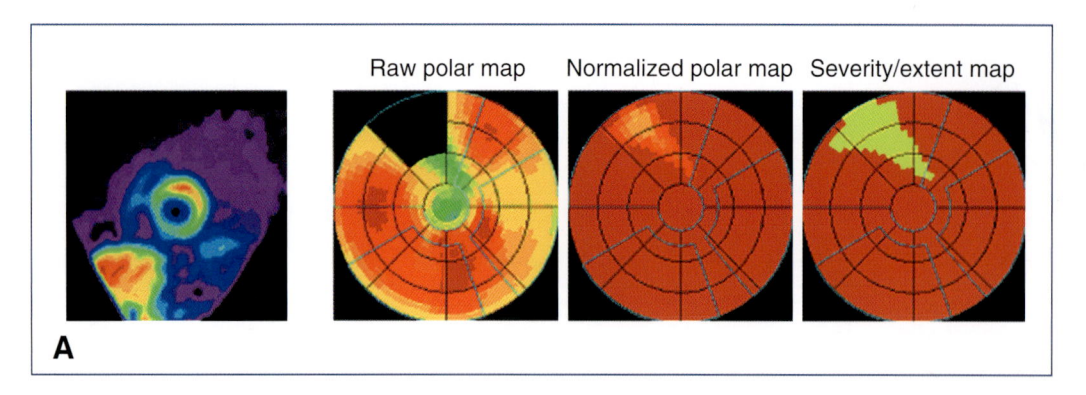

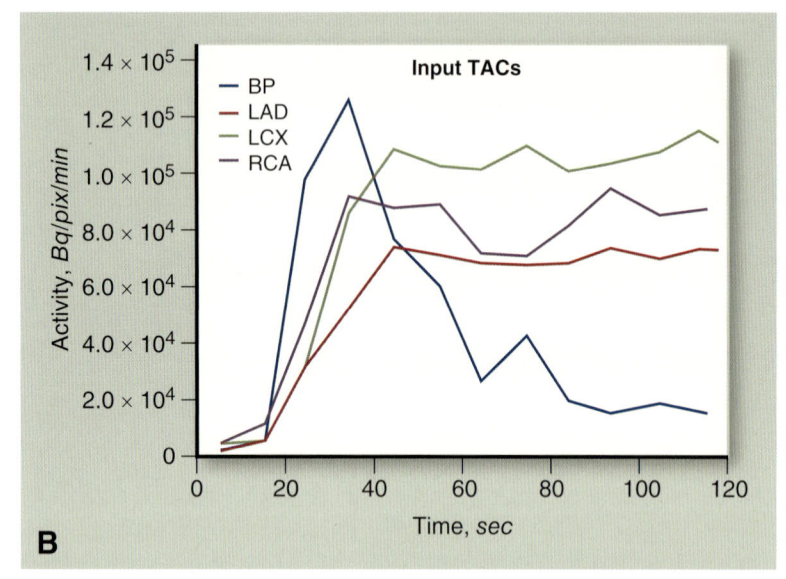

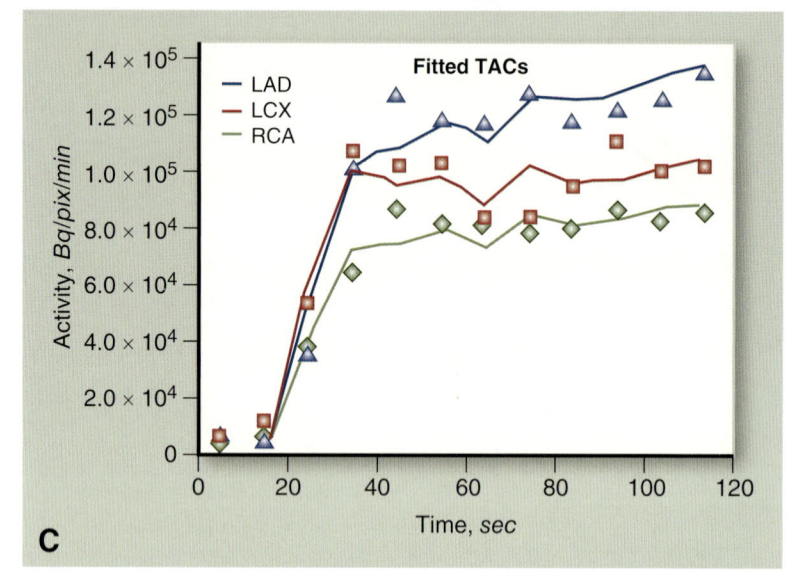

Figure 4-13. **A–C,** Polar map approach for estimating regional myocardial blood flows (MBFs). Software algorithms facilitate determinations of MBF. In the example shown, the last of the serially acquired transaxial images is reoriented into short-axis slices. They are assembled into a polar map of the relative distribution of the flow tracer in the left ventricular myocardium. In this example, regions of interest are assigned to the territories of the three coronary arteries (left anterior descending [LAD], left circumflex [LCX], and right coronary [RCA] arteries) and to the center of the left ventricular cavity (BP). The reorientation parameters are then applied to the serially acquired images. The regions of interest are copied to the serial polar maps. Time activity curves (TACs) for each coronary artery territory are displayed, and are fitted with the tracer compartment model so that estimates of regional MBFs are obtained. In this example, flow is estimated for a region of interest corresponding to a stress-induced flow defect in the territory of the LAD coronary artery and the entire LCX and RCA territories.

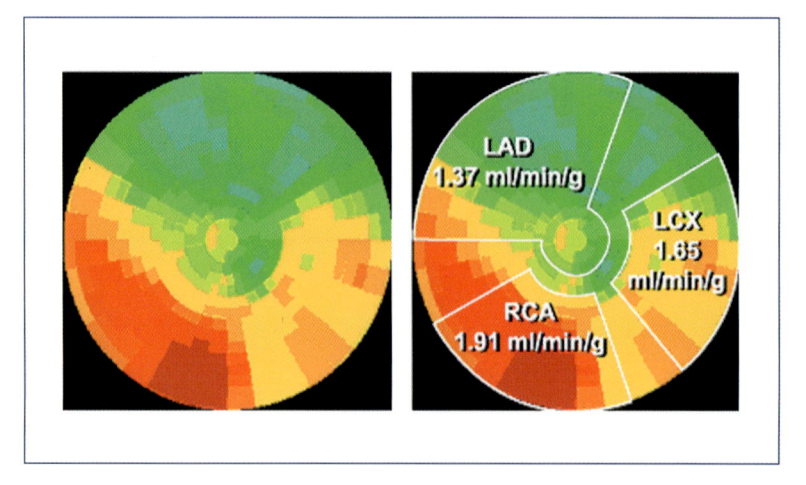

Figure 4-14. Polar map of myocardial tracer activity concentrations and regional myocardial blood flows (MBFs) in a patient with coronary artery disease. The stress myocardial perfusion polar map depicts a flow defect in the territory of the left anterior descending (LAD) and, in part, the left circumflex (LCX) coronary arteries (*green* and *light yellow*). MBF during adenosine hyperemia is 1.37 mL/min/g in the LAD coronary artery territory, 1.65 mL/min/g in the LCX artery territory, and 1.91 mL/min/g in the right coronary artery (RCA) territory. The myocardial flow reserve and the apparently "normal" RCA territory are only 2.2 and thus diminished when compared with flow reserves in healthy volunteers.

Findings in the Normal Human Heart

Myocardial Blood Flows at Baseline

Investigations have reported values of normal for myocardial blood flow (MBF) at rest and during pharmacologically induced hyperemia. Although generally of similar magnitude, regardless of the measurement approach used—for example, ^{13}N-ammonia, rubidium-82, or ^{15}O water—considerable interindividual variations are observed for both rest and hyperemic MBFs. MBF at rest largely depends on oxygen demand and, thus, on cardiac work, estimated by the rate pressure product [RPP] (RPP = heart rate × systolic blood pressure).

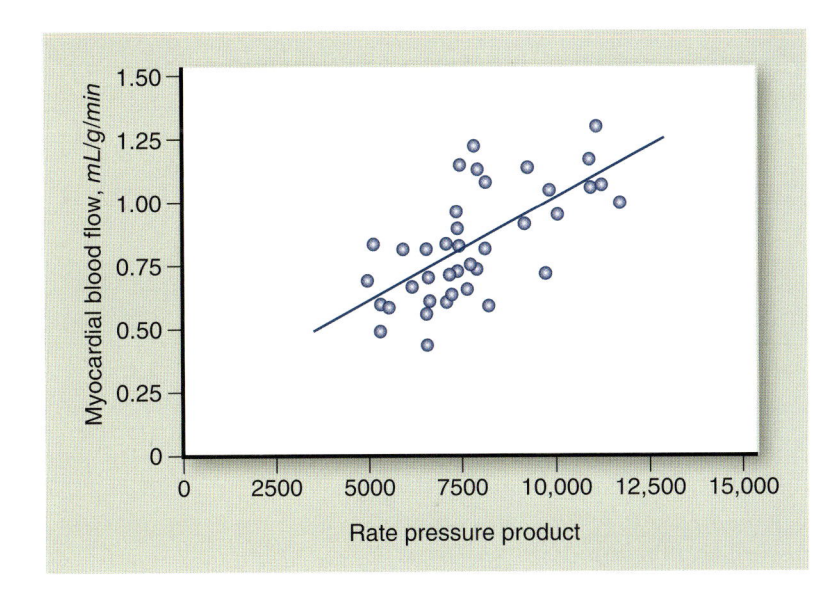

Figure 4-15. Dependency of myocardial blood flow (MBF) at rest on cardiac work. In the normal myocardium, blood flow at rest correlates with the rate pressure product as an index of cardiac work [40,41]. Increases in cardiac work, as for example, with bicycle exercise or induced by intravenous dobutamine infusions, are accompanied by proportionate increases in MBF [42,43].

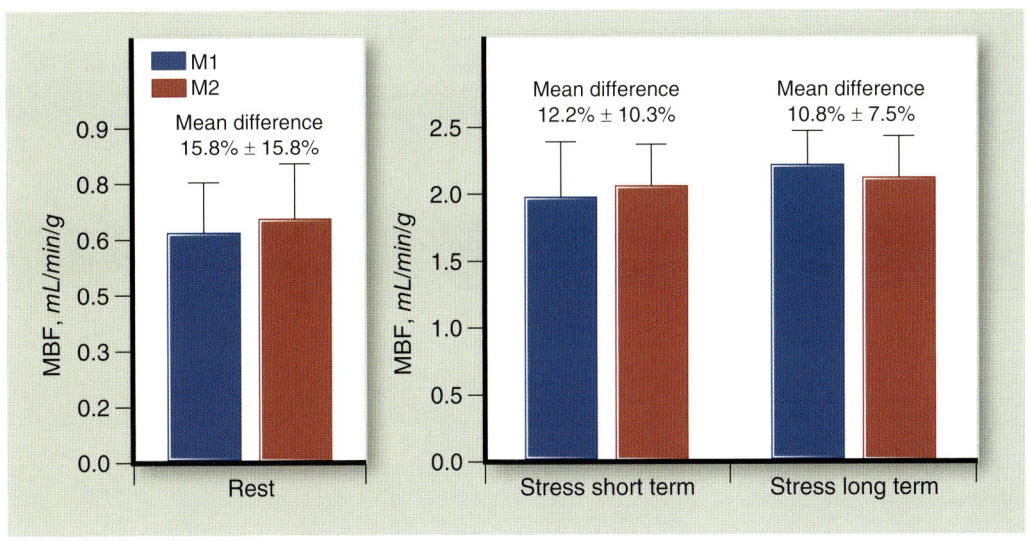

Figure 4-16. Reproducibility of PET measurements of myocardial blood flow (MBF) at rest and during pharmacologic stress. Measurements of resting blood flow were repeated in the same study session (measurement at baseline [M1] and repeat measurement [M2]; *left*) [44]. Mean values of MBF in the 21 healthy volunteers were similar for both measurements; individual measurements differed by an average of 15.8% ± 15.8%. Repeat measurements during adenosine-induced hyperemia in 13 healthy volunteers—again during the same study session (*middle*)—also demonstrated almost identical mean values of hyperemic blood flow. Individual flow values differed between the two measurements by an average of 12.2% ± 10.3%. Long-term repeat measurements during dipyridamole-induced hyperemia are shown on the *right*; again, the mean values in the same seven healthy volunteers are comparable and without statistically significant differences. Individual flow values between the two measurements differed by an average of 10.8% ± 7.5%. (*Adapted from* Nagamachi *et al.* [44].)

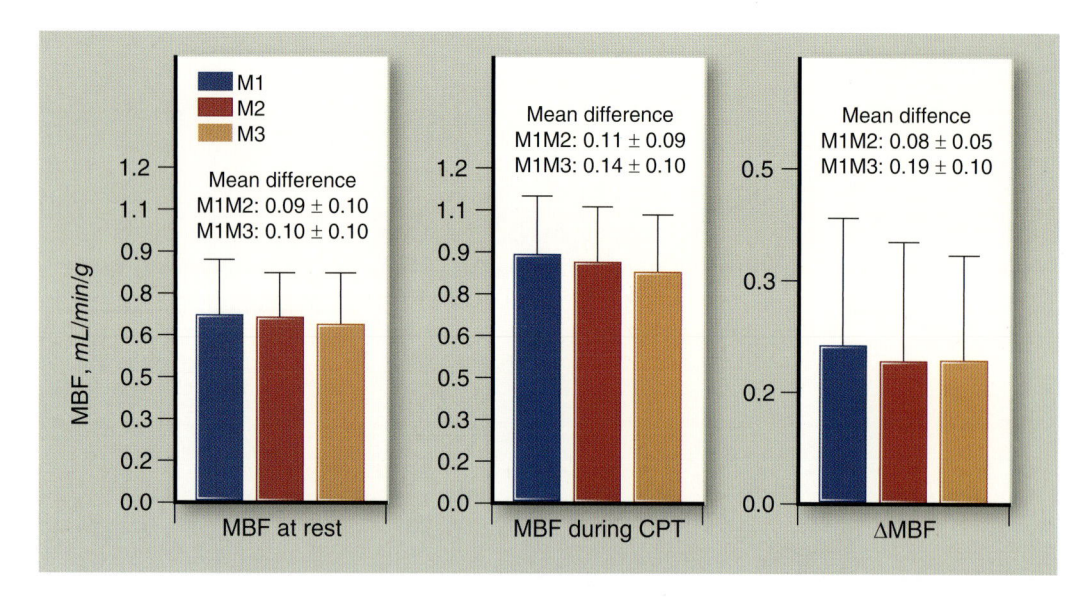

Figure 4-17. Short-term and long-term reproducibility of PET-measured flow responses to cold pressor testing (CPT). Measurements were repeated within the same study session and again in a separate study session 2 to 3 weeks later [45]. The repeat measurements at rest are depicted in the *left panel*, during CPT in the *center panel*, and the endothelium-related increase in myocardial blood flow (MBF) from rest to CPT, defined as ΔMBF, in the *right panel*. There are no statistically significant differences between measurements at rest, during CPT, and for the flow responses ΔMBF. M1—measurement at baseline; M2—repeat measurement during the same study session; M3—repeat measurement 2 to 3 weeks later. (*Adapted from* Schindler et al. [45].)

MBF Values at Rest and With Adenosine-Induced (1-Day Protocol) and Dipyridamole-Induced (2-Day Protocol) Vasodilation Using ¹³N-Ammonia and PET

Protocol	Baseline (t = 1)	Repeated (t = 2)	Mean P value	Difference*, %
Both protocols (n = 21)				
MBF at rest	0.62 ± 0.14	0.66 ± 0.15	NS	15.8 ± 15.8
MBF during hyperemia	2.01 ± 0.39	2.03 ± 0.31	NS	11.8 ± 9.4
1-Day protocol with adenosine (n = 13)				
MBF during hyperemia	1.97 ± 0.45	2.05 ± 0.33	NS	12.2 ± 10.3
2-Day protocol with dipyridamole (n = 7)				
MBF during hyperemia	2.09 ± 0.25	2.00 ± 0.31	NS	10.8 ± 7.5

*Mean difference and standard deviation of values demonstrate within-subject variability (reproducibility).

A

MBF Values at Rest and With Adenosine-Induced Vasodilation Using ¹⁵O Water and PET

Parameter	Baseline (t = 1)	Repeated (t = 2)	P value	Mean difference*, %
MBF at rest	0.89 ± 0.14	0.99 ± 0.15	NS	13 ± 11
MFB during hyperemia	3.51 ± 0.45	3.83 ± 0.49	NS	10 ± 14

*Mean difference and standard deviation of values demonstrate within-subject variability (reproducibility).

B

Figure 4-18. Reproducibility of myocardial blood flow (MBF) at rest, during pharmacologically induced hyperemia, and during sympathetic stimulation with cold pressor testing (CPT). **A**, As demonstrated in this table, pharmacologically induced hyperemia induced reproducible changes in predominantly endothelium-independent MBF increases in healthy volunteers, as measured with ¹³N-ammonia and PET imaging [44]. Because adenosine has a short half-life of less than 8 seconds, it was used to assess the reproducibility of hyperemic flow within the same day (1-day protocol). In contrast, the reproducibility of hyperemic flow with dipyridamole—which has a relatively long half-life of 30 minutes—was determined on different study days (2-day protocol; average time interval, 26.5 ± 18.9 days). Assessment of hyperemic blood flow, induced by dipyridamole, did not differ significantly compared with that achieved with adenosine (P = not significant [NS]). Thus, the short- and long-term reproducibility of pharmacologically induced hyperemic blood flow increases was quite similar.

B, Repeat measurements of MBF at rest and during adenosine-stimulated hyperemia in the same study session of 21 healthy volunteers using ¹⁵O-labeled water and PET resulted in comparable flow estimates, indicating the short-term reproducibility of this technique [46].

Taken together, these observations (**A** and **B**) indicate that MBF can be measured reproducibly with PET and thus, should prove useful as a tool for quantifying effects of pharmaceutical interventions on hyperemic MBF and thus, on the total coronary vasodilatory capacity.

Continued on the next page

Repeat Measurements of MBF Responses to CPT

Parameter	MBF measurement*, mL/min/g			SR absolute mean difference (m = 12), mL/min/g	LR absolute mean difference (m = 13), mL/min/g
	m = 1	m = 2	m = 3		
At rest	0.67 ± 0.19	0.66 ± 0.15	0.63 ± 0.18	0.09 ± 0.10	0.10 ± 0.10
During CPT	0.88 ± 0.21	0.85 ± 0.20	0.82 ± 0.21	0.11 ± 0.09	0.14 ± 0.10
Change to CPT	0.21 ± 0.17	0.19 ± 0.16	0.19 ± 0.14	0.08 ± 0.05	0.19 ± 0.10

*First two measurements (m = 1, m = 2) taken on same day; third measurement (m = 3) taken after 2 weeks.

C

Figure 4-18. *(Continued)* **C**, Repeat measurements of MBF responses to CPT performed within the same study session as well as after 2 weeks in 20 individuals [45]. Assessment of the short-term reproducibility (SR; 1-day session) did not demonstrate a significant absolute difference in MBF at rest, during CPT, or during the endothelium-related change in MBF from rest to CPT (ΔMBF) [45]. Similarly, repeat short-term measurements of hemodynamics at rest and during CPT were comparable. In regard to the long-term reproducibility (LR; 2-week period), the absolute differences in corresponding MBF values and hemodynamics were relatively but nonsignificantly higher. Thus, sympathetic stimulation with CPT induced reproducible changes in the hemodynamic response and in endothelium-related MBFs (ΔMBF) in both the short-term and the long-term. Short- and long-term MBF responses to CPT, as a noninvasive probe for endothelium-related coronary vasomotion, can be measured reproducibly with ^{13}N-ammonia PET [45]. (**A**, adapted from Nagamachi et al. [44]; **B**, adapted from Kaufmann et al. [46]; **C**, adapted from Schindler et al. [45].)

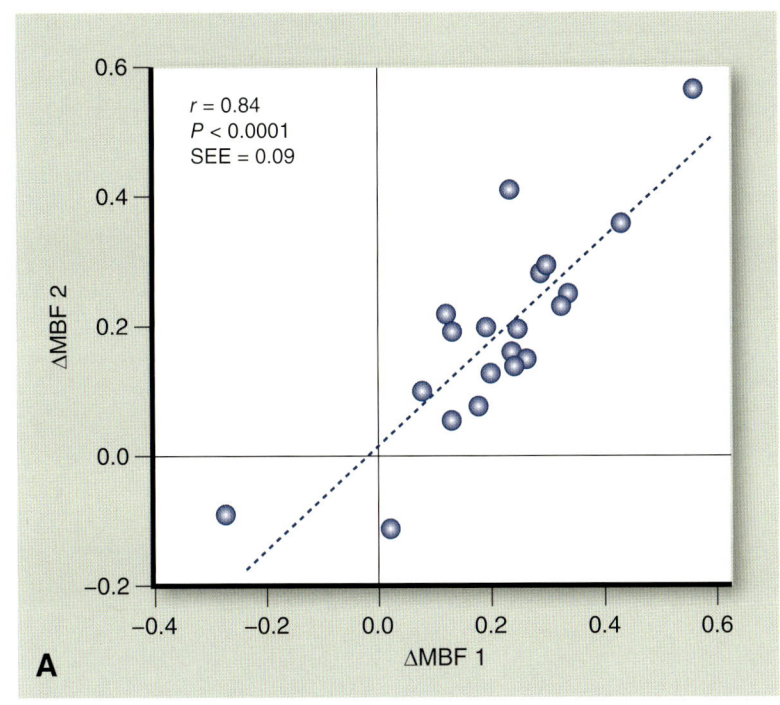

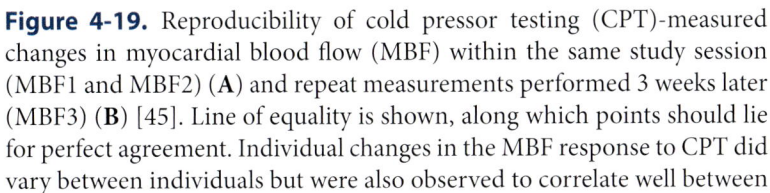

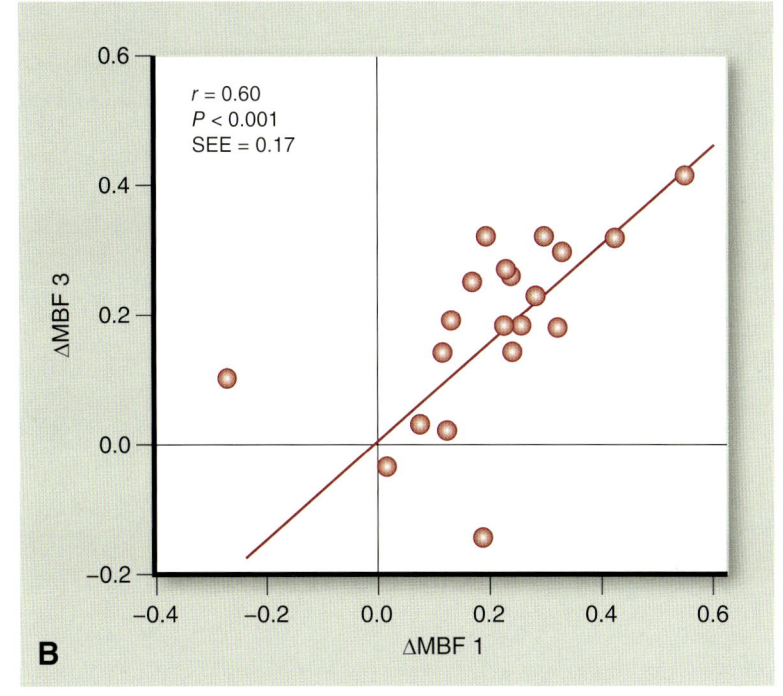

Figure 4-19. Reproducibility of cold pressor testing (CPT)-measured changes in myocardial blood flow (MBF) within the same study session (MBF1 and MBF2) (**A**) and repeat measurements performed 3 weeks later (MBF3) (**B**) [45]. Line of equality is shown, along which points should lie for perfect agreement. Individual changes in the MBF response to CPT did vary between individuals but were also observed to correlate well between short-term and long-term measurements as indicated by the standard error of the estimate (SEE) of the Pearson correlation analysis, which is thought to reflect the range of measurement error. The measurement-related error for change in MBF from rest to CPT (ΔMBF) is 0.09 mL/g/min for short-term and 0.17 mL/g/min for long-term repeat measurements. (*Adapted from* Schindler et al. [45].)

MBF Repeatability Coefficient in Different Studies

Parameter	Schindler et al. [45]	Siegrist et al. [47]	Kaufmann et al. [46]	Wyss et al. [48]	Jagathesan et al. [49]
Radiotracer	^{13}N-ammonia	^{15}O water	^{15}O water	^{15}O water	^{15}O water
Period	Short-term (1 d); long-term (2 wk)	Short-term (1 d)	Short-term (1 d)	Short-term (1 d)	Long-term (24 wk)
MBF					
At baseline	0.26; 0.26	—	0.17	0.26	0.30*/0.26†
During CPT	0.28; 0.31	0.41	—	—	—
ΔMBF to CPT	0.18; 0.27	—	—	—	—
During adenosine	—	—	0.94	1.34	—
To bicycle exercise	—	—	—	0.82	—
During dobutamine	—	—	—	—	0.49*/0.58†

*MBF value in ischemic territory.
†MBF value in remote territory.

Figure 4-20. Myocardial blood flow (MBF) repeatability coefficient (RPC) in different studies [45–49]. The RPC, as proposed by Bland and Altman [50], serves as an index of the agreement between two repeat measurements. Given a normal Gaussian distribution of blood flow estimates, the RPC denotes the expected range of measurement error between repeat MBF measurements. Because of the small sample size of prior MBF repeat studies, ranging from 11 to 25 individuals [46,48,49], the assumption of a normal Gaussian distribution of the MBFs may not be valid. In that case, and as outlined in Figure 4-17, the standard error of the estimate of the Pearson correlation analysis can be used to determine the measurement error in repeat MBF assessments. Notably, the RPC can be used for a direct comparison of the precision of MBF measurements between different studies. As this table shows, the RPC for serial short-term and long-term measurements of MBF responses to cold pressor testing (CPT) is less than it is observed for repeat hyperemic MBF measurements. The RPC for the endothelium-related change in MBF from rest to CPT (ΔMBF) was 0.18 mL/g/min for the short-term and 0.27 mL/g/min for the long-term reproducibility measurements with ^{13}N-ammonia and PET[45]. These values are lower than those for the short-term RPC of CPT-related MBFs with ^{15}O-labeled water [47] as well as for hyperemic MBFs observed in previous studies [46,48,49] ranging between 0.49 mL/g/min and 1.34 mL/g/min. Thus, repeat measurements of MBF responses to CPT appear to be less variable than those for hyperemic MBFs.

Assessment of Coronary Circulatory Function

Responses of myocardial blood flow (MBF) to physiologic or pharmacologic stimulation as measured by PET contain information on the function of the coronary circulation. Hyperemic MBFs as induced by pharmacologic vasodilation with intravenous adenosine, dipyridamole, or, in some laboratories with adenosine triphosphate reflect the total integrated coronary vasodilator capacity. By contrast, flow responses to sympathetic stimulation with, for example, cold pressor testing, contain information on endothelial function. An additional parameter available through PET measurements of regional MBF is the longitudinal base-to-apex myocardial perfusion gradient that contains information on the flow-related vasodilator function of the epicardial coronary conduit vessels.

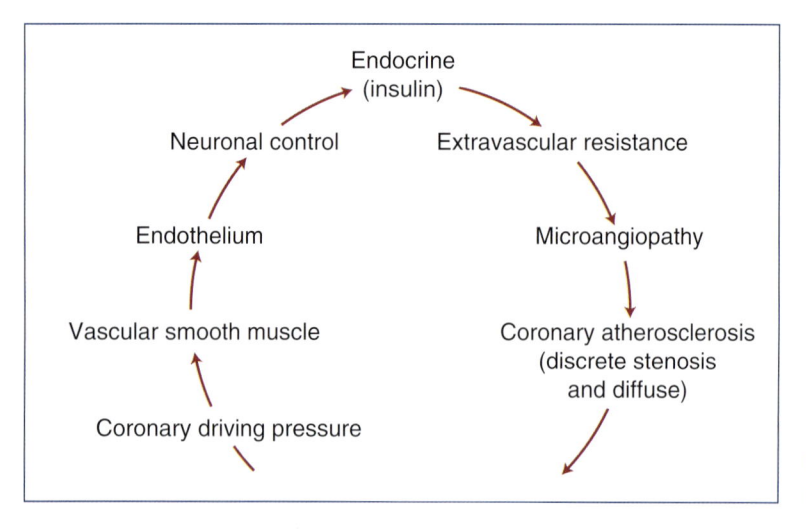

Figure 4-21. Determinants of vasodilator-induced hyperemic myocardial blood flows.

Hyperemic Myocardial Blood Flows and Myocardial Flow Reserve in Healthy Human Volunteers

Study	Patients, n	Age, y	Radiotracer	Agent	MBF, mL/min/g Rest	MBF, mL/min/g Stress	Flow reserve, mL/min/g
Bergmann et al. [10]	11	25.5	H$_2$^{15}O	Dipyridamole	0.90 ± 0.22	3.55 ± 1.15	4.1 ± 1.2
Araujo et al. [51]	11	26 ± 7	H$_2$^{15}O	Dipyridamole	0.84 ± 0.09	3.52 ± 1.12	4.2 ± 1.3
Pitkanen et al. [52]	20	31 ± 8	H$_2$^{15}O	Dipyridamole	0.83 ± 0.13	4.49 ± 1.27	5.4 ± 1.5
Yokoyama et al. [53]	13	56 ± 7	H$_2$^{15}O	Dipyridamole	0.80 ± 0.39	2.92 ± 1.66	3.7 ± 1.4
Kaufmann et al. [46]	21	45 ± 8	H$_2$^{15}O	Adenosine	0.89 ± 0.15	3.51 ± 0.45	NR
Tadamura et al. [54]	20	23 ± 3	H$_2$^{15}O	Dipyridamole	0.67 ± 0.16	4.33 ± 1.23	NR
Hutchins et al. [55]	7	24 ± 4	^{13}NH$_3$	Dipyridamole	0.88 ± 0.17	4.17 ± 1.12	4.8 ± 1.3
Chan et al. [56]	20	35 ± 16	^{13}NH$_3$	Dipyridamole	1.10 ± 0.20	4.3 ± 1.3	4.0 ± 1.3
Kubo et al. [57]	10	36 ± 6	H$_2$^{15}O	ATP	0.79 ± 0.29	3.70 ± 0.67	5.15 ± 1.64
Czernin et al. [40]	18	31 ± 9	^{13}NH$_3$	Dipyridamole	0.76 ± 0.25	3.0 ± 0.8	4.1 ± 0.9

Figure 4-22. Hyperemic myocardial blood flows (MBFs) and myocardial flow reserve in healthy human volunteers. Estimates of MBF in healthy volunteers at rest and during pharmacologically induced hyperemia and myocardial flow reserves as reported in several investigations [10,40,46, 51–57]. ATP—adenosine triphosphate; NR—no ratio.

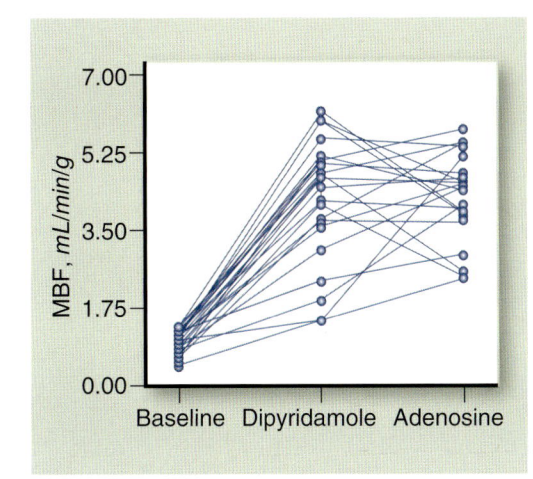

Figure 4-23. Pharmacologic stress and myocardial hyperemia. Vascular smooth muscle–relaxing agents like adenosine (140 µg/min/kg body weight intravenously) or dipyridamole (0.56 mg/kg body weight infused intravenously over 4 minutes) are used for inducing myocardial hyperemia. Both agents induce comparable levels of hyperemic flows as shown in 20 young healthy volunteers [56]. Although the mean group values are virtually identical for both hyperemic agents, individual responses greatly vary between the two vasodilator agents and, further, between individuals. Similar individual variations in the hyperemic flow response to adenosine or papaverine have been observed with independent invasive techniques (eg, intracoronary flow velocity probes) [58]. MBF—myocardial blood flow.

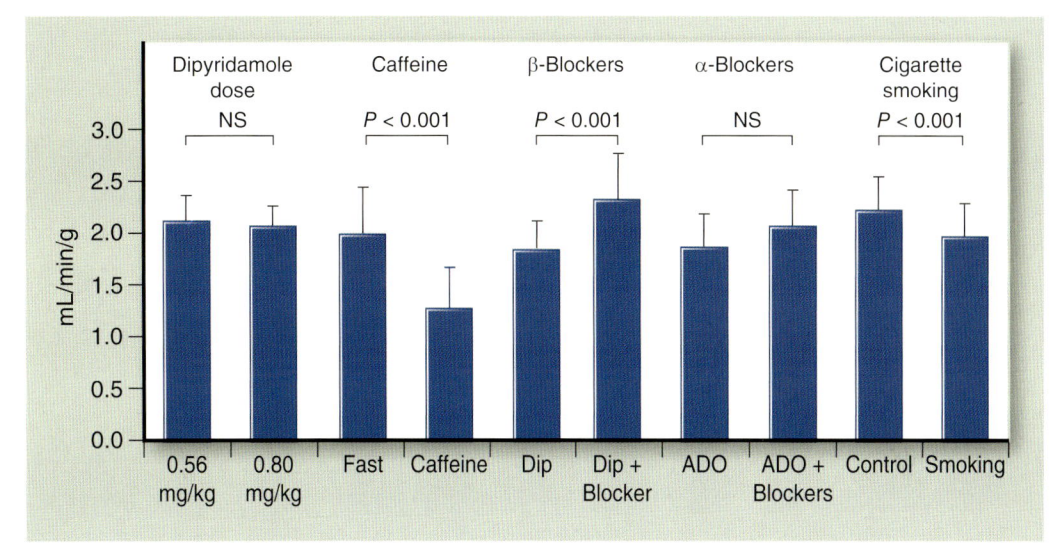

Figure 4-24. Determinants of pharmacologically induced hyperemia. Possible determinants of interindividual variations in the response of myocardial blood flow (MBF) to adenosine (ADO)- or dipyridamole (Dip)-stimulated vasodilation have been explored in several investigations. As depicted by the first two bars on the *left*, standard-dose dipyridamole infusion (0.56 mg/kg body weight) produces a maximum flow response because higher doses (*eg*, 0.80 mg/kg) did not produce higher flows. Caffeine significantly reduces the hyperemic flow response; dipyridamole flows were 35% lower after caffeine intake as compared with those after abstention from caffeine for 24 hours [59]. Indeed, the degree of attenuation of hyperemic blood flow correlates inversely with plasma caffeine concentrations. Adenosine- or dipyridamole-stimulated hyperemia was further augmented by administration of β-adrenergic blockers but not by α-adrenergic receptor blockers [36,60] while, as expected, β$_2$-adrenoreceptor stimulation with intravenous dobutamine raised MBF in a dose-dependent manner and in proportion to cardiac work as defined again by the rate pressure product [43,56,61]. Co-injection of atropine was found to augment dobutamine-induced hyperemia by as much as 36% so that hyperemic MBFs exceeded those observed in the same study after dipyridamole [54]. Further, cigarette smoking during dipyridamole-induced hyperemia significantly reduces the level of hyperemic blood flows, possibly due to an α-adrenergically mediated vasoconstriction [23]. NS—not significant.

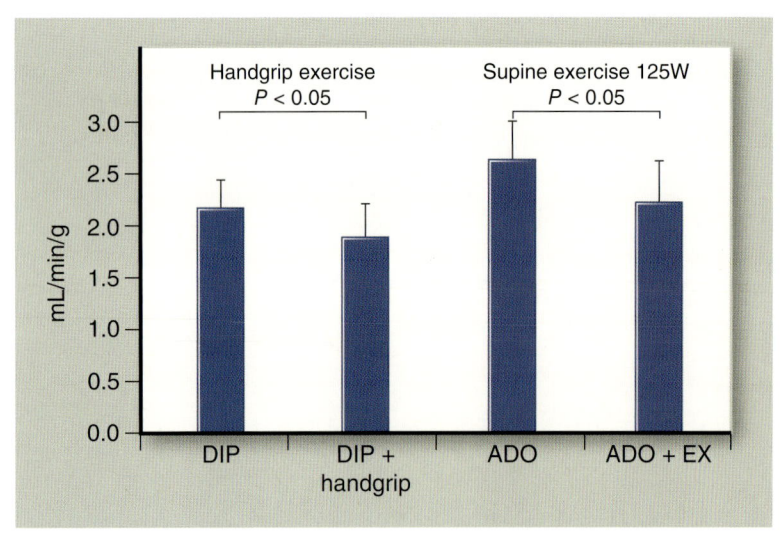

Figure 4-25. Coronary driving pressure and hyperemic myocardial blood flow. Increases in coronary perfusion pressures induced by either sustained handgrip or supine bicycle exercise lowered dipyridamole (DIP)-stimulated blood flows [23,62]. With handgrip, systolic arterial blood pressure rose from 123 ± 8 mm Hg to 147 ± 10 mm Hg and during supine exercise from 125 ± 17 mm Hg to 186 ± 24 mm Hg. Although unexpected, the decline in blood flow most likely resulted from an increase in extravascular resistive forces due to higher systolic blood pressures and heart rates associated with physical exercise. ADO—adenosine.

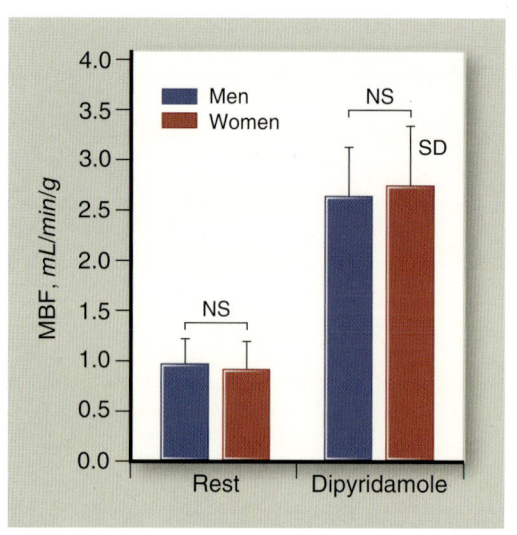

Figure 4-26. Gender and myocardial blood flow (MBF). Average MBFs at rest and during dipyridamole-stimulated hyperemia in 11 healthy males and 11 healthy females [40]. Heart rate, systolic and diastolic blood pressure, and the rate pressure product were similar for the two groups of comparable age. NS—not significant; SD—standard deviation.

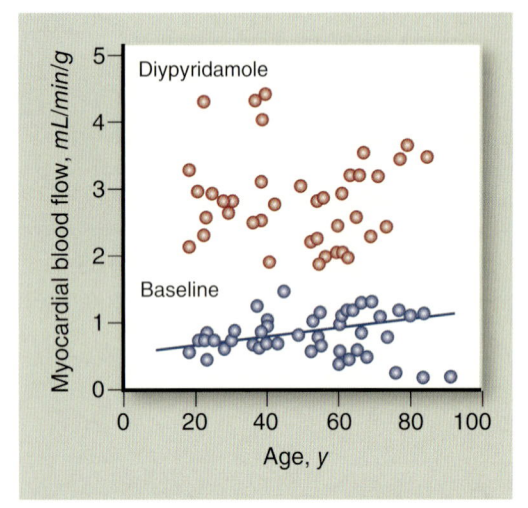

Figure 4-27. Age and myocardial blood flow (MBF) and myocardial flow reserve. MBFs both at rest (*blue*) and during dipyridamole-stimulated hyperemia (*red*) are plotted as a function of age [40]. MBFs at rest progressively increase with age. In this study, cardiac work as defined by the rate pressure product ([RPP] = heart rate × systolic blood pressure) similarly increased with age so that the age dependency of MBF appears most likely explained by an age-dependent increase in cardiac work. However, dipyridamole-stimulated hyperemic blood flows were independent of age in this study.

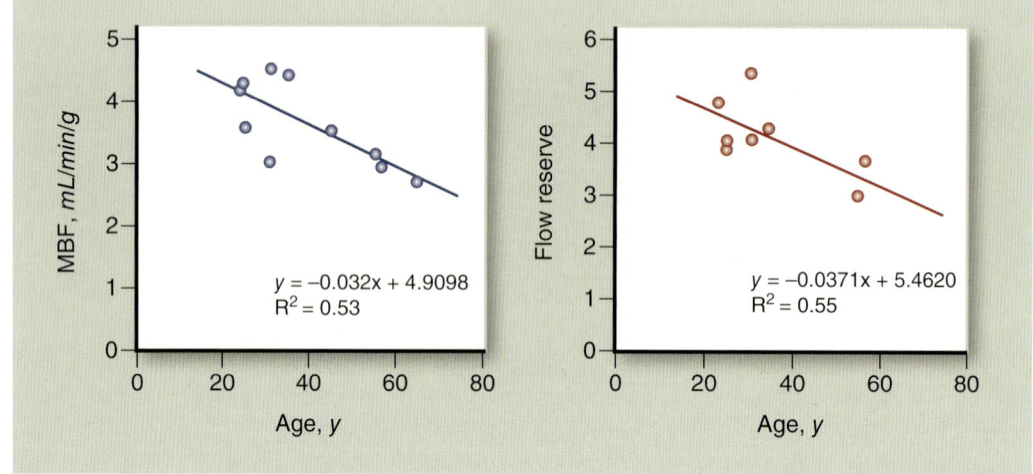

Figure 4-28. Hyperemic myocardial blood flow (MBF) and flow reserve and age. Studies in healthy volunteers report age-related differences in MBFs both at rest and during pharmacologically induced hyperemia and in the myocardial flow reserve. Average values of MBF in several studies are plotted here against age [10,40,46,52,55,56,63,64]. Lower myocardial flow reserves in older, healthy volunteers are attributed by some investigators to higher myocardial flows at rest, whereas others again noticed diminished hyperemic MBFs and, thus, an age-related attenuation of the coronary vasodilator capacity.

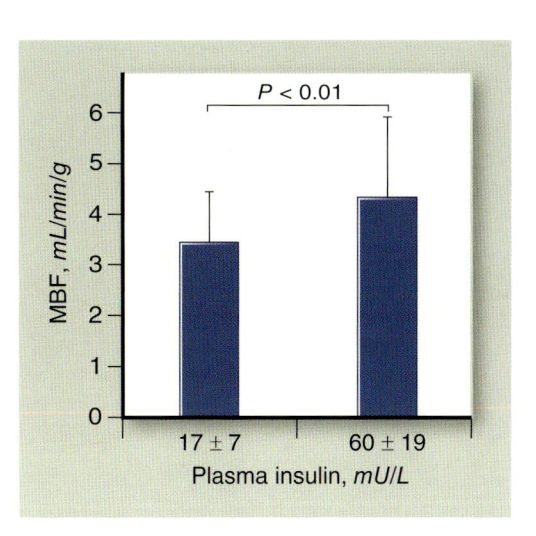

Figure 4-29. Insulin and pharmacologically induced hyperemic myocardial blood flows (MBFs). MBF during pharmacologic vasodilation also depends on plasma insulin concentrations. For example, in 16 healthy volunteers, MBF during standard-dose adenosine infusion was significantly higher during the euglycemic–hyperinsulinemic clamp, which raised plasma insulin concentrations from 17 ± 7 mU/L to 60 ± 19 mU/L, whereas plasma glucose levels remained essentially unchanged [65]. The effect of insulin on hyperemic MBF appears dose dependent as indicated in another study in healthy males with supraphysiological insulin plasma concentrations [64].

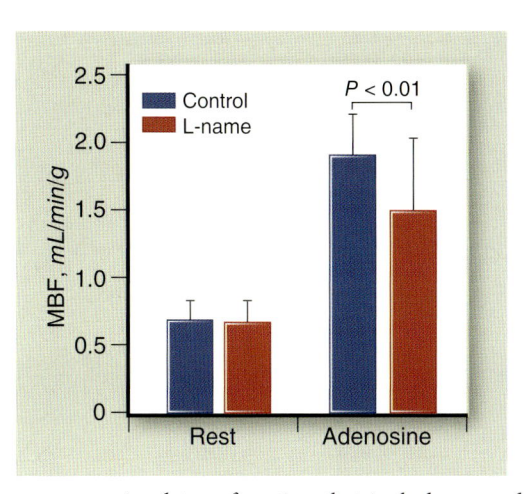

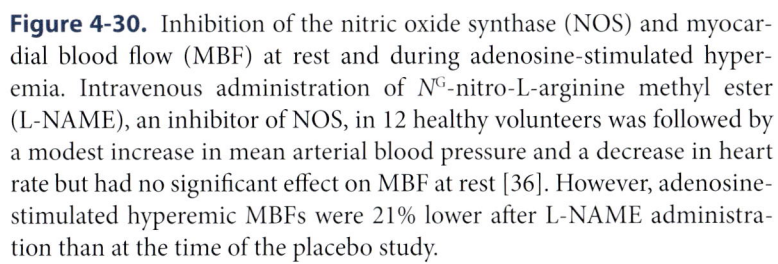

Figure 4-30. Inhibition of the nitric oxide synthase (NOS) and myocardial blood flow (MBF) at rest and during adenosine-stimulated hyperemia. Intravenous administration of N^G-nitro-L-arginine methyl ester (L-NAME), an inhibitor of NOS, in 12 healthy volunteers was followed by a modest increase in mean arterial blood pressure and a decrease in heart rate but had no significant effect on MBF at rest [36]. However, adenosine-stimulated hyperemic MBFs were 21% lower after L-NAME administration than at the time of the placebo study.

Increases in MBF in response to dipyridamole, adenosine, or adenosine triphosphate are related to a decrease in the resistance to flow at the site of the coronary arteriolar vessels. Because the hyperemic flow increases are induced by pharmacologic agents that mediate the relaxation of vascular smooth muscle cells, the resulting increase in hyperemic flow is regarded as a predominantly endothelium-independent flow response. The findings shown in this figure suggest that shear-sensitive components of the endothelium contribute to the total hyperemic response through a flow-related coronary vasodilation. The hyperemic flow response to pharmacologically induced vasodilation can therefore be considered a measure of integrated coronary circulatory function that includes a predominantly endothelium-independent flow increase that is amended by a shear-sensitive and flow-related coronary vasodilation. This contributes about 21% to 25% to the overall hyperemic increase in MBF [35,36].

Probing Coronary Endothelial Function Through Measurements of Myocardial Blood Flow Responses to Sympathetic Stimulation

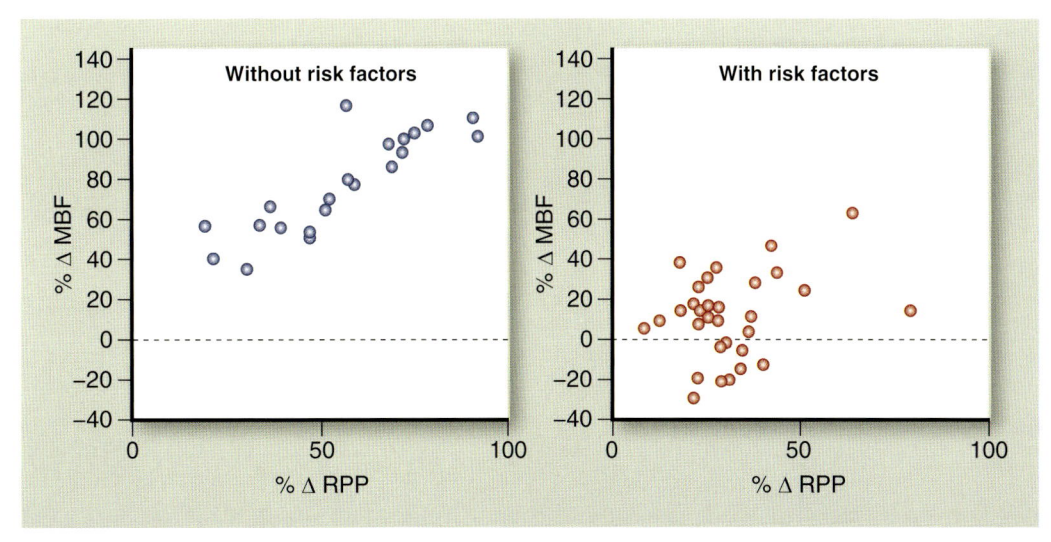

Figure 4-31. Cold pressor–induced increases in cardiac work and responses of myocardial blood flow (MBF). Sympathetic stimulation by exposure to cold (immersion of a hand or foot in a slush of ice water) prompts an increase in heart rate and systolic blood pressure and thus the rate pressure product (RPP). Under normal conditions, the adrenergically mediated increase in cardiac work (defined here as %ΔRPP) is associated with a proportionate, metabolically mediated increase in coronary flow and thus in MBF (defined here as %ΔMBF) [66]. Thus, the normal relationship between cardiac work and MBF is maintained ($y = 0.96x + 19.9$). In individuals with risk factors for coronary artery disease (CAD) or with CAD, the response of MBF to cold pressor testing (CPT) can be significantly attenuated, be absent, or even be paradoxical (*ie*, blood flow actually declines). Thus, in the presence of risk factors for CAD or CAD, the normal blood flow to cardiac work relationship is no longer maintained ($y = 0.36x + 0.10$) [66]. NS—not significant.

PET Perfusion Tracers: Quantitation of Myocardial Blood Flow

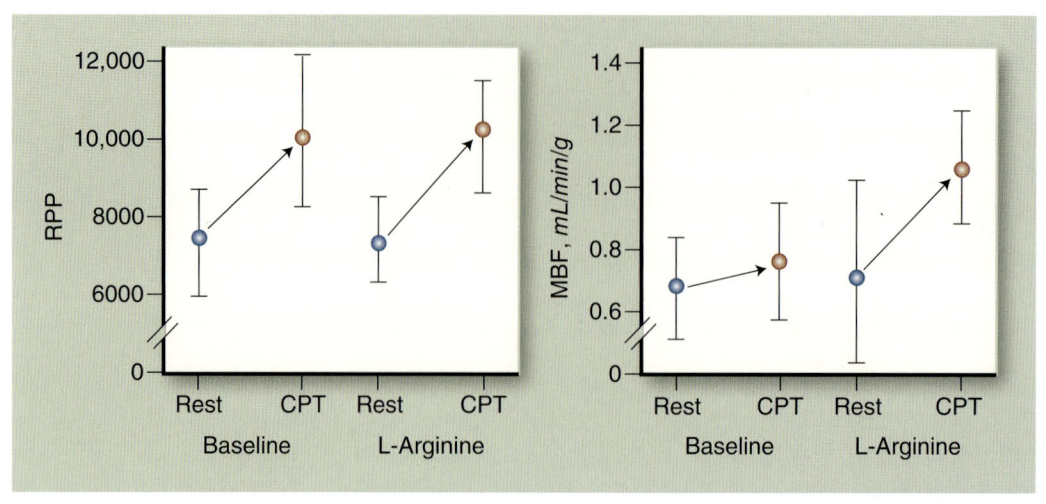

Figure 4-32. Effects of L-arginine as the substrate for nitric oxide synthase (NOS) on the response of myocardial blood flow (MBF) to cold pressor testing (CPT) in long-term smokers. In long-term smokers, MBF failed to increase significantly from rest to CPT despite a significant increase in rate pressure product (RPP). Intravenous administration of L-arginine as the substrate of the endothelial NOS reaction normalizes the response of MBF to CPT without affecting blood flows in an age-matched group of nonsmokers (not shown) [67]. Different from baseline, MBF increased by about 50% after L-arginine and thus, in proportion to the increase in the RPP. The normalization of the flow response after L-arginine implicates endothelial dysfunction and, consequently, diminished nitric oxide bioactivity as a possible reason for the abnormal flow response in long-term smokers. Whether such normalization resulted directly from an increase in nitric oxide synthesis, indirectly by competition of L-arginine with the NOS inhibitor asymmetric dimethyl arginine, or because plasma insulin levels increased during the L-arginine infusion were mediated through insulin remains uncertain.

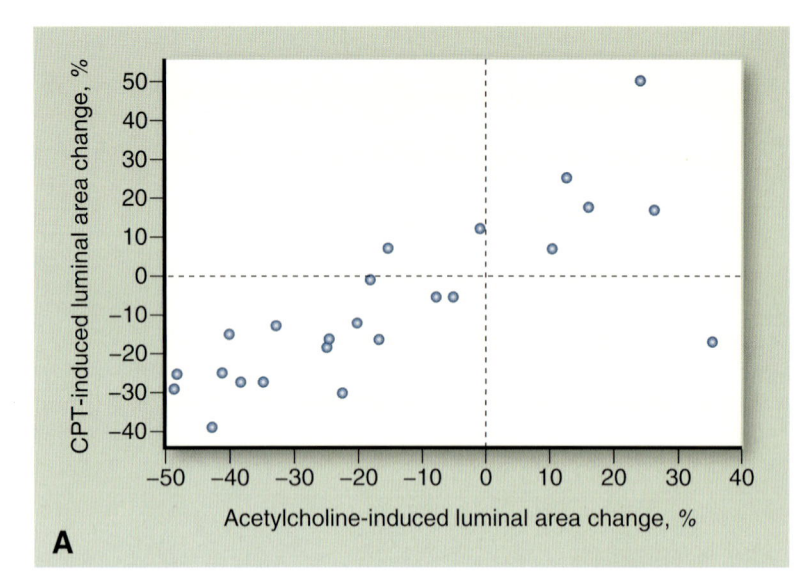

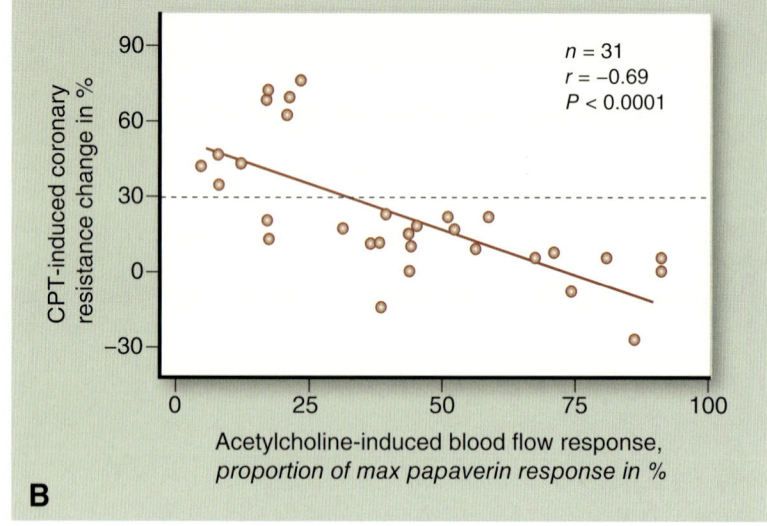

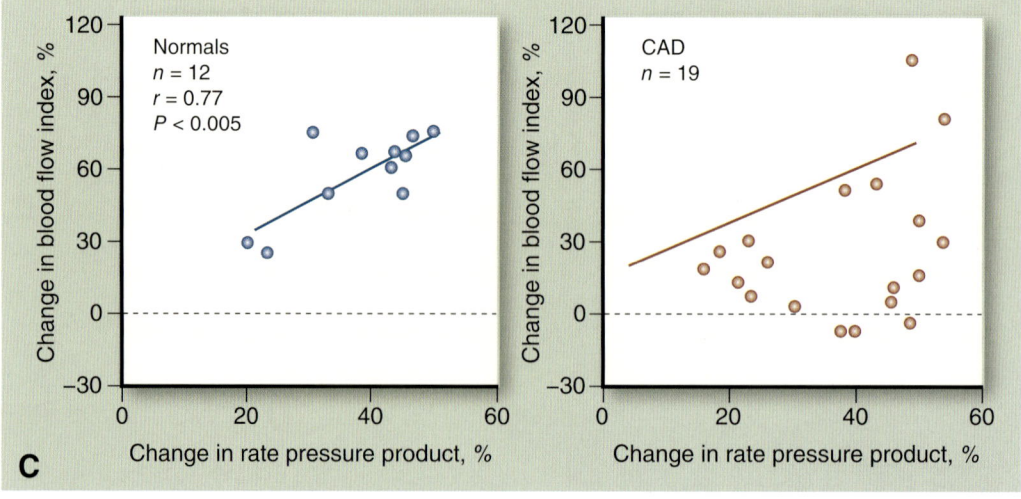

Figure 4-33. Coronary flow responses to cold pressor testing (CPT) as a measure of coronary endothelial function. The adrenergically mediated response of the coronary circulation to cold parallels several features linked directly to stimulation of the coronary endothelium as determined through invasive measurements. For example, increases in coronary flow associated with exposure to cold lead to a flow-dependent dilation of the coronary conductance vessels in the normal circulation. In abnormal states, this flow-dependent dilation is diminished or absent or paradoxical vasoconstriction may occur. These changes and their magnitude correlate directly with those evoked by intracoronary injection of acetylcholine or the flow-dependent, nitric oxide–mediated dilation of the conduit vessel in response to injections of papaverine or adenosine into the distal coronary circulation (**A**) [68]. Secondly, acetylcholine stimulation raises flow in the normal coronary circulation whereas flow responses in the presence of risk factors are diminished or even absent or flow may even decline. Again, flow responses elicited by cold correlate with those in response to intracoronary acetylcholine stimulation (**B**) [69]. Finally, directly measured coronary flows increase in the normal coronary circulation in direct proportion to the increase in the rate pressure product (**C**). In abnormal states, however, responses in coronary blood flow to cold no longer correspond to changes in rate pressure product; as shown in *red*, flow may increase only modestly, remain unchanged, or even decline in response to cold. The invasively determined flow responses to CPT as depicted in **C** are similar to those observed noninvasively with PET measurements of myocardial blood flow (*see* Fig. 4-27). CAD—coronary artery disease.

92 Atlas of Nuclear Cardiology

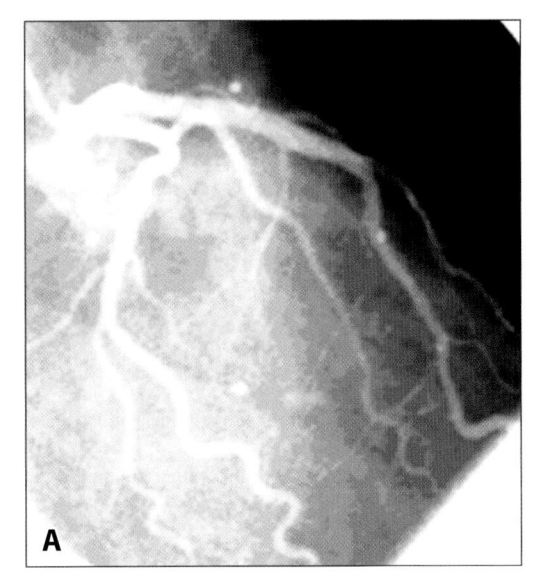

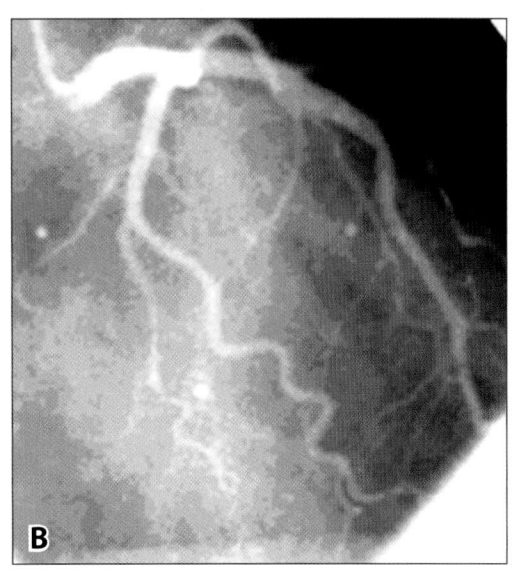

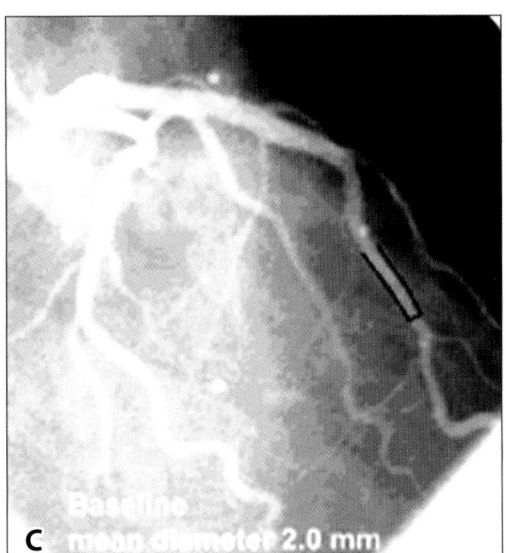

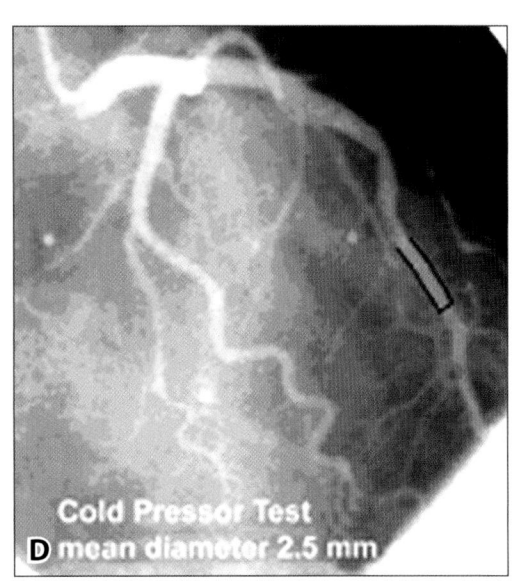

Figure 4-34. Angiographic visualization of normal changes in coronary artery diameter during cold pressor testing (CPT). Exposure to cold leads to a metabolically induced increase in coronary blood flow that is associated in the normal coronary circulation with a flow-related and endothelium-mediated vasodilation [66]. The angiogram of the normal left coronary arteries in the right anterior oblique projection at baseline (**A**) and during CPT (**B**). **C** and **D**, The same angiograms showing the measurements of conduit vessel diameter. At baseline (**C**), the mean diameter was 2.0 mm and increased during CPT (**D**) to 2.5 mm. On PET measurements performed several days later, myocardial blood flow was 0.78 mL/min/g at rest and increased to 1.36 mL/min/g with CPT [66], denoting normal coronary endothelial function. (*From* Schindler *et al.* [66].)

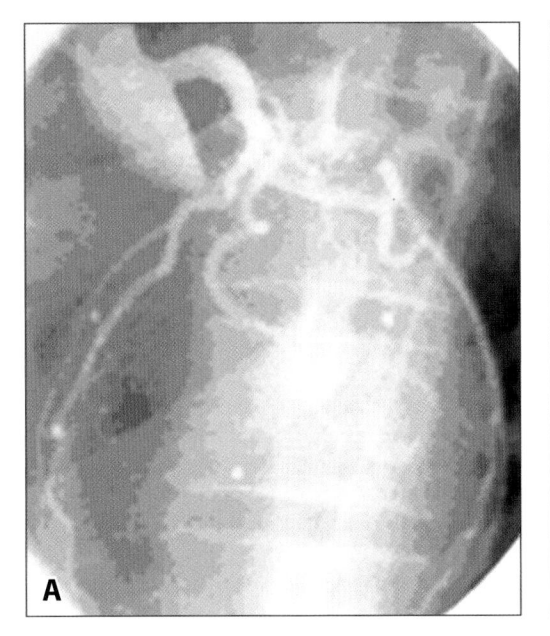

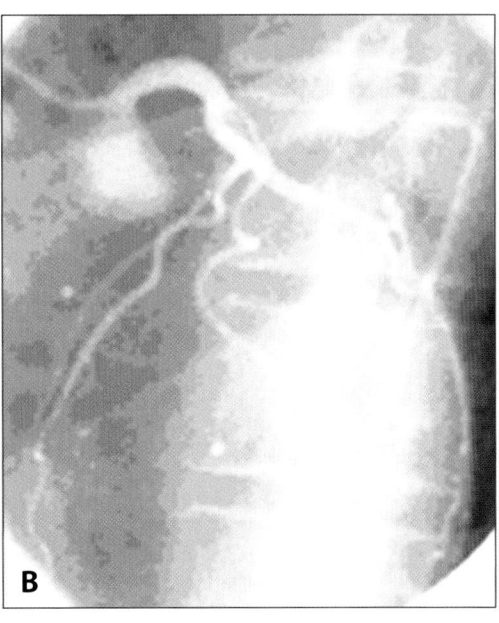

Figure 4-35. Angiographic demonstration of abnormal responses of coronary arterial diameters to cold pressor testing (CPT). In the presence of dysfunctional endothelium, the normal vasodilator response to CPT may be diminished or even absent [66]. The normal coronary angiograms in the left anterior oblique projection at baseline (**A**) and during CPT (**B**). Measurements of the mean diameter of the proximal to mid-segment of the left anterior descending coronary artery indicate a mean diameter of 1.89 mm at rest

Continued on the next page

PET Perfusion Tracers: Quantitation of Myocardial Blood Flow 93

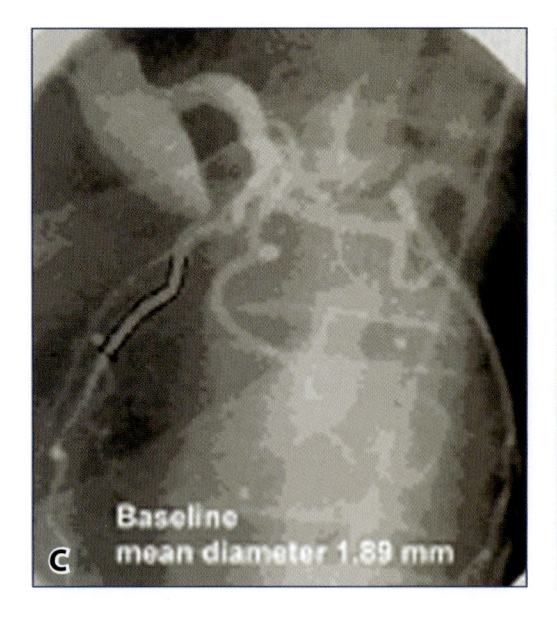

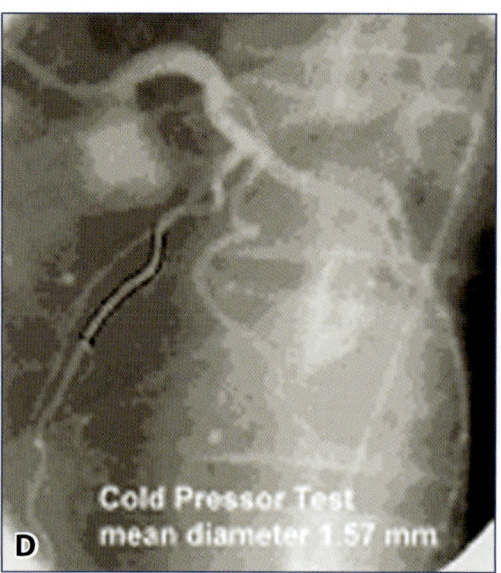

Figure 4-35. *(Continued)* (**C**) and a diameter of 1.57 mm during CPT (**D**). This decrease in the epicardial luminal area corresponded to an attenuated increase of myocardial blood flow during CPT (myocardial blood flow at rest was 0.51 mL/min/g and only 0.68 mL/min/g during CPT) and, thus, indicated coronary endothelial dysfunction. (*From* Schindler *et al.* [66].)

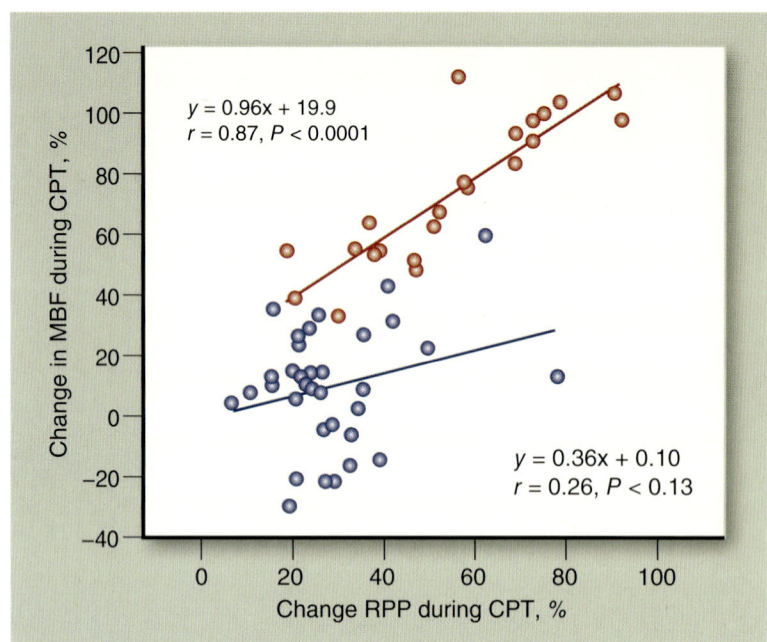

Figure 4-36. Responses of myocardial blood flow (MBF) to cold pressor testing (CPT). Increases in the rate pressure product (RPP) with CPT (defined here in percent from baseline) and changes in PET-measured responses in MBF in healthy volunteers (*blue circles*) and individuals with coronary risk factors but normal coronary angiograms (*red circles*) [66]. MBFs increased in healthy volunteers in proportion to the increase in cardiac work, indicating that the normal relation between cardiac work and thus metabolic demand, and coronary and thus MBF, was maintained. In contrast, this relationship is no longer preserved in individuals with risk factors for coronary artery disease as MBF failed to adequately increase with increases in metabolic demand (*see also* Fig. 4-27). (*Adapted from* Schindler *et al.* [66].)

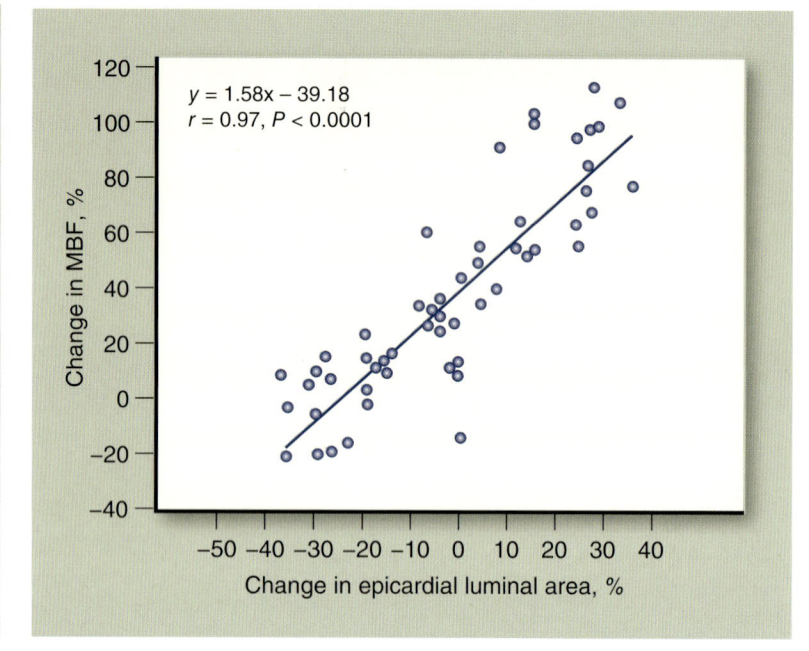

Figure 4-37. Cold pressor–induced changes in myocardial blood flow (MBF) and angiographically determined changes in the luminal area of the coronary conductance vessels. For the same study population shown in Figure 4-34, the cold-induced changes in PET-measured MBFs are compared with changes in conductance vessel diameter [66]. The significant correlation between the two parameters indicates that epicardial vasomotor function during cold pressor testing (CPT) is associated with changes in myocardial and, thus, coronary blood flow, as demonstrated in Figure 4-31 using invasive assay techniques. The correlation further indicates a close association between conductance and resistance vessel function during sympathetic stimulation that can be determined noninvasively with PET measurements of MBF. The correlation further demonstrates that the externally measured change in MBF during CPT corresponds to an established and widely accepted indicator of coronary endothelial function. (*Adapted from* Schindler *et al.* [66].)

Figure 4-38. Interaction between endothelial and vascular smooth muscle cell. Receptor-mediated (*ie*, acetylcholine) and/or receptor-independent shear stress–mediated mechanism related to changes in coronary flow velocities (stimulation of the endothelial cell leads to an increase in nitric oxide synthase [NOS] activity with increased production and release of nitric oxide [NO]) [11,70]. After diffusion of endothelial-derived NO to the vascular smooth muscle cell, guanylate cyclase is activated, with increased production of cyclic guanylate monophosphate (GMP), resulting in vascular smooth muscle relaxation and thus coronary vasodilation.

During cold pressor testing, release of norepinephrine (NE) from adrenergic neuron terminals in response to adrenergic stimulation leads to predominantly α1-adrenoreceptor–mediated vascular smooth muscle constriction. The adrenergically stimulated increase in heart rate and blood pressure and thus, in cardiac work, is associated with an increase in coronary flow velocity, mediated by dilation of the coronary due to a vasodilation of the coronary arteriolar resistance vessel via release of presumably adenosine as metabolic vasodilator. This in turn increases the shear stress–mediated greater availability of endothelial-derived NO and, consequently, vascular smooth muscle relaxation. Secondly, NE-mediated stimulation of β-adrenoreceptors of the endothelium causes release of NO. Both shear stress and adrenergically mediated NO released from the endothelial cell oppose the sympathetically mediated vascular smooth muscle constriction, so that vasodilation prevails. If the endothelium is dysfunctional, release of the vasodilating NO is diminished or even absent so that the sympathetically mediated vasoconstrictor effect on the vascular smooth muscle cell prevails and coronary and myocardial blood flow fails to increase or even declines.

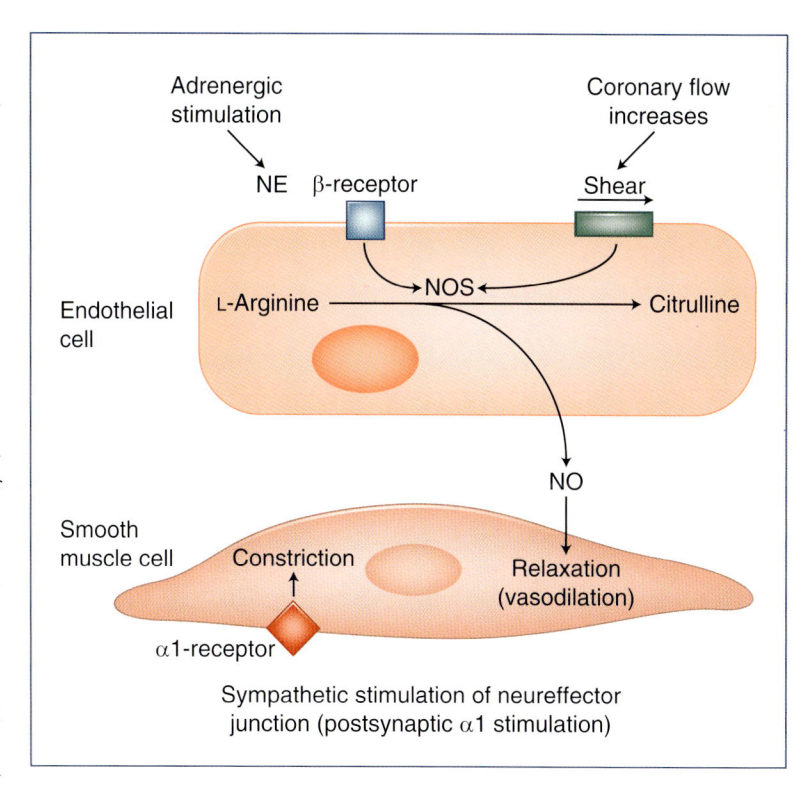

Myocardial Base-to-Apex Perfusion Heterogeneity and Epicardial Conduit Vessel Function

Information on conduit vessel function can also be obtained through comparison measurements of myocardial blood flows in the more basal and in the more apical portions of the left ventricular myocardium. On PET myocardial perfusion images, Gould *et al.* [71] had observed a progressive decrease in tracer activity from the base to the apex of the left ventricle. This gradual decrease in activity in patients without focal coronary stenosis was attributed to diffuse coronary arterial narrowing. The diffuse reduction in luminal diameter was considered to increase the resistance to coronary flow in the conductance vessel so that the intracoronary pressure (and thus, the perfusion pressure) progressively declined from proximal to distal along the epicardial coronary artery. Subsequent investigations with intracoronary pressure measurements did indeed confirm the presence of such a pressure gradient during pharmacologically induced hyperemia in epicardial coronary arteries without flow-limiting stenosis but with diffuse coronary atherosclerosis [72].

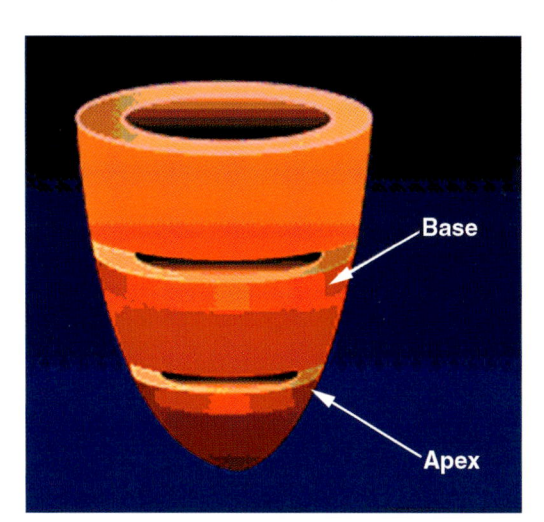

Figure 4-39. Measurements of regional myocardial blood flow in the mid-to-basal portion and the mid-to-apical portion of the left ventricular myocardium.

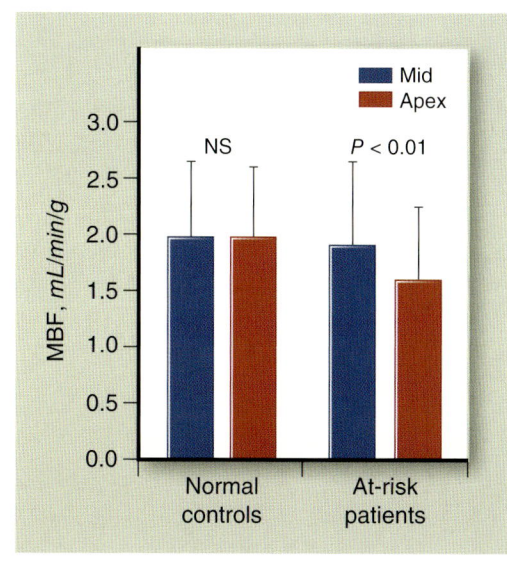

Figure 4-40. Base-to-apex myocardial perfusion at rest and during pharmacologic vasodilation. Myocardial blood flow (MBF) in the mid and apical sectors of the left ventricular myocardium at rest and during pharmacologic vasodilation in individuals with risk factors for coronary artery disease and in healthy, age-matched volunteers [73]. At rest, MBFs were similar in the mid and apical sections of the myocardium in both study groups (not shown). Dipyridamole-stimulated vasodilation in the control group produced comparable flow increases in the mid and the apical myocardium. A similar increase in MBF was observed in the mid left ventricular section in the at-risk individuals. However, hyperemic flows in the apical section of the left ventricular myocardium were significantly lower than in the mid-left ventricle. The diminished hyperemic flow response in the apical portion of the left ventricular myocardium is likely a consequence of the increased resistance to hyperemic flow rates in the epicardial conductance vessels. This increased resistance may have resulted from an inadequate flow-related dilation that may have resulted from endothelial dysfunction and/or diffuse structural changes of the coronary arterial wall. NS—not significant.

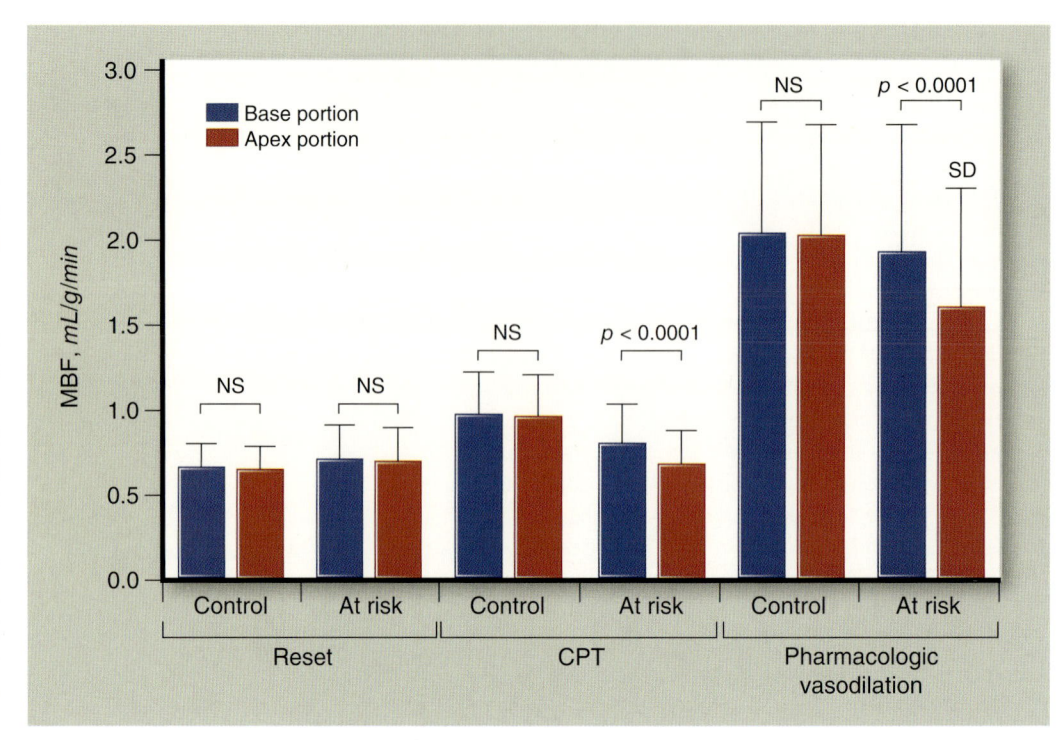

Figure 4-41. Myocardial blood flow (MBF) in the base (*blue bars*) and apex (*red bars*) portions of the left ventricle at rest, during sympathetic stimulation with cold pressor test (CPT), and during pharmacologic vasodilation in asymptomatic individuals without coronary risk factors (controls) and with coronary risk factors (at risk). In the normal controls, MBFs in the base and apex portion of the left ventricular myocardium are similar and remain similar during sympathetic stimulation with CPT and during pharmacologic vasodilation [74]. In the at-risk group, however, CPT and pharmacologic vasodilation induced a heterogeneous flow response with lesser flow increases in the apical than in the base portion of the left ventricle, reflecting a longitudinal perfusion gradient. NS—not significant; SD—standard deviation. (*Adapted from* Schindler et al. [74].)

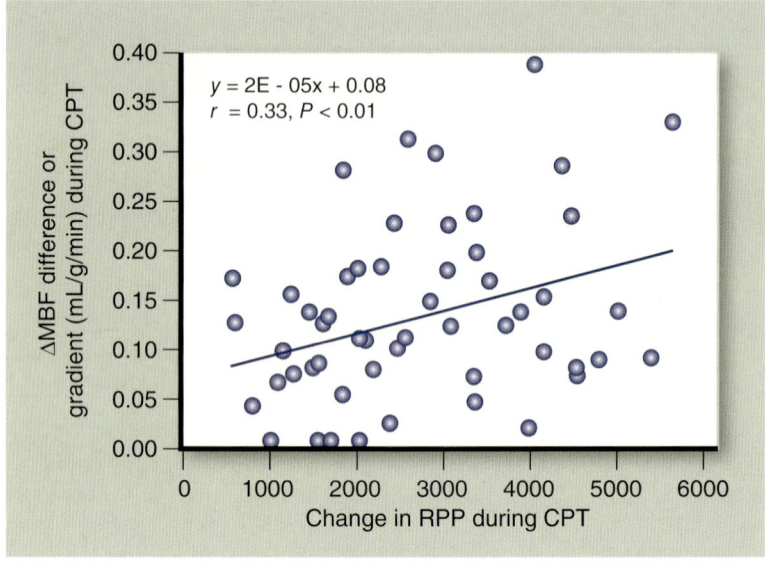

Figure 4-42. Correlation between change in myocardial blood flow (ΔMBF) difference and gradient between base and apical MBF and rate pressure product (RPP) during cold pressor testing (CPT) of the at-risk group [74]. Analogous to pharmacologic vasodilation, sympathetic stimulation with, for example CPT, leads to a longitudinal myocardial perfusion gradient in individuals with risk factors for coronary artery disease (CAD). Different from the pharmacologically stimulated flow increases, CPT elicits in individuals with coronary risk factors a markedly attenuated flow response or no increase in flow at all. Hence, the perfusion gradient cannot be explained by an inadequate dilation of the conduit vessels in response to higher coronary flows. Rather, in the absence of a flow increase, the perfusion gradient likely results from a constriction of the conduit vessels and hence, an increase in resistance to flow. CPT has been shown to cause a decrease in luminal diameter or even paradoxical vasoconstriction of the epicardial conduit vessels in individuals at risk for or with CAD [66,70,75]. If the increase in heart rate and blood pressure with CPT is related to an increase in serum norepinephrine concentrations as a measure of the degree of sympathetic stimulation [76], then an association between increases in RPP, as a noninvasive measure of sympathetic stimulation, and the MBF gradient, as a noninvasive index of epicardial vasoreactivity, should be observed. In the at-risk individuals, higher increases in the RPP during sympathetic stimulation with CPT were associated with a greater magnitude of the perfusion gradient. Thus, a longitudinal MBF or perfusion gradient as measured with PET may indeed reflect early functional and/or structural alterations of the epicardial artery as recent investigations suggest [71,73,74,77–80]. (*Adapted from* Schindler et al. [74].)

Myocardial Blood Flow in Cardiovascular Disease

Anatomical and functional alterations of the coronary circulation profoundly affect myocardial blood flow (MBF) at rest and, even more so, during pharmacologically induced hyperemia. Hyperemic MBFs are markedly attenuated distal to fluid-dynamically significant coronary stenoses. Coronary risk factors including a family history of premature coronary artery disease, hypercholesterolemia, insulin resistance and diabetes, and hypertension may also be associated with an attenuated total vasodilator capacity. The total vasodilator capacity may still be preserved normal in long-term smokers while flow responses to cold as an indicator of the predominantly endothelium-mediated coronary vasomotor function can already be impaired [67,81]. Cardiovascular conditioning and cholesterol lowering improve the total coronary vasomotor function, an effect that can be demonstrated noninvasively through measurements of MBF. Importantly, abnormal flow responses to pharmacologic vasodilation or to sympathetic stimulation contain independent prognostic information on future cardiovascular events [6,18].

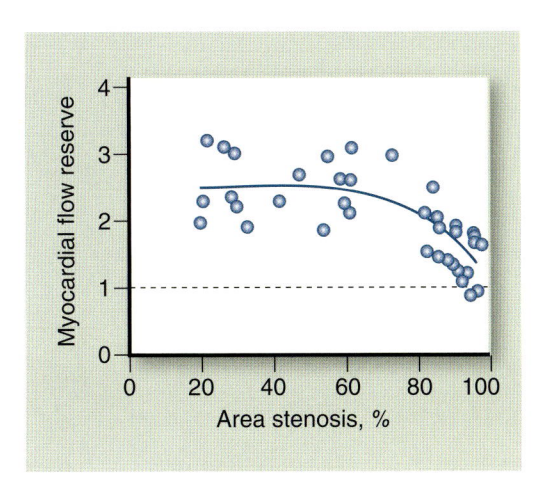

Figure 4-43. Angiographic coronary stenoses and myocardial blood flow (MBF). Comparison between stenosis severity defined as percent cross-sectional area reduction on quantitative angiography and the myocardial flow reserve as examined in 18 patients with coronary artery disease through measurements of regional MBF at rest and during dipyridamole-stimulated hyperemia [28]. The curvilinear correlation is similar to the one observed in chronically instrumented dogs with idealized coronary stenosis [82]. Other investigations report similar reductions in hyperemic flows in the stenosis-dependent myocardial regions [29,30].

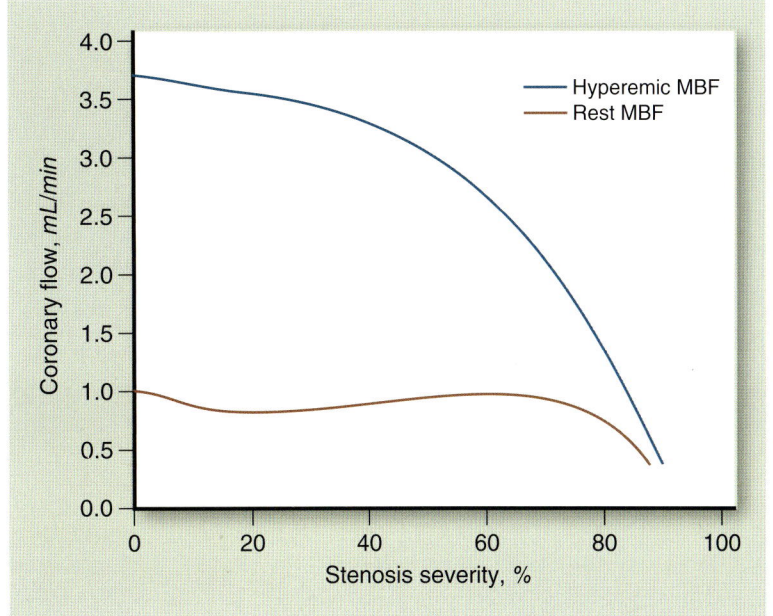

Figure 4-44. Classic correlation between coronary stenosis severity and coronary blood flow velocities in dog experiments. Coronary blood flow in canine hearts was measured at rest and during contrast-induced hyperemia with coronary flow velocity probes. Stenosis severity was determined by quantitative angiography [82]. The findings in human coronary artery disease (shown in Fig. 4-39) confirm the coronary flow–coronary stenosis relationship as established in the experimental animal. Additional clinical studies with PET in patients have reported similar reductions in hyperemic blood in stenosis-dependent myocardium but failed to find a similar curvilinear correlation, most likely because this relationship was observed only for myocardium without collateral blood flow or without prior myocardial infarction and only after vessels with stenosis in series were excluded [29,30]. MBF—myocardial blood flow.

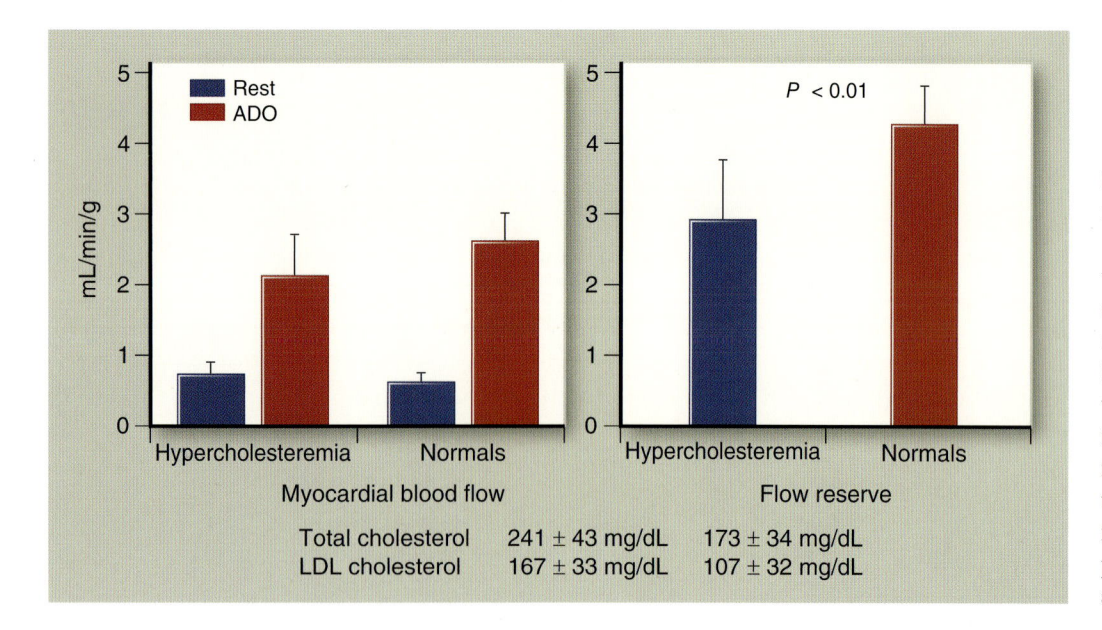

Figure 4-45. Diminished hyperemic blood flows in patients with coronary risk factors. In 16 middle-aged males (49.0 ± 0.5 years of age) with elevated plasma cholesterol levels but without clinical evidence of coronary artery disease, myocardial blood flow at rest was similar to that in an age-matched group of healthy subjects without coronary risk factors. However, during adenosine-induced hyperemia, myocardial flows tended to be lower in the at-risk than in the control group. Importantly, the myocardial flow reserve was significantly lower in the at-risk patients than in normal controls [83]. ADO—adenosine; LDL—low-density lipoprotein.

Reduced Vasodilator Capacity in Patients With Risk Factors but Without Angiographic Coronary Artery Disease

	Patients			Controls				
Study	n	Rest MBF, mL/min/g	Stress MBF, mL/min/g	n	Rest MBF, mL/min/g	Stress MBF, mL/min/g	Difference, %	P value
Dayanikli et al. [83]	16	0.76 ± 0.19	2.18 ± 0.56	11	0.66 ± 0.09	2.84 ± 0.39	-17	< 0.001
Pitkanen et al. [52]	15	0.92 ± 0.24	3.19 ± 1.59	20	0.83 ± 0.13	4.49 ± 1.27	-29	< 0.01
Yokoyama et al. [84]	11 (FH)	0.70 ± 0.21	2.10 ± 0.71	11	0.75 ± 0.35	3.22 ± 1.64	-35	< 0.01
	11 (SH)	0.81 ± 0.31	1.29 ± 0.19				-60	< 0.01
Pitkanen et al. [85]	21	0.79 ± 0.19	3.54 ± 1.59	21	0.88 ± 0.20	4.54 ± 1.17	-22	< 0.025

Figure 4-46. Reduced vasodilator capacity in patients with risk factors but without angiographic coronary artery disease. Rest and hyperemic myocardial blood flow (MBF) in patients without coronary artery disease but with coronary risk factor [52,83–85]. FH—familial hypercholesterolemia; SH—secondary hypercholesterolemia.

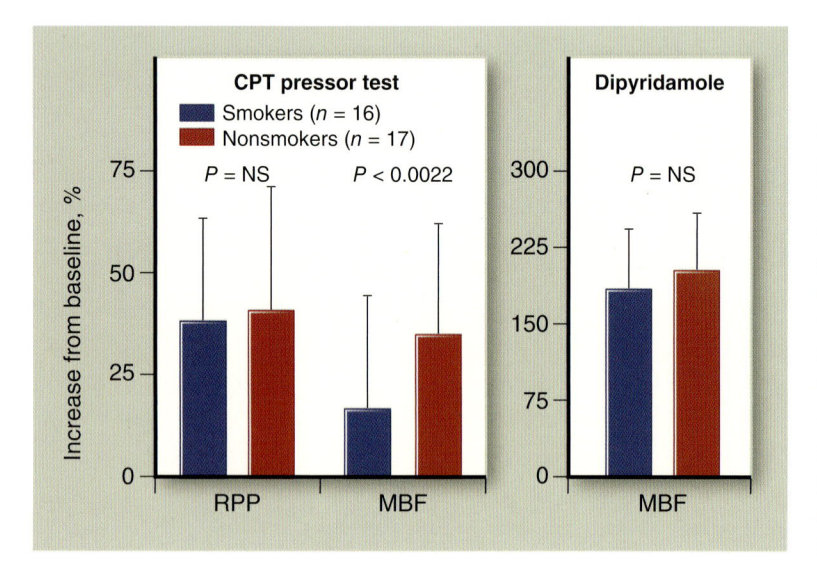

Figure 4-47. Coronary vasomotion in long-term smokers. In long-term smokers without clinical evidence of cardiovascular disease, myocardial blood flow (MBF) both at rest and during dipyridamole-induced hyperemia (shown on the *right*) was similar to that in an age-matched control group of nonsmokers and thus considered to be normal [23]. Because of adverse effects of nicotine and smoking byproducts on the endothelium, the response of MBF to cold pressor testing (CPT) as a means for more selectively examining or evaluating endothelial function was measured. CPT led to a prompt increase in heart rate and systolic blood pressure and thus the rate pressure product (RPP) in both study groups (by approximately 40%–50%). In the age-matched group of nonsmokers, MBF rose in proportion to the increase in cardiac work but not in the long-term smokers despite a normal increase in the RPP, suggesting a smoking-related impairment in coronary endothelial function. NS—not significant.

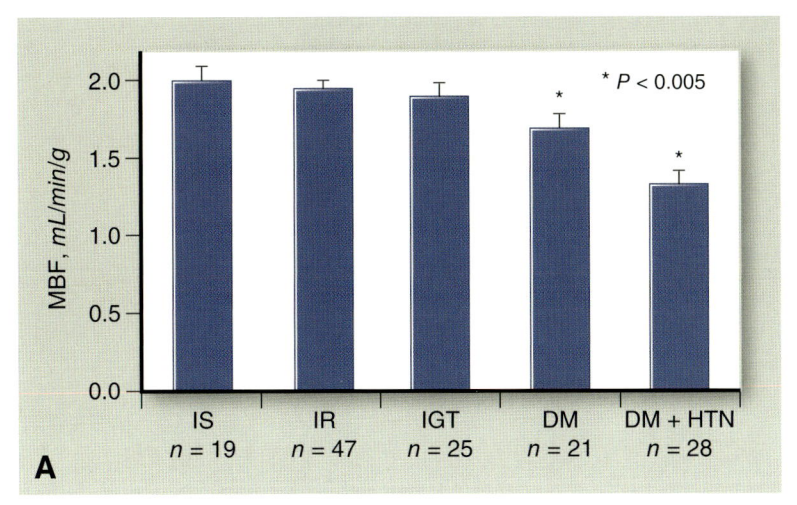

Figure 4-48. A and B, Insulin-resistant states of progressive severity and coronary vasomotor function. Responses of myocardial blood flow (MBF) to cold pressor testing (CPT) (defined as a change in MBF in mL/min/g from rest to cold [B]) and to pharmacologic vasodilation with intravenous adenosine or dipyridamole (A) in insulin-resistant states [32]. PET measurements were obtained in 120 individuals with insulin-resistant states of increasing severity. As depicted in A, the total integrated vasodilator capacity was maintained in euglycemic states of insulin resistance but was diminished in hyperglycemic states. In contrast and as depicted in B, insulin resistance alone was associated with a markedly attenuated flow response to cold (as compared with insulin-sensitive controls) and tended to decline further with more severe states of insulin resistance. The PET-based observations in type 2 diabetic patients in this study are consistent with those by other investigators [86,87] as well as with findings by quantitative angiography and intracoronary flow velocity measurements [88,89]. DM—hyperglycemic type 2 diabetes; HTN—type 2 diabetes with arterial hypertension; IGT—impaired glucose tolerance; IR—euglycemic insulin resistant; IS—insulin-sensitive controls.

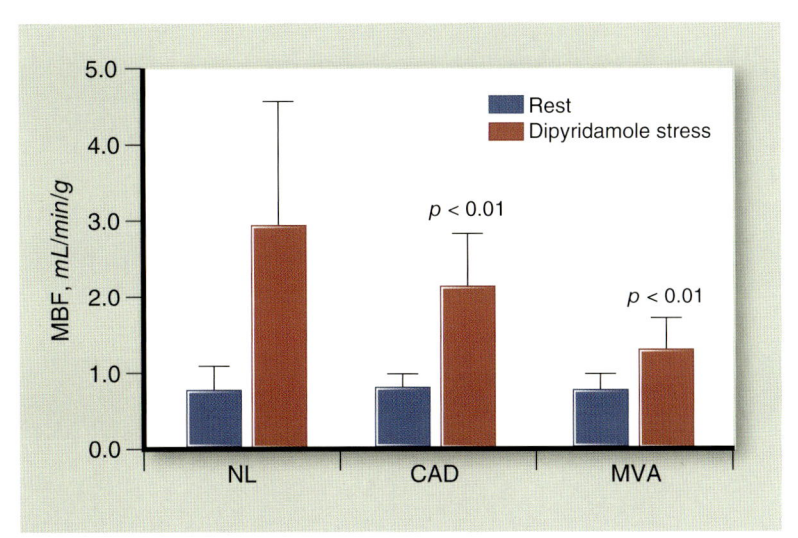

Figure 4-49. Myocardial blood flows (MBFs) at rest and during dipyridamole-induced hyperemia in normal volunteers (NL) and type 2 diabetes mellitus patients with coronary artery disease (CAD) or with microvascular angina (MVA). Resting MBFs do not differ between groups and hence, are normal in type 2 diabetes patients. In contrast, however, hyperemic MBFs are significantly diminished in diabetic patients with CAD and even more so in patients with microvascular disease [90]. (*Adapted from* Yokoyama *et al.* [90].)

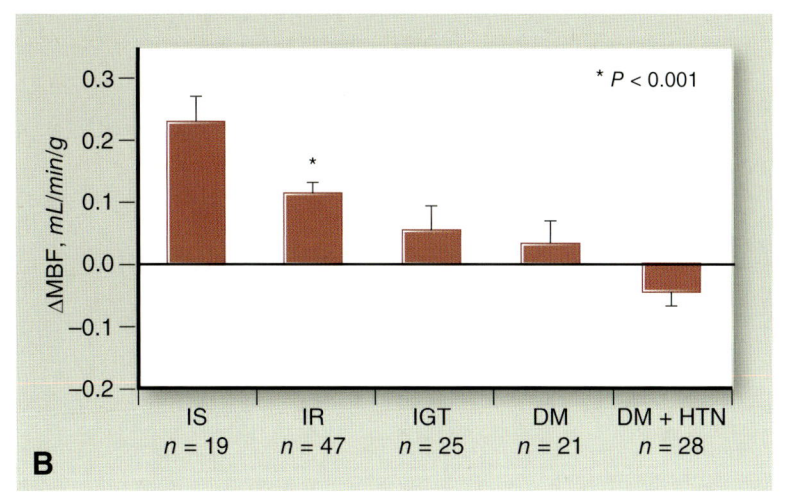

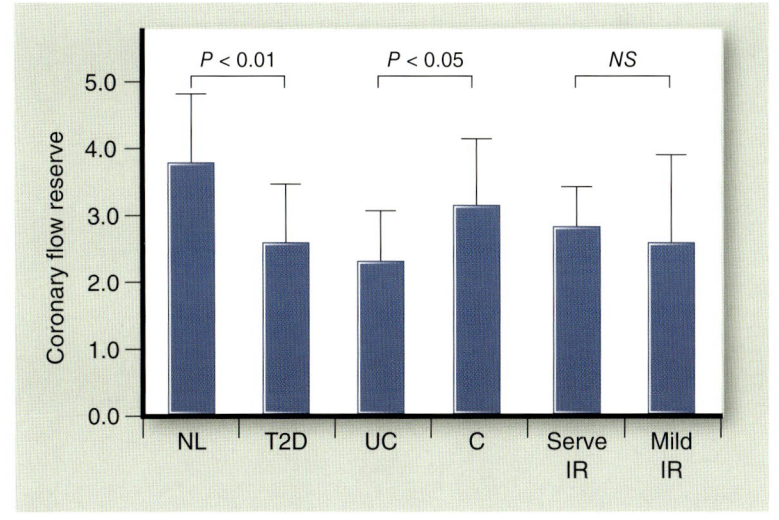

Figure 4-50. Total vasodilator capacity in patients with type 2 diabetes and effect of glycemic control. The pair of bar graphs on the *left* depict the average coronary flow reserve for 31 type 2 diabetes mellitus patients (T2D) [53]. For comparison, average values of coronary flow reserves in 16 normal age-matched control subjects (NL) are shown, indicating a significant reduction in the coronary flow reserve in type 2 diabetic patients.

The *middle* bar graphs depict the average values of the coronary flow reserve in patients with well controlled (C) and poorly controlled (UC) type 2 diabetes patients. Diabetic control was defined by glycosylated hemoglobin (HbA$_{1C}$) less than 8% as compared with poorly controlled diabetes, with an HbA$_{1C}$ greater than 8%.

The bar graphs on the *right* depict the average values of coronary flow reserves for patients grouped by severity of insulin resistance (IR) as determined from the whole body glucose disposal rate during hyperinsulinemic euglycemic clamping. The findings indicate that type 2 diabetes is associated with a significant impairment in the coronary flow reserve and thus, in the total vasodilator capacity. This impairment is related to glycemic control rather than to the severity of insulin resistance. NS—not significant. (*Adapted from* Yokoyama *et al.* [53].)

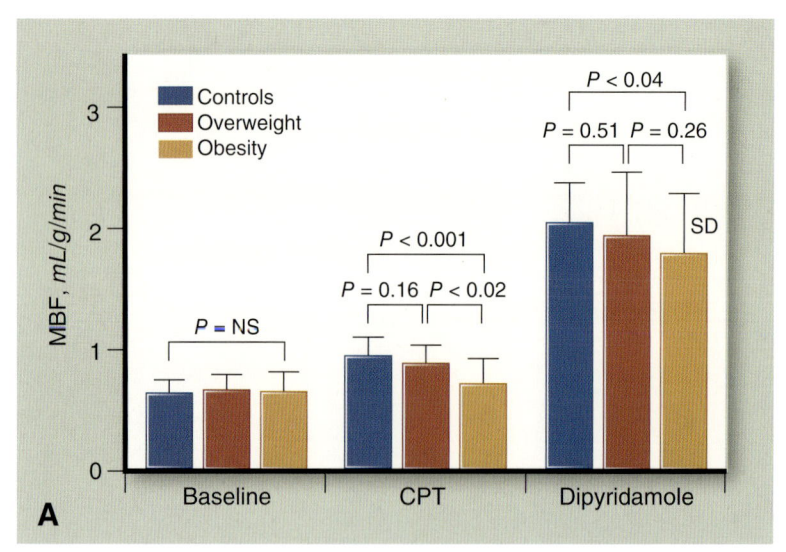

Figure 4-51. Coronary vasomotor function in overweight and obese individuals. Myocardial blood flow (MBF) at rest, during cold pressor testing (CPT), and during pharmacologic vasodilation with dipyridamole in controls (body mass index [BMI] < 25 kg/m^2), overweight (BMI ≥ 25–30 kg/m^2) patients, and obese patients (BMI > 30 kg/m^2) [19]. **A,** The dipyridamole-stimulated hyperemic MBFs tended to be lower in overweight patients than in controls, whereas it further decreased significantly in obesity. **B,** The endothelium-related MBF from rest to CPT (ΔMBF) to CPT progressively decreased from control to overweight and obesity.

The abnormality of coronary vasomotor function in individuals with increasing body weight progresses from an impairment in endothelium-related MBF responses to CPT in overweight individuals to an impairment of predominantly endothelium-independent hyperemic MBFs during pharmacologically induced vasodilation of the coronary arteriolar vessels in obese individuals (**A** and **B**). The latter findings—based on PET flow measurements in individuals with increasing body weight—agree with invasive investigations in the assessment of vasomotor function in the coronary and peripheral circulation [91,92], but extended it to a relatively young study population without traditional coronary risk factors. NS—not significant; SD—standard deviation.

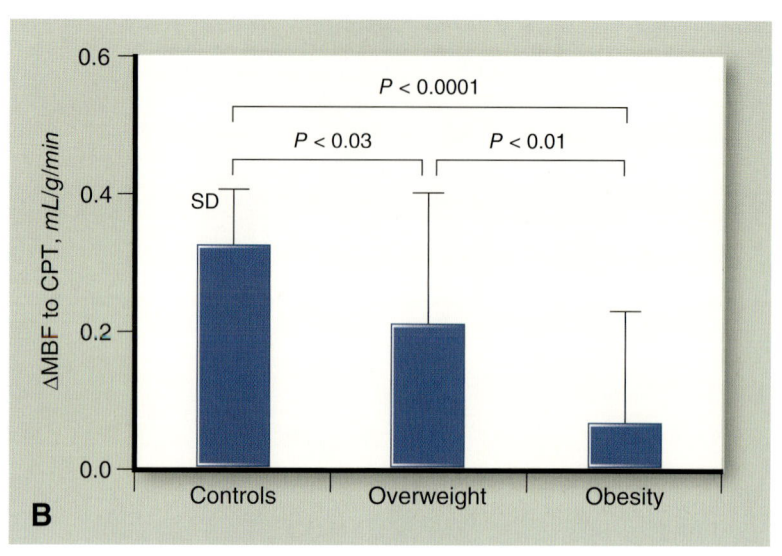

Prognostic Value of PET-Measured Myocardial Blood Flows

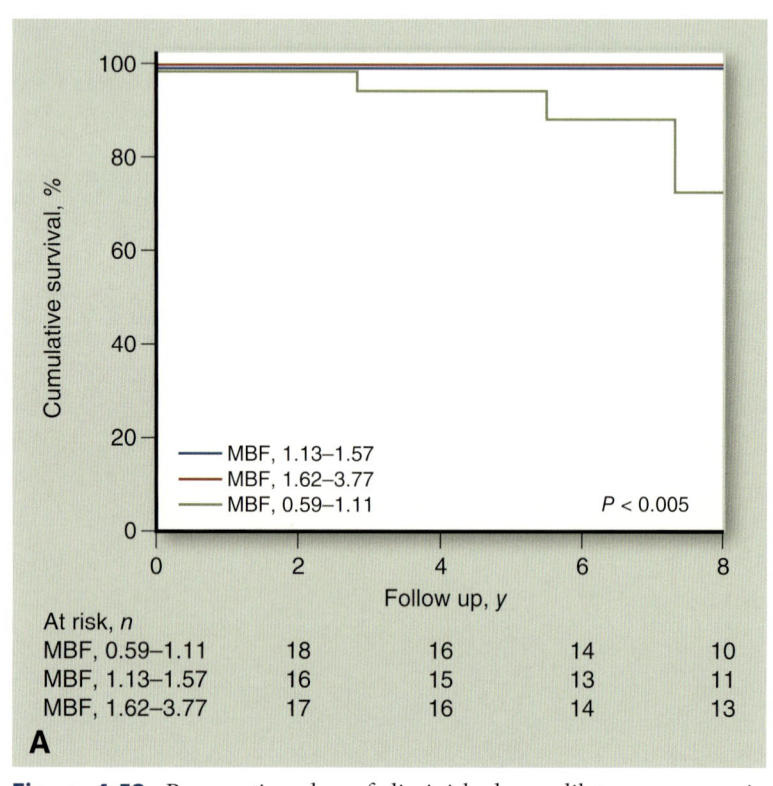

Figure 4-52. Prognostic value of diminished vasodilator responses in patients with hypertrophic cardiomyopathy. Fifty-one patients with hypertrophic cardiomyopathy were submitted to PET measurements of myocardial blood flow (MBF) at rest and during pharmacologic vasodilation and were followed for an average of 8.1 ± 2.1 years [18]. Sixteen patients had cardiovascular events including cardiovascular death, worsening of congestive heart failure symptoms, or implantation of cardioverter/defibrillator for sustained ventricular arrhythmias. Patients were grouped into three approximately equal groups according to the PET estimates of hyperemic MBFs. The overall accumulative survival (**A**) and cumulative survival free from an unfavorable outcome (**B**) were strongly associated with the level of hyperemic MBFs achieved during dipyridamole vasodilation.

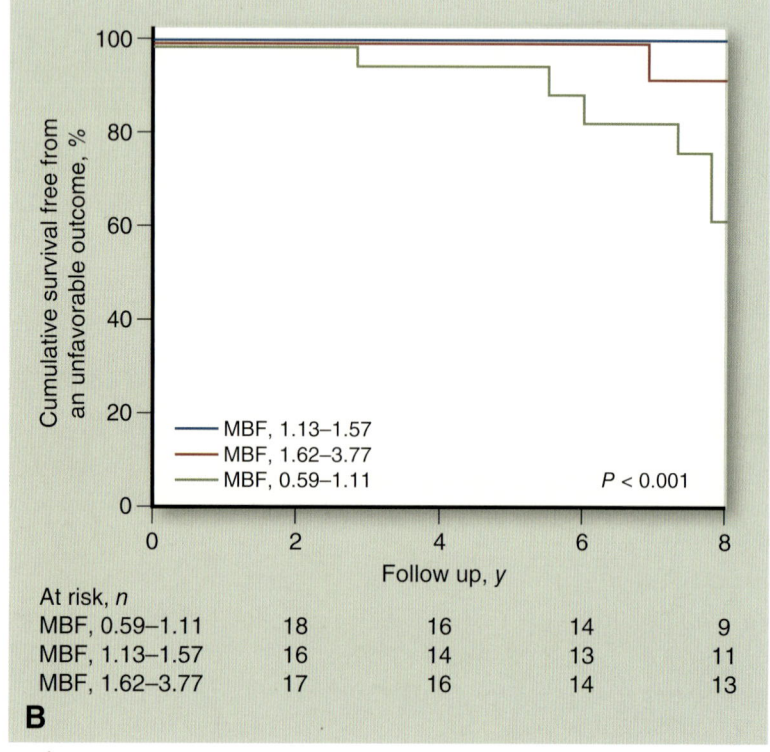

Continued on the next page

Figure 4-52. *(Continued)* The degree of microvascular dysfunction related to functional and/or structural abnormalities of the coronary microcirculation and as reflected by the diminished total vasodilator capacity on PET was thus predictive of future cardiovascular outcome. The observation made in this study with PET is consistent with earlier observations in patients with and without coronary artery disease and in which the coronary vasodilator capacity was assessed with highly invasive quantitative angiographic and flow velocity measurement approaches [2,93].

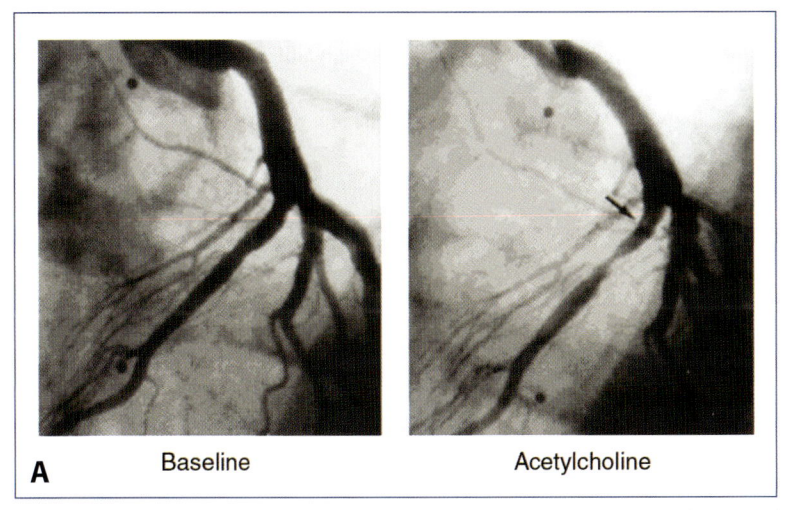

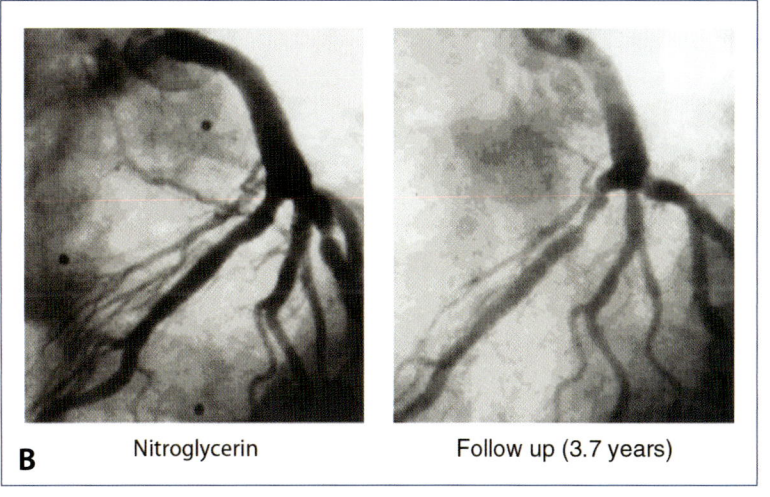

Figure 4-53. Altered coronary vasomotor function as a predictor of future cardiac events. Assessment of endothelium-dependent epicardial coronary vasomotion with intracoronary infusion of acetylcholine and stimulation of endothelial muscarinic receptors as shown by coronary angiograms. Acetylcholine stimulation caused a paradoxical constriction of the proximal left anterior descending coronary artery (*arrow* indicates the tip of the acetylcholine infusion catheter [**A**]) that was relieved by nitroglycerin administration and smooth muscle relaxation (**B**). The acetylcholine-induced vasoconstriction indicates a local reduction of the bioavailability of the atheroprotective endothelial-derived nitric oxide. A similarly diminished vasodilator or even vasoconstrictive effect to acetylcholine may also occur in the coronary arterial resistance vessels as evidenced by the diminished increase in flow velocity and thus reflects the presence of endothelial dysfunction [3–6]. Intracoronary nitroglycerin (**B**, *left*) leads to endothelium-independent vasodilation and reveals some atherosclerotic plaque formation at the site of the paradoxical vasoconstriction to acetylcholine.

During follow-up 3.7 years later, the patient was admitted to the hospital again due to an acute coronary syndrome. Coronary angiography demonstrates a distinct progression of focal atherosclerotic plaque formation (**B**, *right*) at the site of the initial paradoxical vasoconstriction to acetylcholine (**A**). (*From* Schachinger *et al.* [2].)

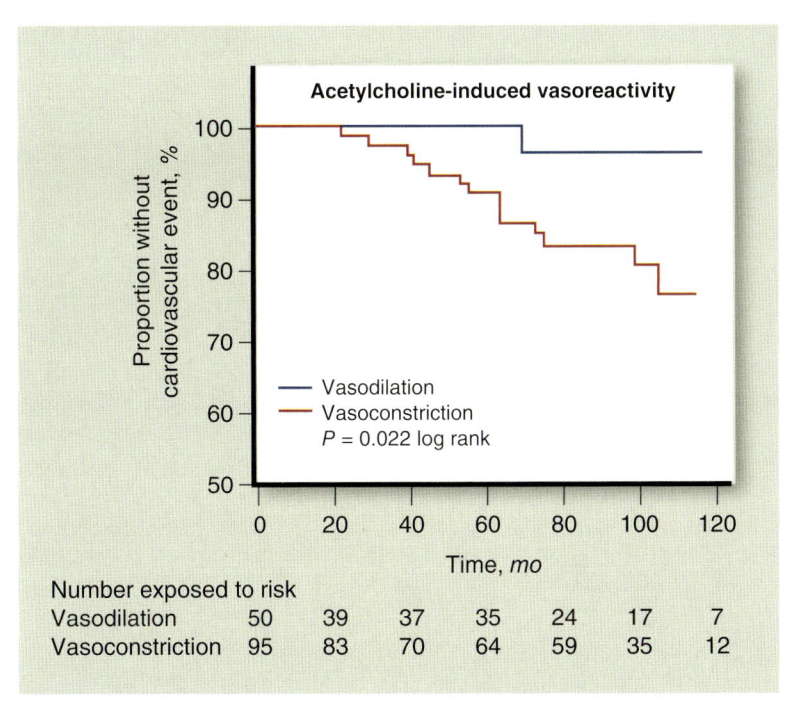

Figure 4-54. Coronary endothelial dysfunction and prediction of cardiovascular events. Kaplan-Meier analysis demonstrating a significantly higher incidence of cardiovascular events in patients without or with only minimal coronary artery disease (CAD) but with a paradoxical vasoconstriction in response to intracoronary acetylcholine [2]. Comparison is made to a group of patients with a normal vasodilator response to acetylcholine. The findings shown in this investigation are similar to those found by other investigators [2–6] and indicate endothelial dysfunction of the coronary circulation at the site of the epicardial artery and coronary arteriolar resistance vessels as an independent predictor for developing future cardiovascular events. The assessment of endothelial dysfunction of the coronary circulation therefore yields important diagnostic and prognostic information in patients without obstructive CAD.

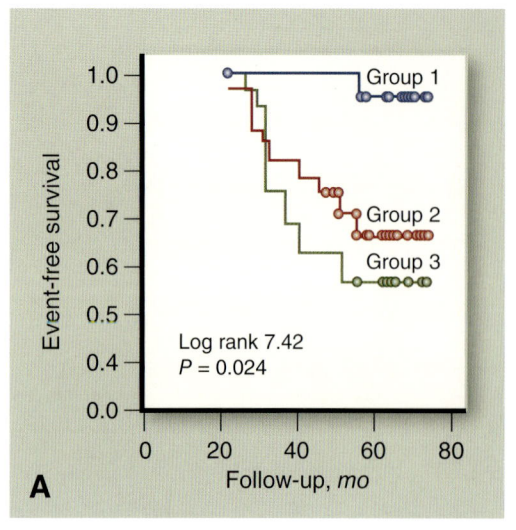

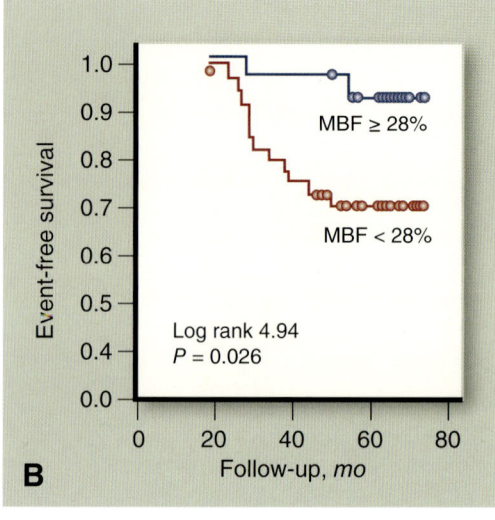

Figure 4-55. Prognostic value of PET-measured flow responses to sympathetic stimulation. Prognostic value of PET-measured, endothelium-related changes in myocardial blood flow (MBF) to cold pressor testing (CPT) (defined as percent change in MBF between rest and CPT) in patients with normal coronary angiograms [6]. **A,** Kaplan-Meier analysis demonstrates an association between the incidence of cardiovascular events and the degree of the attenuation of the flow response to CPT (group 1 with ΔMBF ≥ 40%, group 2 ΔMBF from > 0% and < 40%, group 3 with ΔMBF ≤ 0%). **B,** When patients were grouped by ΔMBF less than 28% or ΔMBF greater than 28%, again patients with a diminished flow response revealed a significantly higher incidence of cardiovascular events. The findings depicted in this figure are consistent with those by angiographic assessment of abnormal endothelium-dependent vasomotion of the coronary circulation in response to sympathetic stimulation [2,5,6,94]. They indicate the predictive value of PET-measured MBF responses during CPT for future cardiovascular events. (*Adapted from* Schindler et al. [6].)

Monitoring Effects of Risk Factor Modification and Therapeutic Interventions

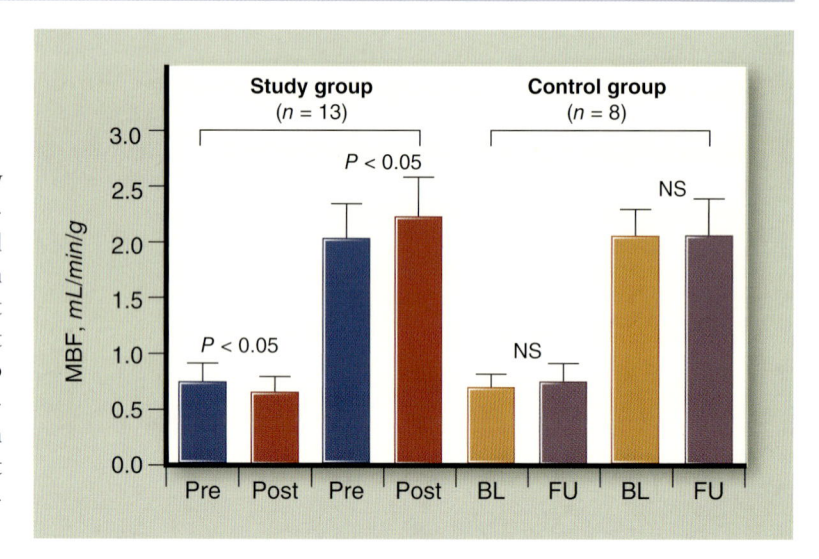

Figure 4-56. Cardiovascular conditioning and myocardial blood flow (MBF). Cardiovascular conditioning with 6 weeks of regular physical exercise, weight loss, and low-cholesterol diet significantly improves myocardial flow reserve [23]. MBF at rest decreased moderately but significantly from baseline (Pre) to treatment (Post) in the study group of 13 patients but not in an age-matched control group (baseline [BL]; follow-up [FU]). This most likely was related to a decrease in the rate pressure product that at follow-up was significantly lower than at baseline. Furthermore, dipyridamole-stimulated hyperemic MBFs increased significantly by an average of 9% from baseline to follow-up, possibly because of lower systolic pressures and heart rates or lower plasma cholesterol levels or, alternatively, an endothelium-related improvement in the total vasodilator capacity. NS—not significant.

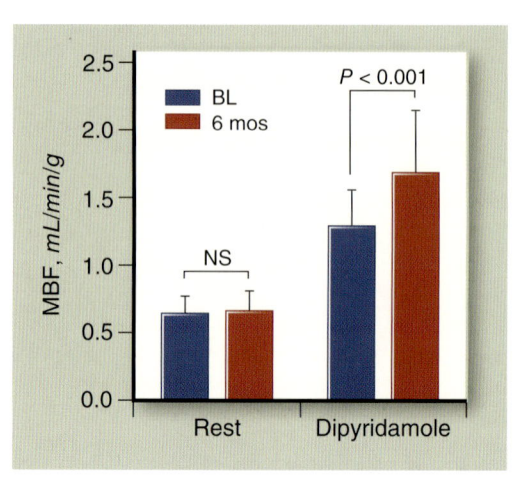

Figure 4-57. Effects of HMG-CoA reductase inhibitors in myocardial blood flow (MBF). In 23 hypercholesterolemia patients with angiographically entirely normal or minimally diseased coronary arteries, treatment with simvastatin for 6 months significantly lowered total and low-density lipoprotein cholesterol levels (by 30% and 42%, respectively), whereas high-density lipoprotein cholesterol increased [95]. At baseline (BL), MBF was normal at rest but markedly diminished during dipyridamole-induced hyperemia. After treatment (6 months), MBF at rest was unchanged but hyperemic blood flows had increased by an average of 31% so that the myocardial flow reserve approached near-normal values (from 2.2 ± 0.6 to 2.64 ± 0.06; $P < 0.01$; or by 20%). NS—not significant.

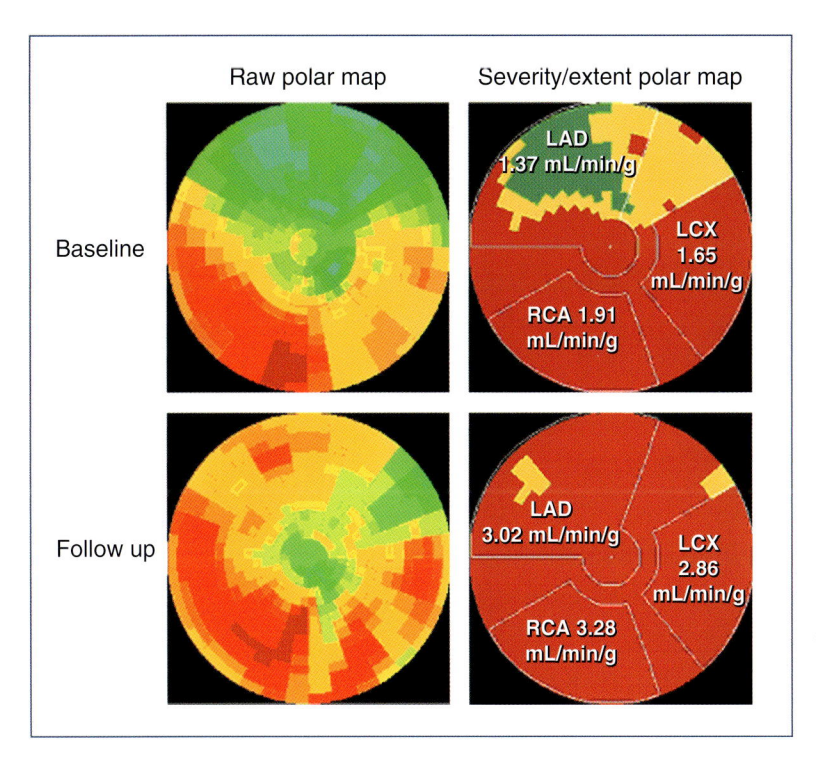

Figure 4-58. HMG-CoA reductase inhibitors and regional myocardial blood flow (MBF). Polar maps of the distribution of MBF during adenosine-stimulated hyperemia in a patient with coronary artery disease at baseline and after 1 year of treatment with pravastatin. The extent of the stress-induced defect declined from 51% of the left anterior descending artery (LAD) territory to only 3%. MBF in each of the three coronary artery territories (as listed in the figure) increased and importantly normalized in the region with a prior stress-induced defect. Only measurements of MBF—not the evaluation of the relative distribution of the radiotracer uptake in the myocardium—demonstrate the improvement in the flow reserve in remote or normally appearing myocardium. LCX—left circumflex artery; RCA—right coronary artery.

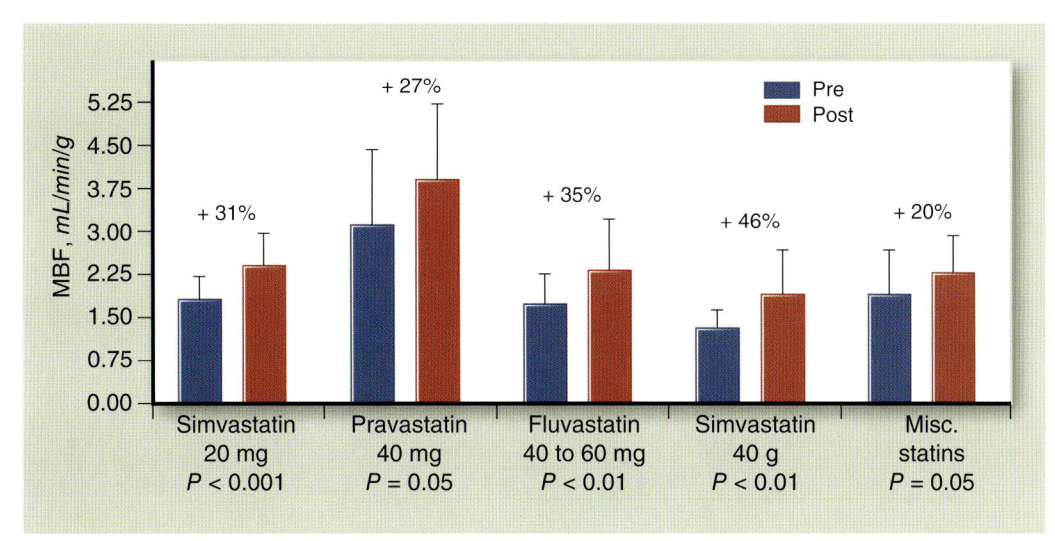

Figure 4-59. HMG-CoA reductase inhibitor treatment and myocardial blood flows (MBFs) in hypercholesterolemia patients. Effects of HMG-CoA reductase inhibitor treatment on MBF during dipyridamole- or adenosine-induced hyperemia in patients with and without coronary artery disease. Hyperemic MBFs after treatment (Post) are compared with those at baseline (Pre) for each study. The daily doses are given in milligrams. The percent improvement in hyperemic MBFs are indicated by the numbers [95–100].

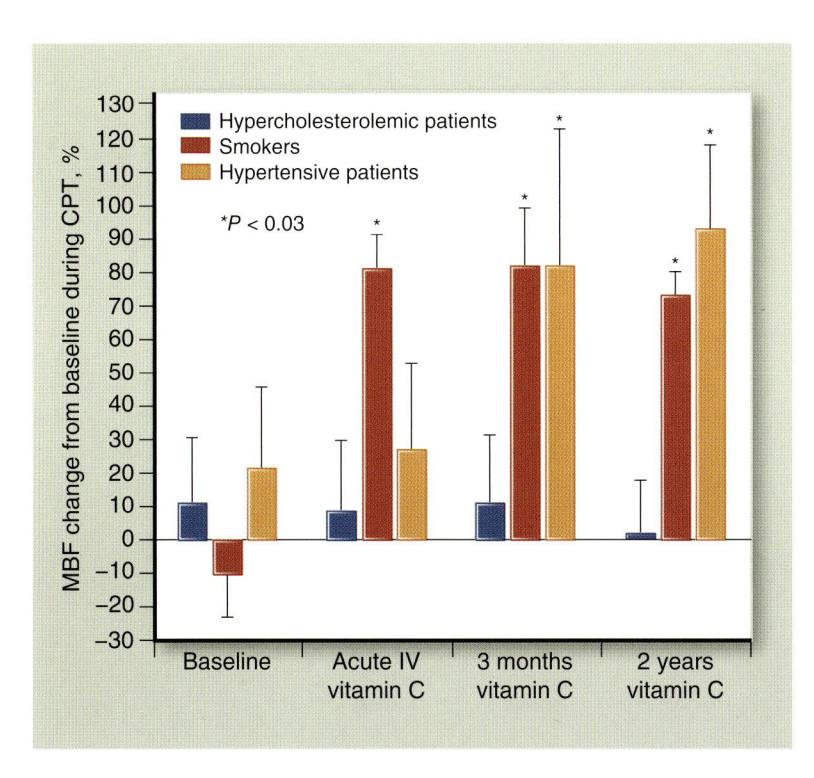

Figure 4-60. Effects of short-term and long-term antioxidant treatment on flow responses to cold pressor testing (CPT). Responses of myocardial blood flow (MBF) to sympathetic stimulation with CPT at baseline, after an intravenous (IV) dose of vitamin C, and after 3 months and 2 years of vitamin C administration are shown from left to right in hypercholesterolemic patients, smokers, and hypertensive patients. Flow responses are defined in percent change from rest [20]. Acute and long-term administration of the antioxidant vitamin C normalized the flow response to CPT in smokers but not in hypercholesterolemic patients. In hypertensive patients, acute vitamin C infusion had no effect on the flow response while long-term administration improved it. These findings may indicate that the abnormal flow response to CPT in smokers is predominantly mediated by increases in reactive oxygen species in the endothelium. In contrast, the delayed beneficial effect of vitamin C on endothelial dysfunction in hypertensive patients may be secondary to an improvement of the redox equilibrium, leading to increased endothelial nitric oxide synthase (eNOS) expression and/or prevention of eNOS uncoupling via enhanced bioavailability of tetrahydrobiopterin (BH_4). Further, the absence of improvement in patients with hypercholesterolemia may be related to mechanisms other than oxidative stress as for example, selective targeting of G-protein–dependent signal transduction by oxidized low-density lipoprotein with diminished flow-mediated stimulation of eNOS. The findings underscore the complex mechanism underlying impaired endothelium-dependent coronary vasomotor function.

Figure 4-61. Effects of insulin-sensitizing therapy with thiazolidinedione on cold pressor–related flow responses in insulin-resistant patients. Effects of thiazolidinedione treatments on endothelium-related coronary vasomotion in euglycemic insulin-resistant individuals [33]. The predominantly endothelium-independent hyperemic myocardial blood flow (MBF) increases to dipyridamole were similar in the insulin-sensitive and insulin-resistant individuals as depicted in Figure 4-48. However, as shown in this figure, the MBF response to cold pressor testing (CPT) was significantly impaired in insulin-resistance individuals when compared with the insulin-sensitive controls. The figure depicts the effects of thiazolidinedione treatment on 16 insulin-resistant individuals for 3 months. PET measurements of blood flow were performed at baseline, at 3 months into treatment, and again 6 months after treatment was discontinued. The markedly improved flow responses to cold at 3 months suggest an improvement or normalization of endothelium-dependent coronary vasomotion that, however, reverts to abnormal after insulin-sensitizing therapy is discontinued. SD—standard deviation.

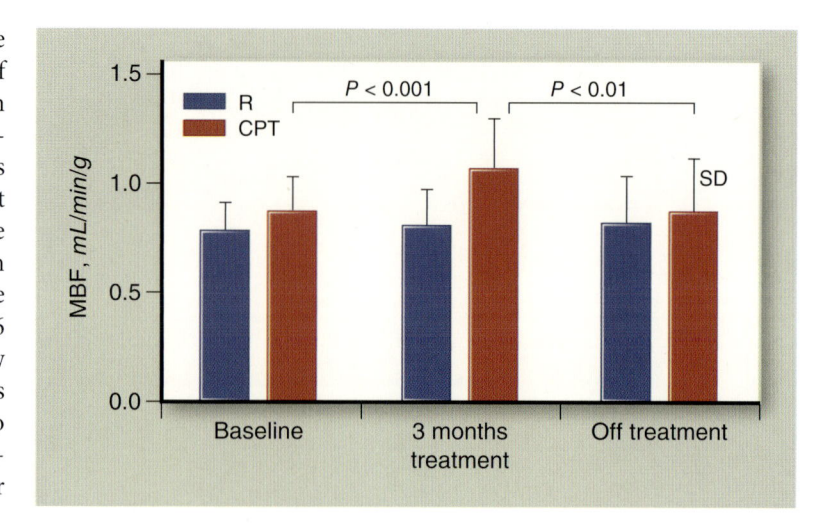

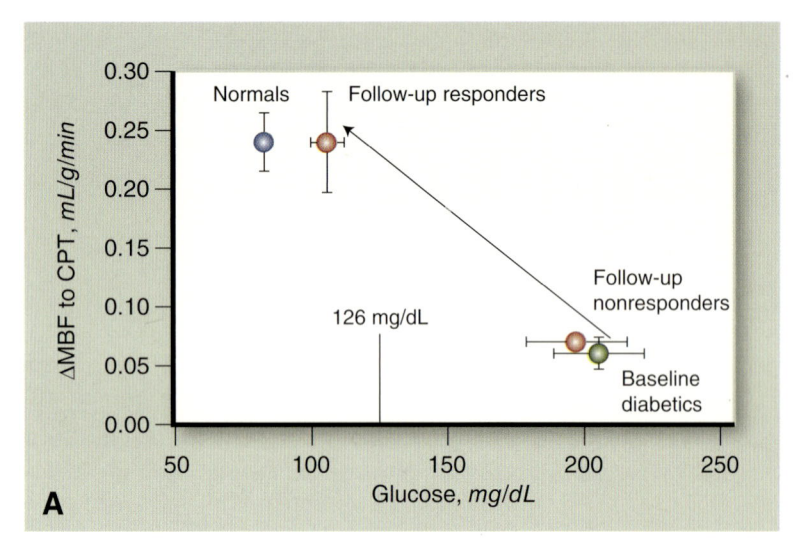

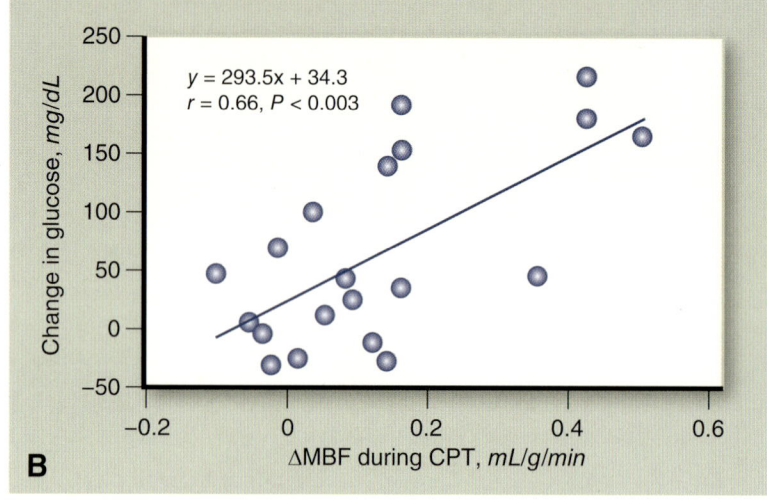

Figure 4-62. Effects of glucose-lowering therapy with glyburide and metformin on endothelium-related alterations in myocardial blood flow (MBF) from rest to cold pressor testing (CPT) (ΔMBF) in type 2 diabetes mellitus [34]. **A,** In type 2 diabetic patients with euglycemic control after 3 months of glucose-lowering treatment with glucose plasma levels 126 mg/dL or less (group of responders), the endothelium-related MBF response to CPT improved and no longer differed from that in normal controls. In patients with glucose plasma levels greater than 126 mg/dL (group of nonresponders), virtually no change in ΔMBF to CPT was observed [34]. **B,** The correlation of the endothelium-related ΔMBF and the change in fasting plasma glucose concentration, defined as difference in ΔMBF and change decrease in glucose levels between 3 months follow-up and baseline. The latter association suggests direct adverse effects of elevated plasma glucose levels, apart from determinants of the insulin resistance syndrome such as body weight, elevated insulin levels, and low high-density lipoprotein cholesterol, on diabetes-related coronary vasomotor dysfunction as precursor of coronary artery disease (CAD). (**A** and **B**, *adapted from* Schindler et al. [34].)

Because coronary vasomotor dysfunction carries important predictive information for CAD-related future cardiovascular events, it remains to be seen whether antidiabetic medical and/or behavioral interventions related to weight, diet, and physical activity, all aiming to improve or restore coronary vasomotor function in patients with type 2 diabetes, will indeed improve the clinical outcome. That such improvement may indeed lower the long-term risk is supported by preliminary observations made with measurements of peripheral vasoreactivity. With such measurements in patients with acute coronary syndromes or in hypertensive postmenopausal women, improvements in endothelium-related vasomotion were associated with a markedly improved long-term outcome [101,102].

Acknowledgments

The authors wish to thank Mary Smith for her assistance in preparing this manuscript. This work was supported in part by the Director of the Office of Energy Research, Office of Health and Environmental Research, Washington D.C., and in part by Research Grant #HL 33177, National Institutes of Health, Bethesda, MD.

References

1. Smith SC Jr: Risk-reduction therapy: the challenge to change. Presented at the 68th Scientific Sessions of the American Heart Association November 13, 1995; Anaheim, California. *Circulation* 1996, 93:2205–2211.

2. Schachinger V, Britten MB, Zeiher AM: Prognostic impact of coronary vasodilator dysfunction on adverse long-term outcome of coronary heart disease. *Circulation* 2000, 101:1899–1906.

3. Halcox JP, Schenke WH, Zalos G, et al.: Prognostic value of coronary vascular endothelial dysfunction. *Circulation* 2002, 106:653–658.

4. Suwaidi JA, Hamasaki S, Higano ST, et al.: Long-term follow-up of patients with mild coronary artery disease and endothelial dysfunction. *Circulation* 2000, 101:948–954.

5. Schindler TH, Hornig B, Buser PT, et al.: Prognostic value of abnormal vasoreactivity of epicardial coronary arteries to sympathetic stimulation in patients with normal coronary angiograms. *Arterioscler Thromb Vasc Biol* 2003, 23:495–501.

6. Schindler TH, Nitzsche EU, Schelbert HR, et al.: Positron emission tomography-measured abnormal responses of myocardial blood flow to sympathetic stimulation are associated with the risk of developing cardiovascular events. *J Am Coll Cardiol* 2005, 45:1505–1512.

7. Lerman A, Zeiher AM: Endothelial function: cardiac events. *Circulation* 2005, 111:363–368.

8. Kuhle WG, Porenta G, Huang SC, et al.: Quantification of regional myocardial blood flow using 13N-ammonia and reoriented dynamic positron emission tomographic imaging. *Circulation* 1992, 86:1004–1017.

9. Schelbert HR, Phelps ME, Huang SC, et al.: N-13 ammonia as an indicator of myocardial blood flow. *Circulation* 1981, 63:1259–1272.

10. Bergmann SR, Herrero P, Markham J, et al.: Noninvasive quantitation of myocardial blood flow in human subjects with oxygen-15-labeled water and positron emission tomography. *J Am Coll Cardiol* 1989, 14:639–652.

11. Schindler TH, Zhang XL, Vincenti G, et al.: Role of PET in the evaluation and understanding of coronary physiology. *J Nucl Cardiol* 2007, 14:589–603.

12. Prior JO, Schindler TH, Facta AD, et al.: Determinants of myocardial blood flow response to cold pressor testing and pharmacologic vasodilation in healthy humans. *Eur J Nucl Med Mol Imaging* 2007, 34:20–27.

13. Kaufmann PA, Camici PG: Myocardial blood flow measurement by PET: technical aspects and clinical applications. *J Nucl Med* 2005, 46:75–88.

14. Camici PG, Crea F: Coronary microvascular dysfunction. *N Engl J Med* 2007, 356:830–840.

15. Di Carli MF, Hachamovitch R: New technology for noninvasive evaluation of coronary artery disease. *Circulation* 2007, 115:1464–1480.

16. Di Carli MF, Dorbala S, Hachamovitch R: Integrated cardiac PET-CT for the diagnosis and management of CAD. *J Nucl Cardiol* 2006, 13:139–144.

17. Vesely MR, Dilsizian V: Nuclear cardiac stress testing in the era of molecular medicine. *J Nucl Med* 2008, 49:399–413.

18. Cecchi F, Olivotto I, Gistri R, et al.: Coronary microvascular dysfunction and prognosis in hypertrophic cardiomyopathy. *N Engl J Med* 2003, 349:1027–1035.

19. Schindler TH, Cardenas J, Prior JO, et al.: Relationship between increasing body weight, insulin resistance, inflammation, adipocytokine leptin, and coronary circulatory function. *J Am Coll Cardiol* 2006, 47:1188–1195.

20. Schindler TH, Nitzsche EU, Munzel T, et al.: Coronary vasoregulation in patients with various risk factors in response to cold pressor testing: contrasting myocardial blood flow responses to short- and long-term vitamin C administration. *J Am Coll Cardiol* 2003, 42:814–822.

21. Naya M, Tsukamoto T, Morita K, et al.: Olmesartan, but not amlodipine, improves endothelium-dependent coronary dilation in hypertensive patients. *J Am Coll Cardiol* 2007, 50:1144–1149.

22. Hattori N, Schnell O, Bengel FM, et al.: Deferoxamine improves coronary vascular responses to sympathetic stimulation in patients with type 1 diabetes mellitus. *Eur J Nucl Med Mol Imaging* 2002, 29:891–898.

23. Czernin J, Barnard RJ, Sun KT, et al.: Effect of short-term cardiovascular conditioning and low-fat diet on myocardial blood flow and flow reserve. *Circulation* 1995, 92:197–204.

24. Bengel FM, Abletshauser C, Neverve J, et al.: Effects of nateglinide on myocardial microvascular reactivity in type 2 diabetes mellitus: a randomized study using positron emission tomography. *Diabet Med* 2005, 22:158–163.

25. Tsukamoto T, Morita K, Naya M, et al.: Myocardial flow reserve is influenced by both coronary artery stenosis severity and coronary risk factors in patients with suspected coronary artery disease. *Eur J Nucl Med Mol Imaging* 2006, 33:1150–1156.

26. Muzik O, Duvernoy C, Beanlands RS, et al.: Assessment of diagnostic performance of quantitative flow measurements in normal subjects and patients with angiographically documented coronary artery disease by means of nitrogen-13 ammonia and positron emission tomography. *J Am Coll Cardiol* 1998, 31:534–540.

27. Parkash R, deKemp RA, Ruddy TD, et al.: Potential utility of rubidium 82 PET quantification in patients with 3-vessel coronary artery disease. *J Nucl Cardiol* 2004, 11:440–449.

28. Di Carli M, Czernin J, Hoh CK, et al.: Relation among stenosis severity, myocardial blood flow, and flow reserve in patients with coronary artery disease. *Circulation* 1995, 91:1944–1951.

29. Uren NG, Melin JA, De Bruyne B, et al.: Relation between myocardial blood flow and the severity of coronary-artery stenosis. *N Engl J Med* 1994, 330:1782–1788.

30. Beanlands RS, Muzik O, Melon P, et al.: Noninvasive quantification of regional myocardial flow reserve in patients with coronary atherosclerosis using nitrogen-13 ammonia positron emission tomography. Determination of extent of altered vascular reactivity. *J Am Coll Cardiol* 1995, 26:1465–1475.

31. Schindler TH, Nitzsche EU, Olschewski M, et al.: Chronic inflammation and impaired coronary vasoreactivity in patients with coronary risk factors. *Circulation* 2004, 110:1069–1075.

32. Prior JO, Quinones MJ, Hernandez-Pampaloni M, et al.: Coronary circulatory dysfunction in insulin resistance, impaired glucose tolerance, and type 2 diabetes mellitus. *Circulation* 2005, 111:2291–2298.

33. Quinones MJ, Hernandez-Pampaloni M, Schelbert H, et al.: Coronary vasomotor abnormalities in insulin-resistant individuals. *Ann Intern Med* 2004, 140:700–708.

34. Schindler TH, Facta AD, Prior JO, et al.: Improvement in coronary vascular dysfunction produced with euglycaemic control in patients with type 2 diabetes. *Heart* 2007, 93:345–349.

35. Tawakol A, Forgione MA, Stuehlinger M, et al.: Homocysteine impairs coronary microvascular dilator function in humans. *J Am Coll Cardiol* 2002, 40:1051–1058.

36. Buus NH, Bottcher M, Hermansen F, et al.: Influence of nitric oxide synthase and adrenergic inhibition on adenosine-induced myocardial hyperemia. *Circulation* 2001, 104:2305–2310.

37. Mosher P, Ross J Jr, McFate PA, Shaw RF: Control of coronary blood flow by an autoregulatory mechanism. *Circ Res* 1964, 14:250–259.

38. Feigl E, Schaper W: Physiology of coronary circulation. In *Cardiology*. Edited by Crawford M, DiMarco J. London: Mosby; 2001:1.1–1.9.

39. Hutchins GD, Caraher JM, Raylman RR: A region of interest strategy for minimizing resolution distortions in quantitative myocardial PET studies. *J Nucl Med* 1992, 33:1243–1250.

40. Czernin J, Muller P, Chan S, et al.: Influence of age and hemodynamics on myocardial blood flow and flow reserve. *Circulation* 1993, 88:62–69.

41. Chareonthaitawee P, Kaufmann PA, Rimoldi O, Camici PG: Heterogeneity of resting and hyperemic myocardial blood flow in healthy humans. *Cardiovasc Res* 200, 50:151–161.

42. Krivokapich J, Smith GT, Huang SC, et al.: 13N ammonia myocardial imaging at rest and with exercise in normal volunteers. Quantification of absolute myocardial perfusion with dynamic positron emission tomography. *Circulation* 1989, 80:1328–1337.

43. Krivokapich J, Huang SC, Schelbert HR: Assessment of the effects of dobutamine on myocardial blood flow and oxidative metabolism in normal human subjects using nitrogen-13 ammonia and carbon-11 acetate. *Am J Cardiol* 1993, 71:1351–1356.

44. Nagamachi S, Czernin J, Kim AS, *et al*.: Reproducibility of measurements of regional resting and hyperemic myocardial blood flow assessed with PET. *J Nucl Med* 1996, 37:1626–1631.

45. Schindler TH, Zhang XL, Prior JO, *et al*.: Assessment of intra- and interobserver reproducibility of rest and cold pressor test-stimulated myocardial blood flow with (13)N-ammonia and PET. *Eur J Nucl Med Mol Imaging* 2007, 34:1178–1188.

46. Kaufmann PA, Gnecchi-Ruscone T, Yap JT, *et al*.: Assessment of the reproducibility of baseline and hyperemic myocardial blood flow measurements with 15O-labeled water and PET. *J Nucl Med* 1999, 40:1848–1856.

47. Siegrist PT, Gaemperli O, Koepfli P, *et al*.: Repeatability of cold pressor test-induced flow increase assessed with H(2)(15)O and PET. *J Nucl Med* 2006, 47:1420–1426.

48. Wyss CA, Koepfli P, Mikolajczyk K, *et al*.: Bicycle exercise stress in PET for assessment of coronary flow reserve: repeatability and comparison with adenosine stress. *J Nucl Med* 2003, 44:146–154.

49. Jagathesan R, Kaufmann PA, Rosen SD, *et al*.: Assessment of the long-term reproducibility of baseline and dobutamine-induced myocardial blood flow in patients with stable coronary artery disease. *J Nucl Med* 2005, 46:212–219.

50. Bland JM, Altman DG: Statistical methods for assessing agreement between two methods of clinical measurement. *Lancet* 1986, 1:307–310.

51. Araujo LI, Lammertsma AA, Rhodes CG, *et al*.: Noninvasive quantification of regional myocardial blood flow in coronary artery disease with oxygen-15-labeled carbon dioxide inhalation and positron emission tomography. *Circulation* 1991, 83:875–885.

52. Pitkanen OP, Raitakari OT, Niinikoski H, *et al*.: Coronary flow reserve is impaired in young men with familial hypercholesterolemia. *J Am Coll Cardiol* 1996, 28:1705–1711.

53. Yokoyama I, Ohtake T, Momomura S, *et al*.: Hyperglycemia rather than insulin resistance is related to reduced coronary flow reserve in NIDDM. *Diabetes* 1998, 47:119–124.

54. Tadamura E, Iida H, Matsumoto K, *et al*.: Comparison of myocardial blood flow during dobutamine-atropine infusion with that after dipyridamole administration in normal men. *J Am Coll Cardiol* 2001, 37:130–136.

55. Hutchins GD, Schwaiger M, Rosenspire KC, *et al*.: Noninvasive quantification of regional blood flow in the human heart using N-13 ammonia and dynamic positron emission tomographic imaging. *J Am Coll Cardiol* 1990, 15:1032–1042.

56. Chan SY, Brunken RC, Czernin J, *et al*.: Comparison of maximal myocardial blood flow during adenosine infusion with that of intravenous dipyridamole in normal men. *J Am Coll Cardiol* 1992, 20:979–985.

57. Kubo S, Tadamura E, Toyoda H, *et al*.: Effect of caffeine intake on myocardial hyperemic flow induced by adenosine triphosphate and dipyridamole. *J Nucl Med* 2004, 45:730–738.

58. Wilson RF, Laughlin DE, Ackell PH, *et al*.: Transluminal, subselective measurement of coronary artery blood flow velocity and vasodilator reserve in man. *Circulation* 1985, 72:82–92.

59. Bottcher M, Czernin J, Sun KT, *et al*.: Effect of caffeine on myocardial blood flow at rest and during pharmacological vasodilation. *J Nucl Med* 1995, 36:2016–2021.

60. Bottcher M, Czernin J, Sun K, *et al*.: Effect of beta 1 adrenergic receptor blockade on myocardial blood flow and vasodilatory capacity. *J Nucl Med* 1997, 38:442–446.

61. Krivokapich J, Czernin J, Schelbert HR: Dobutamine positron emission tomography: absolute quantitation of rest and dobutamine myocardial blood flow and correlation with cardiac work and percent diameter stenosis in patients with and without coronary artery disease. *J Am Coll Cardiol* 1996, 28:565–572.

62. Muller P, Czernin J, Choi Y, *et al*.: Effect of exercise supplementation during adenosine infusion on hyperemic blood flow and flow reserve. *Am Heart J* 1994, 128:52–60.

63. Laine H, Nuutila P, Luotolahti M, *et al*.: Insulin-induced increment of coronary flow reserve is not abolished by dexamethasone in healthy young men. *J Clin Endocrinol Metab* 2000, 85:1868–1873.

64. Sundell J, Nuutila P, Laine H, *et al*.: Dose-dependent vasodilating effects of insulin on adenosine-stimulated myocardial blood flow. *Diabetes* 2002, 51:1125–1130.

65. Laine H, Sundell J, Nuutila P, *et al*.: Insulin induced increase in coronary flow reserve is abolished by dexamethasone in young men with uncomplicated type 1 diabetes. *Heart* 2004, 90:270–276.

66. Schindler TH, Nitzsche EU, Olschewski M, *et al*.: PET-measured responses of MBF to cold pressor testing correlate with indices of coronary vasomotion on quantitative coronary angiography. *J Nucl Med* 2004, 45:419–428.

67. Campisi R, Czernin J, Schoder H, *et al*.: Effects of long-term smoking on myocardial blood flow, coronary vasomotion, and vasodilator capacity. *Circulation* 1998, 98:119–125.

68. Zeiher AM, Drexler H: Coronary hemodynamic determinants of epicardial artery vasomotor responses during sympathetic stimulation in humans. *Basic Res Cardiol* 1991, 86(Suppl 2):203–213.

69. Zeiher AM, Drexler H, Wollschlager H, Just H: Endothelial dysfunction of the coronary microvasculature is associated with coronary blood flow regulation in patients with early atherosclerosis. *Circulation* 1991, 84:1984–1992.

70. Drexler H: Endothelial dysfunction: clinical implications. *Prog Cardiovasc Dis* 1997, 39:287–324.

71. Gould KL, Nakagawa Y, Nakagawa K, *et al*.: Frequency and clinical implications of fluid dynamically significant diffuse coronary artery disease manifest as graded, longitudinal, base-to-apex myocardial perfusion abnormalities by noninvasive positron emission tomography. *Circulation* 2000, 101:1931–1939.

72. De Bruyne B, Hersbach F, Pijls NH, *et al*.: Abnormal epicardial coronary resistance in patients with diffuse atherosclerosis but "normal" coronary angiography. *Circulation* 2001, 104:2401–2406.

73. Hernandez-Pampaloni M, Keng FY, Kudo T, *et al*.: Abnormal longitudinal, base-to-apex myocardial perfusion gradient by quantitative blood flow measurements in patients with coronary risk factors. *Circulation* 2001, 104:527–532.

74. Schindler TH, Facta AD, Prior JO, *et al*.: PET-measured heterogeneity in longitudinal myocardial blood flow in response to sympathetic and pharmacologic stress as a non-invasive probe of epicardial vasomotor dysfunction. *Eur J Nucl Med Mol Imaging* 2006, 33:1140–1149.

75. Nabel EG, Ganz P, Gordon JB, *et al*.: Dilation of normal and constriction of atherosclerotic coronary arteries caused by the cold pressor test. *Circulation* 1988, 77:43–52.

76. Victor RG, Leimbach WN Jr, Seals DR, *et al*.: Effects of the cold pressor test on muscle sympathetic nerve activity in humans. *Hypertension* 1987, 9:429–436.

77. Schindler TH, Zhang XL, Vincenti G, *et al*.: Diagnostic value of PET-measured heterogeneity in myocardial blood flows during cold pressor testing for the identification of coronary vasomotor dysfunction. *J Nucl Cardiol* 2007, 14:688–697.

78. Gould KL: Assessing progression or regression of CAD: the role of perfusion imaging. *J Nucl Cardiol* 2005, 12:625–638.

79. Johnson NP, Gould KL: Clinical evaluation of a new concept: resting myocardial perfusion heterogeneity quantified by markovian analysis of PET identifies coronary microvascular dysfunction and early atherosclerosis in 1,034 subjects. *J Nucl Med* 2005, 46:1427–1437.

80. Sdringola S, Loghin C, Boccalandro F, Gould KL: Mechanisms of progression and regression of coronary artery disease by PET related to treatment intensity and clinical events at long-term follow-up. *J Nucl Med* 2006, 47:59–67.

81. Campisi R, Czernin J, Schoder H, *et al*.: L-Arginine normalizes coronary vasomotion in long-term smokers. *Circulation* 1999, 99:491–497.

82. Gould KL, Lipscomb K, Hamilton GW: Physiologic basis for assessing critical coronary stenosis. Instantaneous flow response and regional distribution during coronary hyperemia as measures of coronary flow reserve. *Am J Cardiol* 1974, 33:87–94.

83. Dayanikli F, Grambow D, Muzik O, Mosca *et al*.: Early detection of abnormal coronary flow reserve in asymptomatic men at high risk for coronary artery disease using positron emission tomography. *Circulation* 1994, 90:808–817.

84. Yokoyama I, Ohtake T, Momomura S, *et al*.: Reduced coronary flow reserve in hypercholesterolemic patients without overt coronary stenosis. *Circulation* 1996, 94:3232–3238.

85. Pitkanen OP, Nuutila P, Raitakari OT, *et al*.: Coronary flow reserve in young men with familial combined hyperlipidemia. *Circulation* 1999, 99:1678–1684.

86. Di Carli MF, Janisse J, Grunberger G, Ager J: Role of chronic hyperglycemia in the pathogenesis of coronary microvascular dysfunction in diabetes. *J Am Coll Cardiol* 2003, 41:1387–1393.

87. Pop-Busui R, Kirkwood I, Schmid H, et al.: Sympathetic dysfunction in type 1 diabetes: association with impaired myocardial blood flow reserve and diastolic dysfunction. *J Am Coll Cardiol* 2004, 44:2368–2374.

88. Nitenberg A, Paycha F, Ledoux S, et al.: Coronary artery responses to physiological stimuli are improved by deferoxamine but not by L-arginine in non-insulin-dependent diabetic patients with angiographically normal coronary arteries and no other risk factors. *Circulation* 1998, 97:736–743.

89. Nitenberg A, Ledoux S, Valensi P, et al.: Impairment of coronary microvascular dilation in response to cold pressor–induced sympathetic stimulation in type 2 diabetic patients with abnormal stress thallium imaging. *Diabetes* 2001, 50:1180–1185.

90. Yokoyama I, Yonekura K, Ohtake T, et al.: Coronary microangiopathy in type 2 diabetic patients: relation to glycemic control, sex, and microvascular angina rather than to coronary artery disease. *J Nucl Med* 2000, 41:978–985.

91. Al Suwaidi J, Higano ST, Holmes DR Jr, et al.: Obesity is independently associated with coronary endothelial dysfunction in patients with normal or mildly diseased coronary arteries. *J Am Coll Cardiol* 2001, 37:1523–1528.

92. Steinberg HO, Chaker H, Learning R, et al.: Obesity/insulin resistance is associated with endothelial dysfunction. Implications for the syndrome of insulin resistance. *J Clin Invest* 1996, 97:2601–2610.

93. Britten MB, Zeiher AM, Schachinger V: Microvascular dysfunction in angiographically normal or mildly diseased coronary arteries predicts adverse cardiovascular long-term outcome. *Coron Artery Dis* 2004, 15:259–264.

94. Nitenberg A, Chemla D, Antony I: Epicardial coronary artery constriction to cold pressor test is predictive of cardiovascular events in hypertensive patients with angiographically normal coronary arteries and without other major coronary risk factor. *Atherosclerosis* 2004, 173:115–123.

95. Baller D, Notohamiprodjo G, Gleichmann U, et al.: Improvement in coronary flow reserve determined by positron emission tomography after 6 months of cholesterol-lowering therapy in patients with early stages of coronary atherosclerosis. *Circulation* 1999, 99:2871–2875.

96. Janatuinen T, Laaksonen R, Vesalainen R, et al.: Effect of lipid-lowering therapy with pravastatin on myocardial blood flow in young mildly hypercholesterolemic adults. *J Cardiovasc Pharmacol* 2001, 38:561–568.

97. Guethlin M, Kasel AM, Coppenrath K, et al.: Delayed response of myocardial flow reserve to lipid-lowering therapy with fluvastatin. *Circulation* 1999, 99:475–481.

98. Huggins GS, Pasternak RC, Alpert NM, et al.: Effects of short-term treatment of hyperlipidemia on coronary vasodilator function and myocardial perfusion in regions having substantial impairment of baseline dilator reverse. *Circulation* 1998, 98:1291–1296.

99. Yokoyama I, Momomura S, Ohtake T, et al.: Improvement of impaired myocardial vasodilatation due to diffuse coronary atherosclerosis in hypercholesterolemics after lipid-lowering therapy. *Circulation* 1999, 100:117–122.

100. Yokoyama I, Yonekura K, Inoue Y, et al.: Long-term effect of simvastatin on the improvement of impaired myocardial flow reserve in patients with familial hypercholesterolemia without gender variance. *J Nucl Cardiol* 2001, 8:445–451.

101. Fichtlscherer S, Breuer S, Zeiher AM: Prognostic value of systemic endothelial dysfunction in patients with acute coronary syndromes: further evidence for the existence of the "vulnerable" patient. *Circulation* 2004, 110:1926–1932.

102. Modena MG, Bonetti L, Coppi F, et al.: Prognostic role of reversible endothelial dysfunction in hypertensive postmenopausal women. *J Am Coll Cardiol* 2002, 40:505–510.

Assessment of Cardiac Function: First-Pass, Equilibrium Blood Pool, and Gated Myocardial SPECT

5

Elias H. Botvinick, Nick G. Costouros, Stephen L. Bacharach, and J. William O'Connell

Radionuclide-based techniques have been used to measure ventricular function for over three decades [1–8]. The methods for measurement of ventricular function can be divided into two basic categories The first category employs any tracer that can directly label the blood pool itself. One then examines the deformity of the cavitary blood pool as it is moved by the thickening and systolic motion of the myocardial walls. With these methods one can directly image the blood pool in the ventricular cavity throughout the cardiac cycle. The second category of methods for measurement of ventricular function uses tracers that label the myocardial walls (eg, ^{99m}Tc-MIBI, [^{18}F]-fluorodeoxyglucose, or others). One then examines how those walls thicken and translate, move, or contract throughout the cardiac cycle. With this method one can directly image the myocardium throughout the cardiac cycle. Active movement or contraction of the inner endocardial wall of the ventricular chamber compresses the blood pool and deforms the ventricular cavity and is the conventional marker for systolic ventricular wall motion or function. Only this method permits the evaluation of myocardial wall thickening, a marker of systolic function and viability which can help separate passive systolic wall motion from active myocardial contraction. This method for measuring ventricular mechanical function simultaneously yields a measurement of myocardial perfusion or of metabolism (depending on the tracer used to label the myocardium). However, this advantage is also a source of one of the methods disadvantages, namely that if perfusion or metabolism is reduced in a particular segment of the myocardium, then that segment is not easily visualized, hampering visualization of wall motion or thickening in that segment. Temporal and spatial resolution of the related functional image data is not as good as the blood pool method.

Both of the above methods may be gated with an electrocardiogram signal. This permits observation of either the blood pool or the myocardium throughout the cardiac cycle. The data can be displayed as a cine to either view or compute left ventricular ejection fraction. The two methods are to some extent complementary, but give slightly different information. The blood pool method directly measures the changing volume of the blood in the cardiac chambers with time. Motion of the adjacent myocardial walls is inferred from the measured regional or global changes/motion in blood pool contour and blood volume. The labeled myocardium methodology directly measures the motion of the walls. One must then infer changes in blood volume from that motion. Each method has its advantages and disadvantages. This chapter explores the advantages and disadvantages of both methods of measuring ventricular function, as well as how each can be applied clinically.

Part I: Blood Pool Imaging of Ventricular Function

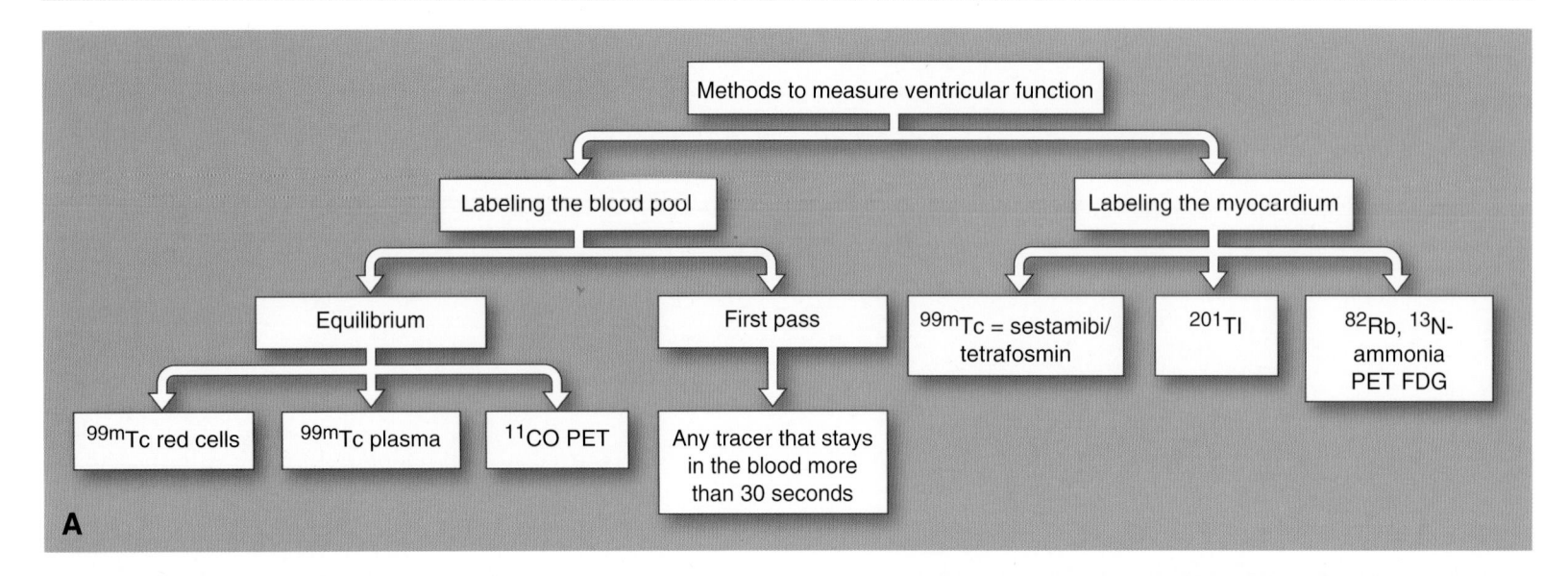

```
                     Methods to measure ventricular function
                    /                                        \
        Labeling the blood pool                      Labeling the myocardium
          /         |                                /         |          \
    Equilibrium   First pass                 99mTc = sestamibi/  201Tl   82Rb, 13N-
       /  |  \         |                        tetrafosmin              ammonia
 99mTc  99mTc  11CO  Any tracer that stays                                PET FDG
 red    plasma PET   in the blood more
 cells                than 30 seconds
```

A

Advantages and Disadvantages of the First Pass Method

Advantages of the First Pass Method

Records and analyzes the transit of a radionuclide bolus through the central circulation.

Allows imaging and physiologic interrogation of individual chambers relatively free of adjacent chamber activity and virtually free of atrial activity.

Records real-time events, which allows the characterization and quantification of individual cardiac beats.

Allows short acquisition times of approximately 30 sec at rest and 10–15 sec at peak exercise. High-quality images can be acquired using a state-of-the-art, high-sensitivity device and, at best, a multicrystal camera. This brief acquisition time is optimal for the study of rapidly changing physiologic states.

Uses most radionuclides appropriate for a conventional gamma camera that can be safely injected intravenously in sufficient dosage for adequate counting statistics. Macroaggregated albumin sequestered in the lungs is not appropriate, as it fails to pass the capillary network.

Can be used in combination with other imaging techniques to enhance diagnostic information.

Disadvantages of the First Pass Method

Can only be used with conventional Anger cameras if they can deliver count rates of 150,000–200,000 counts per sec. Current state-of-the-art cameras are capable. Among other factors, the accuracy of the method varies with the statistics of the study. The greater the count density in the end-diastolic region of interest, the lower the statistical error in the calculation of ejection fraction. Much higher count density is required in patients with abnormal ventricular function than in patients with normal function to derive similar statistical reliability. The statistics applicable to the typical first pass study result in an approximately 3% error in left ventricular ejection fraction calculation.

Measurement requires a separate injection, which limits the number of studies and projections that can be acquired. Serial injections of ^{99m}Tc results in a buildup of background activity.

Study quality depends on the discreteness of the injection bolus. Up to 10% of studies will be compromised by delayed or fractionated boluses.

Patient motion or arrhythmia more easily compromises results than in an equilibrium study.

Cannot avoid structural overlap with planar methods; it is difficult to separate ventricles, especially the right ventricle, from the atria, especially the right atrium.

B

Figure 5-1. A, Measurement of ventricular function. Labeling the blood pool has the advantage of providing a direct measure of left ventricular (LV) volumes. In the ideal circumstance the method provides true quantitatively accurate imaging, and measurement of absolute volume can be obtained directly from the images, since radioactivity per volume (*ie*, the concentration of activity in the ventricular blood pool, or Bq/mL) can be measured within the LV chamber as well as the total Bq within the cavity. LV volume is then (number of Bq in the entire chamber) Bq/mL in the blood. Unfortunately, the ability to make accurate quantitative measurements of Bq/mL from image data is usually limited to PET [9,10]. The more common single photon tomographic measurements can only produce quantitatively accurate results with great difficulty, and actual blood counting. With planar imaging there are even greater inaccuracies. Nonetheless, SPECT blood pool techniques have made considerable progress in recent years [11–14]. Fortunately, for nearly all clinical applications, one is usually content to make relative measurements of ventricular function, *eg*, ejection fraction. These relative measurements, unlike measurements of absolute volumes, depend only on the imaging modality being accurate in a relative, rather than an absolute, sense. For this reason, planar imaging methods can do quite well [15], although for regional measures of function using a blood pool tracer, SPECT offers some advantages [16–19].

There are two methods of blood pool imaging based on the state of radiotracer mixing, first pass (**B**) and equilibrium methods (**C**). The former extracts data during the first passage of the radionuclide through the central circulation. The latter images the heart and calculates functional parameters when the radionuclide is fully mixed and at equilibrium, when each milliliter of blood contains the same amount of activity and blood pool counts are proportional to volume. Both methods may be gated or acquired in synchrony with the cardiac cycle to gain temporal data regarding ventricular contraction for each beat.

Continued on the next page

Figure 5-1. *(Continued)* The most commonly used tracer is ^{99m}Tc-labeled red blood cells. Commercially available kits are available that can easily produce this tracer [20]. For PET, it is possible (but not common) to also do blood pool imaging using ^{11}C-labeled carbon monoxide. This gas is breathed by the patient a few minutes before imaging begins. The quantity of ^{11}C carbon monoxide that must be inhaled is typically no greater than one might breathe in heavy traffic, so there are no deleterious physiologic effects.

Labeling the myocardium provides direct visualization of the myocardial walls throughout the cardiac cycle. It provides only an indirect measurement of the changes in blood volume. These must be inferred from measurement of the endocardial edges, a difficult task given the resolution of nuclear techniques, but one that has proved quite feasible [21]. The method could, in principle, be used to directly measure regional myocardial thickening as well [22,23]. The actual measurement of linear thickening has proven more difficult to accomplish with SPECT than with higher resolution methods such as gated CT or MRI. However, intensity changes can be used to track thickening (as described below) and the gated labeled myocardial methodology has been widely adopted, since it permits measurement of LV function simultaneously with perfusion or metabolism.

Advantages and Disadvantages of the Equilibrium Method

Advantages of the Equilibrium Method

Presents high-resolution images.

Provides excellent assessment of regional wall motion and cardiac structures, with an intraobserver variability of ± 3% and an interobserver variability of ± 4%.

Can be fully automated to yield objective, accurate, and reproducible left and right ventricular ejection fraction.

Can be easily performed with standard, state-of-the-art, single-crystal scintillation cameras.

Can be applied reproducibly for repetitive calculations with interventions.

Is ideally suited for generation of functional images.

Disadvantages of the Equilibrium Method

Must use labeled red cells.

Cannot be used with any ^{99m}Tc-labeled radionuclide passing through the blood pool.

Requires 2 to 33 minutes of acquisition time to gain adequate data with conventional, single-crystal cameras, but about 1 minute using new, high-sensitivity digital cameras.

Risks loss of accuracy or "blurring" of data when applied with brief intervention.

Cannot avoid structural overlap with planar methods; it is difficult to separate ventricles, especially the right ventricle, from the atria, especially the right atrium.

C

Thus, one can perform two measurements with only a single injection and a single imaging session—a great logistical and financial incentive. The method has been used successfully with both SPECT and PET, but not with planar imaging. FDG—fluorodeoxyglucose. (**B** and **C**, *adapted from* Botvinick [24].)

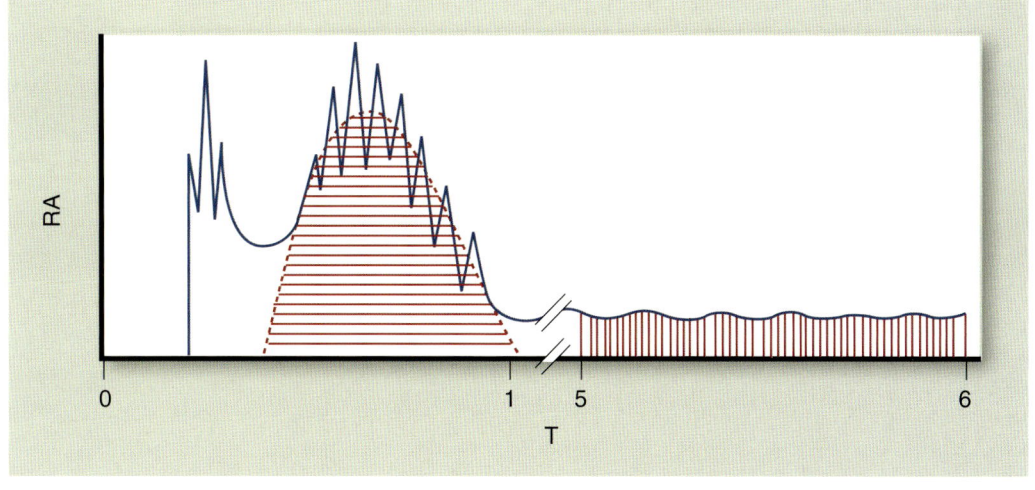

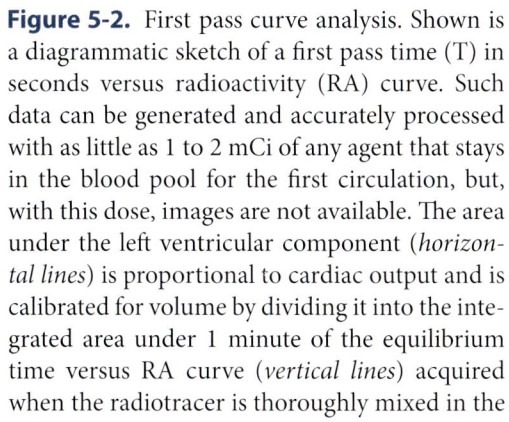

Figure 5-2. First pass curve analysis. Shown is a diagrammatic sketch of a first pass time (T) in seconds versus radioactivity (RA) curve. Such data can be generated and accurately processed with as little as 1 to 2 mCi of any agent that stays in the blood pool for the first circulation, but, with this dose, images are not available. The area under the left ventricular component (*horizontal lines*) is proportional to cardiac output and is calibrated for volume by dividing it into the integrated area under 1 minute of the equilibrium time versus RA curve (*vertical lines*) acquired when the radiotracer is thoroughly mixed in the blood. Alternatively, volumes may be calculated from ventricular outlines using geometric considerations. A unique first pass method of volume calculation is applied with the multicrystal camera where image counts are sampled in a known blood volume at the attenuation distance to the mid-left ventricle and used to standardize ventricular counts during diastole and systole [24,25]. (*Adapted from* Botvinick *et al.* [25].)

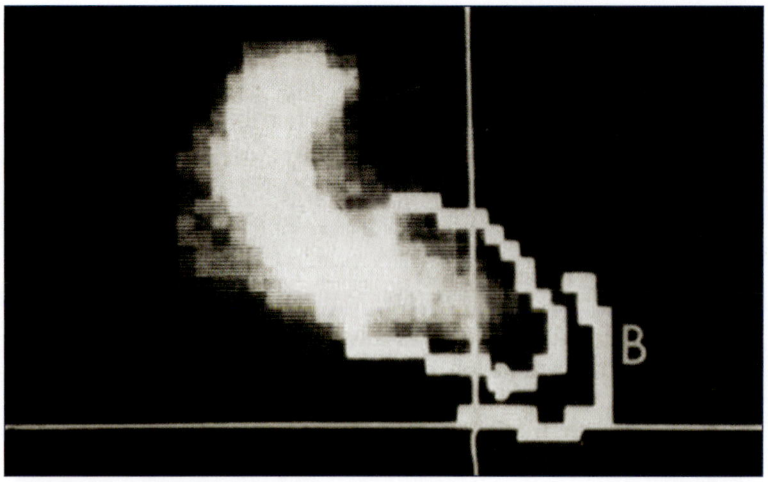

Figure 5-3. First pass analysis of the levophase. An irregular region of interest is drawn on the levophase of the first pass ventriculogram. Correcting for background activity (*B*), the diastolic peaks and systolic valleys are compared to calculate the left ventricular ejection fraction. (*From* Botvinick *et al.* [25]; with permission.)

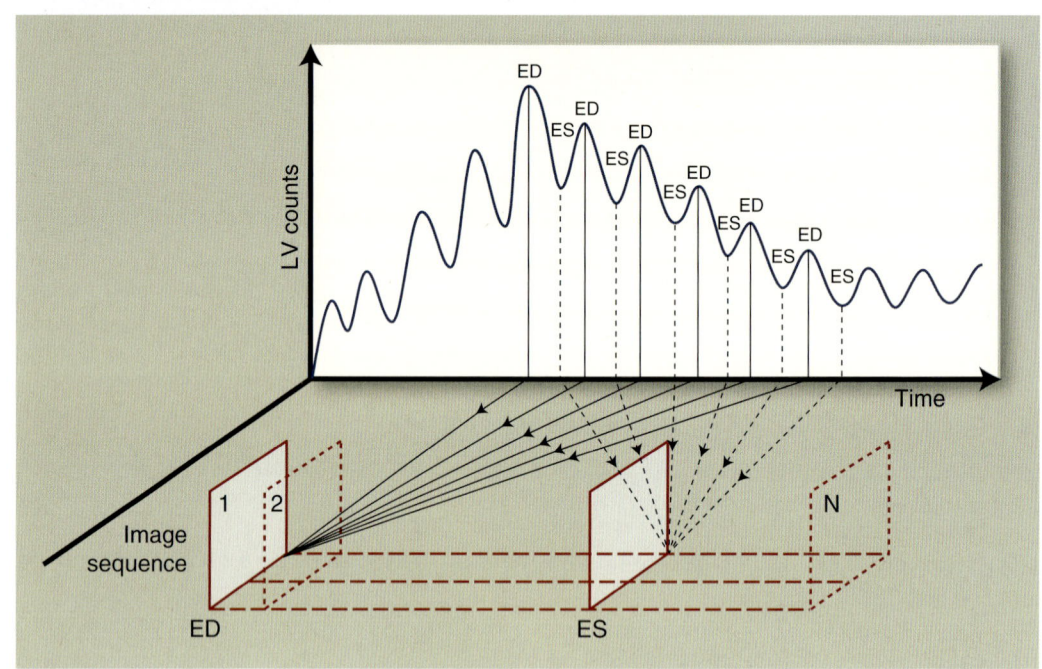

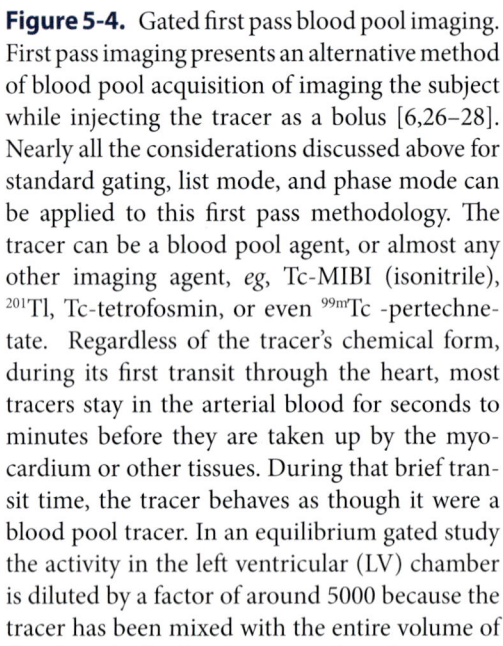

Figure 5-4. Gated first pass blood pool imaging. First pass imaging presents an alternative method of blood pool acquisition of imaging the subject while injecting the tracer as a bolus [6,26–28]. Nearly all the considerations discussed above for standard gating, list mode, and phase mode can be applied to this first pass methodology. The tracer can be a blood pool agent, or almost any other imaging agent, *eg*, Tc-MIBI (isonitrile), ^{201}Tl, Tc-tetrofosmin, or even ^{99m}Tc-pertechnetate. Regardless of the tracer's chemical form, during its first transit through the heart, most tracers stay in the arterial blood for seconds to minutes before they are taken up by the myocardium or other tissues. During that brief transit time, the tracer behaves as though it were a blood pool tracer. In an equilibrium gated study the activity in the left ventricular (LV) chamber is diluted by a factor of around 5000 because the tracer has been mixed with the entire volume of blood in the body. However, when the tracer is injected as a bolus, the concentration of activity in the ventricular chambers is quite large during the tracer's first transit through the heart. This yields count rates that are many fold higher than in equilibrium gated blood pool studies. Despite this much higher count rate, it is still necessary to do some form of gating in order to capture the ejection fraction (EF). For first pass studies only a few beats of data need be added together. This figure illustrates the case of "gating" the first six beats of data to produce one sequence of N images. One of the advantages of first pass imaging is that, as mentioned above, it can be performed with nearly any imaging agent, and thus one can obtain LV function data from studies done for some other purpose, as bone scans. In addition, it is possible to position the gamma camera in a right anterior oblique view and obtain early gated images during the passage of the radioisotope through the right ventricle (RV), prior to contamination by counts from the LV. One of the disadvantages of the first transit is that one usually must obtain all the LV function information from only a small number of beats. This means a rapid bolus injection must be given, resulting in very high count rates during passage of the tracer through the cardiac chambers. Such high count rates often cause unacceptable dead time in many cameras. Therefore, specialized cameras (often not using Anger methodology) have been developed specifically for dealing with these high count rates. However, many standard cameras can perform first pass acquisition with adequate accuracy although the dose may need to be limited. Additionally, the EF, calculated from the average values based on the magnitude of the peak counts proportional to end diastolic (ED) volume, and the valleys, proportional to end systolic (ES) volume, correcting for background activity, is based on a few samples and so is prone to greater variability. The few samples are related to the required tight RV bolus passage.

112 Atlas of Nuclear Cardiology

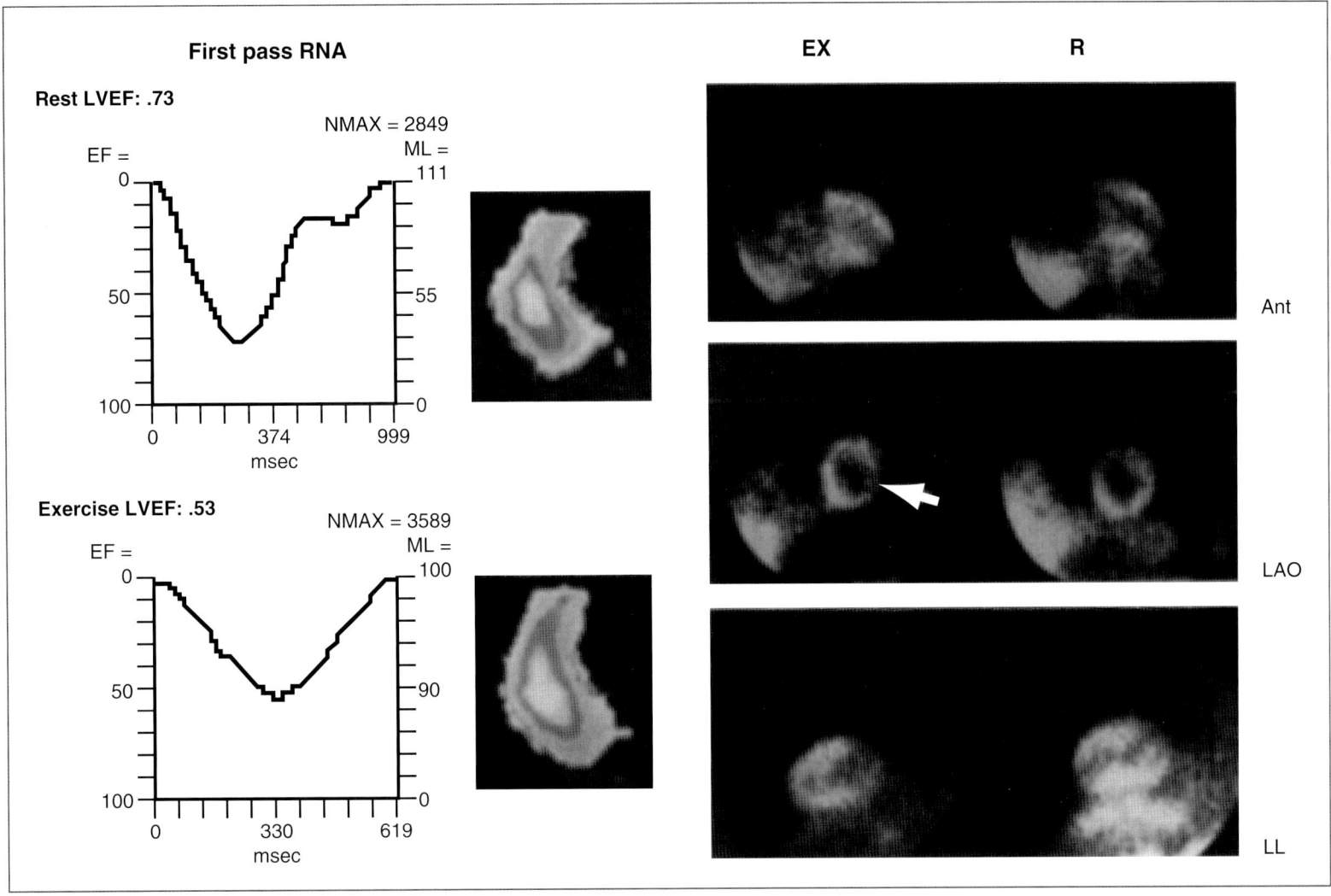

Figure 5-5. The interaction of perfusion and function. This figure demonstrates the perfusion–function interaction [29]. Shown at the *right* are perfusion images in anterior (Ant) (*top*), left anterior oblique (LAO) 40° (*center*), and LAO 70° (*bottom*) with exercise (EX) and at rest (R) in each image pair acquired in a 41-year-old man with a history of coronary disease and prior coronary bypass graft surgery and atypical chest pain. On the *left* are the associated first pass images of the sestamibi bolus administered to evaluate left ventricular function at rest and with exercise. Evident is a reversible inferolateral defect, cavitary dilation, and reduced left ventricular ejection fraction (LVEF) with exercise. (*From* Wackers [29]; with permission.)

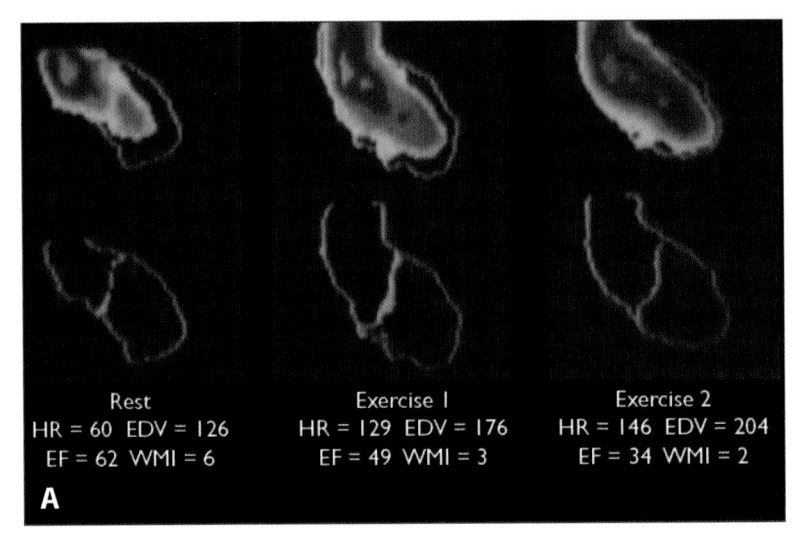

Figure 5-6. Abnormal first pass exercise study. **A,** Examples of baseline (*left*), early exercise (*center*), and peak exercise (*right*) left ventricular function in a patient with coronary disease [30]. In each panel, the end-systolic frame is related to the end-diastolic outline (*top*), while both end-diastolic and end-systolic outlines are presented below. Data including the heart rate (HR), left ventricular ejection fraction (EF), end-diastolic volume (EDV), and wall motion index (WMI) are presented for each period. The ischemic response is characterized, as it is with all methods that evaluate the functional response, by increased EDV and reduced WMI and EF.

Continued on the next page

Assessment of Cardiac Function: First-Pass, Equilibrium Blood Pool, and Gated Myocardial SPECT

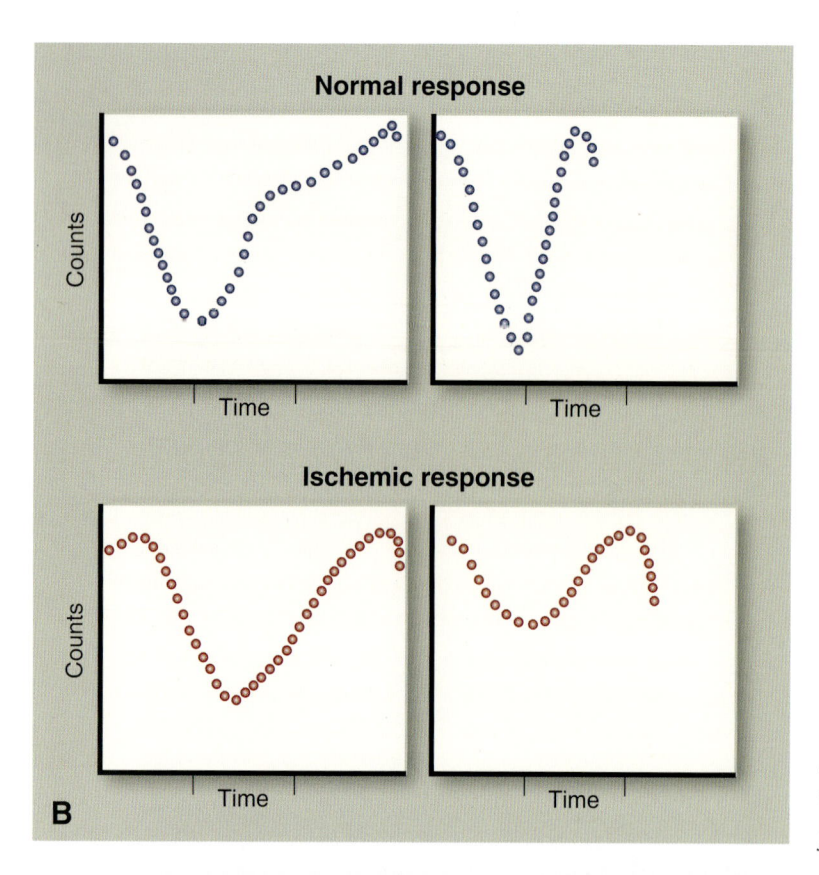

Figure 5-6. *(Continued)* **B,** Typical time versus radioactivity curves related to the normal *(top)* and ischemic *(bottom)* exercise response. In each case the baseline curve is at the *left* and the exercise-related curve is at the *right*. (**A,** *from* Upton *et al.* [30]; with permission; **B,** *adapted from* Botvinick [31].)

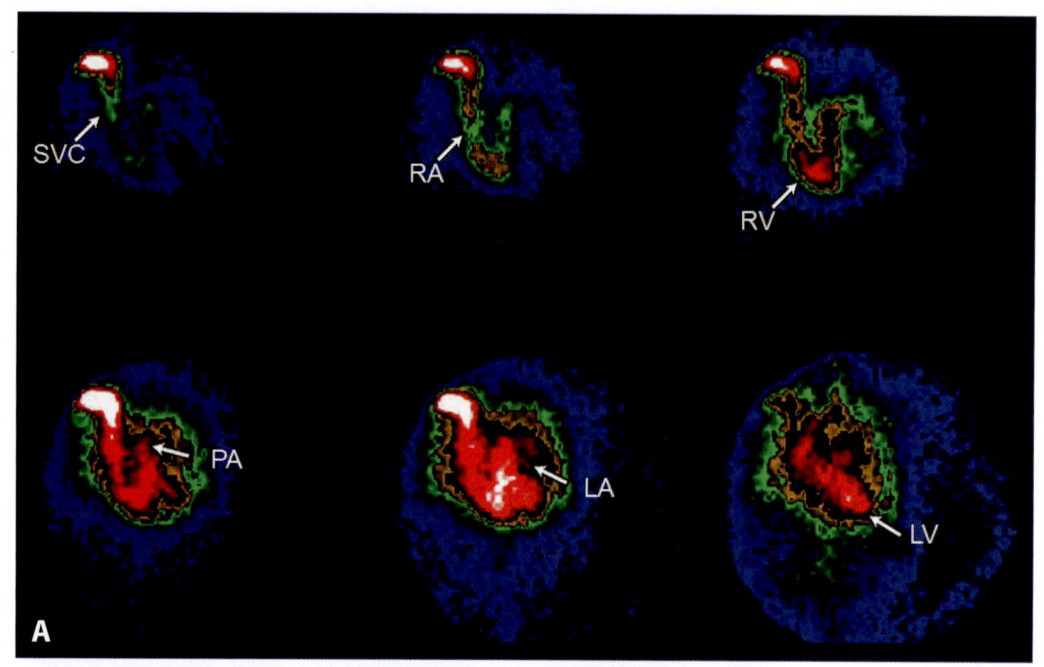

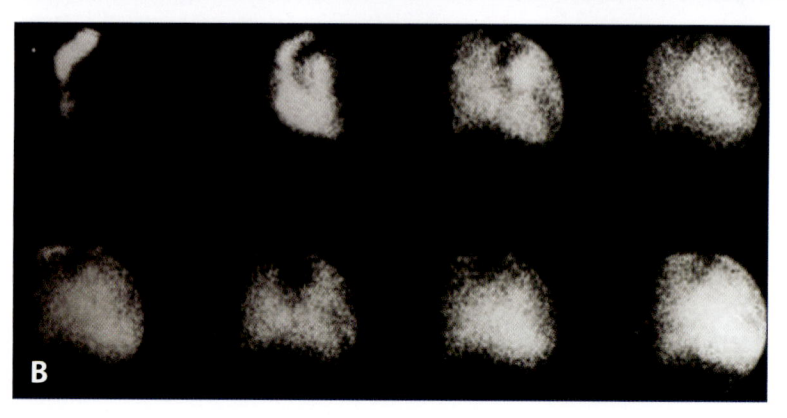

Figure 5-7. First pass images in normal patient and in a patient with left to right shunt. **A,** First-pass radionuclide ventriculography. Individual frames from a first-pass acquisition, illustrating the path of the bolus isotope through the superior vena cava (SVC), the right atrium (RA), the right ventricle (RV), the pulmonary outflow tract and lungs (pulmonary artery [PA]), the left atrium (LA), and the left ventricular (LV) phase, from which the isotope bolus is then distributed systemically. **B,** Similar images taken in a patient with a significant left to right shunt. The lungs never clear due to continued recirculation of the bolus. As a result, the LV teardrop and the levophase is not seen. This "smudge sign" generally relates to a left to right shunt with Qp/Qs ≥ 1.5. (**A,** *from* Udelson *et al.* [32]; with permission; **B,** *from* Botvinick [31]; with permission.)

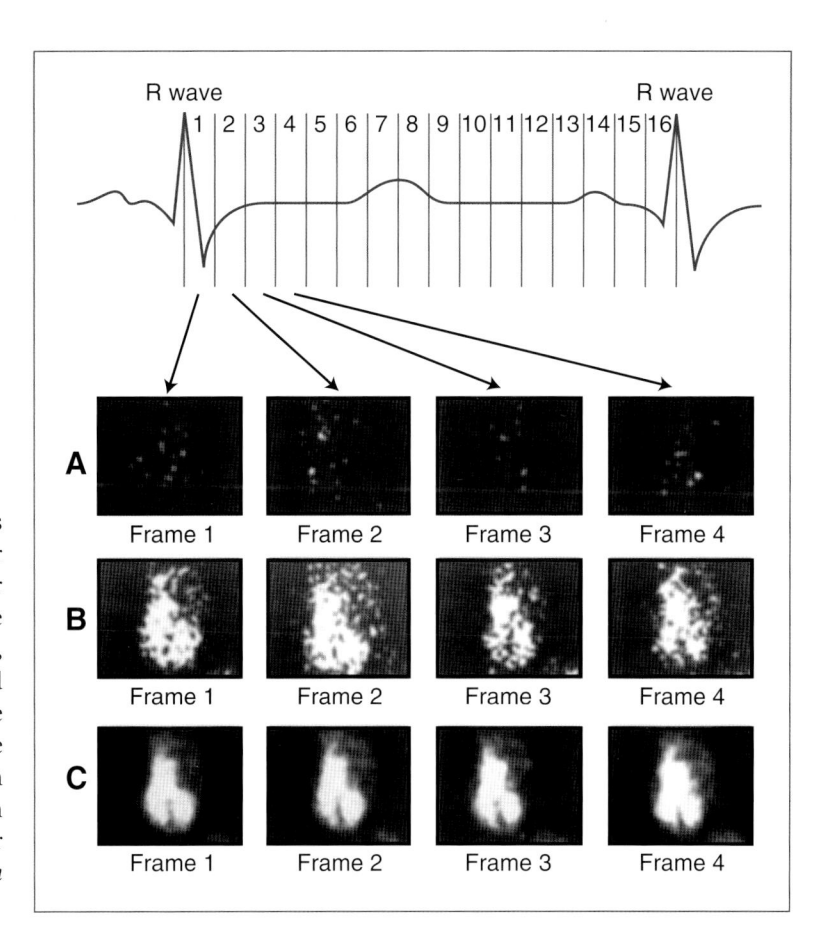

Figure 5-11. Computer acquisition of the equilibrium study. Shown is the relationship between the cardiac cycle or R-R interval acquired over 16 separate frames or intervals, and the related images in each frame over the course of the acquisition [37]. The counts acquired during frame 2 are stored in frame 2, those acquired during frame 3 are stored in frame 3, and so on. Only data accumulated over the first four frames is illustrated here. Owing to the low count rate in this study, 750 counts per frame, there is little to see after acquisition over a single cycle (**A**). However, after the accumulation and addition of the counts from 20 R-R cycles, now with 15,000 counts per frame, the cardiac chambers are taking form (**B**). With the addition of counts acquired over 400 cycles and 300,000 counts per frame, image quality is excellent and the acquisition is over (**C**). (*From* Parker *et al.* [37]; with permission.)

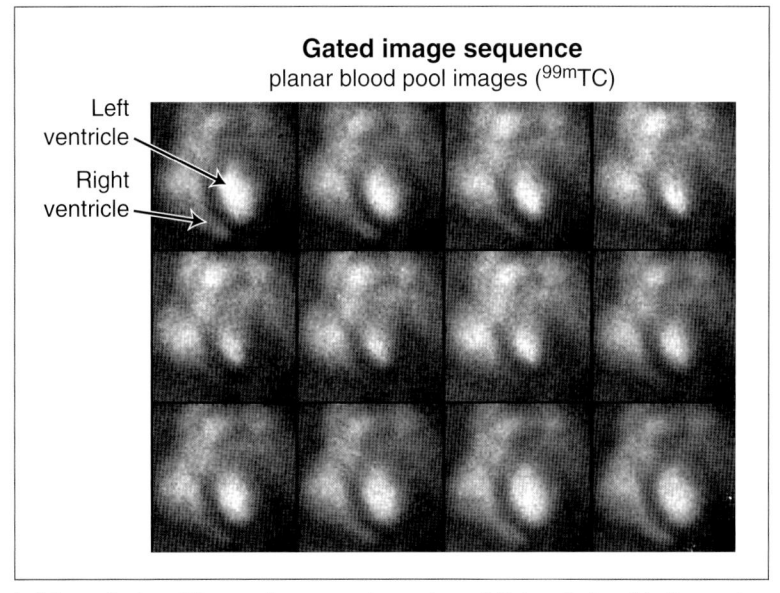

Figure 5-12. Gated imaging sequence This figure illustrates a typical planar gated blood pool sequence of images, 12 in this case, made up of about 300 cardiac cycles "gated" together, as described in the previous figure. The images were taken with ^{99m}Tc-labeled red blood cells. The gamma camera was positioned in a left anterior oblique (LAO) position, approximately 45°, with a 15° caudal tilt. The caudal tilt is used to better separate the left ventricle (LV) from the left atrium. The *top left panel* shows the first image in the gated sequence triggered by the electrocardiographic R wave, at end diastole. The LV is at the right, and the right ventricle (RV) can be seen to the left (*arrow*). Each image (left to right, top row to bottom) represents an additional 60 msec elapsed time from the R wave. By about the fifth or sixth image (300–360 msec), it is clear that the LV has contracted considerably, reaching the end systole. The RV is also much smaller, its apical portion almost disappearing. During the next six images the LV begins filling in the diastolic portion of the cardiac cycle. By the twelfth image, the LV is once again completely full, end diastole, and the cycle begins again. Since there are 12 images of 60 msec each, the average time between beats (the R-R time) is 60 msec × 12 = 720 msec. This corresponds to a heart rate of about 83 beats/min. These images can be played as a cine that will reveal the pattern of contraction. Wall motion defects can clearly be observed from such movie sequences. However, since these are planar images, the effects of motion of the anterior and posterior myocardial walls will be difficult to observe. In this LAO view (with caudal tilt), only the motion of the septal, apical, and lateral LV walls can be observed. For resting studies, two additional views are also usually acquired, an anterior view and a left lateral view. These other two views give additional visual information concerning wall motion. Only the LAO view is used to compute quantitative indices of LV function, since only this view is free from overlapping structures, albeit incompletely. The same technique can be used with gated blood pool SPECT. In this case, however, there is access to all views and cross sections, so that all walls can be observed and there is no difficulty with overlapping structures [11,12,16,38–40].

Assessment of Cardiac Function: First-Pass, Equilibrium Blood Pool, and Gated Myocardial SPECT

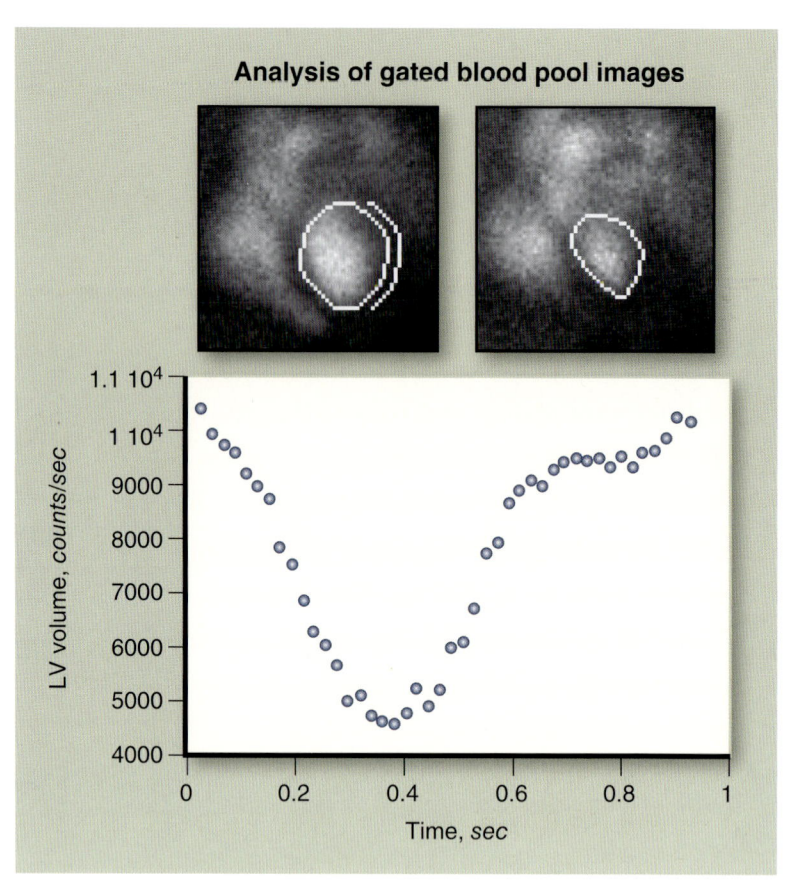

Figure 5-13. Analysis of gated blood pool images. Since the image intensity or counts in the gated image sequence are approximately, or exactly in the case of PET, proportional to the volume of blood, one can create a left ventricular (LV) volume curve from the image set. One can draw a single region of interest (ROI) around the image at end diastole, as shown by the roughly circular ROI in the *upper left image*, and then plot the counts from within this ROI as a function of time represented by the image number against the msec per image. In this figure, the planar gated image set consists of 44 images, each taken for 20 msec, thereby producing a very high temporal resolution LV "volume" curve. The word "volume" is in quotes because in planar studies the counts are only approximately proportional to volume as a quite linear function, and because some of the counts in the planar images arise from the tissues above and below the heart as in the soft tissue between the gamma camera and the heart. In an attempt to correct for these extraneous counts, one usually draws a second ROI adjacent to the LV cavity, and takes this "background" region as a correction indicative of the extraneous counts from above and below the heart [9].

Another method uses not a single region over the LV cavity, but instead a different ROI for each image or frame. This has the advantage of better tracking the LV cavity, and the disadvantage of introducing variability in drawing the numerous regions required. In actual practice both methods give results that correlate quite accurately with one another, although the variable region method gives a consistently "deeper" curve and a higher ejection fraction. Practically images for each frame are used when edges for each ROI can be applied in an automated manner. When edges must be applied manually, regions are drawn on end diastole and end systole. This procedure is semi-automated in many commercial nuclear medicine cardiac analysis packages. It has been shown that 16 frames or more are needed to provide the sampling rate required to capture the extremes of end systole and end diastole in order to gain an accurate ejection fraction and other indices of LV function [41].

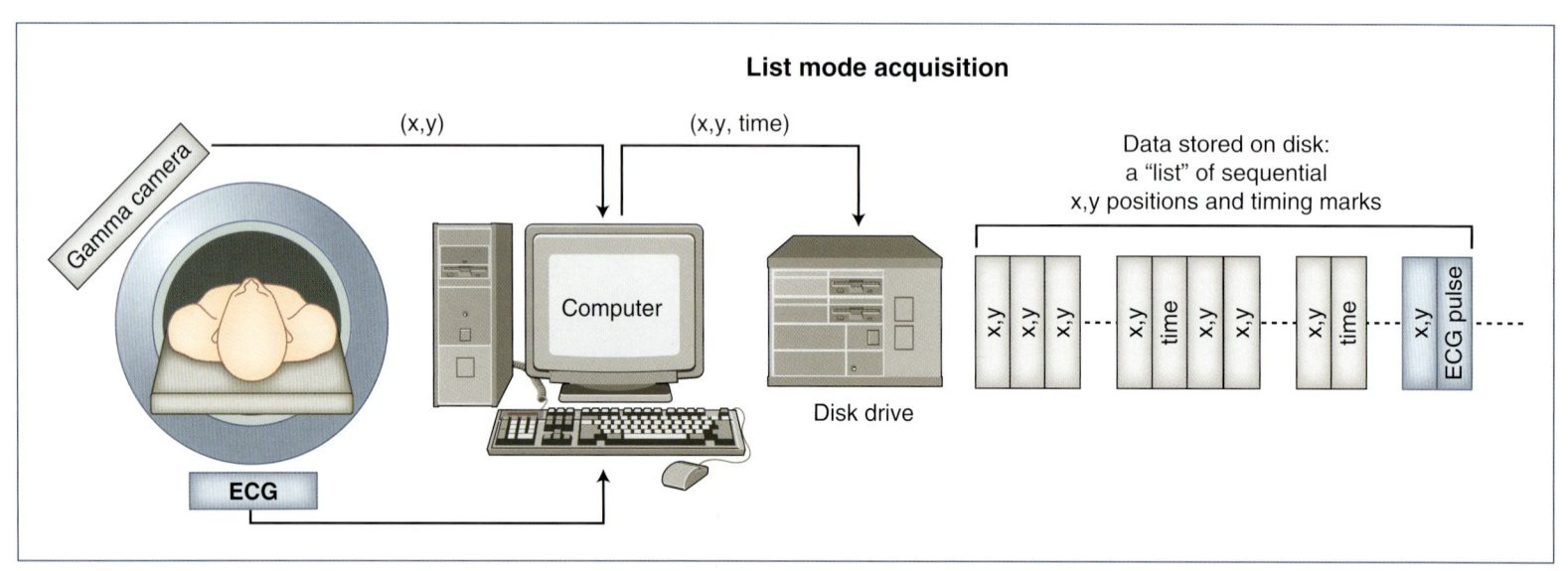

Figure 5-14. List mode acquisition. Shown is a schematic drawing demonstrating the mechanism of list mode acquisition. The equilibrium radionuclide angiography gating method described can be performed in "real time" [7,34], *ie*, the data are sorted into the images on the fly as the photons are registered by the gamma camera. While this is a very convenient method, there are occasions when it is a less than ideal solution. For example, one may wish to retrospectively look only at beats of a certain length. If the data are sorted into the image sequences on the fly, this of course is impossible. To enable "retrospective" analysis of the data, one can use a method called list mode acquisition. In this mode of operation, the computer simply records on disk a "list" of the timing and location of every photon recorded by the camera. Since typically many millions of counts make up a gated blood pool cardiac study, many million words of disk storage are required. On older systems this was a serious problem, as disk space was often both limited and expensive. Obviously, this is no longer an issue. Once the data have been recorded, one can read it back from disk, and perform the gating just as described previously. Why bother to write it to disk then? There are several reasons. First, in frame mode, selecting the beat length window (*ie*, the range of beats to accept and reject) is often problematic. One has to make this decision prior to beginning the acquisition, and it is quite possible and even common for the heart rate to change during the course of the study if the patient becomes more comfortable on the table, or even falls asleep, or conversely, becomes uncomfortable. Thus, the heart rate may slowly shift as the study progresses. Similarly, during exercise studies it is often not possible to accurately predict and hold the heart rate stable. In a list mode study such difficulties are easily overcome, because one is processing the data after the fact, and the computer can first display the progression of heart rates that occurred during the study, and the operator can then select whatever range of heart rates seem most suitable.

Continued on the next page

118 Atlas of Nuclear Cardiology

Figure 5-14. *(Continued)* This method also permits multiple levels of exercise to be studied easily. One can select any combination of heart rates and time periods desired. Finally, list mode acquisition allows the very end of the cycle, atrial contraction, to be reproduced. Again, since processing is retrospective, one can gate "backwards" in time from the R-wave trigger. If the P-wave to R- wave interval is relatively constant from beat to beat, one can then faithfully reproduce the volume increase due to atrial contraction. ECG—electrocardiogram.

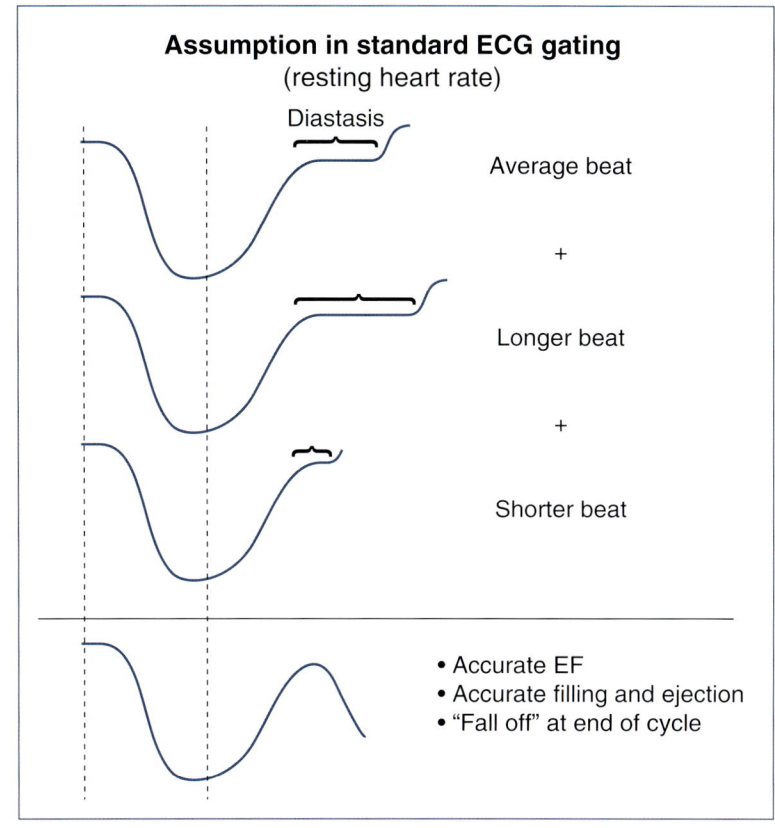

Figure 5-15. Assumptions in standard gated imaging. There is an assumption implicit in the gating process that the heart beats in exactly the same way and has the same contraction and relaxation pattern from one beat to the next [42]. If the subject is in normal sinus rhythm (NSR) this approximation holds quite well. However, owing to the normal sinus arrhythmia, varying beat length requires an adjustment at the end of the cycle. The end of the cycle has to be handled somewhat differently, because not all beats will be of the same length. In fact fluctuations in R to R interval times can be quite large, as much as 100 msec or more for a normal subject in NSR at rest. This means that for beats shorter than average, the last, or last few, frames will not accumulate for the full time, while for beats longer than average, data will be thrown away. Both of these circumstances can easily be accounted for by keeping accurate account of the actual length of each beat and therefore the actual acquisition time for each frame that spans the cardiac cycle. Of course such beat length fluctuations may degrade the ability of the gated data to portray events occurring very late in the cycle as the volume increases due to atrial contraction. Not all computer systems make the compensation for this varying beat length described. If such a correction is not made, the images at the end of the cycle will have an artificially reduced intensity, and quantitative data extracted from these images may be subject to error.

At first one might think that a shorter than average beat might be a "condensed" version of an average length beat and that a long beat is simply a uniformly stretched version of a short beat, scaled temporally, and having a shorter than average time to end systole, and other characteristics. If this were true, then the assumption that all beats are identical would be violated. Fortunately, for subjects in NSR it has been shown that at rest, fluctuations in heart rate are caused primarily by fluctuations in the initiation of the next beat. That is, a "short" beat is shorter only because the next beat begins slightly earlier than average. Thus, at rest in normal individuals, it is only diastasis that is shorter, and the earlier parts of the cycle remain unaltered. This is not true at higher heart rates, where there is no diastasis at all, nor is it necessarily true for subjects who are not in NSR, or for subjects in whom the filling portion of the left ventricular (LV) volume curve is so abnormal that there is no discernable diastasis at all. In these situations, the technique of "beat length windowing" is necessary, in which beats shorter or longer than some predetermined length are not included in the data. However, this may not always make physiologic sense. The short beat itself in all likelihood was functioning like all other beats up until the time it was prematurely terminated. That is, it was too short simply because the next beat began too early. If the next beat began prior to complete LV filling, the beat following the short beat would *not* be identical to all the other beats. It would have a different preload and therefore a different pattern of contraction and filling. Therefore, one may wish to reject the beat following the short beat, not just the short beat itself. In fact, there may be no reason to reject the short beat itself. The user of the computer program for gated acquisition is usually permitted to choose not simply what length beats are unsuitable, but also what to do about the succeeding or even previous beats. ECG—electrocardiogram; EF—ejection fraction.

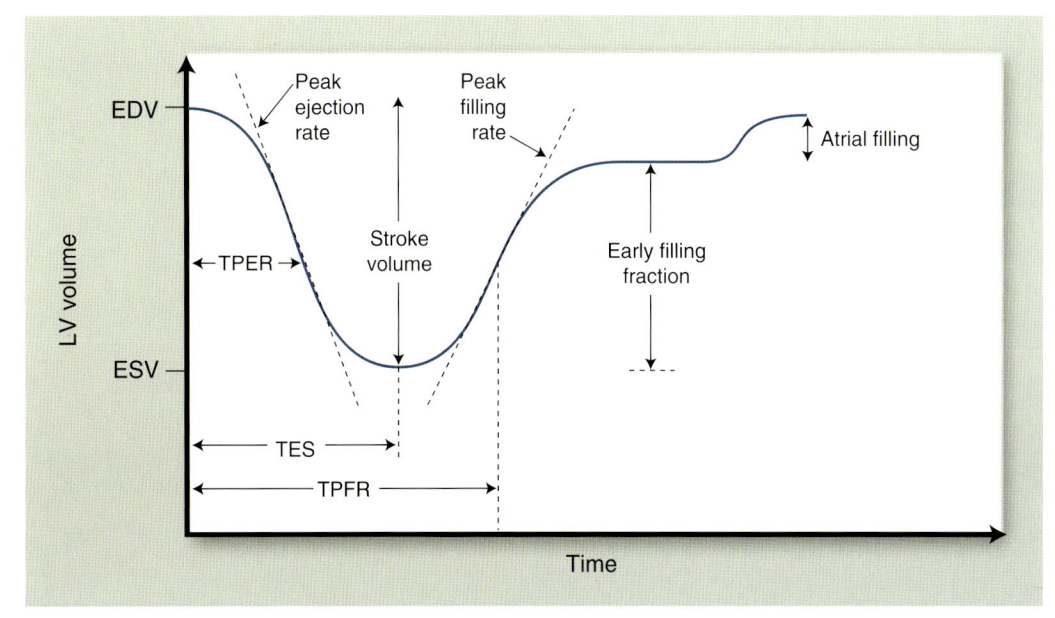

Figure 5-16. Functional measures. Shown here are some of the many useful clinical parameters that can be extracted from the left ventricular (LV) volume curve [34,35]. The most useful measure is ejection fraction, defined as stroke volume/end diastolic volume (EDV) = ED counts - end systolic (ES) counts/ ED counts, where the counts are assumed to have been corrected for background. Note that although the proportionality factor between "counts" and volume is in general unknown, it does not matter, since this factor will cancel out when the ratio defining ejection fraction is computed. Many other parameters can be extracted from this curve. The peak ejection rate (PER) and its time of occurrence (TPER) is usually defined as the maximum negative slope of the LV curve between ED and ES. It characterizes the maximum rate at which blood is ejected by the heart.

Continued on the next page

Assessment of Cardiac Function: First-Pass, Equilibrium Blood Pool, and Gated Myocardial SPECT

Figure 5-16. *(Continued)* The time to end systole (TES) is, of course, defined as the minimum of the LV curve. The peak filling rate (PFR) is the diastolic correlate of the PER. In many diseases impending impairment of systolic function is preceded by slower and later than normal filling. This is thought to be due to poor ventricular compliance. Therefore PFR, a measure of diastolic ventricular function, is often reduced even before the ejection fraction or systolic function is noticeably impaired. ESV—end systolic volume; TPFR—time to peak filling rate.

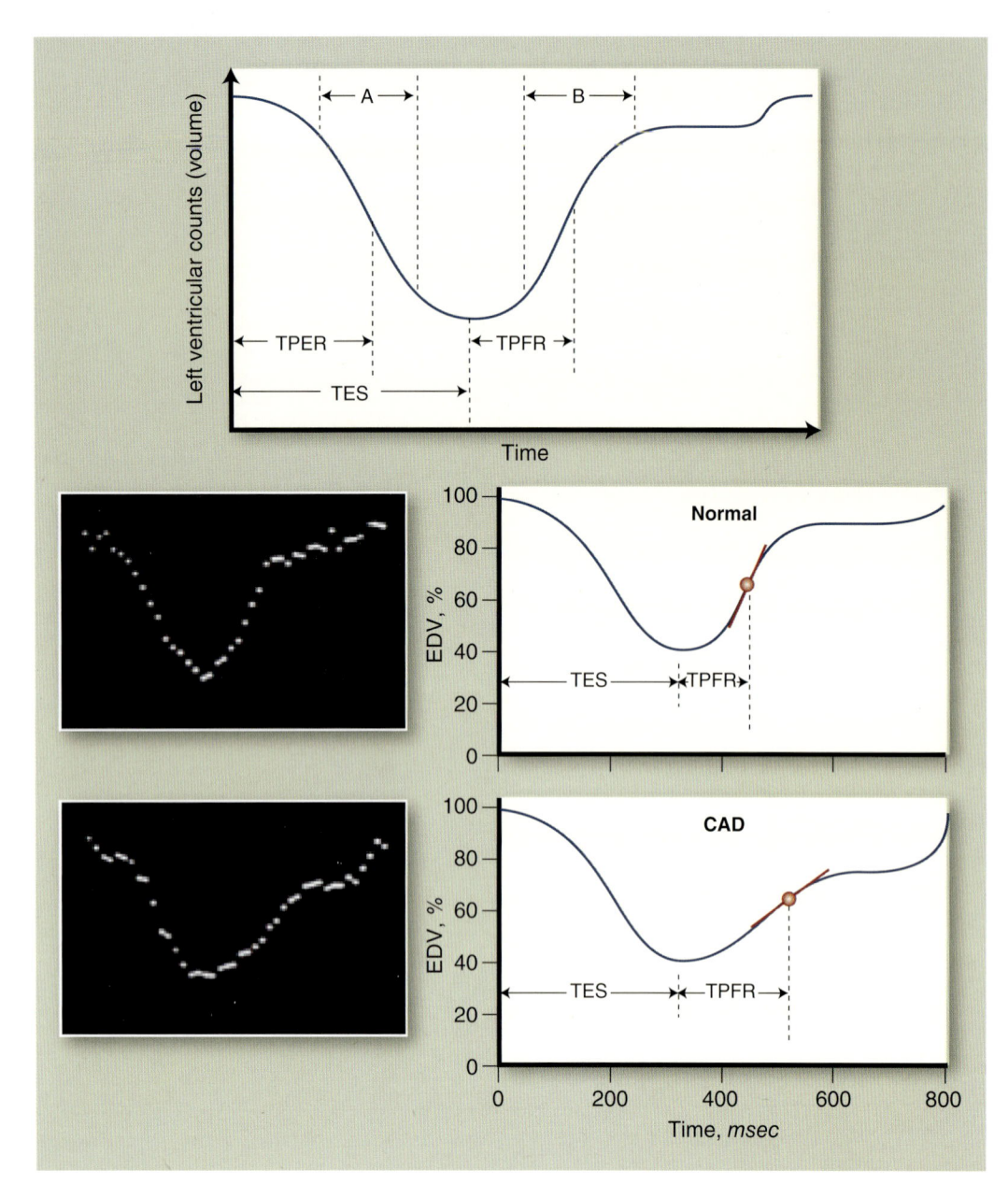

Figure 5-17. Application of filling phase indices. Shown at the *top* is a diagrammatic left ventricular time versus radioactivity curve where time to peak emptying rate (TPER), time to peak filling rate (TPFR), and time to end systole (TES) are shown in systolic (*A*) and diastolic (*B*) periods [43]. At the *bottom*, actual curves (*left*) and diagrammatic representations (*right*) are shown in a normal patient (*top*) and in a coronary patient (*bottom*). The reduced ventricular filling rate in the latter is evident. CAD—coronary artery disease; EDV—end-diastolic volume. (*Adapted from* Bonow et al. [43].)

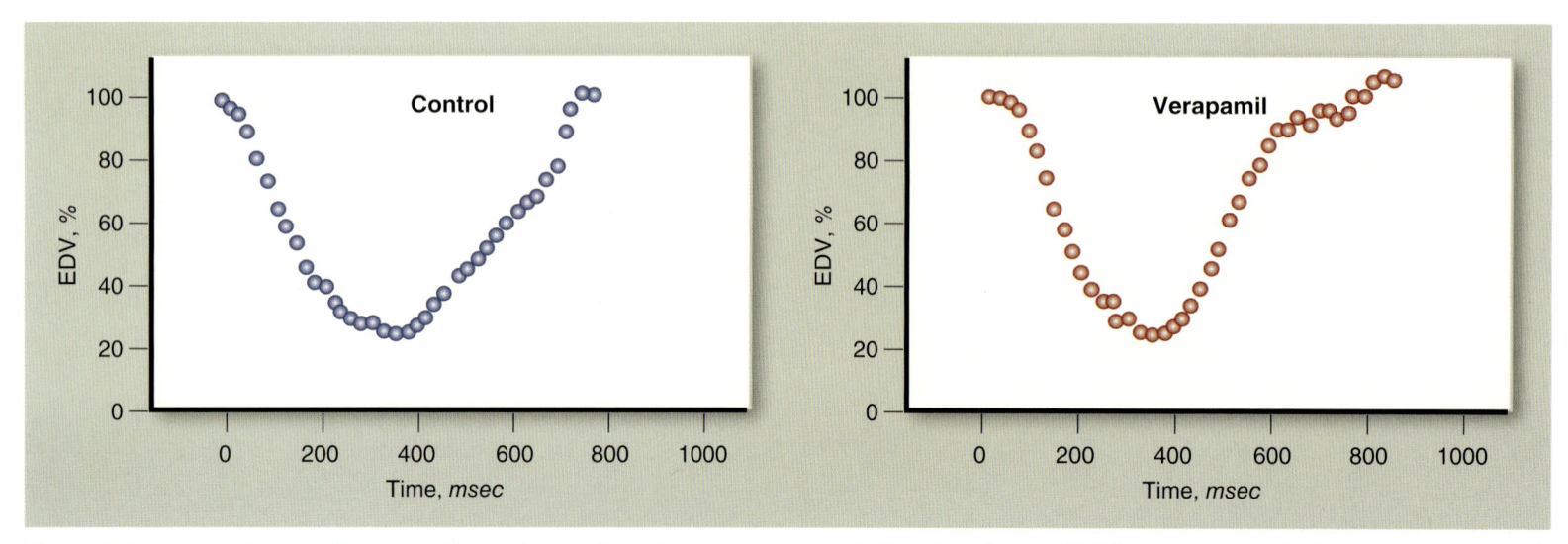

Figure 5-18. Drug effect on filling rate. Shown is the effect of verapamil on left ventricular compliance and filling rate in a patient with left ventricular hypertrophy [43]. The increased slope and filling rate measured in end-diastolic volumes (EDV) per second, is significantly increased with verapamil. (*Adapted from* Bonow et al. [43].)

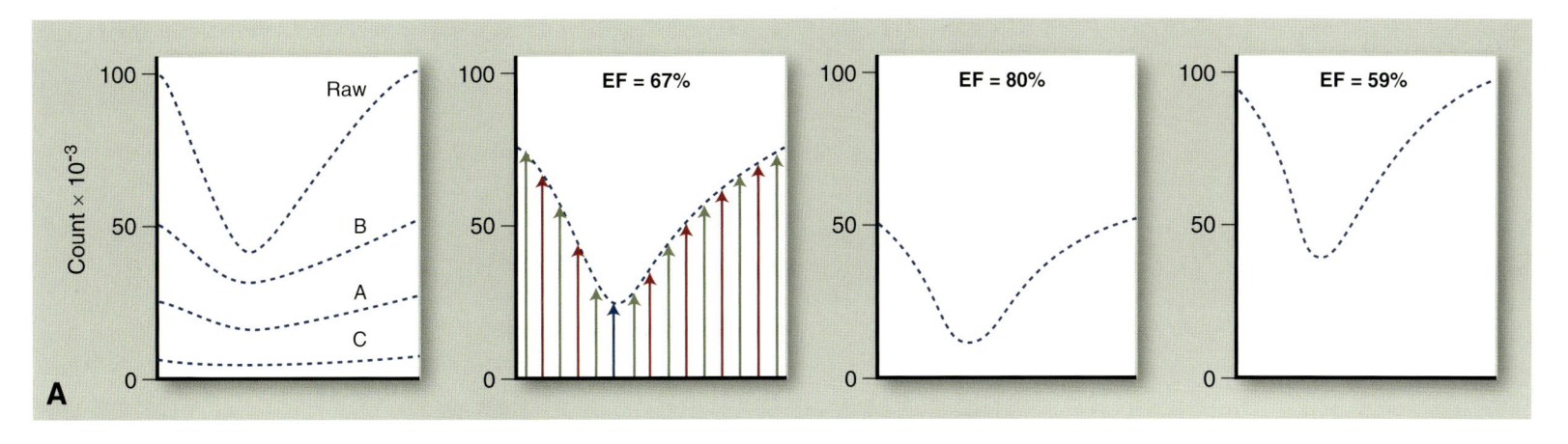

Calculations and Left Ventricular Ejection Fraction Derived from the Varying Background Values in Figure 5-19A

Curve	LV ROI Pixels	Mean Counts Background ROI	ROI Uncorrected Counts	Background Corrected Counts	LVEF, %
A	ED 500	50	100,000	75,000	67
	ES 300		40,000	25,000	
B	ED 500	100	100,000	50,000	80
	ES 300		40,000	10,000	
C	ED 500	10	100,000	95,000	59
	ES 300		40,000	37,000	

B

Figure 5-19. The importance of background in equilibrium blood pool studies. **A,** Shown are three model time versus radioactivity curves, *A, B, C,* which vary only in their background, greatest in *B* and least in *C* as shown in the *left panel* with corresponding background subtracted curves *A, B,* and *C.* The calculations and left ventricular (LV) actual ejection fractions (EF) derived from these varying background values is shown **B**. ED—end diastolic; ES—end systolic; ROI—region of interest. (*Adapted from* Botvinick et al. [44].)

Calculation Method

$$LVEDV = \frac{\text{Count rate from LV in ED frame}/e^{-ud}}{\text{Count rate/mL from blood sample}}$$

where e^{-ud} = attenuation correction

u = average linear attenuation coefficient

d = depth of the center of the LV from the chest wall

LV count rate from ED frame =

$$\frac{\text{Total LV counts in ED frame}}{\text{Time per frame} \times \text{number of cycles acquired}}$$

Blood sample of known volume is withdrawn into small test tube and counted under the same radiation detector (camera) used for radionuclide angiography. The calculated count rate is corrected for decay from the time it was withdrawn during study to the time it was counted.

A

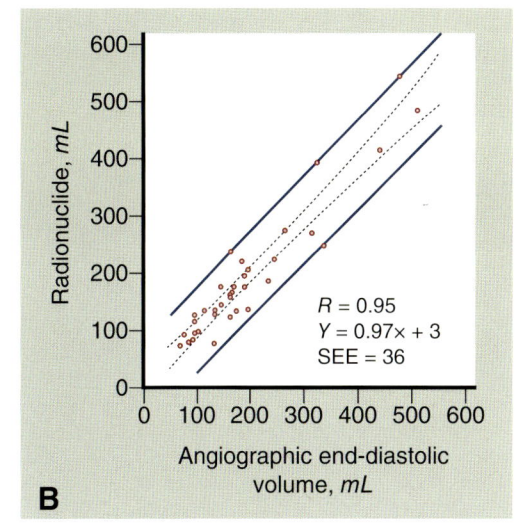

B

$R = 0.95$
$Y = 0.97x + 3$
$SEE = 36$

Figure 5-20. Calculation of left ventricular end-diastolic volume from equilibrium radionuclide angiograms. When corrected for duration of data collection (*ie,* number of beats collected and frame duration), administered dose, and plasma volume, absolute left ventricular (LV) volume can be calculated with relatively high precision from equilibrium radionuclide angiograms (and from first-pass studies). One of the many calculation methods is depicted here (**A**), together with the validating data comparing volumes obtained by equilibrium radionuclide angiography and by contrast angiography at catheterization (**B**). ED—end diastolic; LVEDV—left ventricular end-diastolic volume. (*From* Germano et al., Fig. 5-6, *Atlas of Nuclear Cardiology,* edn 2.)

Radionuclide Angiography in Clinical Cardiology

Useful for patients with
- Chronic stable CAD
  - Diagnosis
  - *Prognostication*
  - Assessment of efficacy of treatment
- Regurgitant valvular diseases
  - *Prognostication and timing of valvular surgery*
  - Assessment of effects of treatment
- Cardiomyopathy
  - *Determination of functional severity, categorization for treatment selection*
  - Assessment of effects of treatment

Useful only for highly selected applications in patients with
- Acute CAD
  - Diagnosis of acute right ventricular infarction
  - Prognostication
- Stenotic valvular diseases
  - Mitral stenosis—may be useful in prognostication

Figure 5-21. Radionuclide angiography in clinical cardiology. Radionuclide angiography can be employed for diagnosis, prognostication, and evaluation of therapy in a variety of situations, as listed here. However, other modalities may be more appropriately applied in specific clinical settings. The most appropriate situations for application of radionuclide angiography are listed, with notation as to whether radionuclide angiography may be considered a primary evaluation method or whether better alternatives clearly exist. *Italicized entities* are those for which radionuclide angiography has the greatest potential applicability in clinical practice. CAD—coronary artery disease. (*From* Germano *et al.*, Fig. 5-1, *Atlas of Nuclear Cardiology*, edn 2.)

Left Ventricular Ejection Fraction During Doxorubicin Therapy

Baseline EF	Perform Equilibrium Radionuclide Angiography	At Risk for CHF
Normal (≈ 50%)	At baseline	≥ 10% EF fall from baseline to < 50%
	At ≈ 450 mg/m²	
	At 250–300 mg/m²	
≥ 30% to < 50%	At baseline	≥ 10% EF fall from baseline or EF < 30%
	Prior to each subsequent dose	
< 30%	Avoid doxorubicin	

Figure 5-22. Directing doxorubicin therapy. Radionuclide angiography (RNA) is the most widely accepted method for serial evaluation of cardiac function in patients undergoing doxorubicin therapy. Left ventricular ejection fraction (LVEF) is an important and universally accepted index of cardiac function. Overt congestive heart failure due to doxorubicin cardiotoxicity is preceded by a progressive fall in LVEF. Serial studies can detect a change in cardiac function over time, and doxorubicin administration can be stopped when a predetermined fall in LVEF is observed. Both the absolute LVEF and the magnitude of fall are important strategic determinants. The guidelines for using serial RNA at rest, during the course of doxorubicin therapy, are standardized and are based upon experience with nearly 1500 patients over a 7-year period. A great than fourfold reduction in the incidence of overt cardiac failure was observed when these guidelines were followed. Moreover, if congestive heart failure (CHF) developed, it was mild and rapidly responsive to medical therapy. A recent study has reestablished the clinical relevance and cost-effectiveness of serial LVEF monitoring with equilibrium RNA for the prevention of congestive heart failure during the course of doxorubicin therapy [15]. Exercise RNA also has been used in patients undergoing treatment with doxorubicin. However, patients with malignancies often are unable to undergo exercise testing because of generalized debility, fever, anemia, or musculoskeletal problems. Moreover, exercise testing does not appear to provide additional information compared with resting RNA. Some caution may be required in interpreting changes in LVEF during the course of chemotherapy, since these values also are affected by several noncardiac conditions such as anemia, fever, and sepsis. Resting RNA continues to be the most practical and effective way of monitoring doxorubicin cardiotoxicity. (*From* Borer, Fig. 9-26, *Atlas of Nuclear Cardiology*, edn 1.)

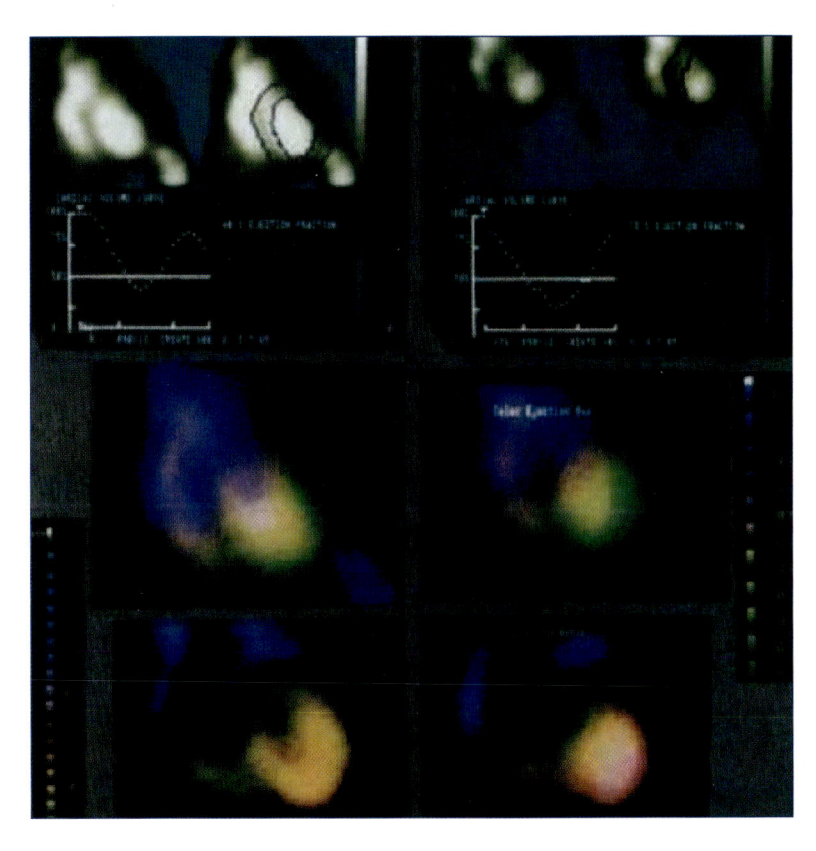

Figure 5-23. Equilibrium blood pool assessment of aortic regurgitation. Shown are left ventricular time versus activity curves derived from a left ventricular region of interest (*top panel*); ejection fraction images, color-coded for regional ejection fraction (*middle panel*); and phase-amplitude images (*bottom panel*) at rest (*left*) and with maximal exercise (*right*) in a young patient with severe aortic regurgitation. Here, the left ventricular edge is derived between the limits of the edges drawn, and background is taken within these geometric boundaries. Dual color and intensity coded images, shown here, permit the integration of multiple parameters in a single image and are an example of the analytic and display potential of the scintigraphic modality. The left ventricular ejection fraction increases with exercise. This is supported by the increased area covered by *yellow* and *green* and high ejection fraction values in the ejection fraction image. Although colors shift to later phase angles as heart rate increases, amplitude and intensity is maintained and apparent ventricular size decreases in all images, consistent with a normal response to exercise. The uniform phase shift, related to increased symmetry of the time versus radioactivity curve with increased heart rate and shortening of end-diastole, represents a normal finding, as do all the image results shown here. (*From* Botvinick *et al.* [44]; with permission.)

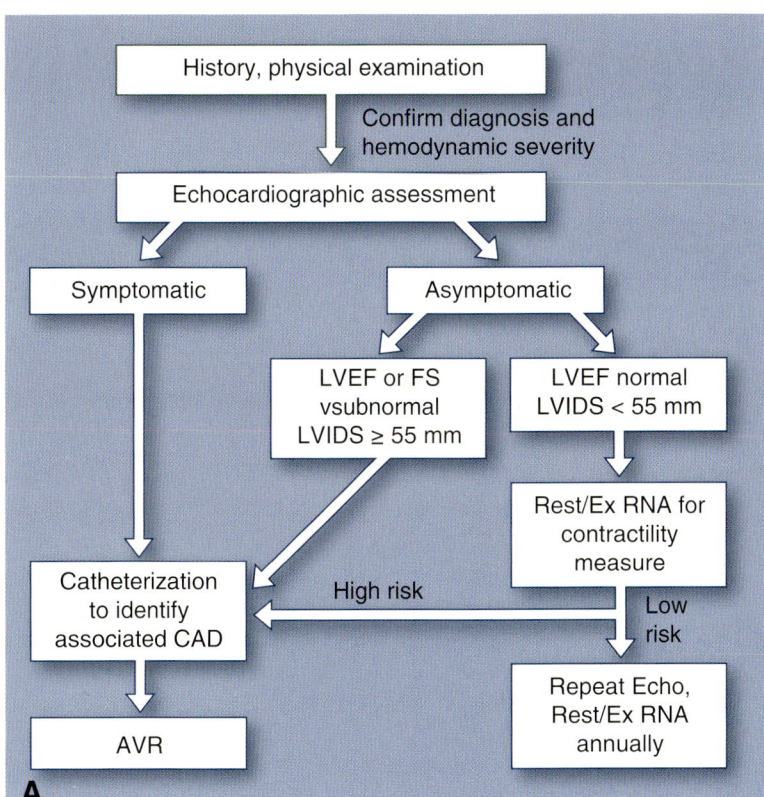

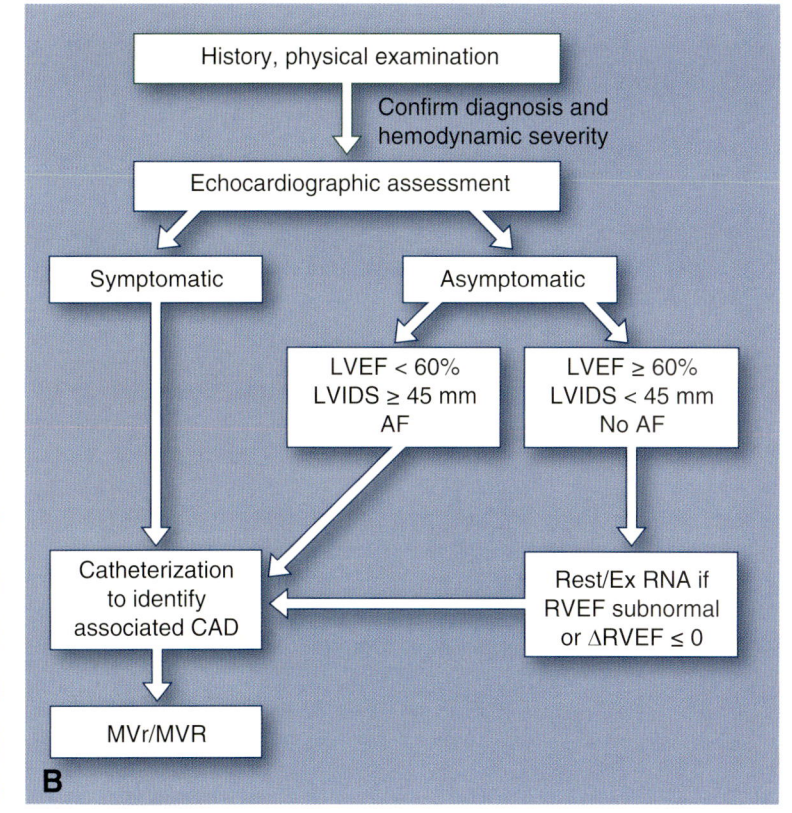

Figure 5-24. Role of radionuclide angiography in patients with aortic regurgitation and mitral regurgitation. For asymptomatic patients with regurgitant valvular diseases, echocardiography (echo) is a primary method for diagnosis and for determination of hemodynamic severity of disease. If echocardiography unequivocally demonstrates subnormal left ventricular ejection fraction (LVEF) at rest, or "high-risk" left ventricular systolic or diastolic dimension descriptors, management decisions can be made with confidence. However, for patients with severe aortic regurgitation (**A**), the geometric irregularity and regional functional variability of the large left ventricle may result in ambiguity of ejection fraction determination, obviated by non–geometry-dependent evaluation with radionuclide angiography (RNA); if echocardiographic results do not indicate high risk, contractility determination by additional RNA with exercise can detect prognostically important disease. For patients with mitral regurgitation (**B**), the unique capacity of RNA to interrogate right ventricular performance adds an important prognostic dimension not available with echocardiography. In patients with mitral stenosis, right ventricular ejection fraction (RVEF) determination by RNA carries prognostically important information, but these data have not yet reached routine use in defining management strategies in this setting. Echocardiography remains the primary evaluative modality for mitral stenosis. AF—atrial fibrillation; AVR—aortic valve replacement; CAD—coronary artery disease; Ex—exercise; FS—echocardiographic fractional shortening; LVIDS—left ventricular internal dimension at end systole; MVr—mitral valve repair; MVR—mitral valve replacement. (*From* Germano *et al.*, Fig. 5-3, *Atlas of Nuclear Cardiology*, edn 2.)

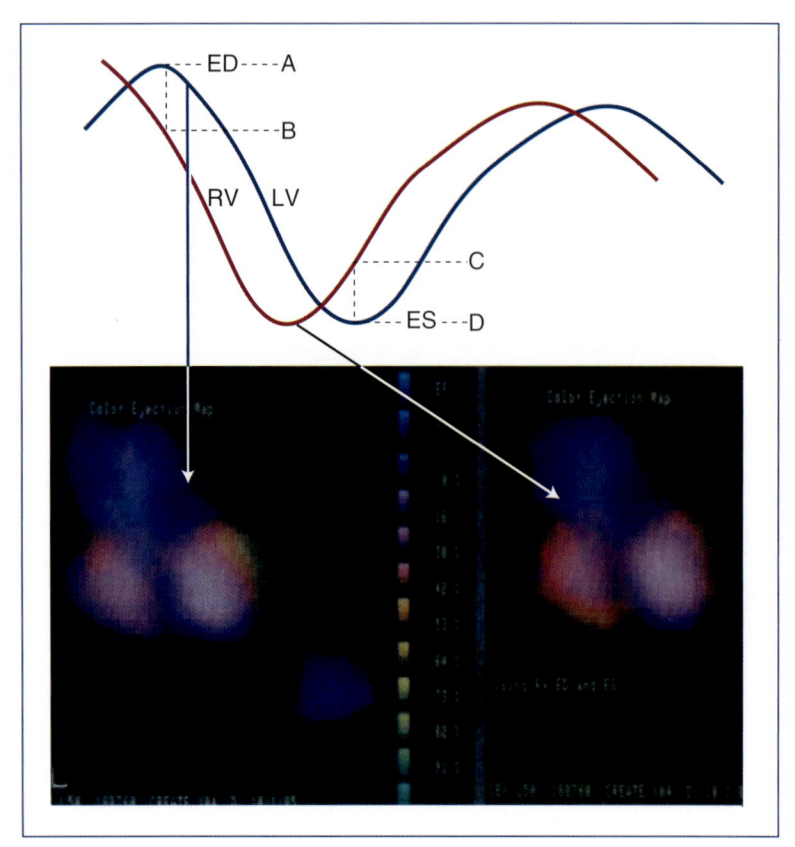

Figure 5-25. Effect of conduction abnormality. Shown are time versus radioactivity curves in a patient with left bundle branch block. The left ventricular (LV) curve lags behind the right ventricular (RV) curve. The ejection fraction (EF) image is derived from frames chosen at LV end-diastole (ED) and end-systole (ES). Owing to the conduction abnormality, LVED (A) and LVES (D) correspond to points at a partially filled (B) and incompletely emptied (C) RV, giving rise to an artificially reduced RVEF. At the *bottom* are color-coded EF images in a patient with left bundle branch block compiled using frames optimized for LVED and ES (*left*) and for RVED and ES (*right*). Note the bright *green-yellow* area at the LV base (*left*) and the augmentation of high EF colors in the RV (*right*) in these images, derived from different aspects of the same data. (*From* Botvinick *et al.* [44]; with permission.)

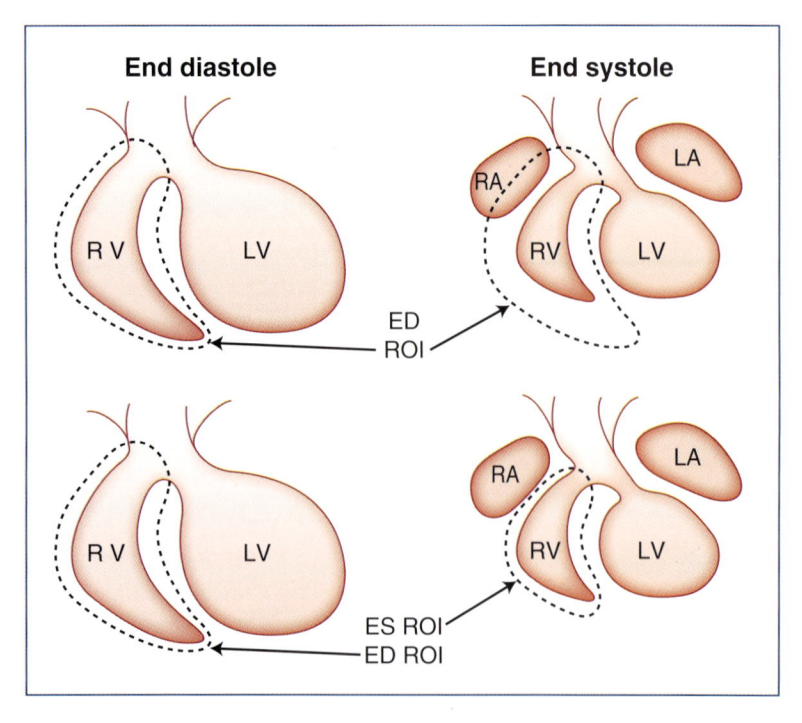

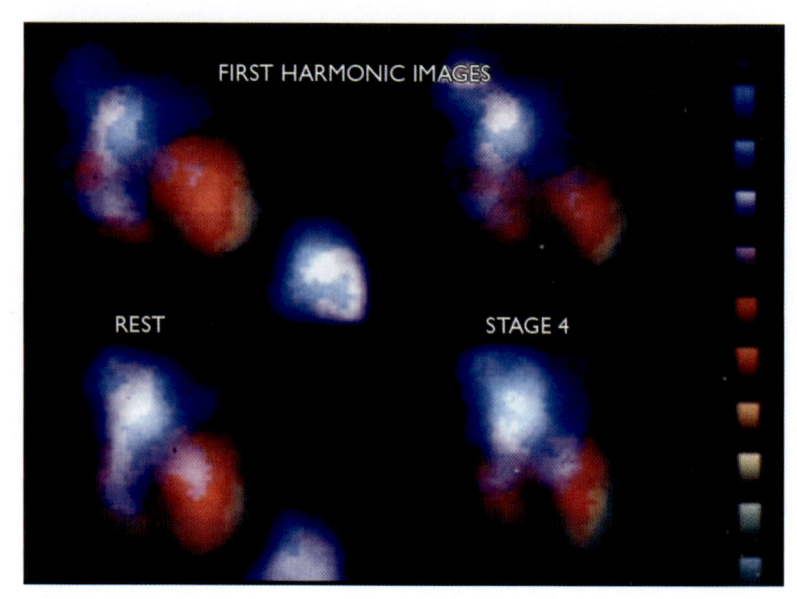

Figure 5-26. Exercise evaluation. Shown are color ejection fraction images at rest (*left*) and with maximal exercise (*right*) in a patient with coronary artery disease (*top*) and with aortic regurgitation (*bottom*). Reduced presence of the "ejection shell," the green and yellow high ejection fraction colors at rest (*left*) demonstrate a decrement in regional function and overall left ventricular ejection fraction (LVEF) at stress (*right*) in the coronary patient, while reduced LV size with an increased green "ejection shell" demonstrates an augmented LVEF in the patient with aortic regurgitation (*bottom*). Such functional images condense a wealth of of information and provide objectivity to the assessment of the effects of intervention on ventricular size and function. (*From* Botvinick *et al.* [44]; with permission.)

Figure 5-27. Right ventricular (RV) ejection fraction. Shown diagrammatically is the application of a RV region of interest (ROI) to an equilibrium blood pool study in end-diastole (ED) (*left*) and in end-systole (ES) (*right*). At *top*, the same ED region is applied in ES with erroneous inclusion of the right atrium (RA), which is largest in ventricular ES below, and ES-specific (ROI is applied with significant improvement, but without total correction for RA overlap on the RV. LA—left atrium; LV—left ventricle. (*Adapted from* Botvinick *et al.* [44].)

124 Atlas of Nuclear Cardiology

Regurgitant index

$$RI = \frac{LVSVC}{RVSVC}$$

RF = Regurgitant fraction

$$RF = \frac{LVSVC - RVSVC}{LVSVC}$$

$$RF = \frac{\frac{LVSVC}{RVSVC} - \frac{RVSVC}{RVSVC}}{\frac{LVSVC}{RVSVC}} = \frac{RI - 1}{RI}$$

Figure 5-28. Regurgitant index (RI)–regurgitant fraction (RF). Shown are the formulas for the RI, the ratio of left ventricular stroke volume (LVSVC) and right ventricular stroke volume (RVSVC) measured in counts, and the RF. These are parameters applied to determine the severity of regurgitant lesions as mitral and aortic regurgitation. The amount that LVSVC exceeds RVSVC is a measure of the regurgitant volume and is expressed as the RI. The RF is that percentage of the LVSV that is regurgitating and adding to the overall LVSVC. However, scintigraphically, both measures fail to correct for right atrial overlap on the right ventricle. This causes an underestimation of RVSV and an exaggeration of the RI, which may be as high as 1.3 in normal subjects.

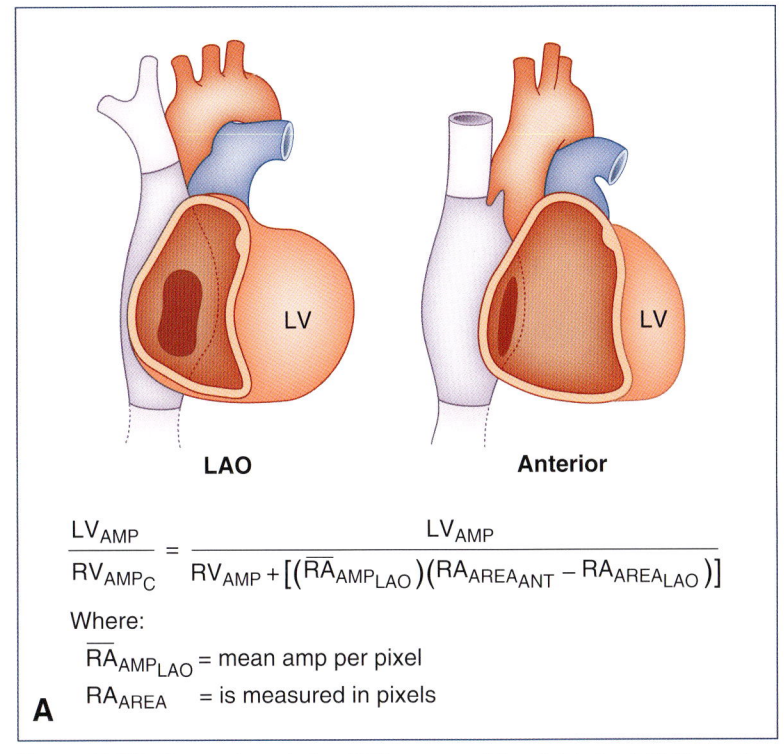

$$\frac{LV_{AMP}}{RV_{AMP_C}} = \frac{LV_{AMP}}{RV_{AMP} + [(\overline{RA}_{AMP_{LAO}})(RA_{AREA_{ANT}} - RA_{AREA_{LAO}})]}$$

Where:
$\overline{RA}_{AMP_{LAO}}$ = mean amp per pixel
RA_{AREA} = is measured in pixels

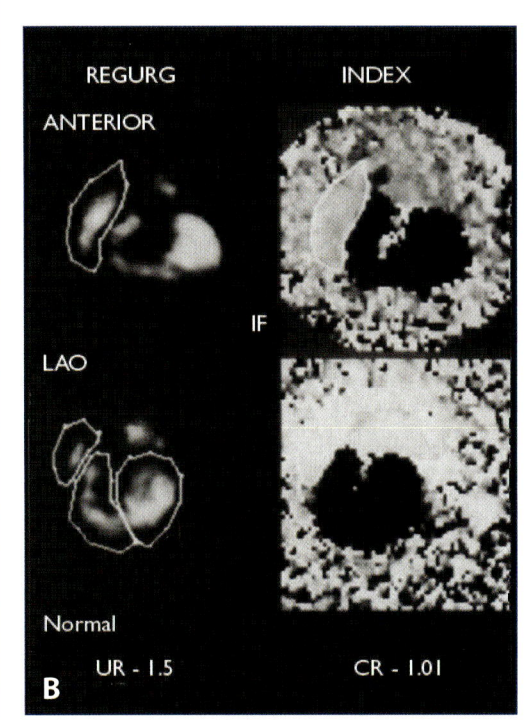

Figure 5-29. Regurgitant index (RI) corrected for right atrial (RA) overlap. **A,** The anatomic basis for the amplitude-based correction of RI for RA overlap [45]. Here right ventricular (RV) amplitude, an analogue of stroke volume, is corrected with the addition of the product of the mean per-pixel amplitude of the RA in the left anterior oblique (LAO) projection and its area, measured in pixels of the RA that are obscured by the RV, the difference in RA area measured on anterior and LAO projections. This correction results in the reduction of the RI to unity in normal subjects and, compared with the uncorrected value, correlates much better with other measures of valvular regurgitation as shown in the clinical example (**B**). Given the ubiquity and capabilities of echocardiography with Doppler evaluation, it is the method of choice for evaluation of regurgitant lesions. (*From* Dae *et al.* [45]; with permission.)

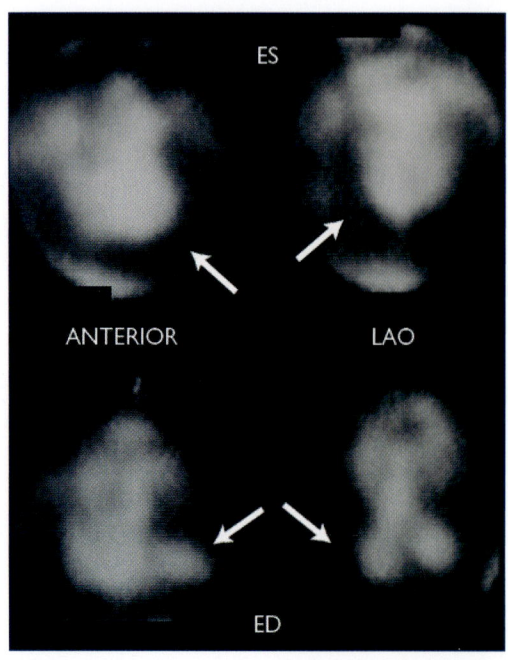

Figure 5-30. Pericardial tamponade. Shown is left anterior oblique (LAO) and anterior views in end systole (ES) (*top*) and end diastole (ED) (*bottom*) in a man with severe fatigability and weakness several weeks after coronary bypass graft surgery. The large "photopenic" region around both ventricles indicates a large pericardial effusion. The small, volume-starved left ventricle is consistent with tamponade, which was the eventual diagnosis.

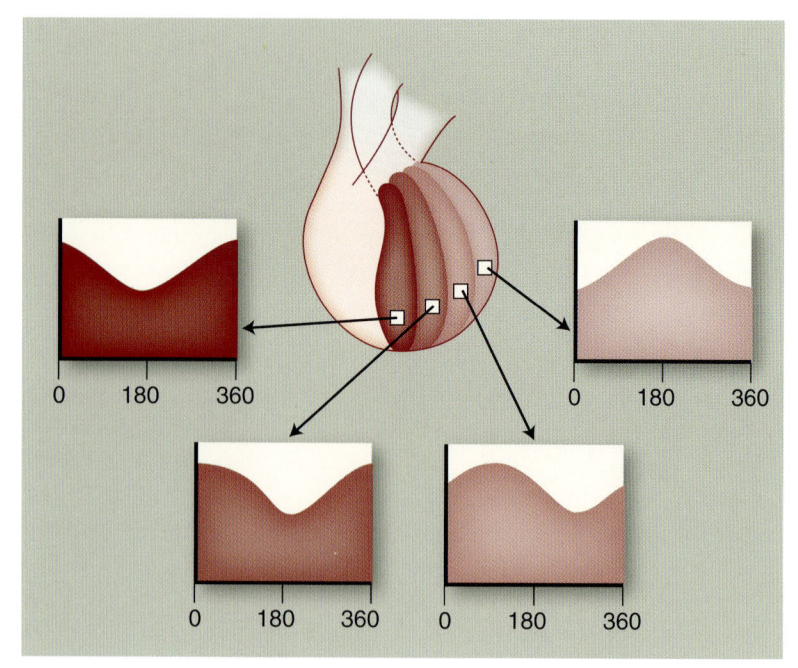

Figure 5-31. Phase analysis. This diagram presents a ventricle that is grayscale coded for increasing delay in contraction sequence, from septum to lateral wall. The resultant cosine curves, fitted to the regional time-versus-radioactivity curve, are shown below. The septum and its corresponding curve begin contraction at the R wave. The region has a phase angle of 0° and is coded dark gray. The lateral wall and its related cosine curve fill when the ventricle should empty. This wall would demonstrate paradoxical motion, and the curve would have a phase angle of 180°. (*Adapted from* Frais *et al.* [46].)

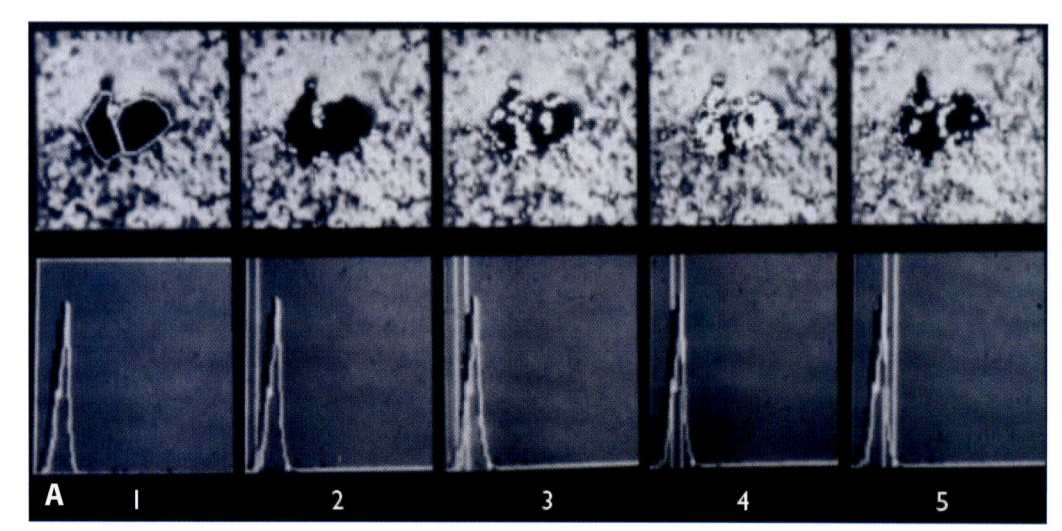

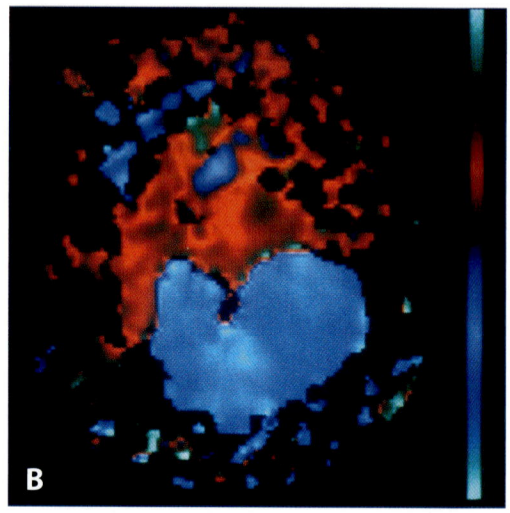

Figure 5-32. Phase image with normal conduction. **A,** Phase image (*top*) and left (*white*) and right (*black*) ventricular histograms (*bottom*) plotting phase angle on the abscissa and its frequency of occurrence on the ordinate in the "best septal" left anterior oblique projection in a patient with normal conduction. Serial phase angle is sampled in the intervals of the vertical gray bars setting the histogram windows, and the corresponding spatial location is indicated by a progressive white highlight of associated pixels on the phase image, from left to right. Earliest phase angle is seen at the base of the septum. **B,** A background subtracted color composite image of the sequential phase angle in this patient reveals symmetric phase distribution and contraction of the two ventricles.

126 Atlas of Nuclear Cardiology

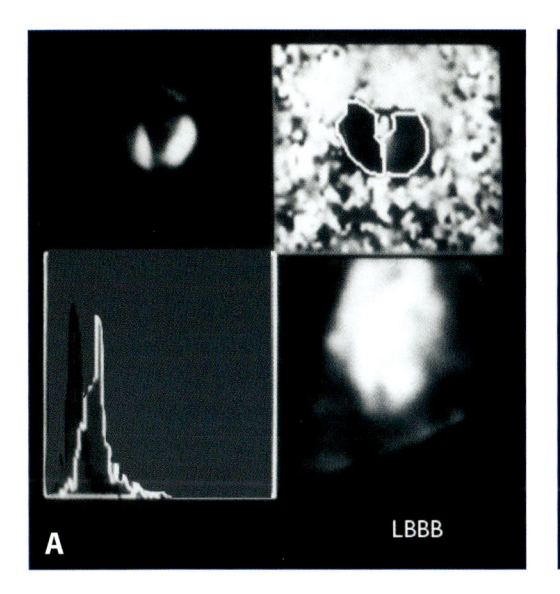

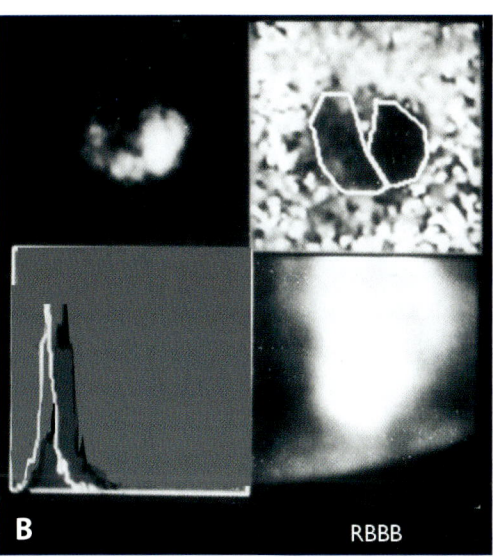

Figure 5-33. Phase images in bundle branch block. Shown are amplitude images (*upper left*), phase images with right and left ventricular regions of interest (*upper right*), phase histograms (*lower left*), and summed blood pool images in the "best septal" left anterior oblique projections in patients with left bundle branch block (LBBB) (**A**) and right bundle branch block (RBBB) (**B**) [46]. The phase histogram plots left (*white*) and right (*black*) ventricular histograms, with phase angle on the abscissa and its frequency on the ordinate. The right ventricular phase histogram and right ventricular activation are earliest in LBBB, while the left ventricular histogram and activation are earliest in RBBB. (*From* Frais *et al.* [46]; with permission.)

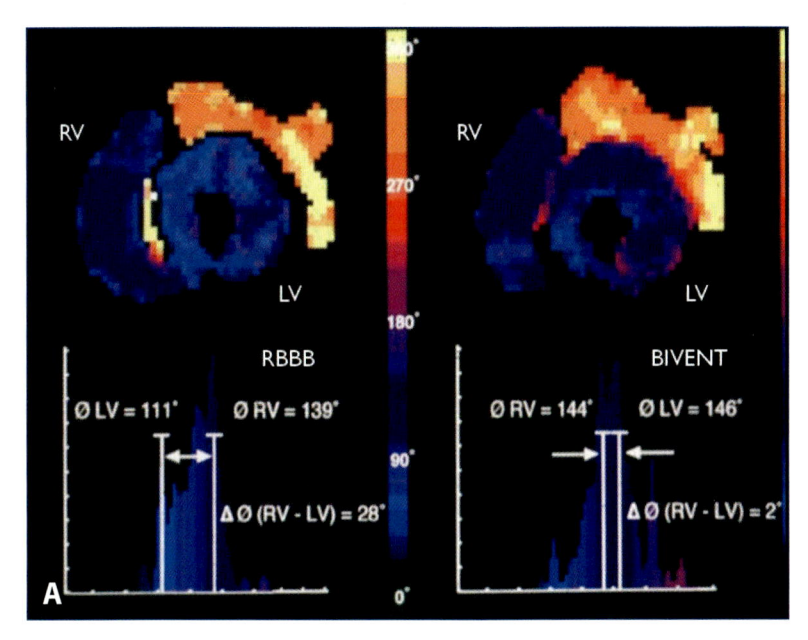

Figure 5-34. The effects of biventricular (BIVENT) pacing. **A**, Phase images and right ventricular (RV) and left ventricular (LV) phase histograms from a heart failure patient with baseline right bundle branch block (RBBB), before and after placement of a biventricular pacemaker [47]. The difference in mean ventricular phase angle is reduced with increased interventricular synchrony. **B**, The inverse relationship between left ventricular ejection fraction (LVEF) (*left*) and right ventricular ejection fraction (RVEF) (*right*) and interventricular phase difference. That is, the greater the reduction brought by biventricular pacing in the difference between the mean phase angles of RV and LV, the greater the subsequent improvement in LVEF. (*From* Kerwin *et al.* [47]; with permission.)

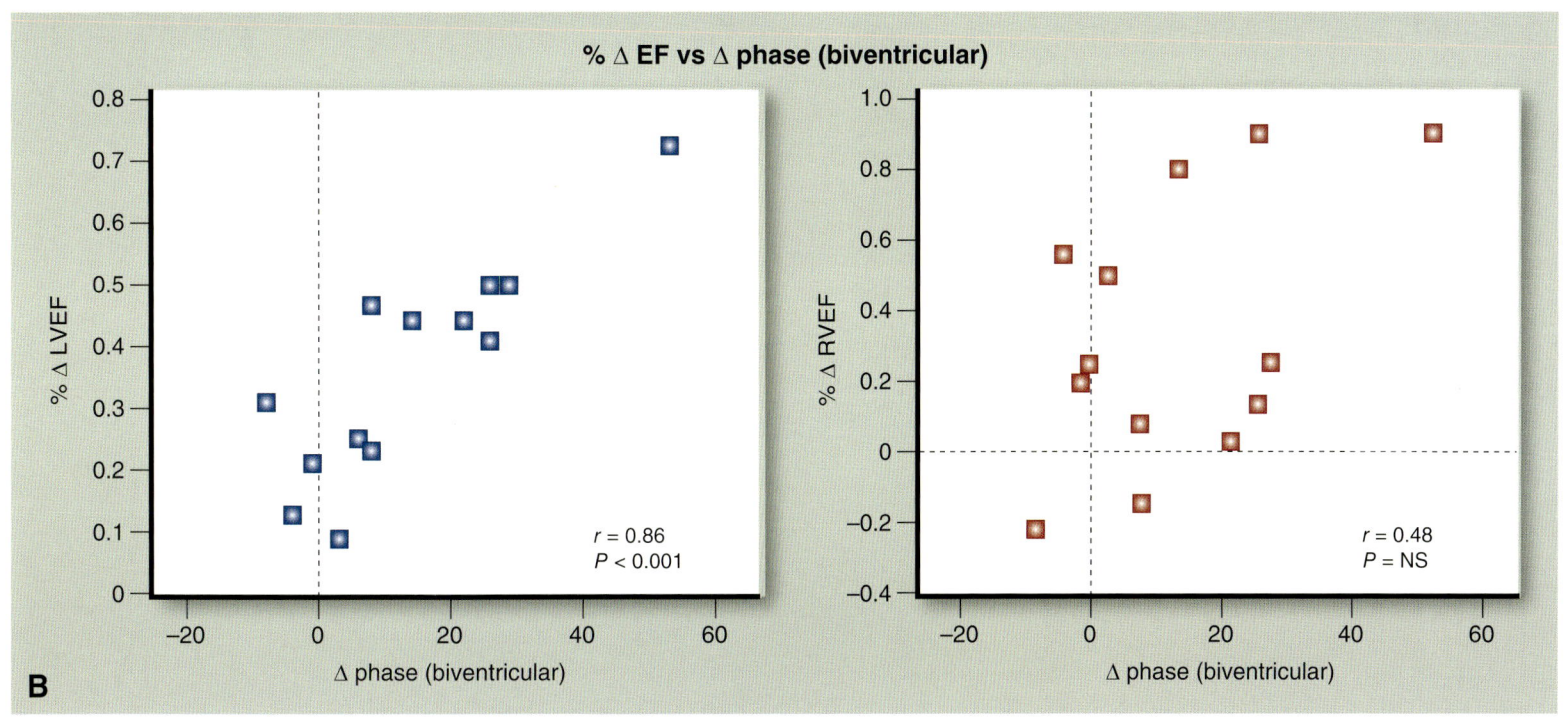

Assessment of Cardiac Function: First-Pass, Equilibrium Blood Pool, and Gated Myocardial SPECT

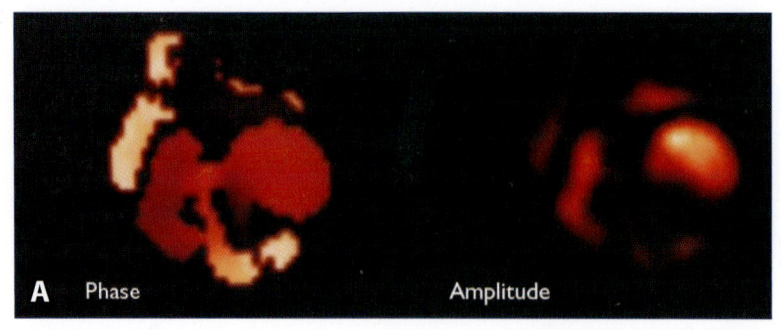

Figure 5-35. Phase image analysis of synchony before and after biventricular pacing. Shown are examples of phase and amplitude images derived from gated equilibrium blood pool scintigrams in a patient with heart failure [48]. **A,** Images from the patient acquired at baseline, with evidence of gross regional dyssynchrony in the phase image at *left* (white color in the septum and apex) and with reduced amplitude in most of the distal left ventricle, as shown by the low intensity regions of the amplitude image at *right*. **B,** Color is more homogeneous and phase is more synchronous, with much improvement in the intensity of the amplitude image following biventricular pacemaker insertion. Not surprisingly, the patient was much improved clinically following the procedure. (*From O'Connell et al.* [48]; with permission.)

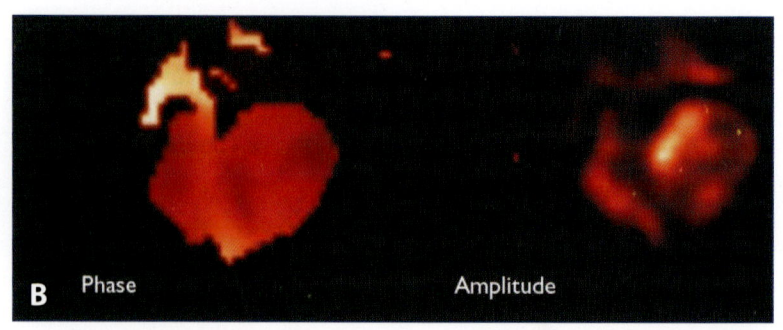

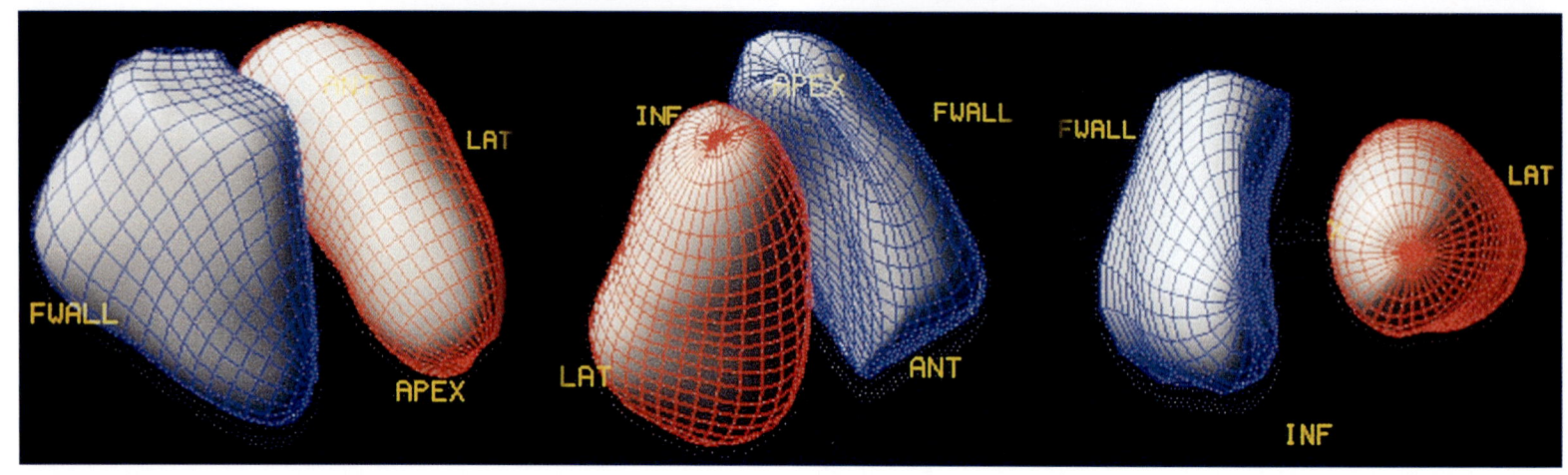

Figure 5-36. Gated blood pool SPECT: left ventricle (LV) and right ventricle (RV). With the increase in the use of echocardiographic procedures and the widespread acceptance of gated myocardial perfusion SPECT, gated planar blood pool imaging has decreased to less than 10% of all nuclear cardiac studies performed in the United States, although the percentage may be substantially higher in other countries. Conversely, the case for gated blood pool SPECT has considerably strengthened owing to the increase in computer speed, the greater diffusion of multidetector cameras, and the general acceptance of state-of-the art three-dimensional analysis and display techniques. We believe that gated blood pool SPECT will become the most commonly utilized nuclear cardiology method for blood pool scintigraphy, the main rationale for its use being its ability to assess both LV and RV function parameters, without need for background subtraction. Gated blood pool SPECT images can be displayed in parametric three-dimensional format, much like gated perfusion SPECT; because the epicardium is not visualized in blood pool imaging, a standard display will represent the LV and RV endocardium as shaded surfaces and their location at end-diastole as wire grids.

The clinical circumstances in which this procedure is likely to become effective are the same as those in which resting blood pool scintigraphy is currently applied, chief among them the assessment of adriamycin cardiotoxicity. Blood pool scintigraphy is also commonly employed in serial assessment of patients with aortic insufficiency, congestive heart failure, and patients who have undergone cardiac transplantation. Promising recent data have suggested that phase analysis from blood pool scintigraphy may be of clinical value in selecting patients who might benefit from biventricular pacing for resynchronization. ANT—anterior LV wall; FWALL—free RV wall; INF—inferior LV wall; LAT—lateral LV wall. (*From Germano et al.*, Fig. 5-33, *Atlas of Nuclear Cardiology*, edn 2.)

128 Atlas of Nuclear Cardiology

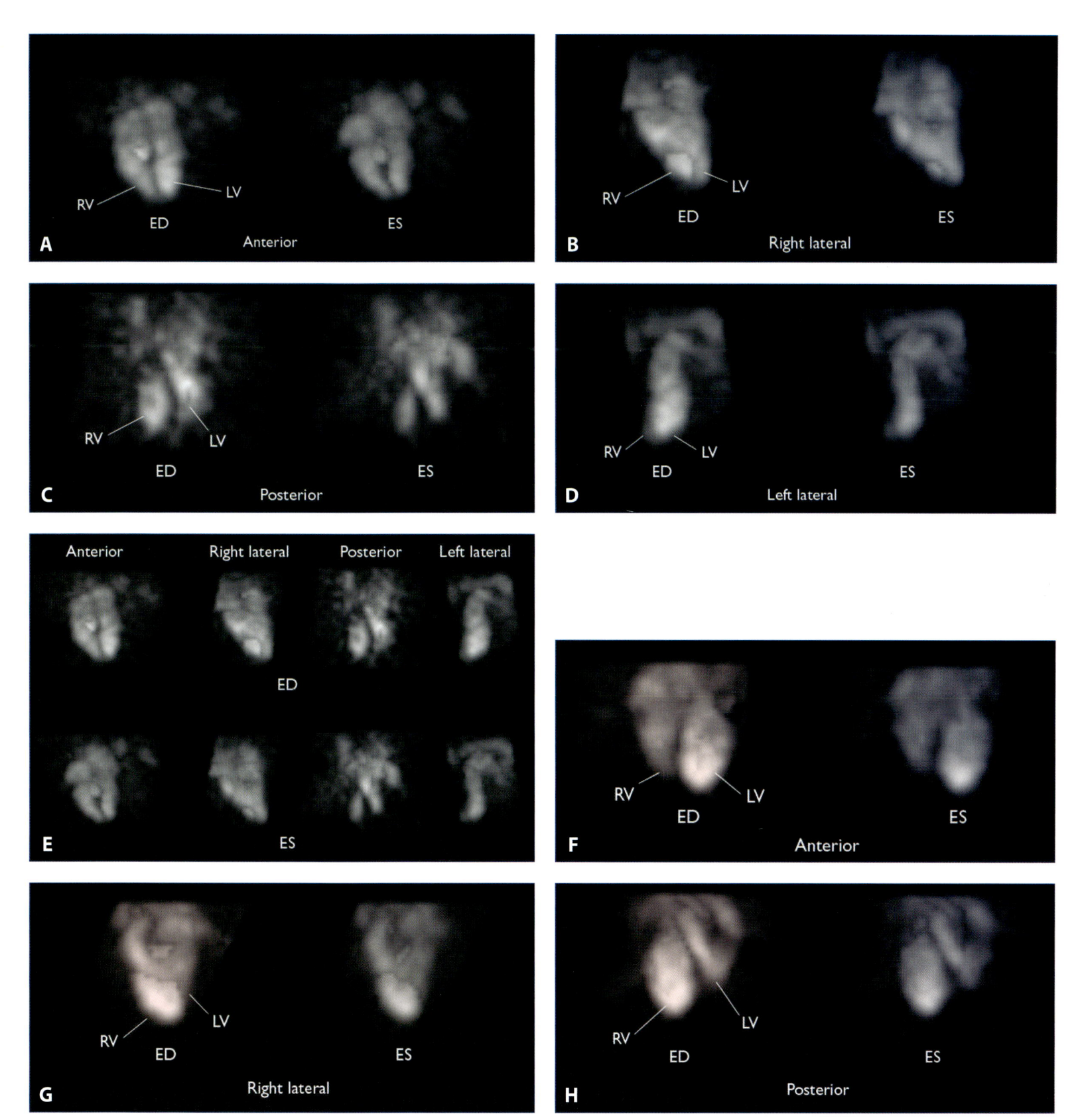

Figure 5-37. SPECT blood pool imaging. Three-dimensional reconstruction of SPECT gated equilibrium images of a normal ventricle in end-diastole (ED) and end-systole (ES) viewed from multiple angles counterclockwise around a 360° orbit, from anterior (**A**), to right lateral (**B**), to posterior (**C**), and left lateral (**D**) views. The *arrow* points to the left atrium and the *arrowhead* identifies the right atrium. **E**, ED and ES images in all views of this normal heart in a single panel. **F–I**, The same views as in **A–D**, the 3-D reconstruction of ED and ES gated blood pool images in a patient with an anterior, apical, and septal left ventricular (LV) aneurysm.

Continued on the next page

Assessment of Cardiac Function: First-Pass, Equilibrium Blood Pool, and Gated Myocardial SPECT

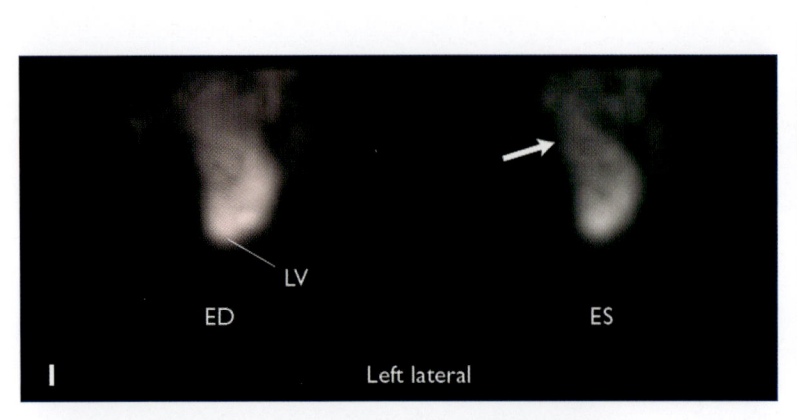

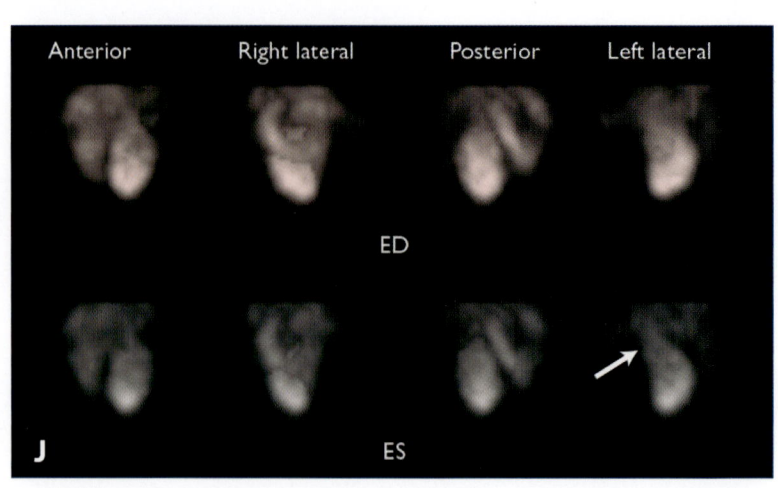

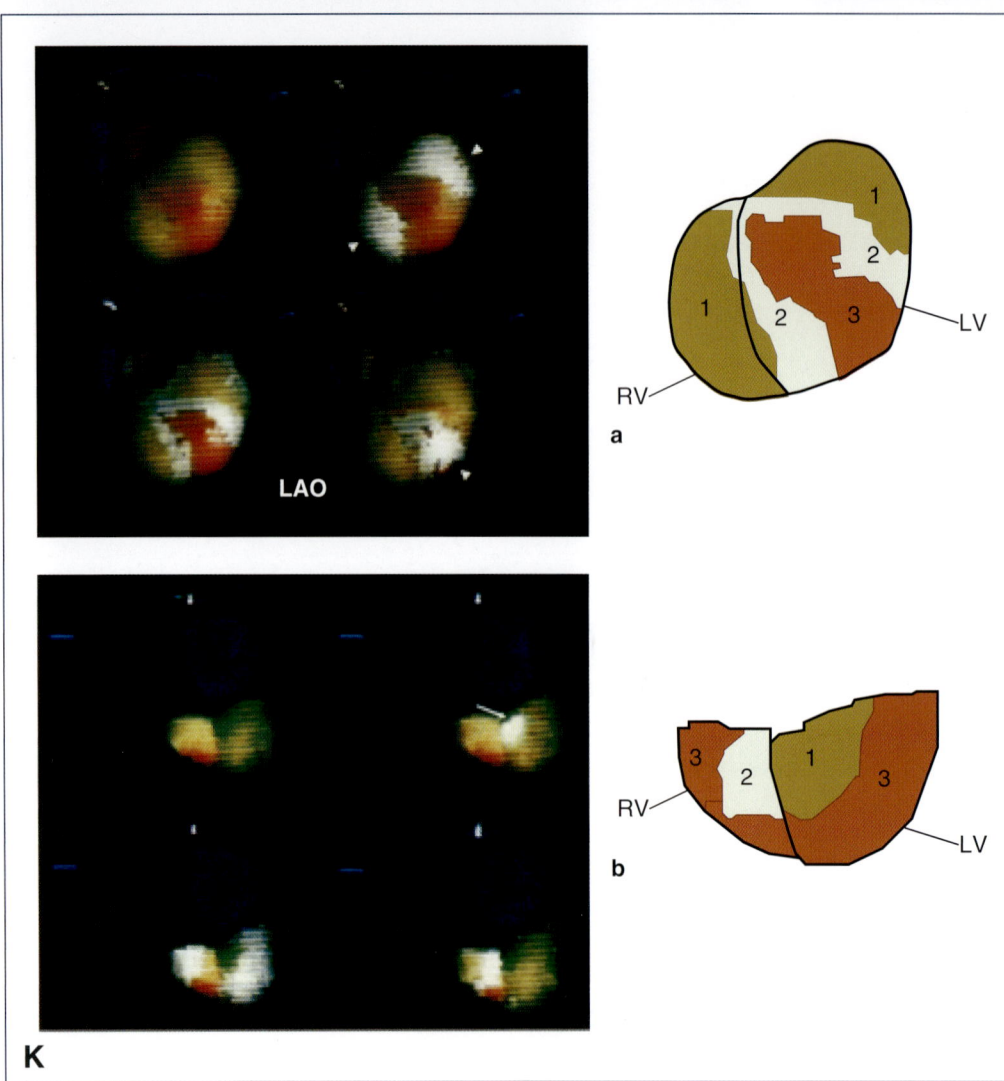

Figure 5-37. *(Continued)* The *arrow* in **I** points to the dynamic base of the LV where the distal aspects are essentially akinetic. This is not well appreciated in other views. **J,** The ED and ES images in all views of this aneurysmal heart in a single panel. **K,** A reconstructed gated 3-D blood pool study in a patient with pre-excitation and a posterior septal bypass pathway in the left anterior oblique (LAO) projection *(top)* and the posterior view *(bottom)*. The sequential phase progression is sequentially highlighted in *white* from upper left to lower right in each panel, as shown in the adjacent diagrams from *1* through *3*. In the *top panel*, the *arrowheads* show the phase progression from the lateral left and right ventricular (RV) walls (above), progressing toward the middle of the image (below). However, in the *bottom* panel, the focus is really shown to be the posterior septum *(arrow)*. (**K,** *from* Oeff *et al.* [49]; with permission.)

130 Atlas of Nuclear Cardiology

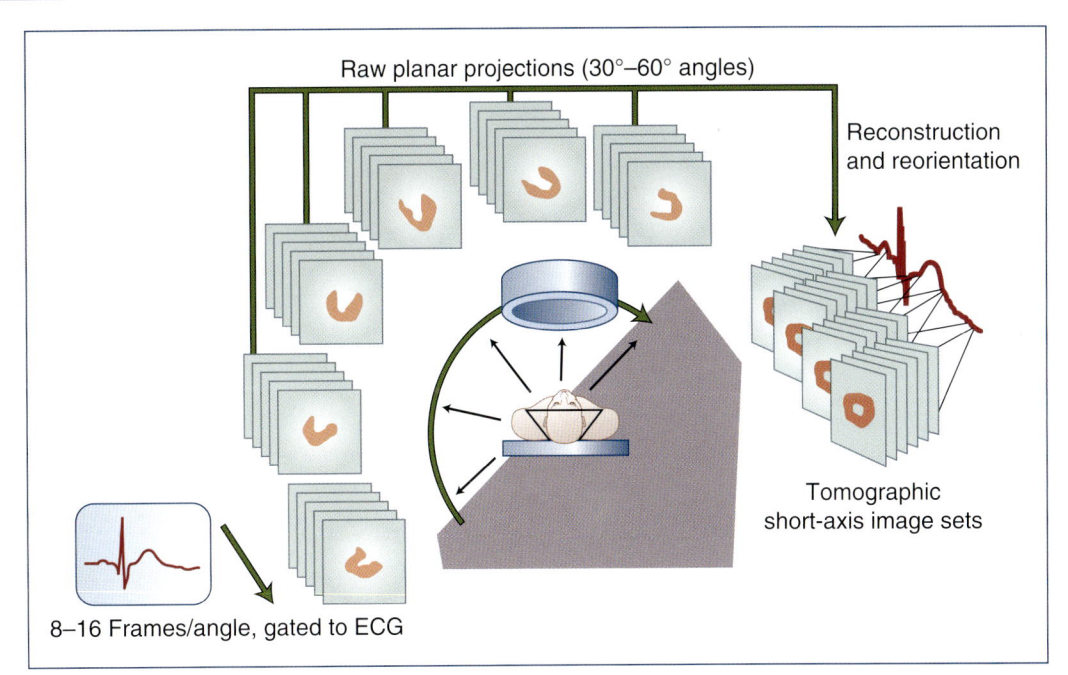

Part II: Gated Myocardial Perfusion SPECT

Figure 5-38. Gated myocardial perfusion SPECT: acquisition. It is estimated that over 90% of myocardial perfusion SPECT studies performed in the United States in 2004 used electrocardiographic (ECG) gating, which makes it possible to provide both perfusion and function information with a single radiopharmaceutical injection and a single acquisition sequence. A gated cardiac SPECT acquisition proceeds almost exactly like an ungated one: the camera detector(s) rotate around the patient, collecting projection images at equally spaced angles along a 180° or 360° arc, and these projections are then filtered and reconstructed into tomographic short- and long-axis images [50,51]. Gated SPECT imaging's distinguishing feature is that at each angle, not one but several (eight, 16, or even 32) projection images are acquired, each corresponding to a specific phase of the cardiac cycle. Reconstruction of all same-phase projections produces a three-dimensional "snapshot" of the patient's heart, frozen in time at that particular phase, and doing so for all phases results in four-dimensional image volumes (x, y, z, and time) from which cardiac function can be readily assessed.

In our laboratory, we do not increase the injected dose or the acquisition time when gating a myocardial SPECT study: typical parameters used are low-energy high-resolution collimator(s), patient weight–based injection of 25 to 40 mCi of ^{99m}Tc-sestamibi/tetrofosmin or 3 to 4.5 mCi of ^{201}Tl, 3° spacing between adjacent projections, and 25 seconds (^{99m}Tc) or 35 seconds (^{201}Tl) acquisition time per projection [52]. The resulting total acquisition time can be as short as 12.5 minutes (^{99m}Tc) or 17.5 minutes (^{201}Tl) if a dual-detector camera with the detectors at a 90° angle is used. (*Adapted from* Germano and Berman [52].)

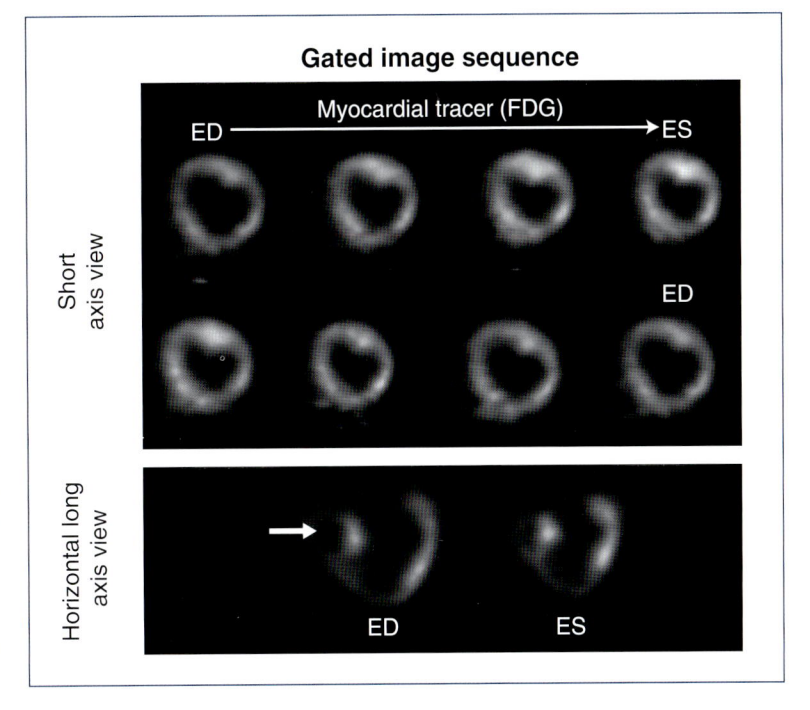

Figure 5-39. Gated myocardial perfusion images. This sequence shows the gated set of eight images obtained from imaging a tracer that labels the myocardium, in this case 18-fluorodeoxyglucose (FDG). The small number of images and reduced sampling rate tends to slightly blur true end-systolic (ES) with late systolic and early diastolic data, overestimating ES volume and underestimating ejection fraction. However, it has been shown that this effect is not too severe on ejection fraction calculations [41] as long as heart rate is not too low. Using only eight images greatly distorts diastolic and systolic parameters such as peak ejection and filling rates, however. Note too the small right ventricle (*arrow*). ED—end diastolic.

Assessment of Cardiac Function: First-Pass, Equilibrium Blood Pool, and Gated Myocardial SPECT

Figure 5-40. Ejection fraction (EF) measurement. Left ventricular function can be computed from the series of gated myocardial uptake images to give a similar curve to that obtained from a gated blood pool study. Unfortunately, the resolution and noise of most SPECT perfusion studies is far worse than that shown in this gated fluorodeoxyglucose image sequence, leading to greater difficulties in accurately determining the endocardial edges, and computing EF. Unlike the gated blood pool images, counts are no longer proportional to blood volume. Instead, one must define the endocardial border from each image in the sequence for every slice, or at least end-diastolic (ED) and end-systolic (ES) frames for EF, and compute the volume from the sum of the enclosed areas of the endocardial surfaces. Short axis slices do not give good endocardial border information near the apex, so long axis views must be used as well. This procedure has been successfully semiautomated in many commercial nuclear medicine cardiac analysis packages [53,54]. However, the results one obtains depend to some extent on the resolution (see partial volume effect discussion later) and noise in the images, so can vary from one site to another and from one SPECT system to another [55]. However, measurements from rest to stress should be more reliable, as the same filtering, imaging system, and other parameters are used for both. In the images shown here, the epicardial surface has also been outlined.

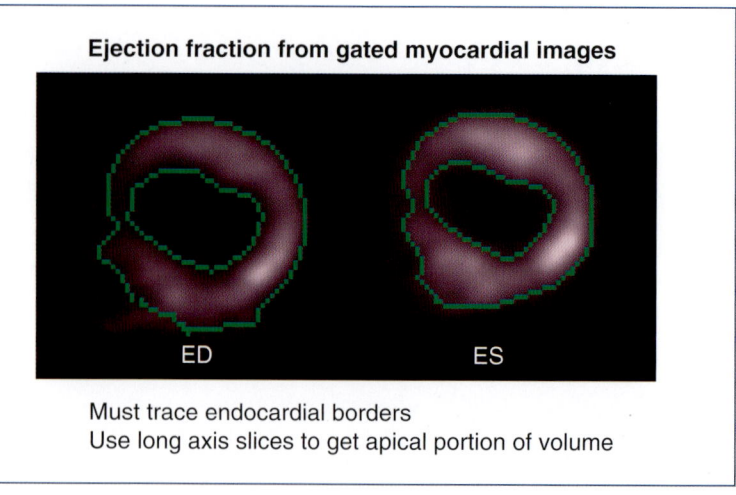

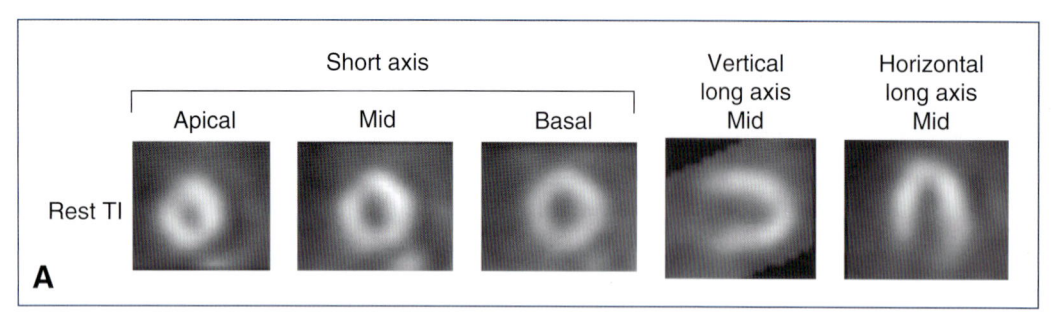

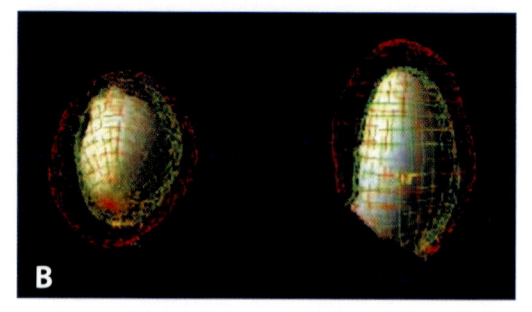

Figure 5-41. A and B, Display of left ventricular function. The epi- and endocardial borders at end-diastolic (ED) and end-systolic (ES) and at the other points in the cardiac cycle can be put together to form the "wire cage" image as shown in this figure, or even a pseudo volumetric surface display. The epicardial and endocardial surfaces at ED are shown in *orange* and *yellow/green* in **B**. Here the ES surface is shown in *gray*. Two different pseudo-three-dimensional views are shown. These data were obtained from ^{99m}Tc-MIBI images where typical short axis and long axis images are shown in **A**. Obviously, when there are severe perfusion defects this methodology is problematic, and one must assume what the contours would have looked like had those segments of the myocardium been visible. Similarly, three-dimensional displays have been used to great effect in gated blood pool imaging [56–59].

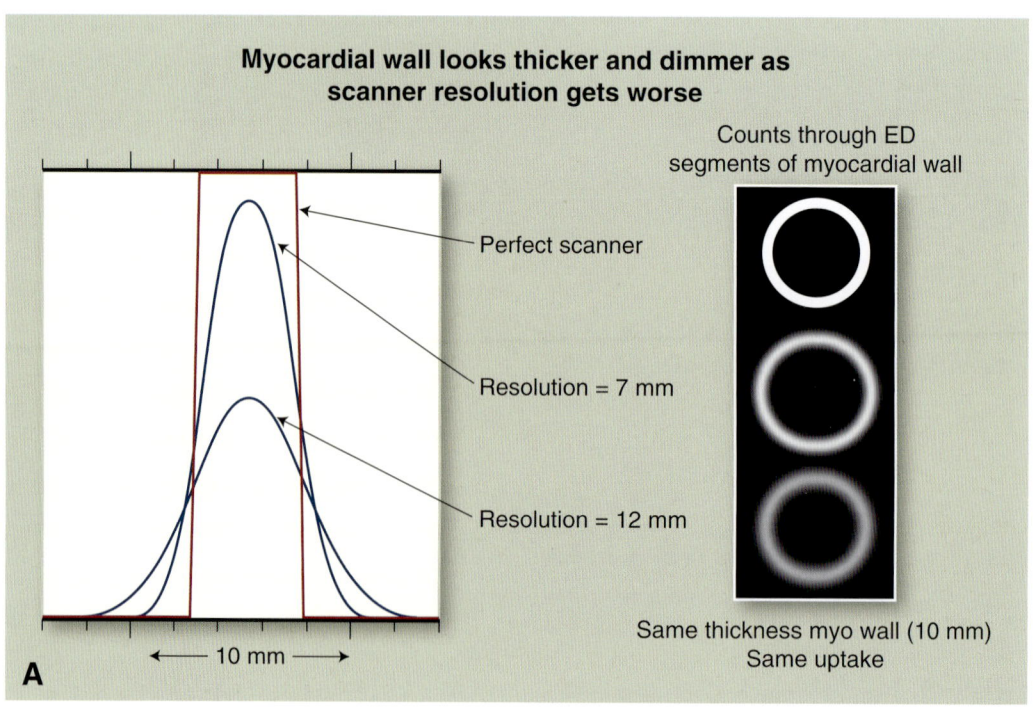

Figures 5-42. Partial volume effect. Changes in myocardial wall thickening may be inferred from gated perfusion or metabolism images, using the so-called "partial volume effect" [60]. This term is somewhat misleading, in fact referring to two different phenomena that alter the relationship between image counts and intensity. The first effect is simply that related to imaging an object using a scanner with less than perfect resolution. The effect becomes noticeable whenever the scanner resolution is comparable to the object being imaged.

For example, the *top right* image in **A** is a simulated image of one short axis slice of a 10-mm thick myocardial wall imaged at end-diastole (ED) with a "perfect" scanner, *ie*, one with 0-mm resolution. The profile of counts through the line shown across the myocardial wall gives the square curve on the *left*. The width of this curve is exactly 10 mm. When the same myocardium is imaged with a scanner with 7-mm resolution (typical of a PET scanner), the *middle right* image is obtained. It is somewhat blurrier and looks dimmer and wider, as shown on the corresponding profile on the *left*. Finally, when the 10-mm thick myocardial wall is imaged with a 12-mm full width at half maximum (FWHM) scanner (typical of a very good SPECT scanner), the image at the *bottom right* results—still dimmer and apparently wider. In fact, all three images have the same total counts, the same "uptake" of tracer. As the resolution gets worse and worse, the counts get blurred more and more, giving the appearance of decreasing brightness and increasing width. If one were to add up all the counts under the three profiles, they would give exactly the same number of counts.

Continued on the next page

132 Atlas of Nuclear Cardiology

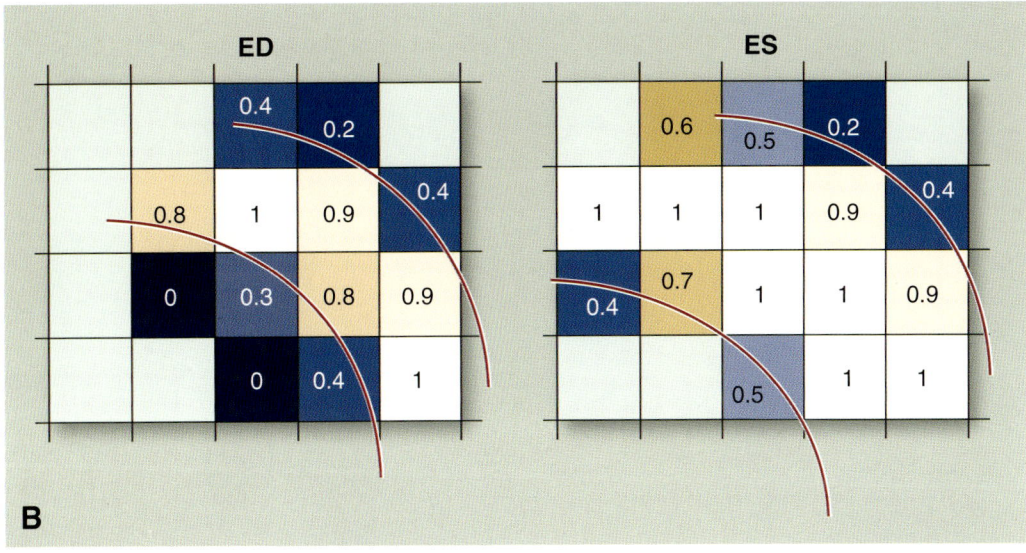

Figures 5-42. *(Continued)* Insufficient image sampling is the second phenomenon related to partial volume effect (**B**). Shown diagrammatically is a myocardial region in ED and end-systole (ES) superimposed on a pixel grid, in which only a small number of pixels span the myocardial wall (a situation typical of cardiac SPECT imaging). The *squares* represent pixels which are color coded for and labeled with the percentage of the pixel occupied by the myocardium. Thickening brings a larger fraction of the pixels fully within the myocardial walls, producing a brighter (lighter) intensity response. Of course, the magnitude of this effect will depend on the matrix size used, *ie*, on the mm/pixel. As long as the pixel size is much smaller than the size of the object being imaged (*eg*, the myocardial wall thickness), the effect is small. However, in cardiac SPECT imaging, this is frequently not the case. While insufficient sampling can be considered a separate phenomenon from the "partial volume effect" described in **A**, the consequences are quite similar. Systolic thickening, *eg*, from 8 to 12 mm, translates into increased pixel intensity, as is illustrated in **B**. Visually, the contracting, thickening wall appears to brighten or move up the color scale in systole. Thickening or brightening then is gross evidence of regional myocardial viability, but cannot exclude a nontransmural infarction. The relationship between regional pixel intensity and thickening has been documented in phantoms and in correlations with echocardiography and MRI. Evidence of wall motion and thickening may be important for coronary disease diagnosis and appears to add to diagnostic specificity [61] from 84% to 92%. Here, motion and thickening in the presence of a "fixed" defect suggest an artifact of motion or attenuation rather than a true infarction [62]. (*Adapted from* Botvinick [60].)

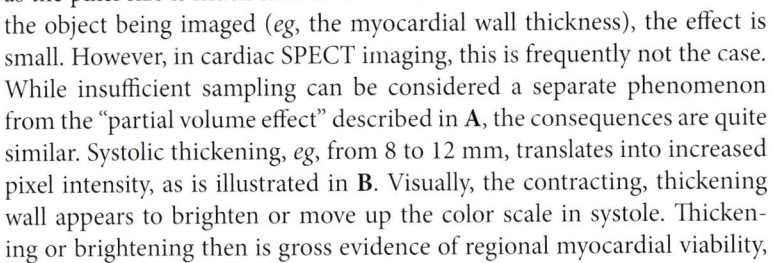

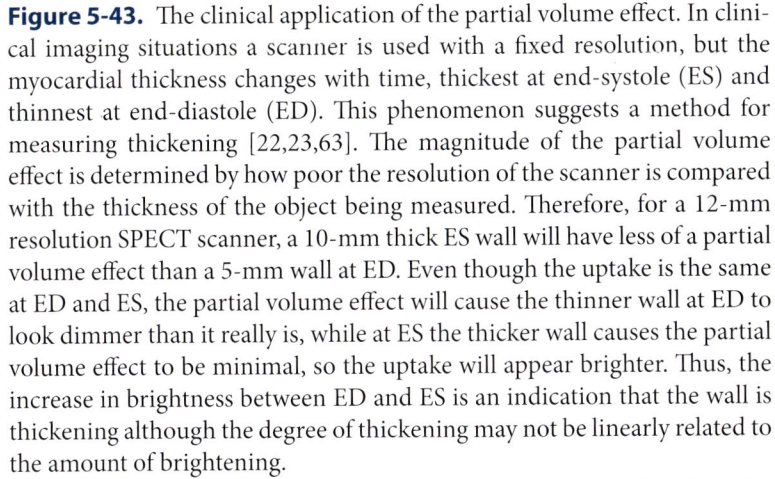

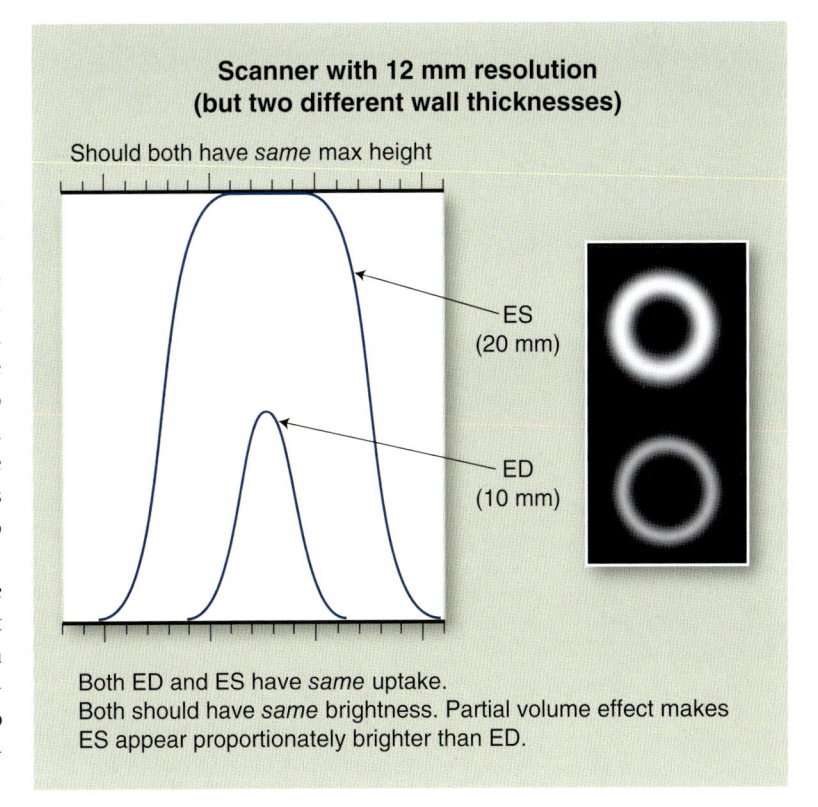

Figure 5-43. The clinical application of the partial volume effect. In clinical imaging situations a scanner is used with a fixed resolution, but the myocardial thickness changes with time, thickest at end-systole (ES) and thinnest at end-diastole (ED). This phenomenon suggests a method for measuring thickening [22,23,63]. The magnitude of the partial volume effect is determined by how poor the resolution of the scanner is compared with the thickness of the object being measured. Therefore, for a 12-mm resolution SPECT scanner, a 10-mm thick ES wall will have less of a partial volume effect than a 5-mm wall at ED. Even though the uptake is the same at ED and ES, the partial volume effect will cause the thinner wall at ED to look dimmer than it really is, while at ES the thicker wall causes the partial volume effect to be minimal, so the uptake will appear brighter. Thus, the increase in brightness between ED and ES is an indication that the wall is thickening although the degree of thickening may not be linearly related to the amount of brightening.

Note that when the myocardial wall at ED is much thicker than the resolution (*eg*, 20 mm or more thick), the partial volume blurring effect will be small and little brightening will occur between ED and ES, even though the wall does thicken. Therefore, although brightening always indicates thickening, lack of brightening does not necessarily indicate that no thickening is occurring. This must be kept in mind when clinical interpretations of brightening are made.

Assessment of Cardiac Function: First-Pass, Equilibrium Blood Pool, and Gated Myocardial SPECT

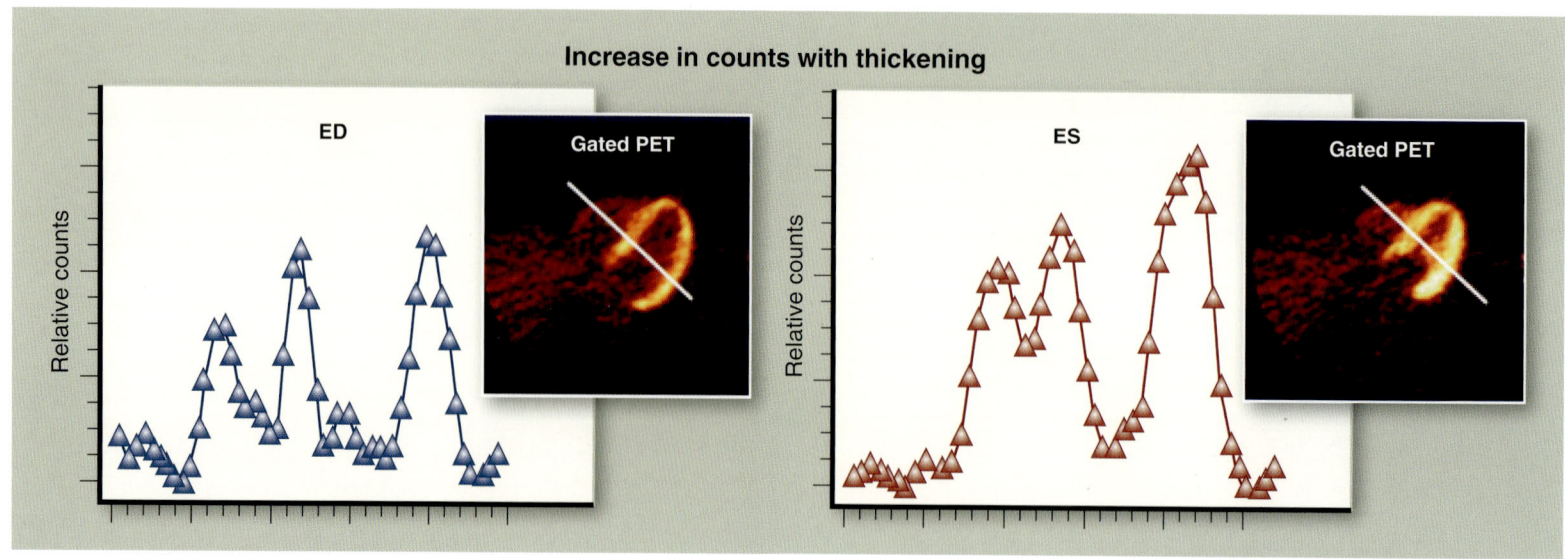

Figure 5-44. Myocardial thickening. A clinical example of how the partial volume effect can be used to indicate whether thickening is occurring is illustrated here. The *upper left* image shows a transaxial myocardial uptake image, in this case [^{18}F]-fluorodeoxyglucose at end-diastole (ED). The curve below this image is the profile of counts through the *line* shown in the image. The *upper right* image is the same transaxial slice, but at end-systole (ES). Again the profile through the image, as indicated, is shown below. Note that the myocardial walls in the *upper right* image appear uniformly brighter than in the *upper left* image. This is a definitive indication that thickening has occurred. This increase in brightness is clearly shown in the profiles. Note that the right ventricular wall also shows an increase in counts. This is clearly seen in the profile of counts, but is harder to appreciate visibly in the image. Again it is important to remember that brightening always indicates thickening, but lack of brightening does not necessarily indicate that no thickening is occurring. This, and the related causes of thickening in the absence of brightening, must be kept in mind when clinical interpretations of brightening are made.

Figure 5-45. Partial volume effect: ambiguities and misleading effects. Although the partial volume effect can be useful to determine whether thickening is occurring, it also can cause difficulties in myocardial perfusion imaging. Thin myocardial walls, those that are thin compared with the resolution of the system, will appear to have less activity than they really do. If it is a fluorodeoxyglucose (FDG) scan, the reader may erroneously think that the region is nonviable, when in reality it is just thin. Similarly if it is a perfusion scan, thin walls will erroneously appear to have reduced perfusion. If one compares two studies taken some months apart, and a portion of the myocardial wall has thinned, that portion will erroneously appear to have less uptake. Of course wall thinning is related to infarction and scar, which are also causes of reduced perfusion and uptake. Similarly, owing to their different physical properties and related associated spatial resolution, the same myocardial wall could appear broader with different intensity and erroneously appear to have relative less activity when imaged by ^{201}Tl compared with ^{99m}Tc radiotracers. All these factors must be taken into consideration when interpreting scans of myocardial uptake.

Partial Volume Effect: Ambiguities and Misleading Effects

Thin myocardial walls may erroneously appear to be nonviable in FDG imaging
Thin myocardial walls erroneously appear to have lower perfusion for Tl and MIBI or other perfusion agents
Walls imaged with ^{201}Tl erroneously appear to be thicker with lower perfusion compared with ^{99m}Tc perfusion agents
Changes in myocardial thickness cause you to think activity has changed

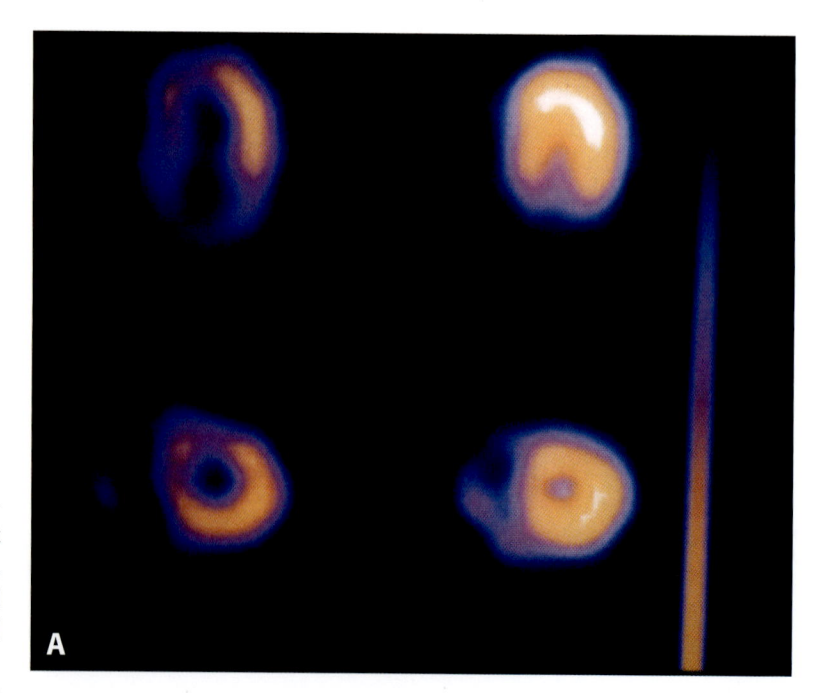

Figure 5-46. Gated perfusion imaging. **A**, End-diastolic (*left*) and end-systolic (*right*) gated ^{99m}Tc-sestamibi perfusion images in a normal heart in selected short axis (*top*) and horizontal long axis (*bottom*) SPECT slices. Inward systolic motion is evident, as well as brightening, or increased intensity during systole. The latter, a result of partial volume effect, is well correlated with myocardial thickening.

Continued on the next page

Practical Comparison of First Pass and Gated Perfusion Methods for Evaluation of Ventricular Function

First pass

- Needs ^{99m}Tc-based agents
- Needs state-of-the-art, high-sensitivity cameras (detectors)
- Technically demanding camera requirements/protocol
- Performed with radionuclide administration
- Can be performed with stress but not always possible
- May be performed with rest and stress
- Left ventricular wall motion, volumes, and ejection fraction
- Can provide right ventricular ejection fraction and wall motion
- Evaluates features of background-free blood pool

Gated

- May be performed with ^{201}Tl or ^{99m}Tc-based agents
- Uses conventional cameras
- Always delayed after radionuclide injection and after stress
- May be performed with rest and stress
- Left ventricular wall motion, volumes, and ejection fraction
- Provides left ventricular wall thickening
- Accuracy dependent on endothelial border definition

B

Technical Considerations in Gated SPECT Perfusion Imaging

- Acquisition and reconstruction of a 16-frame gated SPECT study requires 16 times as much random access memory (RAM) and takes 16 times as long for reconstruction
- For clinical utility, gated SPECT perfusion imaging needs a fast computer with 8 Mb of RAM and 500 Mb of hard disk space
- Vendor software should:
  - Permit acquisition of up to 16 frames SPECT
  - Display time at each camera stop in seconds or in accepted beats within a user-defined R-R interval
  - Permit collapse of the study to an ungated study or image including only specified frames, for example, an end-diastolic image
  - Display of dynamic beating short-axis slices, selected long-axis slices, and three-dimensional rendering of the beating heart
  - Calculate quantitative measures of regional perfusion, contraction, and wall thickening

C

Figure 5-46. *(Continued)* **B** and **C**, Such functional data may be derived from the perfusion study by either first pass or postlocalization gated methods. (*Adapted from* Botvinick et al. [64].)

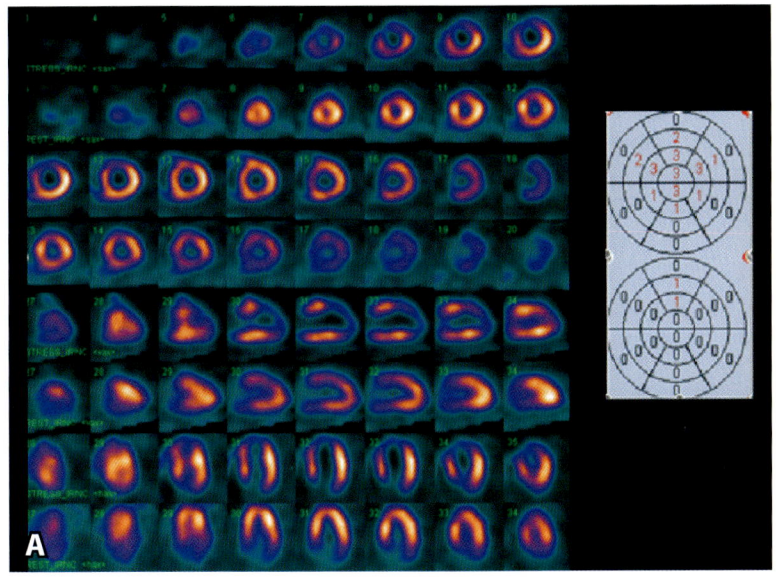

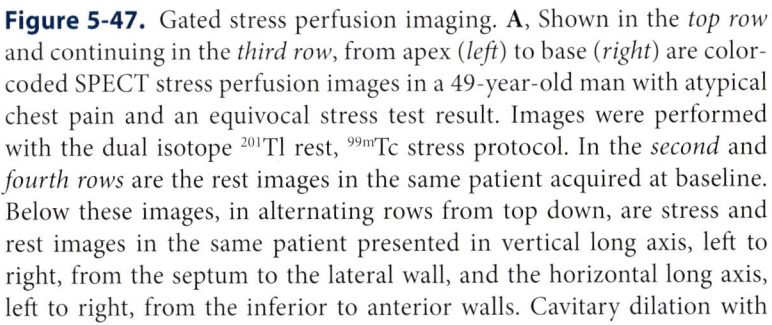

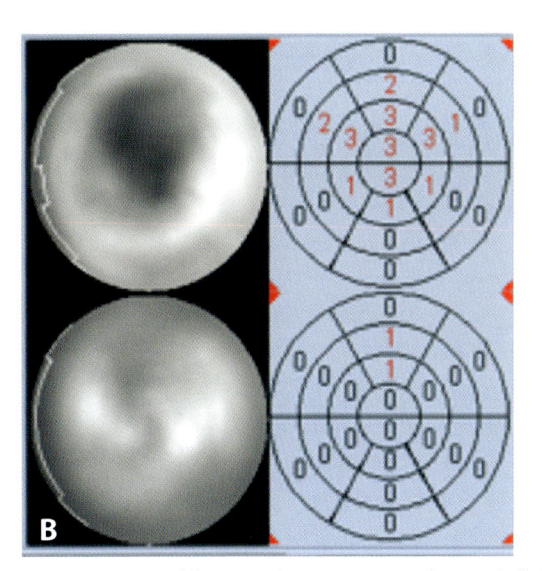

Figure 5-47. Gated stress perfusion imaging. **A**, Shown in the *top row* and continuing in the *third row*, from apex (*left*) to base (*right*) are color-coded SPECT stress perfusion images in a 49-year-old man with atypical chest pain and an equivocal stress test result. Images were performed with the dual isotope ^{201}Tl rest, ^{99m}Tc stress protocol. In the *second* and *fourth rows* are the rest images in the same patient acquired at baseline. Below these images, in alternating rows from top down, are stress and rest images in the same patient presented in vertical long axis, left to right, from the septum to the lateral wall, and the horizontal long axis, left to right, from the inferior to anterior walls. Cavitary dilation with a gross, reversible, apical, anterior, and septal defect is evident, consistent with significant flow limiting disease in the left anterior descending coronary artery. The summed stress score of 20 confirms the high related coronary risk. **B**, Shown is the quantitative perfusion SPECT or quantitative perfusion AutoQuant (Cedars Sinai Hospital, Los Angeles, CA) display with the *left panel* showing segmented stress slices, above, at *far left*, followed by rest slices, below, and polar maps in the *right panels*, with stress above and rest below. Here the display is calibrated for the percentage of relative regional intensity. In the *right panel*, color coded defect is painted on a model left ventricle.

Continued on the next page

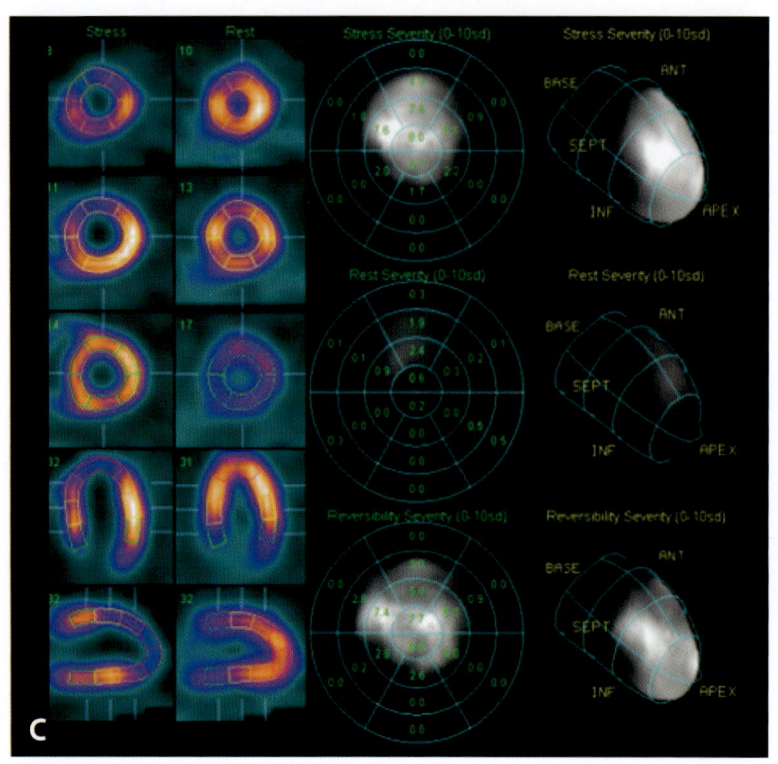

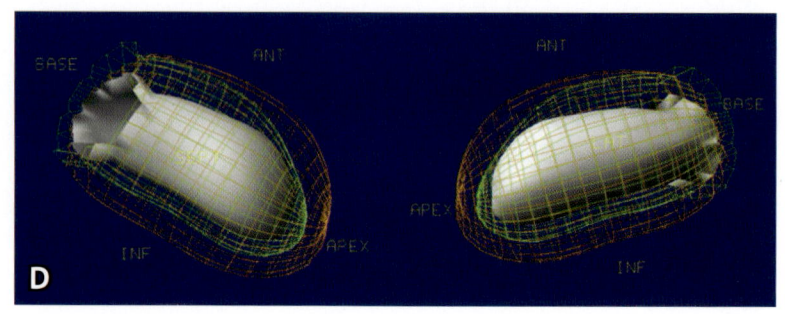

Figure 5-47. *(Continued)* **C**, A similar display as in **B**, but now showing, from above down, stress, rest, and difference polar maps with intensity scaled to the standard deviation derived from the normal rest-stress male activity distribution using this dual isotope protocol. **D**, Models of the epicardium (*orange mesh*), endocardium at end-diastole (*green mesh*), and at end-systole (*solid orange*) in anterior (*left*) and left lateral (*right*) projections taken from the gated myocardial perfusion images in this case at peak stress. Evident are anterior, apical, and septal wall motion abnormalities. Rest function was normal. Evidence of stress-induced dysfunction adds significant prognostic risk to any perfusion abnormalities induced. ANT—anterior; INF—inferior; SEPT—septal.

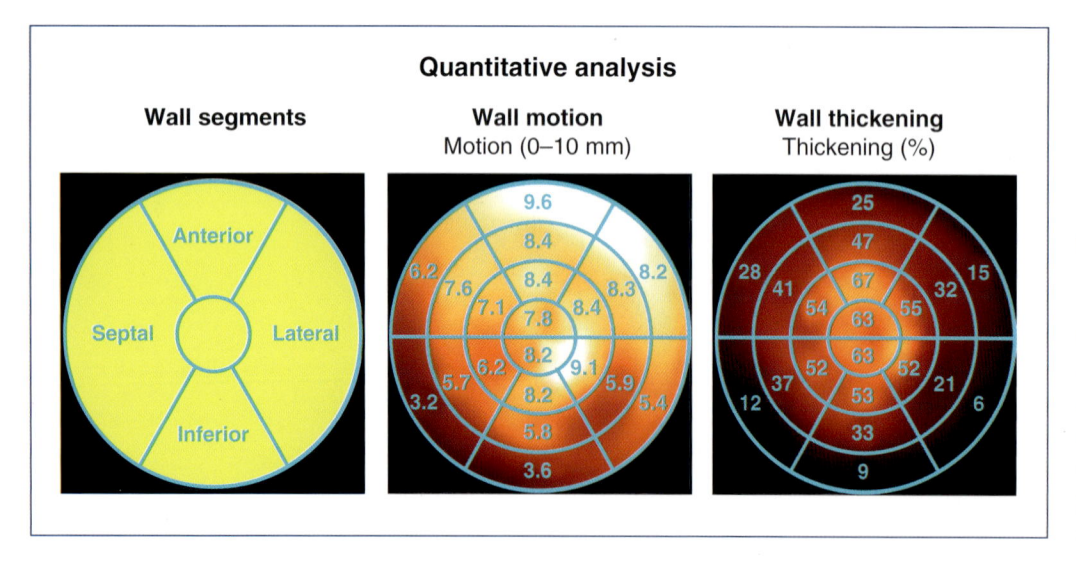

Figure 5-48. Normal quantitative wall motion and thickening on gated perfusion imaging. Shown are AutoQuant (Cedars Sinai Hospital, Los Angeles, CA) polar maps demonstrating wall segments (*left*), normal wall motion (*center*), and normal wall thickening (*right*) [65]. Thickening is accurately measured as percent increase from end-diastole by the linear relationship to the percentage increase in wall intensity. (*From* Yun *et al.* [65]; with permission.)

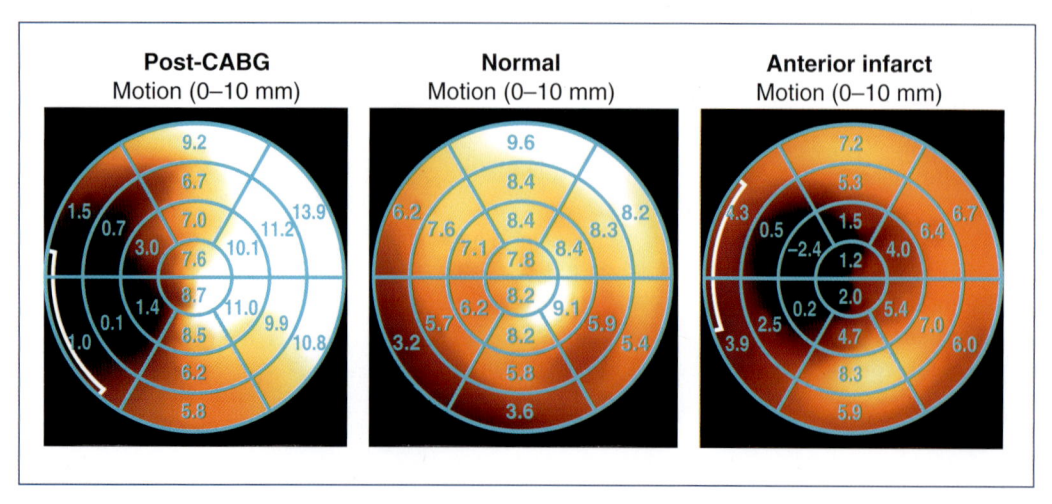

Figure 5-49. Abnormal quantitative wall motion on gated perfusion imaging. Shown are AutoQuant (Cedars Sinai Hospital, Los Angeles, CA) polar maps demonstrating wall motion patterns in a patient after coronary artery bypass graft (CABG) surgery (*left*), in a normal patient (*center*), and in a patient with a prior anterior infarction (*right*). Abnormal septal wall motion is evident in post-CABG and postinfarct patients. (*From* Yun *et al.* [65]; with permission.)

136 Atlas of Nuclear Cardiology

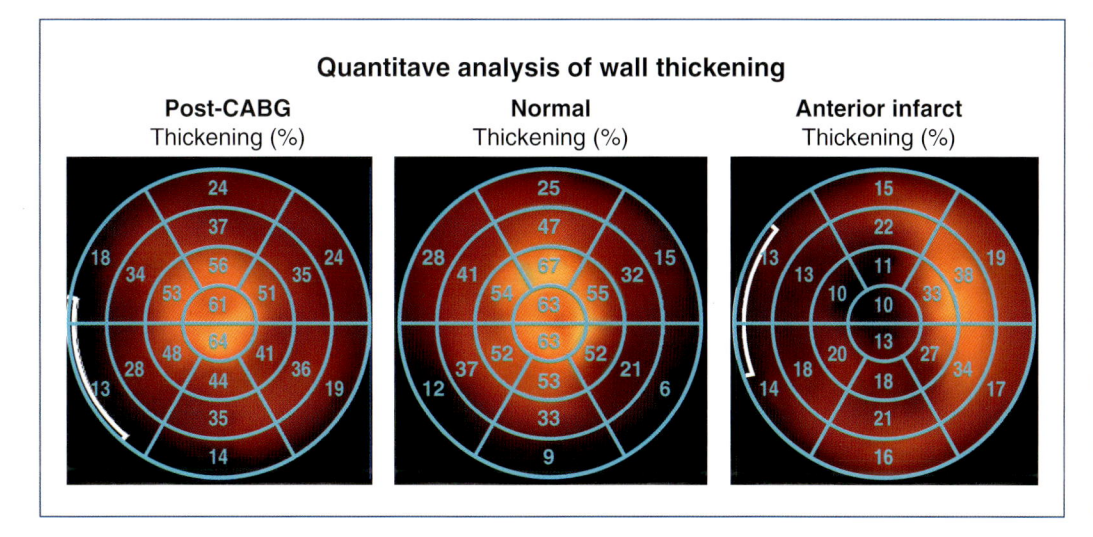

Figure 5-50. Abnormal quantitative wall thickening on gated perfusion imaging. Shown are AutoQuant (Cedars Sinai Hospital, Los Angeles, CA) polar maps demonstrating wall thickening patterns in the same three patients after coronary artery bypass graft (CABG) surgery (*left*), in a normal patient (*center*), and in a patient with a prior anterior infarction (*right*). Abnormal septal and apical wall thickening is evident only postinfarction. The abnormal wall motion after CABG is not accompanied by abnormal thickening since there is no intrinsic wall pathology. The abnormal wall motion post-CABG relates to the absence of the pericardial restraint with a resulting anterior swing of the epicardium, seen on dynamic images. (*From* Yun *et al.* [65]; with permission.)

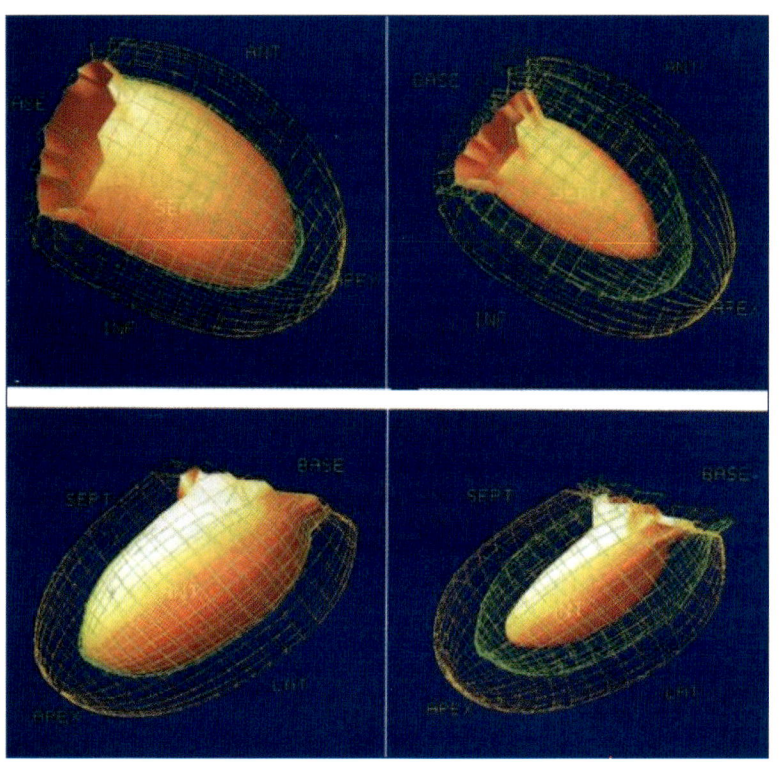

Figure 5-51. Normal wall motion and thickening: ventricular model. Shown on the AutoQuant (Cedars Sinai Hospital, Los Angeles, CA) display of gated perfusion images is normal wall motion and thickening in anterior (*top*) and lateral (*bottom*) projections, where end-diastolic frames are on the *left* and end-systolic frames are on the *right*. Here again the epicardium is represented by the *green mesh*, the endocardium at end-diastole is the *orange mesh*, and the endocardium at end-systole (*right*) is the *solid orange* surface. Note the symmetrical inward motion of the endocardium. ANT—anterior; INF—inferior; LAT—lateral; SEPT—septal. (*From* Yun *et al.* [65]; with permission.)

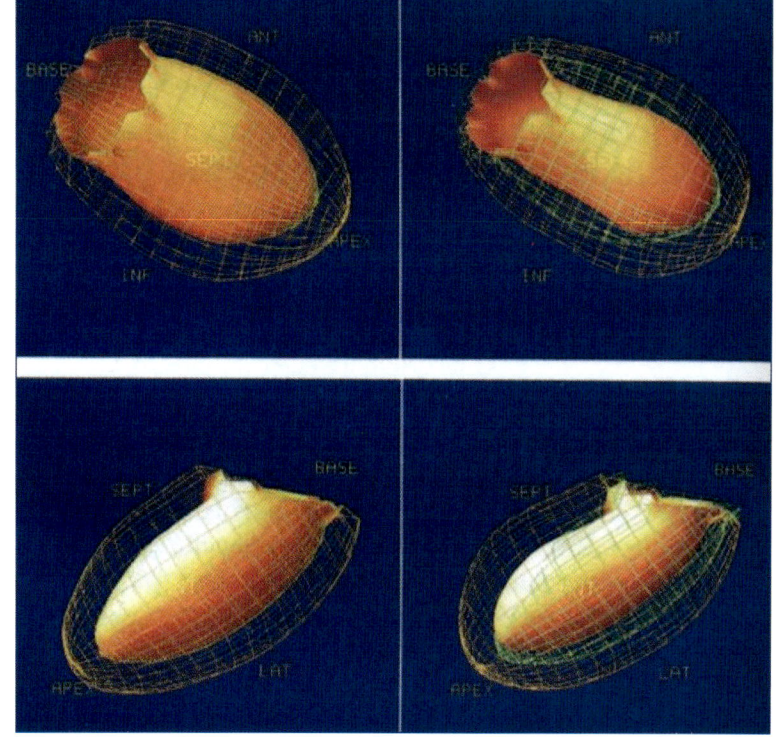

Figure 5-52. Abnormal wall motion and thickening with anterior infarction: ventricular model. Shown on the same AutoQuant (Cedars Sinai Hospital, Los Angeles, CA) display of gated perfusion images as Figure 5-47 is akinesis of the apex, septum, and distal anterior wall in anterior (*left*) and lateral (*right*) projections in a patient with a prior anterior myocardial infarction. The perfusion image showed a dense anterior, septal, and apical defect. ANT—anterior; INF—inferior; LAT—lateral; SEPT—septal. (*From* Yun *et al.* [65]; with permission.)

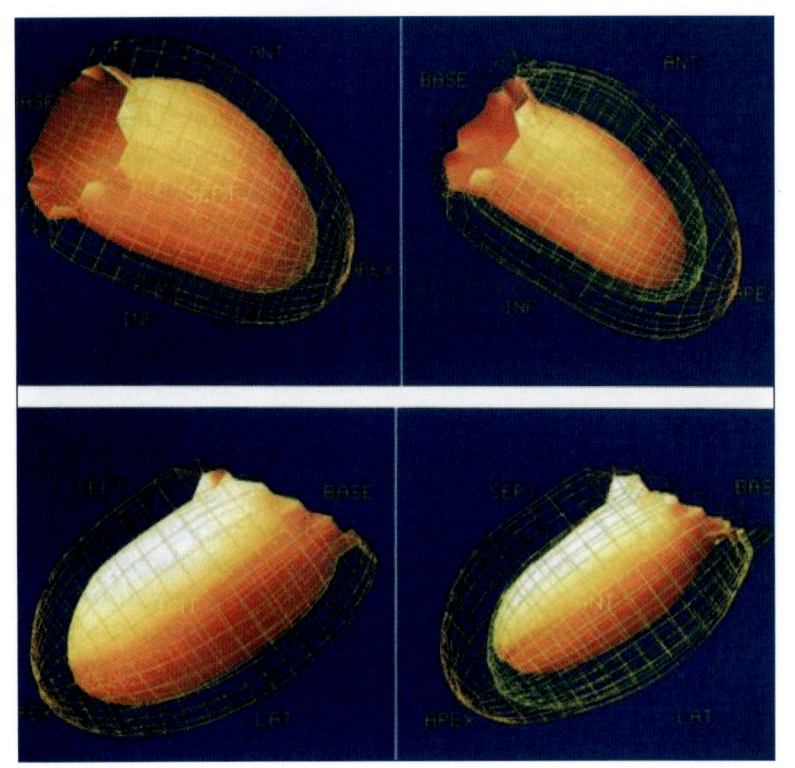

Figure 5-53. Anterior swing post–coronary artery bypass graft (CABG): ventricular model. Shown on the same AutoQuant (Meyer Instruments, Houston, TX) display of gated perfusion images as the prior figures is the pattern of abnormal wall motion seen after CABG or any cardiac surgery in anterior (*left*) and lateral (*right*) projections. Here the anterior swing of the epicardium is well seen in the lateral projection where the septum appears to be akinetic but demonstrates normal wall thickening and is associated with preserved anterior wall motion, differentiating this pattern from that seen in patients after anterior infarction. ANT—anterior; INF—inferior; LAT—lateral; SEPT—septal. (*From* Yun *et al.* [65]; with permission.)

References

1. Hoffmann G, Klein N: Die methode der radiokardiographischen funktions analyse. *Nuklearmedizin* 1968, 7:350–370.

2. Strauss HW, Zaret BL, Hurley PJ: A scintiphotographic method for measuring left ventricular ejection fraction in man without cardiac catheterization. *Am J Cardiol* 1971, 28:575–580.

3. Zaret BL, Strauss HW, Hurley PJ: A noninvasive scintiphotographic method for detecting regional ventricular dysfunction in man. *N Engl J Med* 1971, 284:1165–1170.

4. Parker JA, Secker-Walker R, Hill R.: A new technique for the calculation of left ventricular ejection fraction. *J Nucl Med* 1972, 13:649–651.

5. Green MV, Ostrow HG, Douglas MA, et al.: High temporal resolution ECG-gated scintigraphic angiocardiography. J. Nucl. Med 1975;16:95-98.

6. Steele P, Kirch D, LeFree M, et al.: Measurement of right and left ventricular ejection fractions by radionuclide angiocardiography in coronary artery disease. *Chest* 1976, 70:51–56.

7. Bacharach SL, Green MV, Borer JS: A real-time system for multi-image gated cardiac studies. *J Nucl Med* 1977, 18:79–84.

8. Borer JS, Bacharach SL, Green MV: Real-time radionuclide cineangiography in the noninvasive evaluation of global and regional left ventricular function at rest and during exercise in patients with coronary-artery disease. *N Engl J Med* 1977, 296:839–844.

9. Freedman NMT, Bacharach SL, Cuocolo A, et al.: ECG gated PET C-11 monoxide studies: an answer to the "background" question in planar Tc-99m gated bloodpool imaging. *J Nucl Med* 1992, 33:938.

10. Boyd HL, Gunn RN, Marinho NVS, et al.: Left-ventricular volumes and wall-motion with gated positron emission tomography - comparison with radionuclide ventriculography. *Circulation* 1994, 90:364–364.

11. Fischman AJ, Moore RH, Gill JB, et al.: Gated blood pool tomography - a technology whose time has come. *Semin Nucl Med* 1989, 19:13–21.

12. Underwood SR, Walton S, Laming PJ, et al.: Left ventricular volume and ejection fraction determined by gated blood pool emission tomography. *Br Heart J* 1985, 53:216–222.

13. Ishino Y: Assessment of cardiac function and left ventricular regional wall motion by 99mTc multigated cardiac blood-pool emission computed tomography. *Kaku Igaku* 1992, 29:1069–1081.

14. Bartlett ML, Srinivasan G, Barker WC, et al.: Left ventricular ejection fraction: comparison of results from planar and SPECT gated blood-pool studies. *J Nucl Med* 1996, 37:1795–1799.

15. Borer J, Supino P: Radionuclide angiography part II: equilibrium imaging. In *Nuclear Cardiac Imaging: Principles and Applications*. Edited by Iskandrian AE, Verani MS. New York: Oxford University Press; 2003:323–367.

16. Botvinick EH, O'Connell JW, Kadkade PJ, et al.: The potential added value of three-dimensional reconstruction and display of SPECT gated blood pool images. *J Nucl Card* 1998, 25:509–514.

17. Gill JB, Moore RH, Tamaki N, et al.: Multigated blood-pool tomography: new method for the assessment of left ventricular function. *J Nucl Med* 1986, 27:1916–1924.

18. Groch MW, Marshall RC, Erwin WD, et al.: Quantitative gated blood pool SPECT for the assessment of coronary artery disease at rest. *J Nucl Card* 1998, 5:567–573.

19. Groch MW, Marshall RC, Schippers D, et al.: Three dimensional analysis of gated blood pool SPECT: applicability of multiple reference models. *J Nucl Med* 1998, 39:45P–145P.

20. Garcia, E, Bacharach SL, Mahmarian JJ, et al.: Imaging guidelines for nuclear cardiology procedures: part 1. *J Nucl Med* 1996, 3:G3–G46.

21. Germano G, Kavanagh PB, Wachter P: A new algorithm for the quantitation of myocardial perfusion SPECT. *J Nucl Med* 2000, 41:712–719.

22. Bartlett ML, Buvat I, Vaquero JJ, et al.: Measurement of myocardial wall thickening from PET/SPECT images: comparison of two methods. *J Comput Assist Tomogr* 1996, 20:473–481.

23. Cooke CD, Garcia EV, Cullom SJ, et al.: Determining the accuracy of calculating systolic wall thickening using a fast Fourier transform approximation: a simulation study based on canine and patient data. *J Nucl Med* 1994, 35:1185–1192.

24. Topic 7, Radionuclide angiography: equilibrium and first pass methods. Self-study program III. In *Nuclear Medicine: Cardiology*. Edited by Botvinick E. Reston, VA: Society of Nuclear Medicine; 2007.

25. Botvinick EH, Glazer H, Shosa D: What is the relationship and utility of scintigraphic methods for the assessment of ventricular function? *Cardiovasc Clin* 1983, 13:65–78.

26. Bodenheier MM, Banka FS, Fooshee CM: Quantitative radionuclide angiography in the right anterior oblique view: comparison with contrast ventriculography. *Am J Cardiol* 1978, 41:718–725.

27. Marshall RC, Berger HJ, Costin JC: Assessment of cardiac performance with quantitative radionuclide angiocardiography. *Circulation* 1977, 56:820–829.

28. VanDyke D, Anger HO, Sullivan RW: Cardiac evaluation from radioisotope dynamics. *J Nucl Med* 1972, 13:585–592.

29. Wackers JF: New horizons for myocardial perfusion imaging with technetium -99m labeled isonitriles. In *New Concepts in Cardiac Imaging*. Edited by Pohost GM, Higgins CB, Nanda NC, *et al*. Chicago: Year Book Medical Publishers; 1989:93–108.

30. Upton MT, Rerych SK, Newman GE, *et al*.: Detecting abnormalities in left ventricular function during exercise before angina and ST segment depression. *Circulation* 1980, 62:341–349.

31. Topic 1, Physical and technical aspects of nuclear cardiology. Self-study program III. In *Nuclear Medicine: Cardiology*. Edited by Botvinick E. Reston; VA: Society of Nuclear Medicine; 2003.

32. Udelson JE, Dilsizian V, Bonow RO: Nuclear cardiology. In *Braunwald's Heart Disease: A Textbook of Cardiovascular Medicine*, edn 8. Edited by Libby P, Zipes DP, Mann DL, Bonow RO. Philadelphia: WB Saunders; 2007:287–331.

33. Maltz OL, Treves S: Quantitative radionuclide angiocardiography. Determination of Qp/Qs in children. *Circulation* 1973, 76:1049.

34. Bacharach SL, Green MV, Borer SJ: Instrumentation and data processing in cardiovascular nuclear medicine: evaluation of ventricular function. *Semin Nucl Med* 1979, 9:257–274.

35. Bacharach SL, Green MV: Data processing in nuclear cardiology: measurement of ventricular function. *IEEE Transact Nucl Sci* 1982, 29:1343–1354.

36. Strauss HW, Zaret BW, Hurley PJ: A scintigraphic method for measuring left ventricular ejection fraction in man without cardiac catheterization. *Am J Cardiol* 1971, 28:575–583.

37. Parker DA, Karvelis KC, Thrall JH, Froelich JW: Radionuclide ventriculography: methods. In *Cardiac Nuclear Medicine*, edn 2. New York: McGraw Hill; 1997.

38. Groch MW, Marshall RC, Erwin WD, *et al*.: Quantitative gated blood pool SPECT imaging: Sensitivity dependence on region definition. *J Nucl Med* 1996, 37:656–656.

39. Links JM, Frank TL, Engdahl JC, *et al*.: Cardiac single-photon emission tomography with a 90-degrees dual-head system. *Eur J Nucl Med* 1995, 22:548–552.

40. Underwood, SR, Walton S, Ell PJ, *et al*.: Gated blood-pool emission tomography: a new technique for the investigation of cardiac structure and function. *Eur J Nucl Med* 1985, 10:332–337.

41. Bacharach SL, Green MV, Borer JS, *et al*.: Left-ventricular peak ejection rate, filling rate, and ejection fraction - frame rate requirements at rest and exercise. *J Nucl Med* 1979, 20:189–193.

42. Bacharach SL, Green MV, Borer JS, *et al*.: Beat-by-beat validation of ECG gating. *J Nucl Med* 1980, 21:307–313.

43. Bonow R, Bacharach SL, Green MV: Impaired left ventricular diastolic filling in patients with coronary artery disease assessment with radionuclide angiography. *Circulation* 1981, 64:315–323.

44. Botvinick EH, Dae MW, O'Connell JW: Blood pool scintigraphy. *Clin Cardiol* 1989, 7:537–563.

45. Dae MW, Botvinick EH, O'Connell JW: Atrial corrected Fourier amplitude ratios for the scintigraphic quantitation of valvar regurgitation. *Am J Noninvas Cardiol* 1987, 1:155–162.

46. Frais M, Botvinick E, Shosa D, O'Connell JW: Phase image characterization of ventricular contraction in left and right bundle branch block. *Am J Cardiol* 1982, 50:95–103.

47. Kerwin W, Botvinick EH, O'Connell JW. Ventricular contraction abnormalities in dilated cardiomyopathy: acute effects of dual chamber simultaneous biventricular pacing to correct interventricular dyssynchrony. *J Am Coll Cardiol* 2000, 35:1221–1227.

48. O'Connell JW, Schreck C, Moles M, *et al*.: A unique method by which to quantitate synchrony with equilibrium radionuclide angiography. *J Nucl Cardiol* 2005, 12:441–450.

49. Oeff M, Scheinman MM, Abbott JA, *et al*.: Phase image triangulation of accessory pathways in patients undergoing catheter ablation of posteroseptal pathways. *PACE* 1991, 14:1072–1080.

50. Germano G: Technical aspects of myocardial SPECT imaging. *J Nucl Med* 2001, 42:1499–1507.

51. The Cardiovascular Imaging Committee, American College of Cardiology; The Committee on Advanced Cardiac Imaging and Technology, Council on Clinical Cardiology, American Heart Association; and Board of Directors, Cardiovascular Council, Society of Nuclear Medicine: Standardization of cardiac tomographic imaging. *J Am Coll Cardiol* 1992, 20:255–256.

52. Germano G, Berman D: Acquisition and processing for gated perfusion SPECT: technical aspects. In *Clinical Gated Cardiac SPECT*. Edited by Germano G, Berman D. Armonk, NY: Futura Publishing Company; 1999:93–113.

53. Botvinick EH, O'Connell JW, Kadkade PJ, *et al*.: The potential added value of three-dimensional reconstruction and display of SPECT gated blood pool images. *J Nucl Cardiol* 1998, 25:509–514.

54. Nakajima K, Higuchi T, Taki J, *et al*.: Accuracy of ventricular volume and ejection fraction measured by gated myocardial SPECT: comparison of 4 software programs. *J Nucl Med* 2001, 42:1571–1578.

55. Schaefer WM, Lipke CSA, Standke D, *et al*.: Quantification of left ventricular volumes and ejection fraction from gated Tc-99m-MIBI SPECT: MRI validation and comparison of the Emory Cardiac Tool Box with QGS and 4D-MSPECT. *J Nucl Med* 2005, 46:1256–1263.

56. Nakajima K, Nishimura T: Inter-institution preference-based variability of ejection fraction and volumes using quantitative gated SPECT with Tc-99m-tetrofosmin: a multicentre study involving 106 hospitals. *Eur J Nucl Med Molec Imaging* 2006, 33:127–133.

57. Honda N, Machida K, Mamiya T, *et al*.: Two-dimensional polar display of cardiac blood pool SPECT. *Eur J Nucl Med* 1989, 15:133–136.

58. Links JM, Devous MD: 3-Dimensional display in nuclear medicine: a more useful depiction of reality, or only a superficial rendering? *J Nucl Med* 1995, 36:703–704.

59. Metcalfe MJ, Cross S, Norton MY, *et al*.: Polar map or novel three-dimensional display technique for the improved detection of inferior wall myocardial infarction using tomographic radionuclide ventriculography. *Nucl Med Commun* 1994, 15:330–340.

60. Topic 5, Myocardial perfusion scintigraphy-technical aspects. Self-study program III. In *Nuclear Medicine: Cardiology*. Edited by Botvinick E. Reston, VA: Society of Nuclear Medicine; 2003.

61. Indovina AG: Three-dimensional surface display in blood pool gated SPECT. *Angiology* 1994, 45:861–866.

62. Taillefer R, DePuey EG, Udelson JE, *et al*.: Comparison between the end-diastolic images and the summed images of gated Tc-99m sestamibi SPECT perfusion study in detection of coronary artery disease in women. *J Nucl Card* 1999, 6:169–176.

63. Mok DY, Bartlett ML, Bacharach SL, *et al*.: Can partial volume effects be used to measure myocardial thickness and thickening? *IEEE Comp Cardiol* 1992, 19:195–198.

64. Botvinick EH, Dae MW, O'Connell JW: The scintigraphic evaluation of the cardiovascular system, In *Cardiology*. Edited by Parmley WW, Chatterjee KC. Philadelphia: JB Lippincott; 1983.

65. Yun J, Block M, Botvinick EH: Unique contraction pattern in patients after coronary bypass graft surgery by gated SPECT myocardial perfusion imaging. *Clin Nucl Med* 2003, 28:18–24.

Risk Stratification and Patient Management

Daniel S. Berman, Rory Hachamovitch, and Guido Germano

Since its beginnings in the early 1970s, clinical nuclear cardiology has evolved substantially, gaining both technical sophistication and enhanced imaging capabilities. Importantly, in parallel to these developments, an extensive literature supporting the clinical and cost effectiveness of this modality has developed. Today, state-of-the-art nuclear cardiology allows for the objective measurement of both myocardial function and relative regional myocardial perfusion at rest and stress, providing accurate risk assessment in a wider variety of patient subsets. This chapter will highlight stress myocardial perfusion SPECT (MPS), which currently comprises approximately 95% of the procedures performed in this field.

The chapter is organized as follows: first, there is a discussion of the general concepts of risk assessment in chronic coronary artery disease (CAD), including evidence for the cost-effective characteristics of stress MPS compared with alternative strategies without MPS, as well as data supporting the selection of MPS in specific patient populations. This discussion is followed by the largest section of the chapter dealing with the current evidence for the use of MPS for risk stratification. This is followed by a brief section dealing with the importance of parameters other than stress myocardial perfusion defects that impact post-MPS patient risk and estimates of risk. The final portion of this chapter deals with the role of MPS in identifying whether patients will have enhanced survival with medical therapy versus revascularization based on the results of the MPS study. In this context, the role of gated SPECT ejection fraction and the potential importance of validated scores to estimate patient risk will be mentioned as well. The conclusion of the chapter addresses the need for integration of SPECT results with other clinical data in guiding inpatient management decisions.

This chapter will be limited to the consideration of stable patients with known or suspected chronic coronary artery disease and will focus primarily on stress myocardial perfusion abnormalities, since myocardial viability (predominantly assessed by resting studies) is addressed in another chapter.

The main use of nuclear cardiology studies for guiding management decisions is determining which patients with suspected or known coronary artery disease require catheterization with consideration of revascularization. In patients who have "limiting" chest pain symptoms, which despite medical therapy affect their well being, nuclear cardiology studies play a limited role, chiefly being useful for identifying the culprit coronary lesion and determining which vessel or vessels might be most appropriate for revascularization. Since revascularization has been shown to relieve anginal symptoms in patients with CAD, it would not be cost effective to study all patients with limiting symptoms with MPS, and direct invasive coronary angiography is generally indicated.

If revascularization is being considered for purposes of improving prognosis, MPS can be helpful in determining whether the patient's risk is high enough to warrant revascularization. Risk stratification is the most rapidly growing area of application of MPS. The use of MPS for this purpose provides a widely accepted new paradigm in patient management, which is endorsed by clinical guidelines. A risk-based approach to patients with known or suspected CAD is well suited to the current environment, in which cost containment is of great importance and in which dramatic improvements in medical therapy have been developed. In contrast, the approach focusing on simple diagnosis, in which patients with suspected disease undergo invasive coronary angiography and then are frequently revascularized based on coronary anatomic findings, has been shown to be less cost effective. With the risk-based approach, the focus is not on predicting who has anatomic CAD, but on identifying and separating patients at higher risk for a major adverse cardiac event from those who are at lower risk.

Pathophysiologic Basis for Risk Assessment in Myocardial Perfusion SPECT

The basis for the power of nuclear testing for risk stratification is found in the fact that the major determinants of prognosis in CAD can be assessed by measurements of stress-induced perfusion or function. These measurements include the amount of infarcted myocardium, the amount of jeopardized myocardium (supplied by vessels with hemodynamically significant stenosis), and the degree of jeopardy (tightness of the individual coronary stenosis). An additional important factor in prognostic assessment is the stability (or instability) of the CAD process. This last consideration may help explain what appears to be a clinical paradox: nuclear tests, which in general are expected to be positive only in the presence of hemodynamically significant stenosis, are associated with a very low risk of either cardiac death or nonfatal myocardial infarction when normal. In contrast, it has been observed that most myocardial infarctions occur in regions with premyocardial infarction coronary plaques causing less than 50% stenosis [1,2]. It has been postulated that this paradox may be explained by the different response to stress of mild stenosis associated with stable and unstable plaque. For example, it has been shown that mild coronary narrowings associated with unstable plaque manifest a vasoconstrictive response to acetylcholine stimulation due to abnormal endothelial function, whereas stable, mild coronary lesions respond to acetylcholine with vasodilation [1]. It is possible that factors released during exercise or vasodilator stress may be similar to acetylcholine in terms of stimulation of a differential endothelial response in stable and unstable plaque. Thus, beyond the ability to define anatomic stenosis, nuclear tests (by virtue of their assessment of physiology) would be able to discern abnormalities of endothelial function associated with high risk, even in the absence of significant stenosis.

Differentiating Outcome Type by Nuclear Test Results

Recent evidence in large patient cohorts has revealed that factors estimating the extent of left ventricular dysfunction (left ventricular ejection fraction, the extent of infarcted myocardium, transient ischemic dilation of the left ventricle, and increased lung uptake) are excellent predictors of cardiac mortality. In contrast, measurements of inducible ischemia are better predictors of the development of acute ischemic syndromes. These include exertional symptoms, electrocardiographic changes, as well as the extent of perfusion defect reversibility and stress-induced ventricular dyssynergy. Several recent reports have shown that nuclear testing yields incremental prognostic value over clinical information with respect to cardiac death, or the combination of cardiac death and nonfatal myocardial infarction as isolated endpoints. By understanding how clinical information and nuclear test markers can be used to estimate varying outcomes, it is now possible to tailor therapeutic decision making for an individual patient based on the combination of clinical factors and nuclear scan results. For example, a patient with severe perfusion abnormalities on their stress imaging may have a five- to 10-fold higher likelihood of cardiac death compared with a patient with a normal MPS. If the defects are stress induced (reversible), therapies known to improve survival might be chosen in order to result in an optimized outcome for that patient.

Figure 6-1. Definition of nuclear variables. In order to optimize the prognostic performance of stress myocardial perfusion SPECT, it is crucial to maximize the information extracted from the images at the time of interpretation. Previous studies have shown that the extent and severity of reversible hypoperfusion are independent variables in predicting subsequent cardiac events in patients with suspected coronary artery disease [2]. To this end, it is necessary to consider the full extent and severity of the abnormality, either quantitatively [3–5] or semiquantitatively [6], rather than simply determining that the nuclear study is normal or abnormal. While a 20-segment model was initially widely used [7], a 17-segment model is currently recommended for all forms of tomographic myocardial imaging [8]. This figure provides a diagrammatic representation of the segmental division of the SPECT slices and assignment of individual segments to individual coronary arteries using a 17-segment model. The numbers refer to the individual segments. Each segment is scored from 0 normal, to 4 absent uptake of radioactivity. In order to circumvent these issues, we have recently proposed normalizing these variables [9] by dividing by the model-dependent maximum potential score and multiplying by 100. The result is the % myocardium abnormal with stress, fixed (nonreversible), and ischemic (reversible) defects, providing intuitively useful information that will apply to any segmental scoring system. C—left circumflex coronary artery; L—left anterior descending coronary artery; R—right coronary artery.

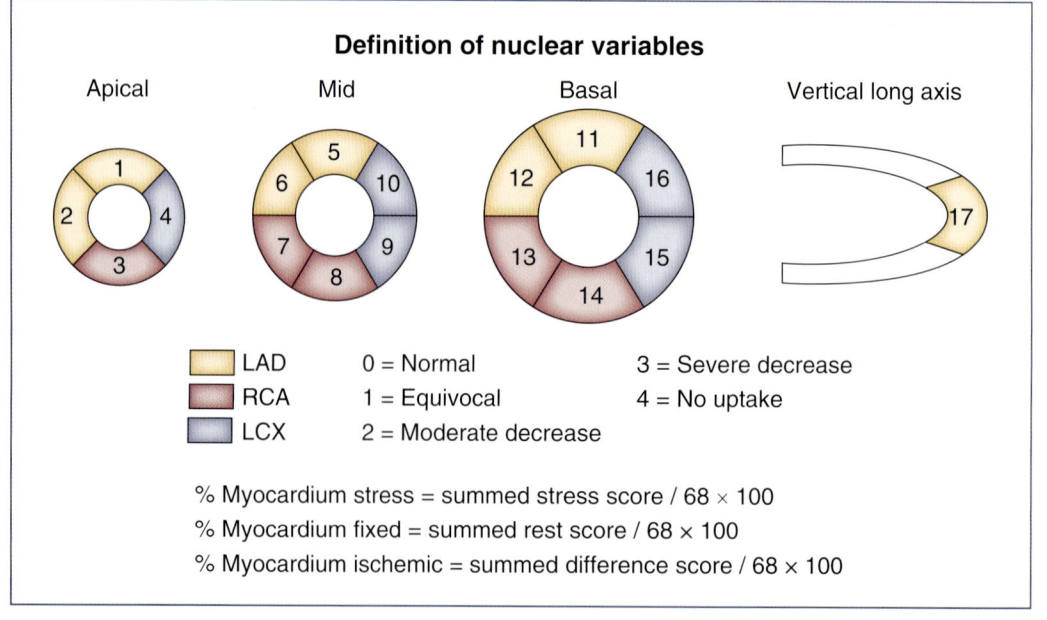

Definition of nuclear variables

- LAD
- RCA
- LCX

0 = Normal
1 = Equivocal
2 = Moderate decrease
3 = Severe decrease
4 = No uptake

% Myocardium stress = summed stress score / 68 × 100
% Myocardium fixed = summed rest score / 68 × 100
% Myocardium ischemic = summed difference score / 68 × 100

Figure 6-2. Semiquantitative global indicies of hypoperfusion. Scoring perfusion defects in each individual segment is useful in deriving summed perfusion parameters, which incorporate the global extent and severity of perfusion abnormality [6]. The summed stress score (SSS) reflects the extent and severity of perfusion defects at stress, and is affected by prior myocardial infarction as well as by stress-induced ischemia. The summed rest score (SRS) reflects the amount of infarcted or hibernating myocardium. The summed difference score (SDS) is a measure of the extent and severity of stress-induced ischemia. These global perfusion parameters can be considered the perfusion analogs of left ventricular ejection fraction, the most commonly employed global ventricular function parameter. By incorporating the extent and severity of perfusion defect, these global parameters allow assessment of the variables shown in Figure 6-1 to be incrementally important in assessing risk from perfusion scintigraphy. The principal problem of these summed scores is that their implications depend on the particular scoring system employed and these implications are not intuitive.

Semiquantitative Global Indicies of Hypoperfusion

Summed scores

SSS = sum of 20/17 stress scores

SRS = sum of 20/17 rest scores

SDS = SSS–SRS

Degree of abnormality by % myocardium (myo) stress

Normal: SSS* 0–3 (< 5% myo)

Mildly abnormal: SSS* 4–7 (5%–10% myo)

Moderately to severely abnormal: SSS* > 8 (> 10% myo)

*17-Segment model.

Figure 6-3. Comparison of the percent myocardium with abnormal perfusion at stress (% myocardium stress) derived from myocardial perfusion SPECT analyzed with either 20-segment or 17- segment approaches. In a population of 16,020 patients with known or suspected coronary artery disease followed up for 2.1 years, equally effective prognostic assessment regarding cardiac death was shown with the two models. The summed stress score values shown for normal, mildly abnormal, and moderately to severely abnormal were those used in prognositic studies using the 20-segment model. Slight modification would be appropriate for the 17-segment model. (*Adapted from* Berman et al. [6].)

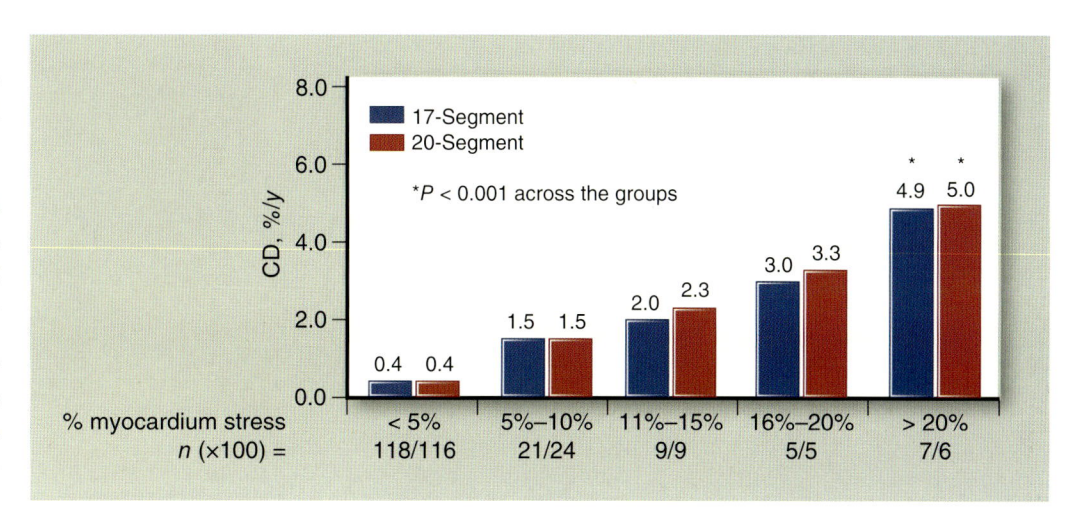

Figure 6-4. Total perfusion deficit (TPD). Being intrinsically three dimensional and digital, myocardial perfusion abnormalities with SPECT or PET lend themselves to automated quantitative analysis. Several software packages for quantitative analysis are commercially available. This figure illustrates the TPD that is a computer-derived analogue of the visual percent myocardium abnormal by visual analysis, representing both defect extent and severity of perfusion defect. TPD is calculated as the percentage of the total surface area of the left ventricle below the predefined uniform average deviation threshold [10] using quantitative perfusion SPECT software (*see* Fig. 6-1) [11]. A circumferential profile for one short axis slice is shown with corresponding normal limits [9,10]. The area below the normal limit curve but above the circumferential profile curve for a given slice defines perfusion deficit in a given slice. These areas are computed for all circumeferential profiles in the myocardium and summed forming TPD. TPD is measured at stress and rest, and ischemic TPD is calculated from the difference (stress TPD minus rest TPD).

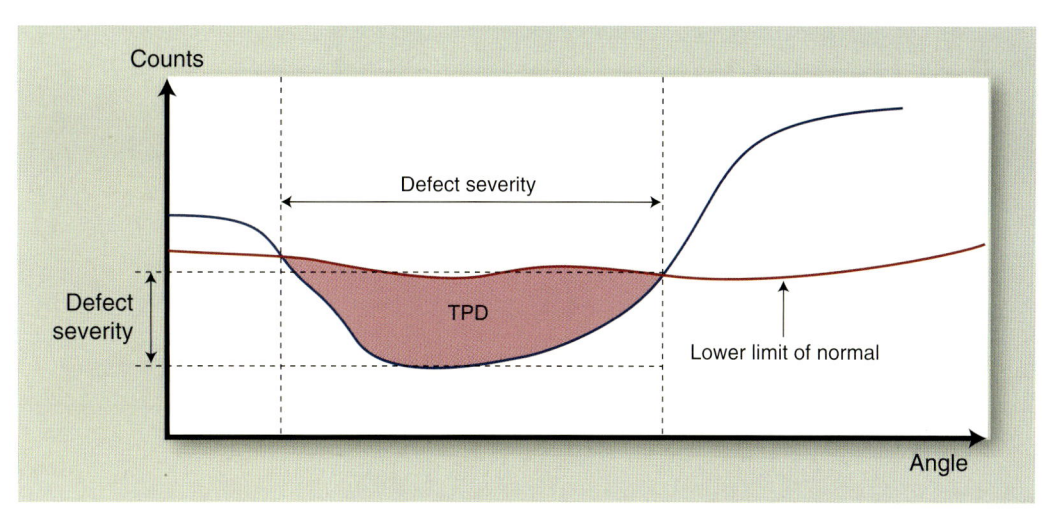

The reproducibility thresholds for quantitative stress, rest, and ischemic TPD have been reported to all be less than 7% and smaller than the thresholds for visual percent myocardium abnormal (10%–13%) [12], suggesting that this type of objective, quantitative assessment of ischemia may be more effective in assessing the effects of therapy in individual patients than visual analysis alone. Ischemic TPD was the variable used in the Clinical Outcomes Utilizing Revascularization and Aggressive Drug Evaluation (COURAGE) nuclear substudy to evaluate baseline ischemia and the change in ischemia after therapy (*See* Figs. 6-45A and B). (*Adapted from* Berman et al. [9].)

Risk Stratification and Patient Management

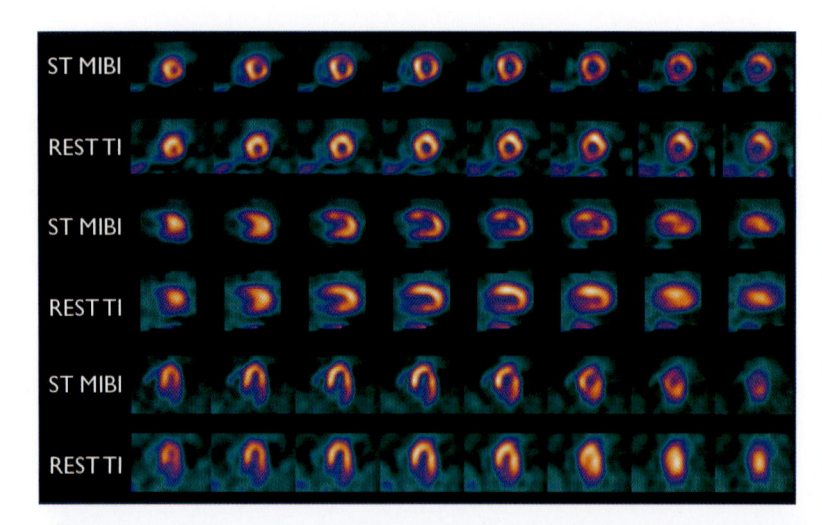

Figure 6-5. Example of a patient with a small stress perfusion defect resulting in a mildly abnormal summed stress score. The patient is a 69-year-old man with atypical angina. The only risk factor for coronary disease was hypercholesterolemia. The patient exercised for 7 minutes and 20 seconds to a heart rate of 139 (92% of maximal predicted) and had a normal blood pressure response. He developed minimal chest discomfort during stress, which was considered equivocal for an ischemic response. The electrocardiogram response to stress was normal. Exercise stress ^{99m}Tc-sestamibi (ST MIBI) and rest ^{201}Tl (rest TI) images are interlaced in the alternate rows, which show short axis images (*top two rows*), vertical long axis images (*middle two rows*), and horizontal long axis images (*bottom two rows*). The images reveal a small to moderate size defect in the distal anterior left ventricular wall with sparing of the interventricular septum and the apex. This pattern is classic for the territory of the mid to distal portion of the diagonal branch of the left anterior descending coronary artery.

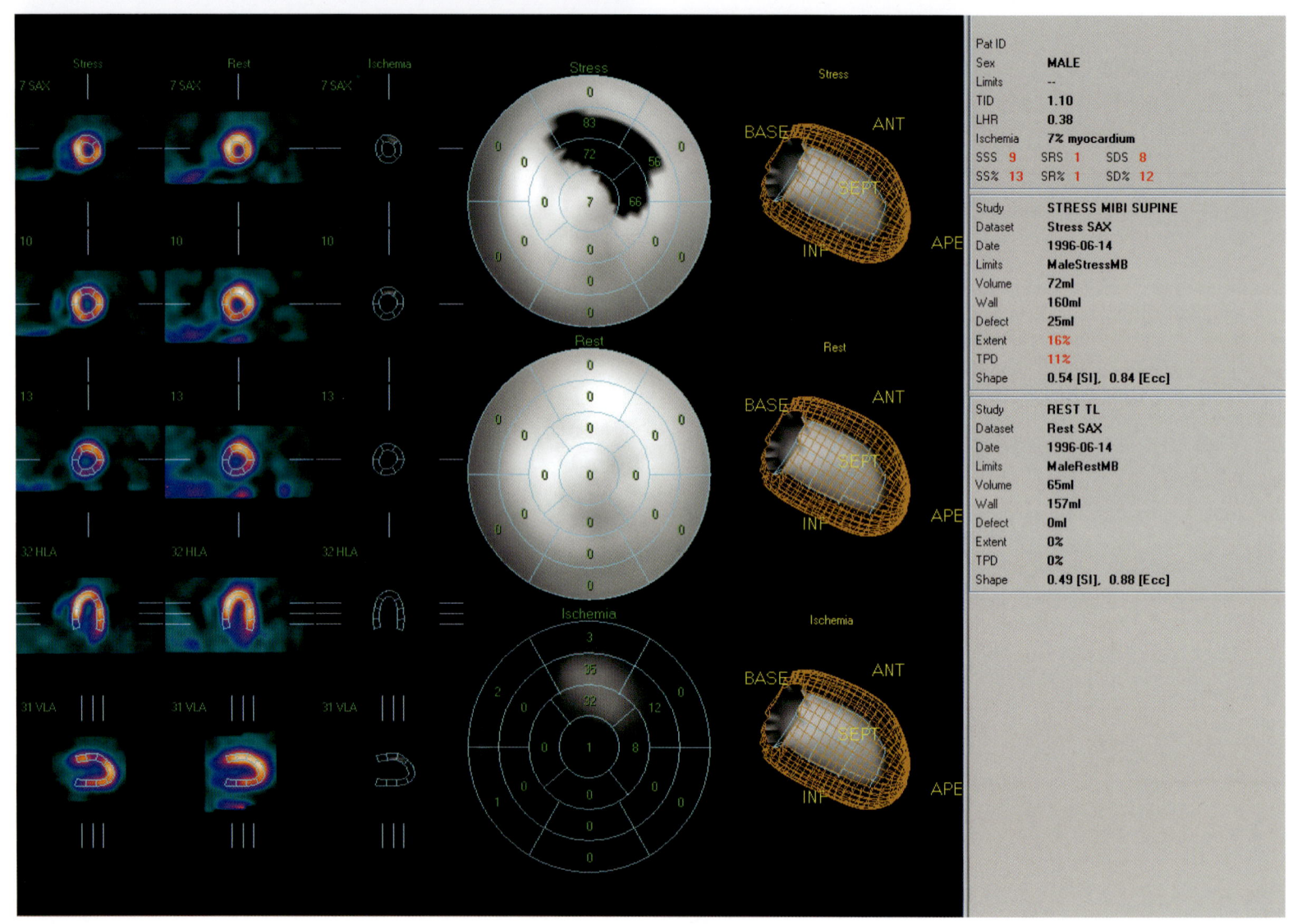

Figure 6-6. Quantitative perfusion SPECT analysis of the patient shown in Figure 6-5 indicating the presence of a small perfusion defect in the diagonal coronary territory. The summed stress score (SSS) attributed to the images in this figure is illustrated in the *upper right corner*. The SSS of 9 indicates a moderate abnormality (*see* Fig. 6-2). The quantitative total perfusion deficit is 11%. The typical diagonal territory location is shown in the two-dimensional (*middle panel*) and three-dimensional (*right panel*) images at stress with a normal quantitative pattern at rest.

144 Atlas of Nuclear Cardiology

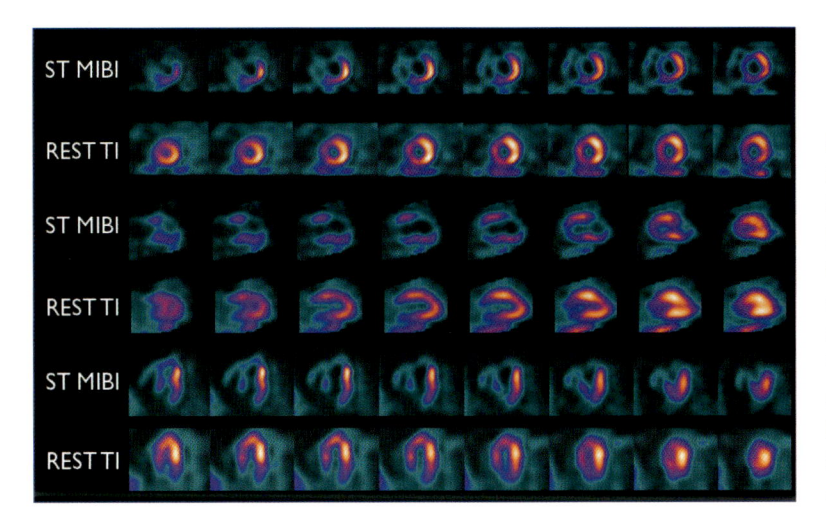

Figure 6-7. Example of a patient with a severe and extensive stress-induced perfusion defect. A 69-year-old man with atypical chest pain who had hypertension and diabetes as risk factors as well as left ventricular hypertrophy on resting electrocardiogram (ECG) exercised for 5 minutes to heart rate 139 (87% of maximal predicted). The patient did develop chest discomfort and had an ischemic ECG response to stress. There was no exercise hypotension. Exercise stress ^{99m}Tc sestamibi (ST MIBI) and rest ^{201}Tl (rest Tl) images are interlaced in the alternate rows, which show short axis images (*top two rows*), vertical long axis images (*middle two rows*), and horizontal long axis images (*bottom two rows*). The myocardial perfusion SPECT study reveals a severe perfusion defect throughout the distribution of the left anterior descending coronary artery.

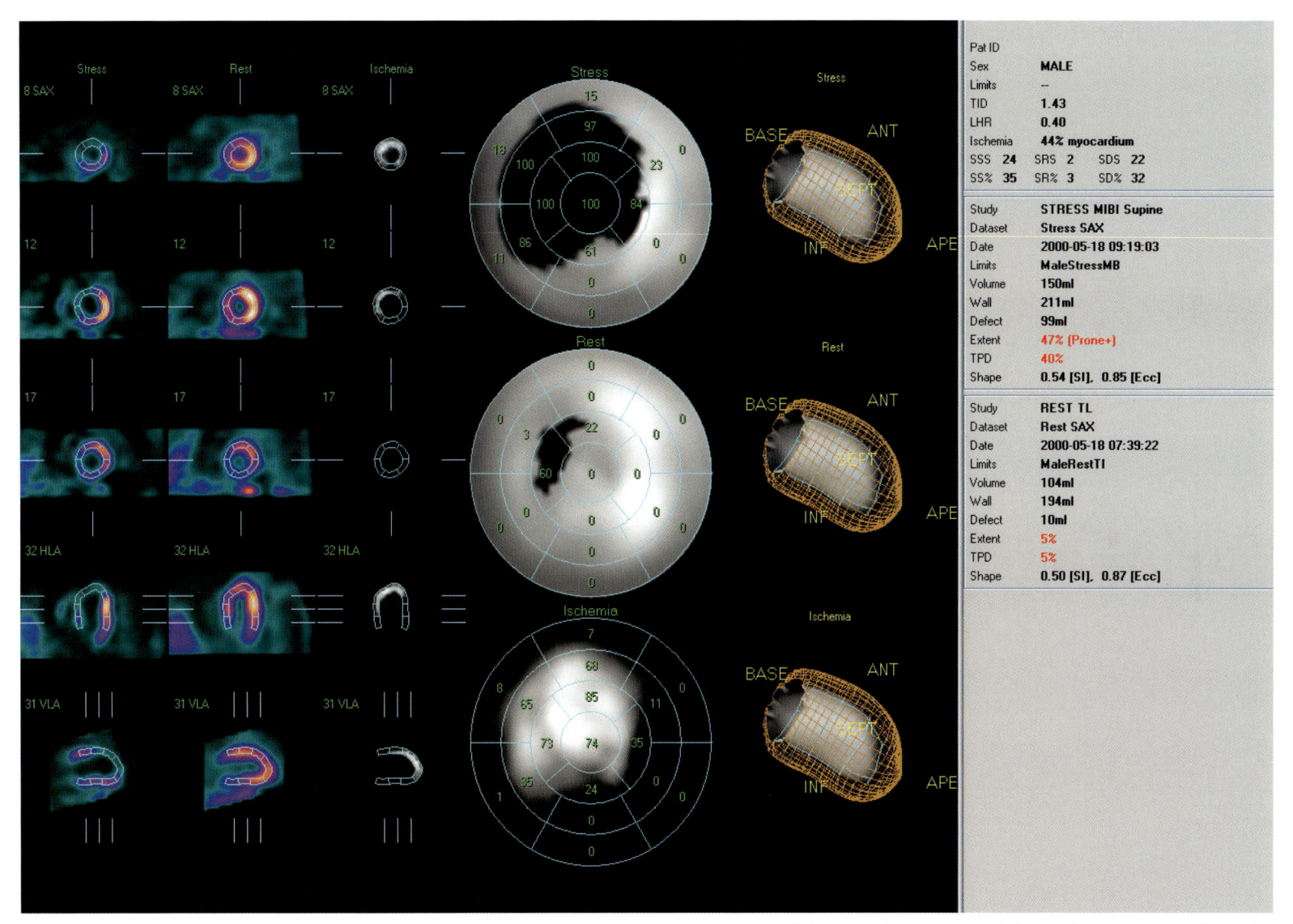

Figure 6-8. Quantitative perfusion SPECT analysis of the patient in Figure 6-7. The summed stress score is very high at 24, the summed rest score is low at 2, and the summed difference score is 22. The total perfusion deficit (TPD) measurements revealed that 40% of the left ventricle is abnormal after stress, corresponding to the entire left anterior descending coronary artery (LAD) territory. The resting TPD was 5%. Note 40% is generally considered the proportion of the myocardium supplied by the LAD. Thus, the findings are predictive of a proximal stenosis of the LAD, and the severity of the perfusion defect allows the interpreter to state that the proximal LAD is likely to have a critical stenosis (> 90%) [13,14]. In this study, the finding of transient ischemic dilation of the left ventricle, measured at 1.43 [11], is an ancillary finding associated with severe and extensive coronary artery diesase. At catheterization the patient was found to have a 100% proximal stenosis of the LAD, a 60% circumflex lesion, and a 50% to 60 % mid right coronary artery stenosis.

Risk Stratification and Patient Management 145

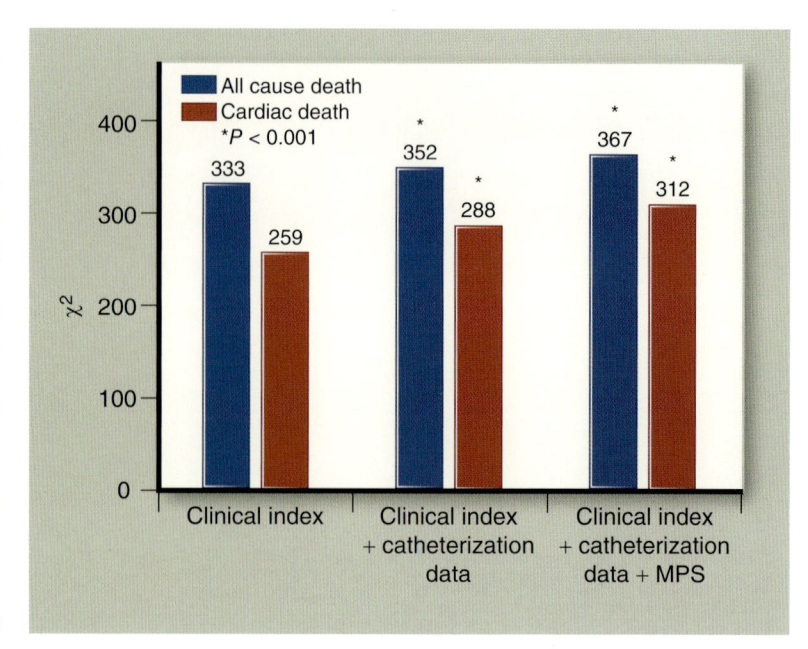

Figure 6-9. Incremental prognostic value of myocardial perfusion SPECT (MPS) results over anatomic and clinical data. Borges-Neto et al. [15] examined the incremental value of stress MPS over clinical and catheterization data in 3275 patients who were followed up for 3.1 years for death, cardiovascular death, and a composite of cardiovascular death or nonfatal myocardial infarction. This study constitutes the largest dataset accumulated with both anatomic and MPS data with follow-up. Using these patients, Cox proportional hazards regression models were developed for the prediction of all cause death, cardiovascular death, and hard events (cardiovascular death or nonfatal myocardial infarction). Based on these models, a one unit change in summed stress score was found to be associated with increased risks of 4%, 7%, and 5% for death, cardiovascular death, and death or nonfatal myocardial infarction, respectively.

With respect to incremental value, the results of Cox proportional hazards modeling of all cause death and cardiac death is shown, with the strength of various models depicted by their global chi-square. First, the addition of anatomic data from catheterization added incremental prognostic value over clinical data alone in the setting of both endpoints. Further, even after adjustment for clinical and anatomic data, the addition of stress MPS results added further incremental value with respect to prediction of both of these endpoints.

Importantly, these results support the concept that the physiologic data contributed by MPS yields additive information not available from assessment of anatomic data alone. Thus, a patient management strategy of direct referral to catheterization, or an approach of revascularization without consideration of physiologic data, would result in some patients undergoing unnecessary and inappropriate procedures, while other patients who, on the basis of MPS data, may benefit from an intervention may not receive one. (*Adapted from* Borges-Netl *et al.* [15].)

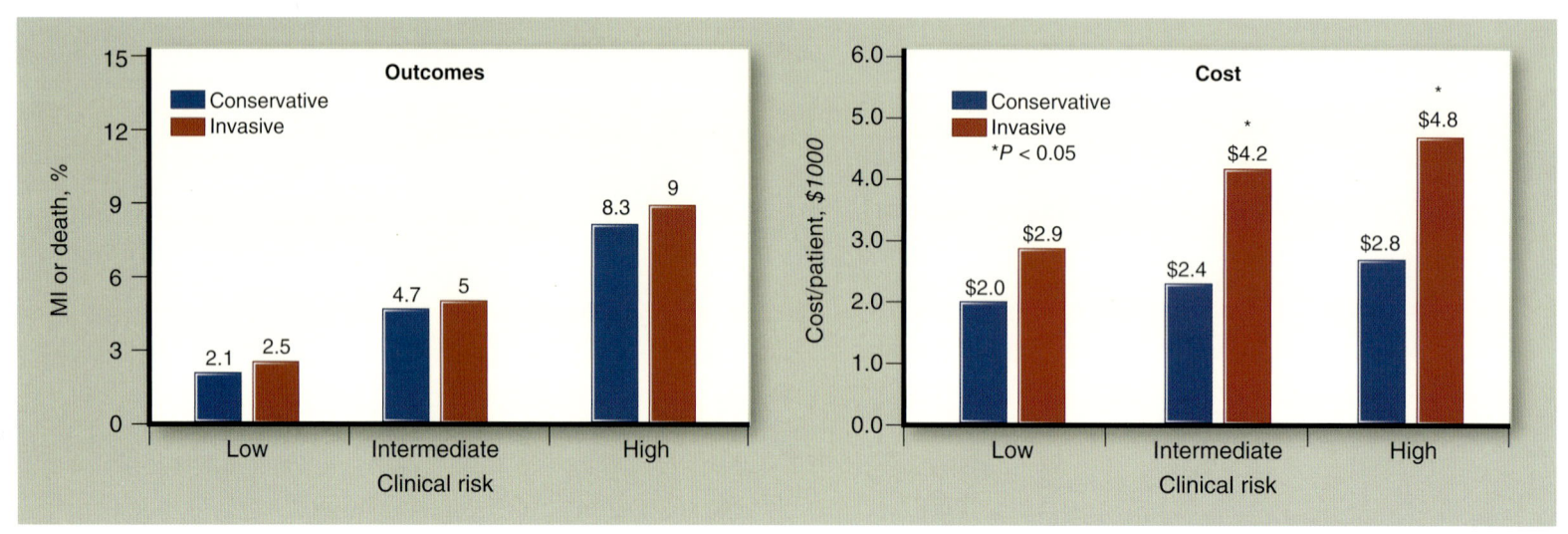

Figure 6-10. Outcomes and referral rates to catheterization in patients with stable chest pain from the Economics of Noninvasive Diagnosis (END) study group [12]. In this study of 11,372 consecutive stable angina patients who were referred for stress myocardial perfusion tomography or cardiac catheterization, composite 3-year costs of care and patient outcomes were compared as a function of two strategies: aggressive (direct referral to cardiac catheterization without stress imaging) versus conservative (initial stress myocardial perfusion tomography and selective catheterization of high-risk patients). After matching patients referred to these two procedures by their pretest clinical risk of coronary disease, comparisons of aggressive and conservative testing strategies revealed that no difference in the rates of cardiac death or nonfatal myocardial infarction (MI) was present between these two groups, suggesting similar quality care. Significantly, the costs of care were higher for direct cardiac catheterization in all clinical risk subsets compared with the costs associated with stress myocardial perfusion imaging plus selective catheterization. Importantly, note that the difference in cost between the strategies did not reach significance in the low-risk patient subset.

The cost savings identified in the intermediate- and high-risk patient subsets was accrued predominantly by preventing referral to catheterization in patients without significant myocardial perfusion SPECT (MPS) abnormalities. This is borne out by significant differences in normal catheterization rates (in the subset of patients referred to catheterization) between the two strategies examined, suggesting that MPS aids in the identification of the appropriate candidate for the catheterization laboratory. Hence, the use of a strategy incorporating MPS as an initial test results in improved cost effectiveness without compromise of patient outcomes. This supports the use of MPS as a reasonable alternative to catheterization in patients presenting with stable angina. (*Adapted from* Shaw *et al.* [12].)

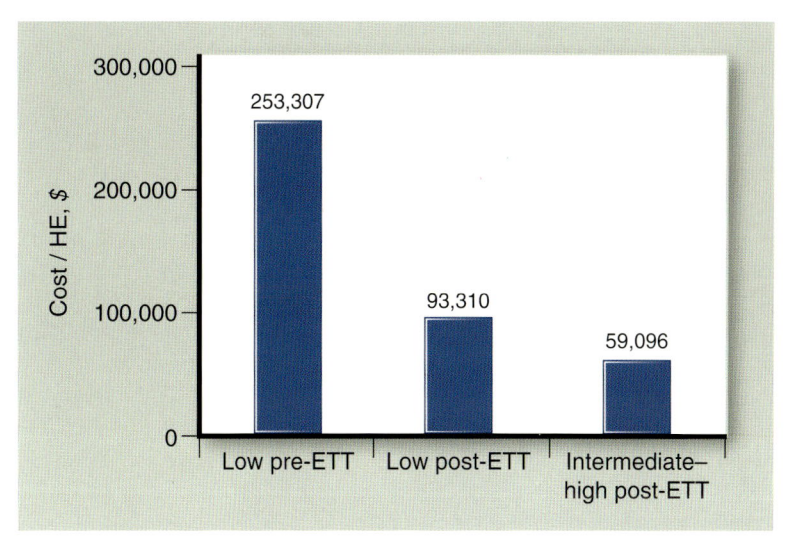

Figure 6-11. Cost-effectiveness ratios (costs of testing per hard event [HE] identified) in patients with low pre–exercise tolerance test (ETT) likelihood of coronary artery disease (CAD), patients with low post-ETT likelihood of CAD, and patients with intermediate to high post-ETT likelihood of CAD. While the previous figures support the role of myocardial perfusion SPECT (MPS) as providing added prognostic value to clinical and catheterization data, as well as cost savings when utilized before catheterization, which patients should be referred to MPS is also important to examine. In a seminal study, Berman et al. [16] examined the incremental prognostic implications of normal and equivocal exercise MPS results, its incremental prognostic value, and cost implications in 1702 patients without prior revascularization who were followed up for 20 ± 5 months. When the complete spectrum of MPS results were considered, MPS yielded incremental prognostic value, as demonstrated by enhanced risk stratification, in all patient subgroups analyzed (low, intermediate, and high likelihood of CAD) (results not shown). However, MPS was cost effective only in patients with interpretable exercise electrocardiogram (ECG) responses and an intermediate to high post-ETT likelihood of CAD and in those with uninterpretable exercise ECG responses and an intermediate to high pre-ETT likelihood of CAD. This study demonstrates the impact of patient selection for MPS on the clinical and cost-effectiveness of testing. The referral of patients identified as low risk by clinical evaluation (low pre-ETT likelihood of CAD) or by ETT (low post-ETT likelihood of CAD) results in excess costs with minimal impact on identification of at risk patients (since so few patients are reclassified with respect to risk in these patient subsets). On the other hand, MPS can be a cost-effective test if patients at adequate risk are referred. (*Data from* Berman et al. [16].)

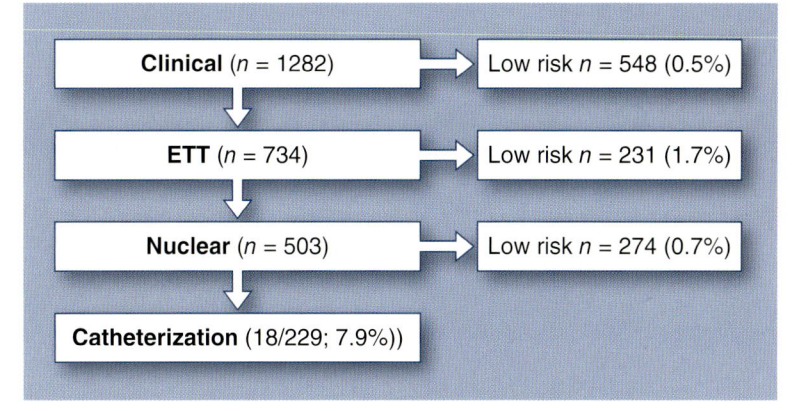

Figure 6-12. Successive testing to optimize outcomes and cost. Based on the data from Berman et al. [16] presented above, a potential strategy of successive testing can be hypothesized to optimize outcomes and cost. As shown in the figure, a significant number of patients presented to clinical evaluation (*n* =1282). Clinical evaluation alone would have identified 43% of the patients in this cohort as low risk (0.5% hard event rate over 20 months) and not in need of further testing. Similarly, the use of exercise tolerance testing (ETT) as the second-line test in the intermediate to high clinical risk patients would have identified an additional 231 patients as not needing further testing (31% of the intermediate- to high-risk patients, 18% of total). This approach would have reduced the number of patients referred to myocardial perfusion SPECT (MPS) from 1282 to 503, as shown. The low risk associated with a normal study would have identified an additional 274 patients (54% of MPS patients) as low risk and not in need of further evaluation. Thus, of 1282 patients originally referred to MPS, a successive testing strategy may have avoided 39% of all the MPS performed in these patients (the 779 patients identified as low risk by pre-MPS assessment). As importantly, only 229 patients, who were at greater risk (7.9% hard event rate) would be referred on to catheterization, resulting in a considerable potential cost saving.

Thus, a strategy of successive evaluations, with the evaluations of increasing sophistication and cost at each step, results in reduced cost with adequate identification of at risk patients. This approach ensures both the cost effectiveness of MPS as a modality within a strategy, as well as that of the testing strategy as a whole. (*Data from* Berman et al. [16].)

Risk Stratification and Patient Management 147

Figure 6-13. Cost effectiveness of myocardial perfusion SPECT (MPS) in reclassifying patients' likelihood of high-risk coronary artery disease (CAD). Although risked-based patient management strategies have gained widespread acceptance, many studies still focus on anatomic endpoints for the assessment of MPS. While it is generally assumed that the two are reasonable alternatives, the test performance characteristics of stress MPS are distinctly different when assessed using an anatomic versus a prognostic endpoint. In 1994, the Mayo Clinic group examined the cost-effectiveness of stress MPS for identifying patients with high-risk anatomic CAD in a cohort of 411 patients with normal resting electrocardiograms (ECGs) and no prior CAD who underwent exercise MPS and were subsequently referred to catheterization [17]. The analytic approach they utilized was to determine each patient's likelihood of having high-risk anatomic CAD (left main [LM] or three-vessel [3VD] CAD) on the basis of pre-MPS data, and assess how many patients' likelihood were reclassified on the basis of MPS data [17]. These investigators found that although there was a significant reclassification achieved by SPECT over pre-SPECT data, the number of patients reclassified by SPECT (3% of all patients) did not justify the cost accrued, as evidenced by an unacceptably high cost-effectiveness ratio. They concluded that although MPS could reclassify patients' likelihood of high-risk CAD, it failed to do so in a cost-effective manner, hence, should not be used in patients with normal rest ECG without prior CAD. Interestingly, the Cedars-Sinai group examined this same population (no prior CAD, normal rest ECG), using the same analytic approach (the ability of MPS data to reclassify patients' likelihood of an outcome), but used outcomes (cardiac death, nonfatal myocardial infarction) rather than an anatomic endpoint [18]. With respect to this prognostic endpoint, the investigators found that SPECT reclassified a far greater proportion of patients with respect to their risk of adverse outcomes (40%), thus doing so at less than one third the cost of an anatomic-based approach. Hence, stress SPECT appears to have far greater clinical and cost effectiveness in the context of an outcome than an anatomic endpoint. Of note, the cost effectiveness of SPECT with respect to this prognostic endpoint demonstrated this superiority only when patients with intermediate to high risk were examined. The inclusion of low-risk patients, as described previously, compromised the clinical and cost effectiveness of SPECT.

Figure 6-14. Identification of the appropriate candidate for stress imaging. This figure shows the initial decision node in the evaluation of patients with known or suspected coronary artery disease (CAD). The first clinical step is the determination of a patient's pretest likelihood of CAD or their pretest risk of adverse events. In patients with low likelihood or risk, the clinical question is primarily whether the patient is a candidate for primary versus secondary prevention, and whether further testing (eg, atherosclerosis assessment) would be necessary. Patients at intermediate or high likelihood of risk are appropriate candidates for ischemia evaluation.

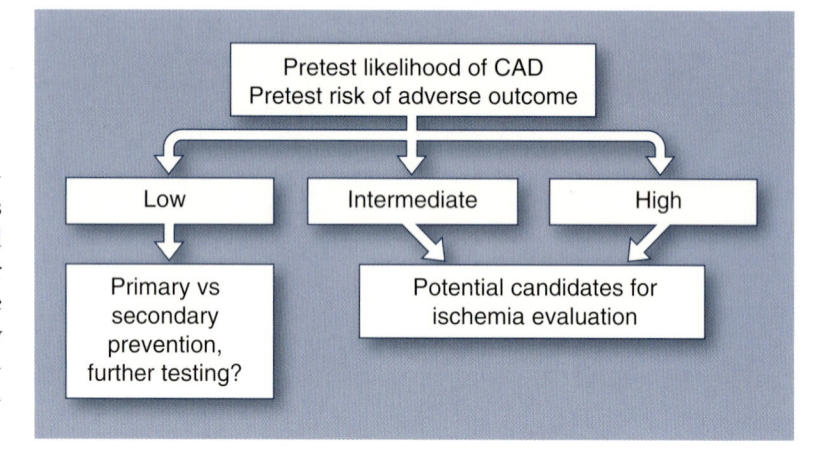

148 Atlas of Nuclear Cardiology

Figure 6-15. Hard event rates after normal myocardial perfusion SPECT (MPS) (*line*) and relative risks associated with abnormal versus normal MPS in the 12 prognostic studies cited by the 2003 Radionuclide Guidelines. To date, there is an extensive literature base for examining risk after a normal stress MPS, with most studies reporting rates of hard events (cardiac death or nonfatal MI) of less than 1% per year of follow-up [19,20]. This level of risk has been described to be independent of gender, age, symptom status, past history of coronary artery disease (CAD), presence of anatomic CAD, imaging technique, or isotope (^{201}Tl or ^{99m}Tc-sestamibi) [15]. Two important concepts in understanding how well MPS fulfills the basic requirements of risk stratification are shown in this figure. First, the risk of hard events after a normal MPS is relatively low (*right Y axis*; < 1% in 10 of the 12 studies cited). Indeed, these guidelines also pool data from 16 studies finding that in over 27,000 patients followed for a mean of 26.8 months the annualized hard event rate was only 0.6%. The relative risk associated with an abnormal MPS ranges from 3 to 14 in these studies (*left Y axis*), indicating that MPS successfully aggregates or concentrates risk in patients with abnormal studies relative to normal studies, resulting in the former being of far greater risk than the latter. The identification of low risk with a normal study, and the reclassification of higher risk patients with abnormal studies are two of the most basic characteristics of risk stratification with tests. (*Data from* Klocke et al. [19].)

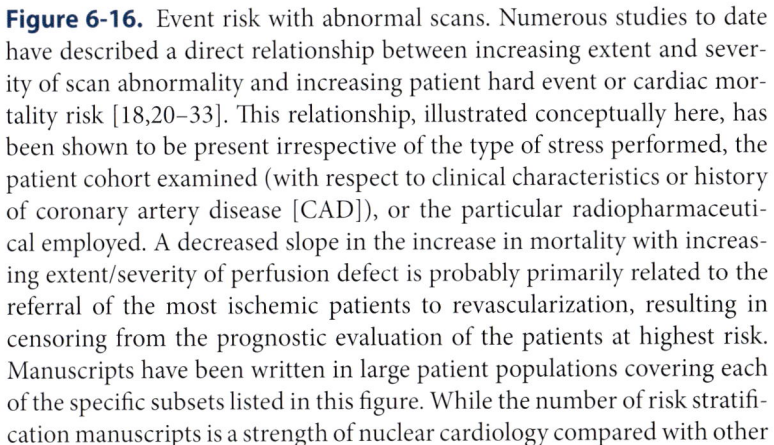

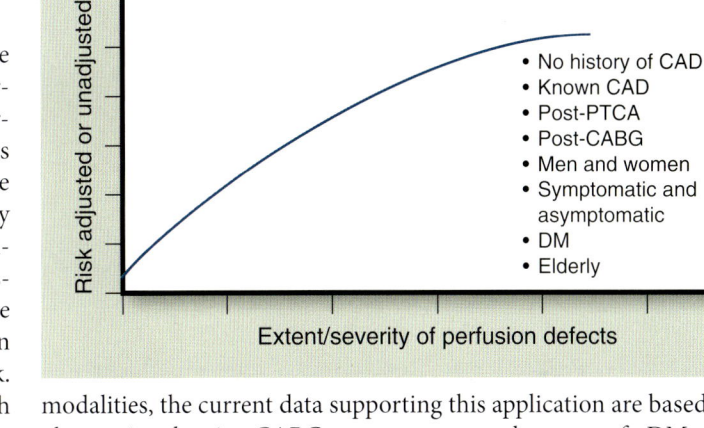

Figure 6-16. Event risk with abnormal scans. Numerous studies to date have described a direct relationship between increasing extent and severity of scan abnormality and increasing patient hard event or cardiac mortality risk [18,20–33]. This relationship, illustrated conceptually here, has been shown to be present irrespective of the type of stress performed, the patient cohort examined (with respect to clinical characteristics or history of coronary artery disease [CAD]), or the particular radiopharmaceutical employed. A decreased slope in the increase in mortality with increasing extent/severity of perfusion defect is probably primarily related to the referral of the most ischemic patients to revascularization, resulting in censoring from the prognostic evaluation of the patients at highest risk. Manuscripts have been written in large patient populations covering each of the specific subsets listed in this figure. While the number of risk stratification manuscripts is a strength of nuclear cardiology compared with other modalities, the current data supporting this application are based on large observational series. CABG—coronary artery bypass graft; DM—diabetes mellitus; PTCA—percutaneous transluminal coronary angioplasty.

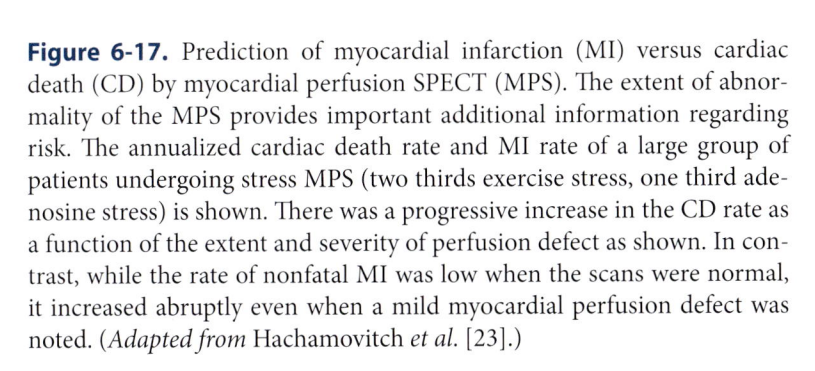

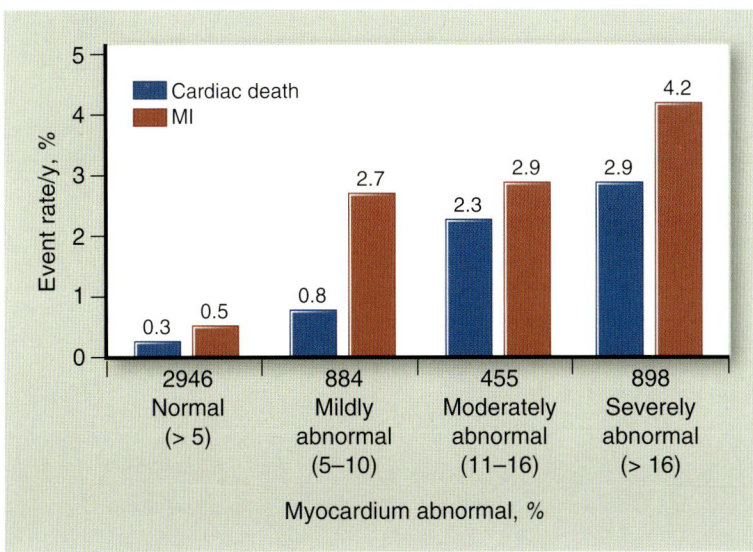

Figure 6-17. Prediction of myocardial infarction (MI) versus cardiac death (CD) by myocardial perfusion SPECT (MPS). The extent of abnormality of the MPS provides important additional information regarding risk. The annualized cardiac death rate and MI rate of a large group of patients undergoing stress MPS (two thirds exercise stress, one third adenosine stress) is shown. There was a progressive increase in the CD rate as a function of the extent and severity of perfusion defect as shown. In contrast, while the rate of nonfatal MI was low when the scans were normal, it increased abruptly even when a mild myocardial perfusion defect was noted. (*Adapted from* Hachamovitch et al. [23].)

Figure 6-18. Risk stratification in patients with a high pretest likelihood of coronary artery disease (CAD). Appropriate patient selection is the first important step in cost-effective risk stratification. Traditionally, anatomic endpoints have served as the basis of patient management strategies. In this context, the principle guiding the decision to use noninvasive testing in patients with suspected CAD was that the patient's pretest likelihood of angiographically significant CAD [34]. For diagnostic purposes, in accordance with Bayes' theorem, only patients with an intermediate likelihood of CAD are considered candidates for exercise treadmill testing, because in this range, the results would reclassify patients as having either a low likelihood (not in need of further testing) or a high likelihood (in need of angiography to determine the suitability for revascularization). This approach is embodied in multiple American College of Cardiology/American Heart Association guidelines in which stress testing, with and without stress imaging, is considered a class IIb indication (usefulness/efficacy is less well established by evidence/opinion) for diagnostic testing in patients with either a high or low pretest probability of CAD [24,35,36]. In an outcomes- or risk-based strategy, intermediate-risk patients would be referred to testing in a similar pattern to referral of intermediate likelihood of CAD patients in an anatomic-based strategy. In an anatomic strategy, patients with a high likelihood of CAD would be referred for invasive coronary angiography. However, in an outcomes-based strategy, such patients would be referred for stress imaging rather than catheterization, based on the assumption that 1) a normal myocardial perfusion SPECT (MPS) result would identify them as low risk despite the high likelihood of anatomic CAD, and 2) a sufficient majority of patients with high pre-MPS likelihood of CAD would have normal MPS so that the use of SPECT in this scenario would be cost effective.

A validation of an outcomes-based approach to the use of MPS was first evaluated in 1270 consecutive patients with no previous revascularization or myocardial infarction who had a pre–exercise tolerance test (ETT) likelihood of CAD less than 0.85 and were followed up for 2.2 ± 1.2 years [37]. As shown the figure, a normal MPS was associated with low risk (0.3% cardiac death [CD] per year, 0.7% hard event [HE] rate per year), with a significant increase in risk with worsening MPS results. Further, 630 of the 1028 patients (61%) included in the survival analysis had normal MPS despite their high likelihood of CAD. A strategy of initial MPS in patients able to exercise was more cost effective than a strategy of initial ETT followed by MPS only in the patients with intermediate to high post-ETT likelihood of CAD. Also, although the subset of patients with interpretable rest electrocardiograms were risk stratified by ETT without imaging, only a small proportion of these patients were reclassified as sufficiently low risk that no further testing was required. Hence, ETT without imaging was considered to be unlikely to be clinically efficient in practice. Finally, MPS was also a superior strategy to initial catheterization in these patients. Hence, it appears that a risk-based strategy is valid and probably more clinically effective and cost effective than a traditional anatomic-based strategy. NL—normal. (*Adapted from* Hachamovitch *et al.* [37].)

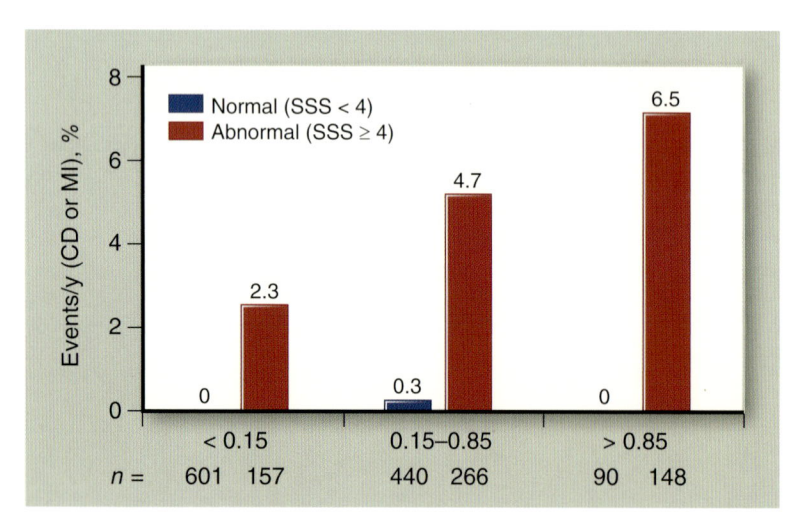

Figure 6-19. Incremental prognostic value of stress myocardial perfusion SPECT (MPS) as a function of prescan likelihood of coronary artery disease (CAD). In a study of 1702 patients undergoing ^{99m}Tc-sestamibi imaging, a normal scan was associated with a very low (0.2%) likelihood of cardiac death (CD) or myocardial infarction (MI) over a 20-month period. The figure illustrates the rate of CD or nonfatal MI throughout the follow-up period as a function of SPECT results and pre-MPS likelihood of CAD (low likelihood, < 0.15; intermediate likelihood, 0.15–0.85; high likelihood, > 0.85). These results demonstrate that MPS could be used for prognostic purposes throughout the range of likelihood of CAD, and that the greatest impact was in the patients with a high likelihood of CAD. SSS—summed stress score. (*Adapted from* Berman *et al.* [16].)

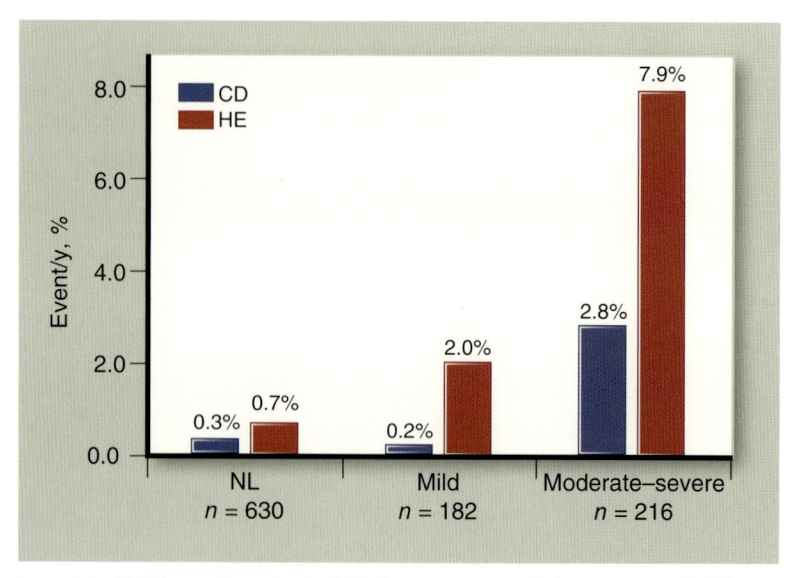

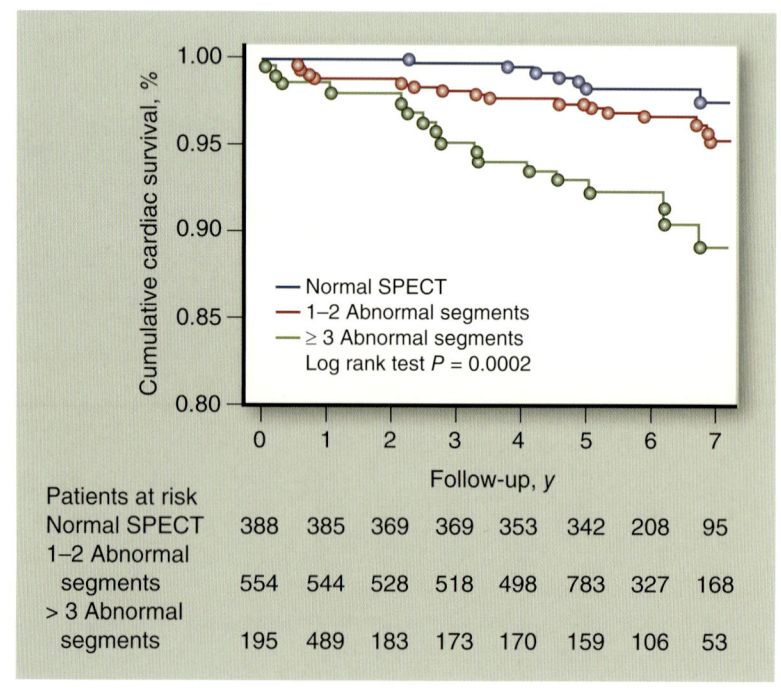

Figure 6-20. Long-term prognostic value of ^{201}Tl SPECT. Vanzetto *et al.* [33] reported the results of a large series of patients who were followed for long-term cardiac events. In the presence of a normal ^{201}Tl SPECT study, the event-free survival was excellent. A progressive worsening of event-free survival was noted as a function of the number of abnormal segments on stress myocardial perfusion SPECT studies. (*Adapted from* Vanzetto *et al.* [33].)

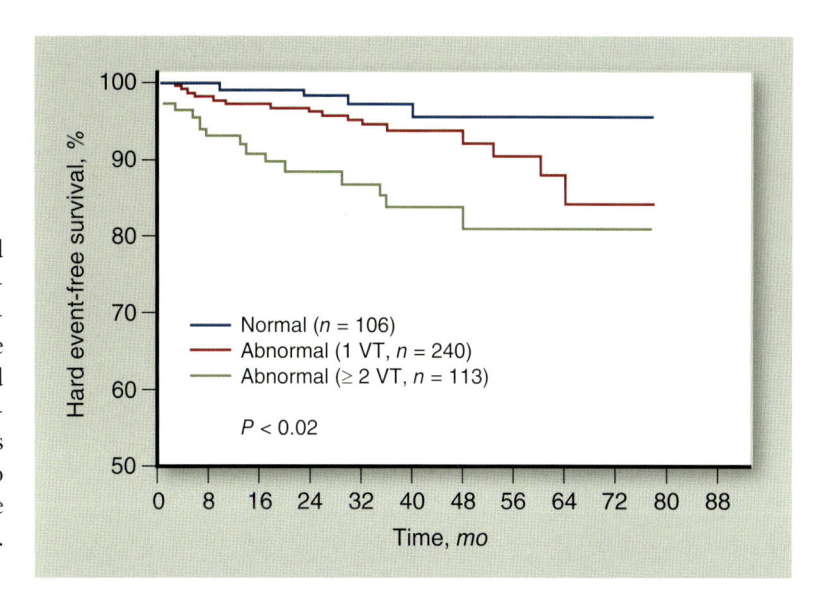

Figure 6-21. Hard event-free survival rate in patients with normal and abnormal ^{99m}Tc-tetrofosmin SPECT from a series of 459 patients. Similar to the results of the previously illustrated studies, the normal tetrofosmin SPECT study was associated with an excellent hard event-free survival, while the patients with abnormal tetrofosmin SPECT studies had lower hard event-free survival in proportion to the extent of abnormality observed. Although the greatest amount of prognostic information is available in the literature regarding the use ^{99m}Tc-sestamibi, there is also extensive prognostic literature based on ^{201}Tl SPECT. Recent studies have demonstrated excellent prognostic stratification with ^{99m}Tc-tetrofosmin. VT—vascular territories. (*Adapted from* Stratmann *et al.* [38].)

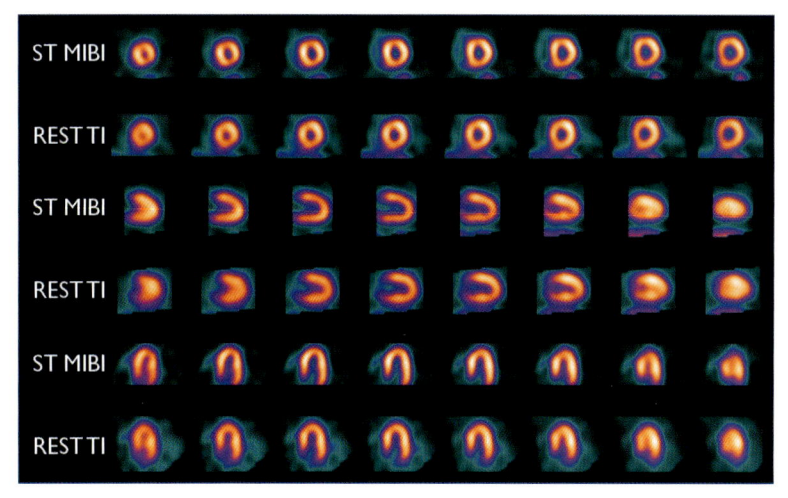

Figure 6-22. Stress myocardial perfusion SPECT (MPS) in a patient with a high likelihood of coronary artery disease. The patient, a 71-year-old woman, had chronic, mild typical angina pectoris and a history of hypertension. Being unable to exercise, she had an adenosine stress for the MPS and showed normal clinical and electrocardiographic responses. Stress ^{99m}Tc-sestamibi (ST MIBI) and rest ^{201}Tl (rest Tl) images are interlaced in the alternate rows, which show short axis images (*top two rows*), vertical long axis (*middle two rows*), and horizontal long axis (*bottom two rows*). The MPS images are entirely normal. With this result, the patient was treated medically. Eleven years following the initial stress imaging study, the patient remained free from cardiac catheterization and free from cardiac events, and a repeat adenosine MPS remained normal.

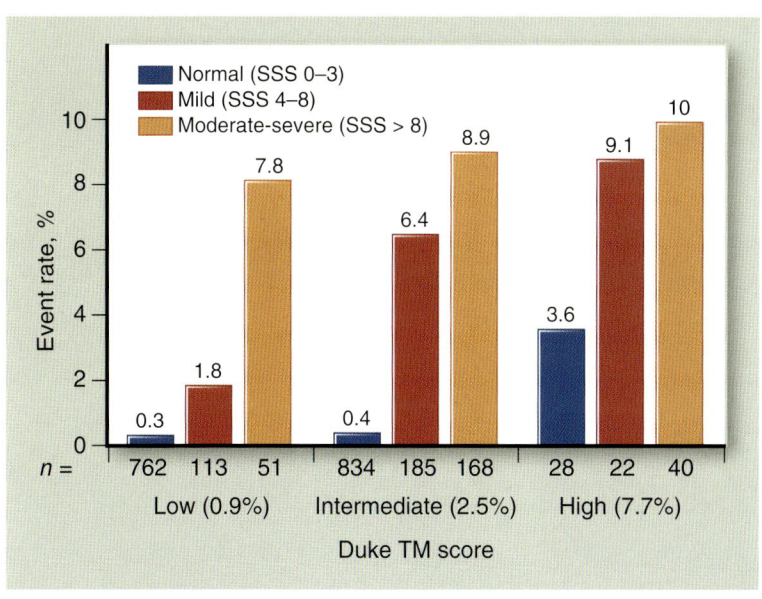

Figure 6-23. Hard event rate as a function of summed stress score (SSS) and Duke treadmill (TM) score. In patients with interpretable stress electrocardiograms (ECGs), it has been demonstrated that the Duke TM score can separate patients into low, intermediate, and high risk of cardiac events. Thus, current guidelines suggest beginning with a stress ECG in these patients [39]. However, nuclear testing is recommended as useful in the patients with intermediate- or high-risk Duke TM scores. Stress myocardial perfusion SPECT (MPS) studies further risk stratify patients within each of these Duke TM score categories [22]. All patients examined had no known coronary artery disease (patients with prior catheterization, myocardial infarction [MI], or revascularization were excluded). The hard event (cardiac death or MI) rate as a function of the Duke TM score category and the nuclear scan results (summed stress score [SSS]) are illustrated. The normal, mild, and severe SSS categories are based on the subgroups of percent myocardium abnormality at stress described in Figure 6-2. For purposes of this study due to small patient numbers, those patients with moderate to severe SSS were categorized as severe. Overall, patients with a low-risk Duke TM score had such a low rate of cardiac events that it would not be cost effective to study them for prognostic purposes. Additionally, since patients with a high-risk Duke TM score usually undergo catheterization, these patients are generally not sent for further nuclear testing. However, 55% of the population had the intermediate-risk Duke TM score with a cardiac event rate of 2.5%. Thus, MPS provided excellent stratification of these patients with respect to risk of hard event [22]. (*Adapted from* Hachamovitch *et al.* [22].)

Risk Stratification and Patient Management 151

Nuclear Cardiology for Risk Stratification in Chronic CAD: Specific Patient Subsets

Nuclear testing has been shown to be effective for risk stratification in several relevant subsets:

- Women
- Elderly
- Diabetes
- LBBB, LVH
- Intermediate Duke Treadmill Score
- After coronary angiography
- Post MI
- After PCI, CABG

Figure 6-24. Nuclear cardiology for risk stratification in chronic coronary artery disease (CAD). Nuclear cardiology has been shown to be effective for risk stratification in several relevant clinical subsets. Several randomized trials in progress should provide a higher level of evidence for this risk stratification application. CABG—coronary artery bypass grafting; LBBB—left bundle branch block; LVH—left ventricular hypertrophy; MI—myocardial infarction; PCI—percutaneous coronary intervention. (*Data from* Klocke *et al.* [19].)

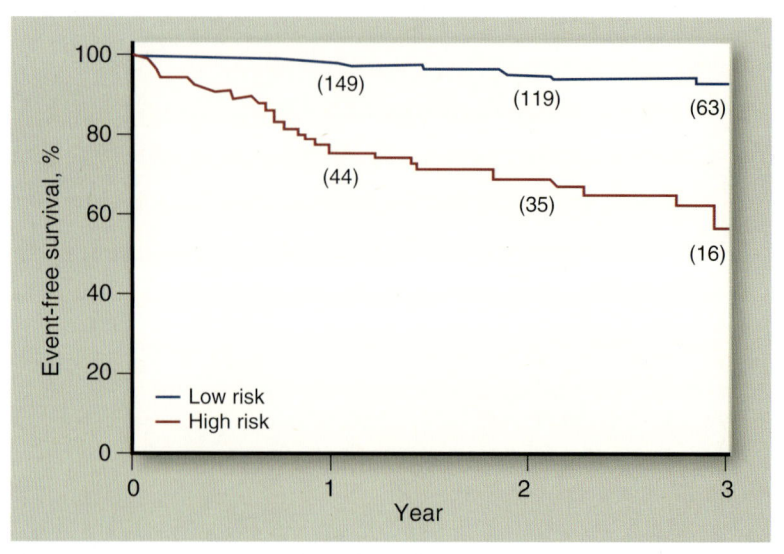

Figure 6-25. Prognostic value of vasodilator SPECT in left bundle branch block (LBBB). When patients with LBBB are considered for testing, vasodilator SPECT is the preferred form of stress in order to avoid the frequent stress-induced septal perfusion defect associated with high heart rates during exercise. This figure illustrates the effectiveness of vasodilator myocardial perfusion SPECT for risk stratification of patients with LBBB. In a relatively large group of patients with LBBB undergoing vasodilator ^{201}Tl SPECT, survival free of cardiac death or myocardial infarction or of needing cardiac transplantation in patients with low-risk myocardial perfusion scans is much higher compared with those with high-risk myocardial perfusion scans. (*Adapted from* Wagdy *et al.* [40].)

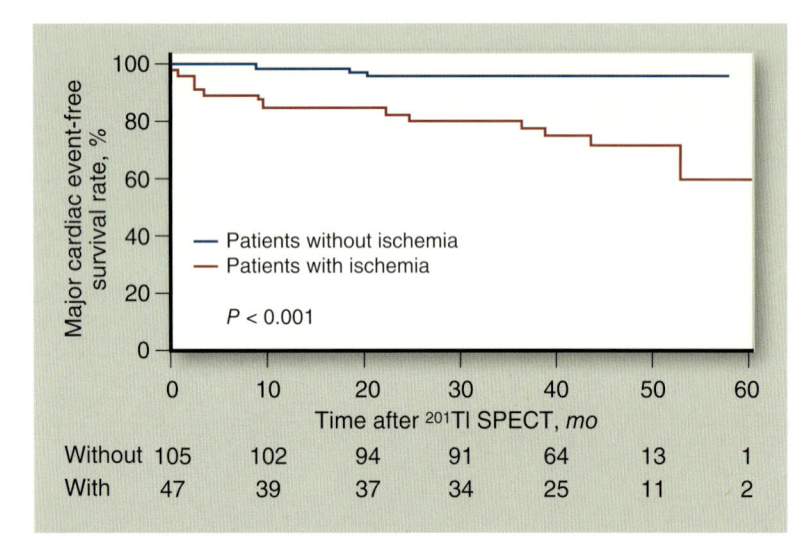

Figure 6-26. Long-term prognostic value of ^{201}Tl myocardial perfusion SPECT (MPS) after coronary stenting. MPS has been demonstrated to be useful in risk stratification following percutaneous coronary intervention. In patients without ischemia on MPS, the likelihood of a major cardiac event is very low, and clearly distinct from the event-free survival rate of patients demonstrating ischemia following stenting. (*Adapted from* Cottin *et al.* [41].)

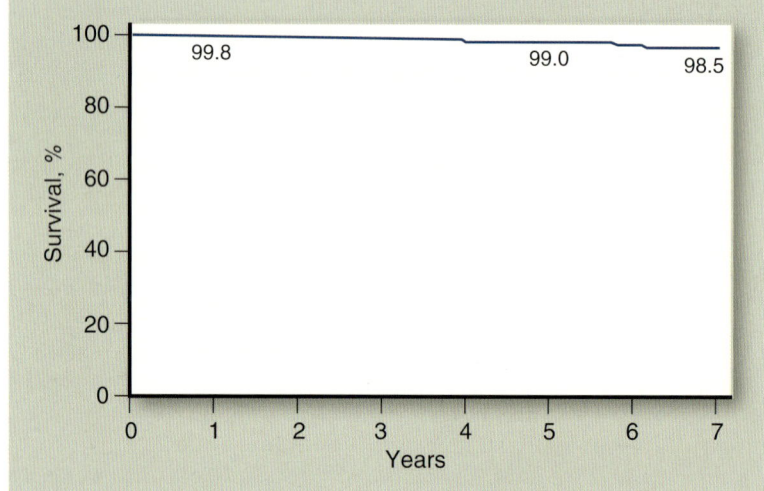

Figure 6-27. Long-term outcome of 4649 patients (pooled from four institutions) with an intermediate-risk exercise electrocardiogram based on the Duke treadmill score and no or minimal stress myocardial perfusion defects. The mortality rate is extremely low for patients with no stress myocardial perfusion defect. (*Adapted from* Gibbons *et al.* [42].)

152 Atlas of Nuclear Cardiology

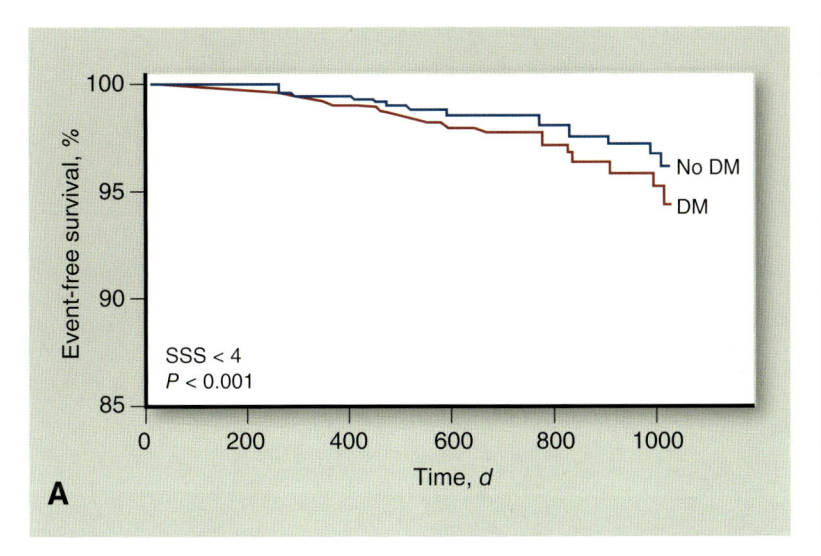

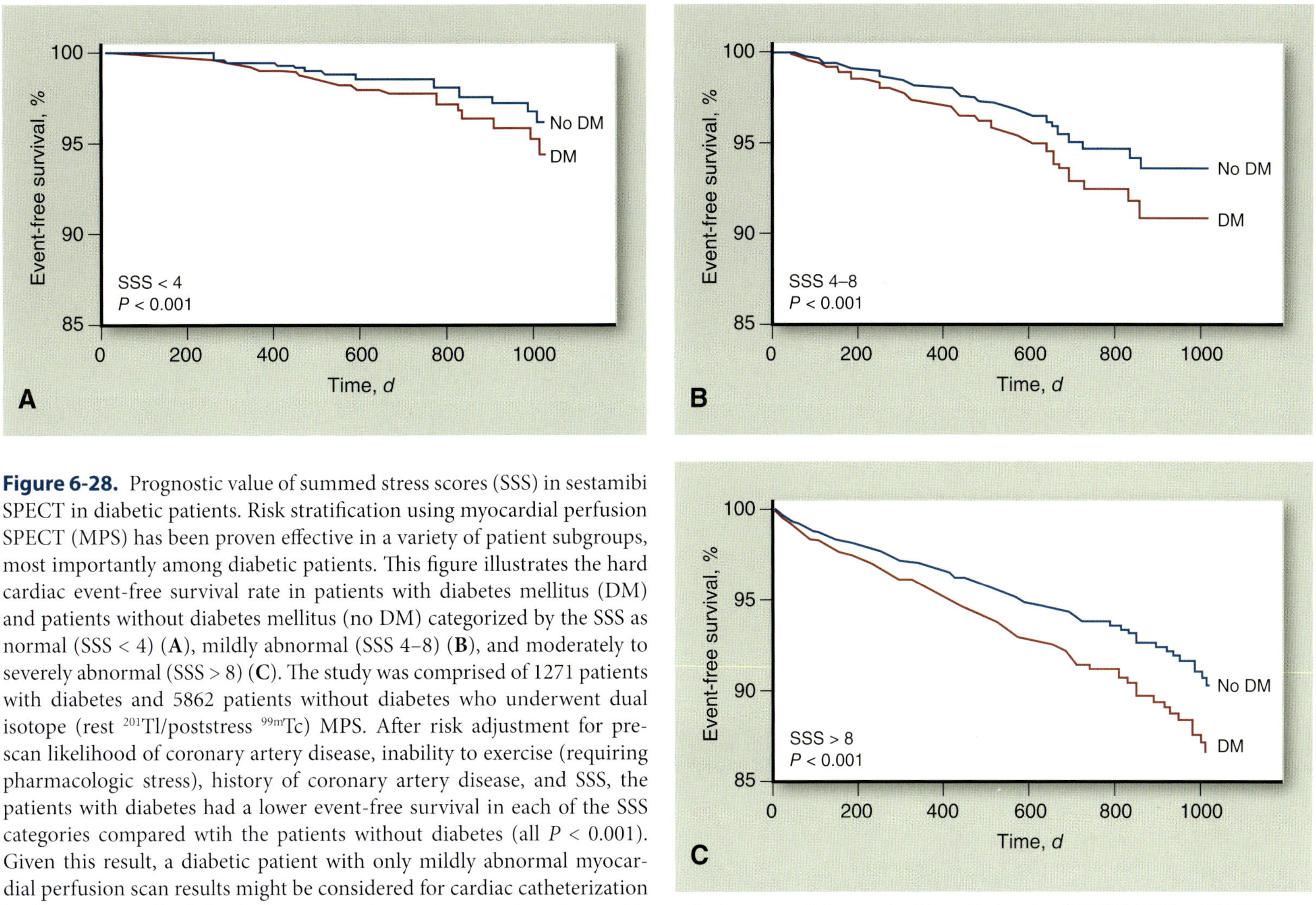

Figure 6-28. Prognostic value of summed stress scores (SSS) in sestamibi SPECT in diabetic patients. Risk stratification using myocardial perfusion SPECT (MPS) has been proven effective in a variety of patient subgroups, most importantly among diabetic patients. This figure illustrates the hard cardiac event-free survival rate in patients with diabetes mellitus (DM) and patients without diabetes mellitus (no DM) categorized by the SSS as normal (SSS < 4) (**A**), mildly abnormal (SSS 4–8) (**B**), and moderately to severely abnormal (SSS > 8) (**C**). The study was comprised of 1271 patients with diabetes and 5862 patients without diabetes who underwent dual isotope (rest ^{201}Tl/poststress ^{99m}Tc) MPS. After risk adjustment for pre-scan likelihood of coronary artery disease, inability to exercise (requiring pharmacologic stress), history of coronary artery disease, and SSS, the patients with diabetes had a lower event-free survival in each of the SSS categories compared wtih the patients without diabetes (all $P < 0.001$). Given this result, a diabetic patient with only mildly abnormal myocardial perfusion scan results might be considered for cardiac catheterization in the presence of minimal symptoms, whereas in general, patients with only mildly abnormal scans might be considered appropriate for aggressive medical management without catheterization [23,39]. Similar results were obtained in a smaller diabetic population from a multicenter registry [32]. More recent data from the Detection of Ischemia in Asymptomatic Diabetics (DIAD) study [35] and the Clinical Outcomes Utilizing Revascularization and Aggressive Drug Evaluation (COURAGE) trial [43], however, would suggest that such a referral might not be appropriate unless there is extensive and severe ischemia. Data from the BARI 2D Bypass Angioplasty Revascularization Investigation will provide important information regarding the use of MPS in risk stratification in diabetic patients. (*Adapted from* Kang *et al.* [31].)

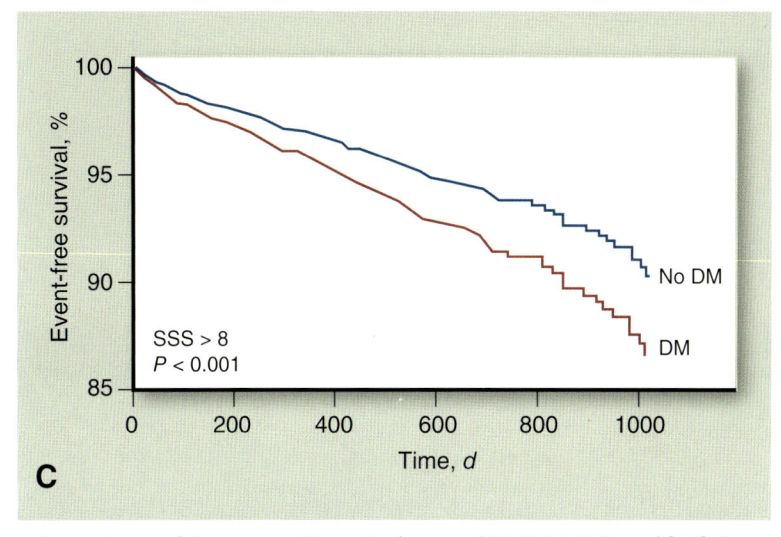

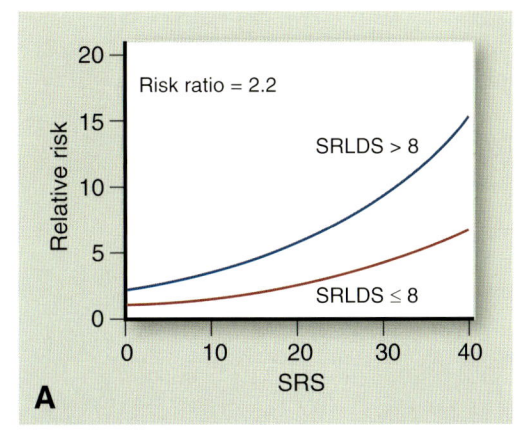

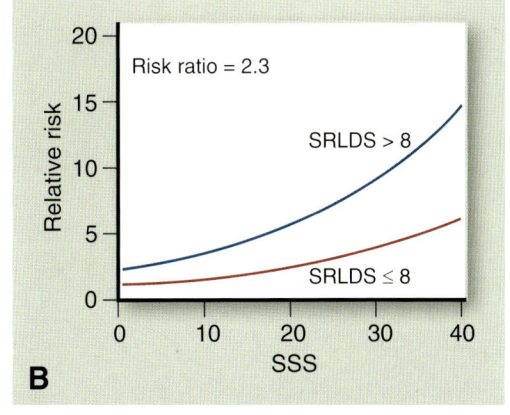

Figure 6-29. **A** and **B**, Resting ^{201}Tl reversibility added value over summed stress score (SSS) and summed rest score (SRS). In patients with chronic coronary artery disease, the added prognostic value of resting ^{201}Tl reversibility in dual isotope myocardial perfusion SPECT is shown. The two curves represent differing amounts of resting reversibility as measured by the summed rest late difference score (SRLDS). When this score is greater than 8 (extensive resting ischemia), the relative risk with respect to subsequent cardiac events is clearly higher than when less resting reversibility is present. The incremental prognostic value of resting reversibility persists when either the SRS or the SSS is considered. These data suggest that a combination of assessing both stress-induced ischemia and resting ischemia (presumably hibernating myocardium) might be more effective than stress-induced ischemia alone in evaluating risk of patients with chronic coronary artery disease. (*Adapted from* Sharir *et al.* [36].)

Risk Stratification and Patient Management

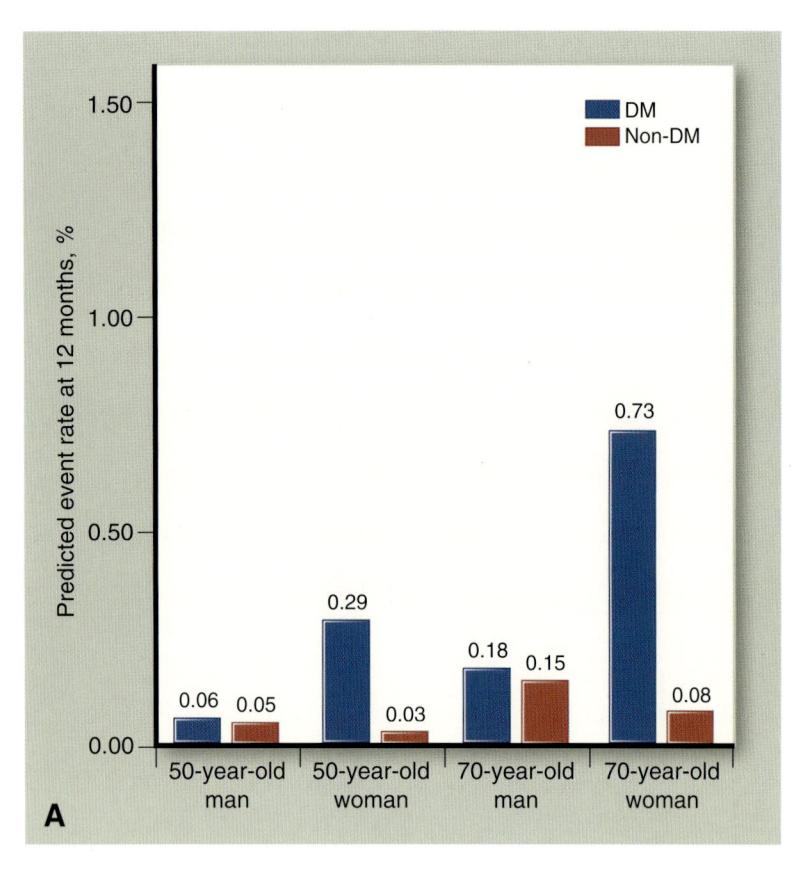

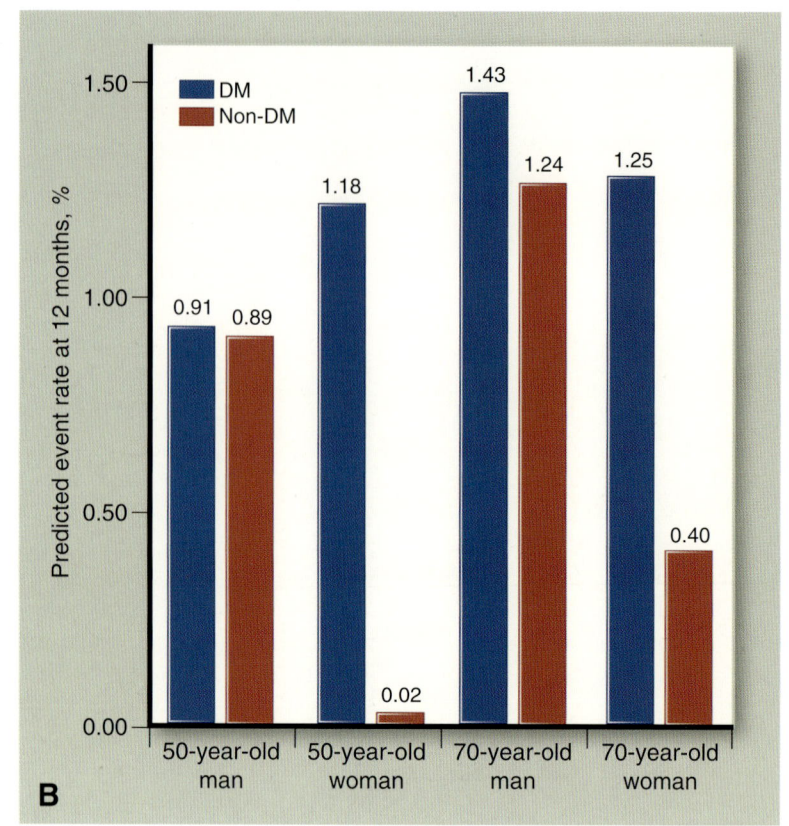

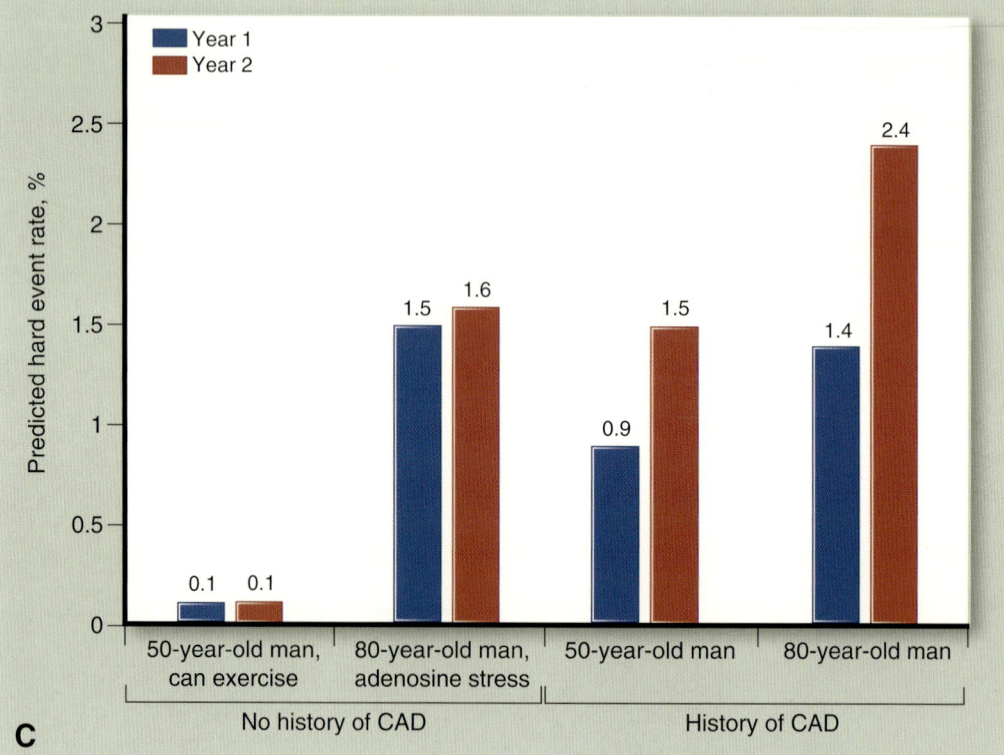

Figure 6-30. Risk of adverse events after a normal myocardial perfusion SPECT (MPS) study: variation with underlying patient characteristics. More recently, published prognostic studies performed in patients undergoing pharmacologic stress, a population with more comorbidities and at higher risk than patients undergoing exercise stress, have reported hard event rates of 1.3% to 2.7% per year with a normal MPS, suggesting that underlying clinical risk and prior coronary artery disease (CAD) may influence event rates even when the perfusion scan is normal [30,31,38,43–45]. Key higher risk subsets have been defined such as those with known CAD or its risk equivalent, which include diabetic patients as well as those with a clustering of risk factors (*eg*, metabolic syndrome), noncardiac atherosclerotic disease (*eg*, peripheral arterial disease or cerebrovascular disease or high-risk subclinical disease), or those with extensive comorbidity and/or functional disability. Along these lines a recent study reported a series of 7376 patients with normal stress MPS, addressing the predictors and temporal characteristics of risk [46].

This study identified a number of variables—the need for pharmacologic stress, the presence of known CAD, diabetes mellitus (DM) (in particular, female diabetic patients), and advanced age as markers of increased risk and shortened time to risk (*eg*, risk in the first year of follow-up was less than in the second year). **A** and **B** illustrate the increased event rate in diabetic patients and the elderly, particularly in the diabetic women. While confirming that as a whole, patients with normal MPS are at very low risk, several additional insights were revealed by this study. First, baseline patient risk after a normal MPS varied widely as a function of the patient's clinical characteristics, as described above. In certain patients, for example elderly patients who were unable to exercise with known CAD or DM, risk of cardiac death or myocardial infarction exceeded 1% even in the first year of follow-up. This study also showed that in patients with known CAD who had normal MPS, the temporal component of risk increased rapidly, as shown in **C**. Hence, even patients who had low risk in the first year after normal MPS may no longer be at low risk in the second year. Little is known regarding this concept of accelerated risk over time, and further studies are needed to delineate this "warranty period" after a normal MPS in various patient subsets. Thus, to date there is little information currently available to guide the need for and timing of retesting after a normal scan. (*Adapted from* Hachamovitch *et al.* [46].)

154 Atlas of Nuclear Cardiology

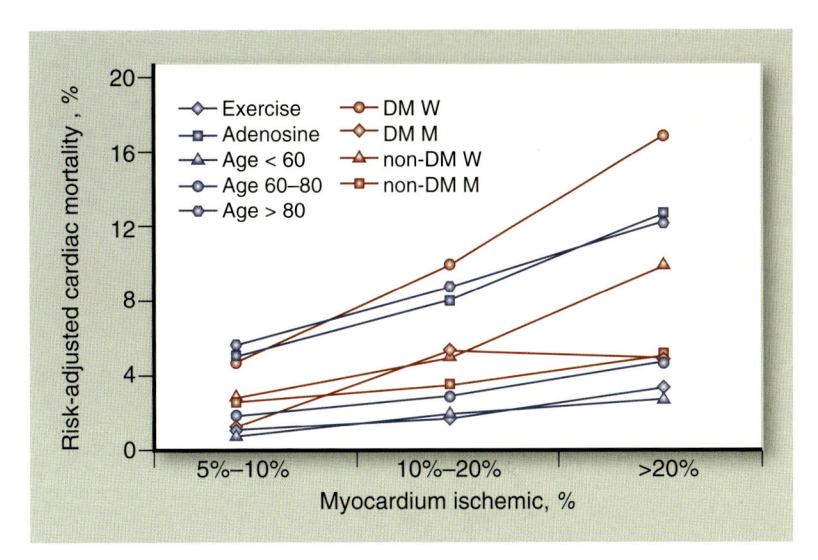

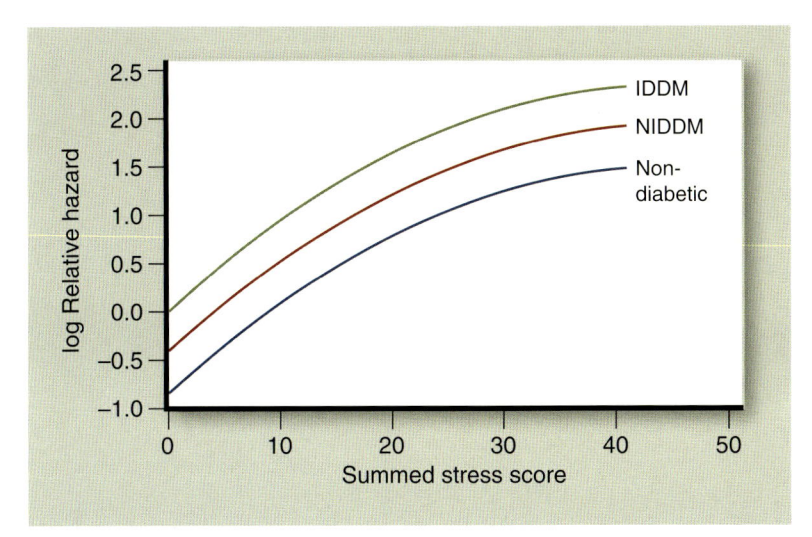

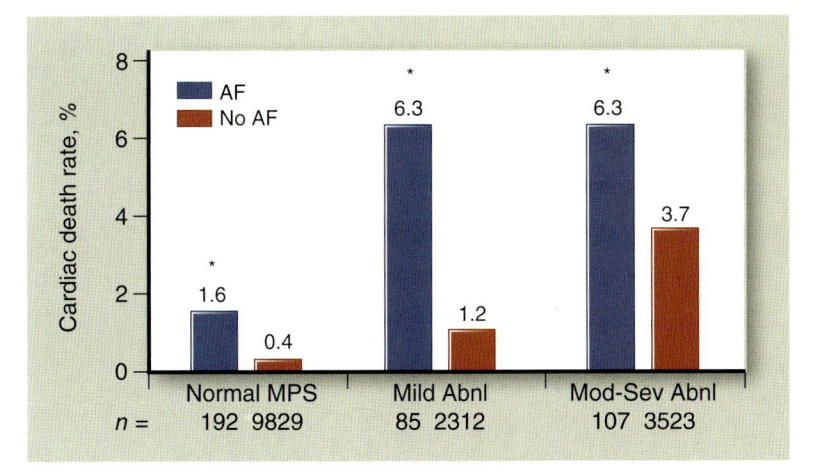

Figure 6-31. Variability in risk-adjusted cardiac mortality as a function of myocardial perfusion SPECT (MPS)-detected ischemia in medically treated patients. The dependence of post-normal MPS risk on the patients' underlying clinical, demographic, and historical characteristics also extends to patients with abnormal MPS results. In a large study of 10,627 patients with follow-up, while there is an increase in risk-adjusted cardiac mortality rates with increasing ischemia in the subset of medically treated patients, the precise level of risk associated with mild (5%–10% myocardium ischemic), moderate (10%–20% myocardium ischemic), or large (> 20% myocardium ischemic) amounts of ischemia varies widely. For example, in moderately ischemic patients, the cardiac death risk may be as low as 2% or as high as 10% depending on the patient subgroup. Hence, patients who cannot exercise, who are older, or who are diabetic will have far greater risk than those patients who are younger, able to exercise, or are not diabetic, despite similar extent and severity of ischemia on their stress MPS study. DM—diabetes mellitus; M—men; W—women. (*Data from* Hachamovitch et al. [47].)

Figure 6-32. Risk-adjusted analysis. Although the shape of the relationship between the degree of perfusion abnormality and risk appears to be the same across populations, the precise level of risk for any scan abnormality has been shown to vary with the underlying clinical characteristics of the patients examined. For example, in a recent large study, for any level of defect extent and severity, risk-adjusted analysis demonstrated that risk of cardiac death was greater in patients with insulin dependent diabetes mellitus (IDDM) than in those with non–insulin dependent diabetes mellitus (NIDDM), who in turn had greater risk than nondiabetics [48]. Along these lines, several studies have now shown that not only does scan data provide incremental prognostic information over prescan information, but prescan data also yields incremental prognostic information over myocardial perfusion SPECT results [9,27,47,49,50]. Further, the type of event likely to occur on follow-up varies as a function of the type of defect found, with myocardial infarction more likely in the setting of reversible defects and cardiac death more likely in the setting of fixed defects [51]. (*Adapted from* Berman et al. [48].)

Figure 6-33. Cardiac death rates in patients with and without atrial fibrillation (AF) as a function of myocardial perfusion SPECT (MPS) results: an example of how prescan information affects risk. In patients with mildly abnormal MPS, those with chronic AF have been shown to have a high risk of cardiac death, whereas those without AF do not. While patients with mildly abnormal MPS results are generally at low risk of cardiac death, this is not the case in patients with significant comorbidities (*eg*, advanced age, prior coronary artery disease, diabetes mellitus [31], AF [52], pharmacologic stress). In this light, the decision whether or not to catheterize a patient with a mildly abnormal perfusion scan becomes a function of the underlying patient condition. *$P = 0.001$; follow-up 2.2 ± 1.2 years. (*Adapted from* Abidov et al. [52].)

Risk Stratification and Patient Management

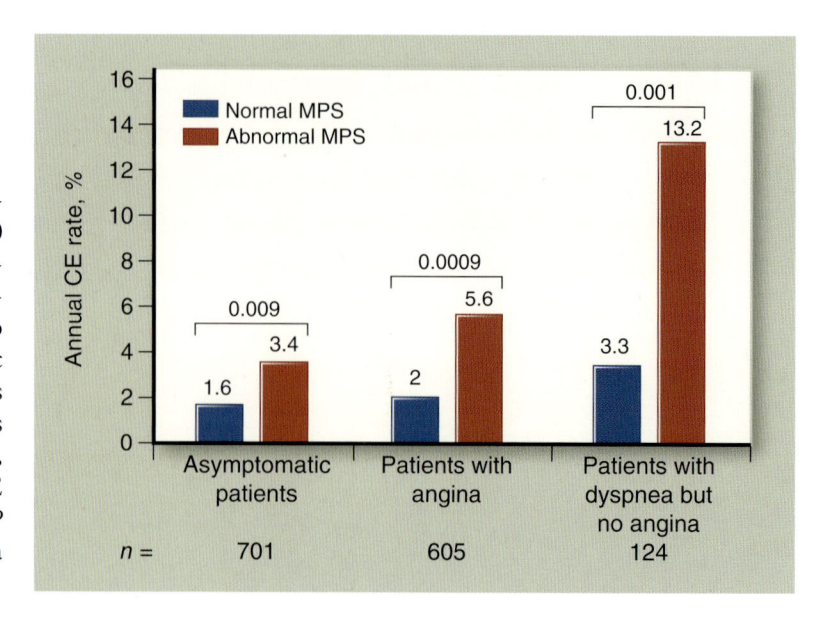

Figure 6-34. Relationship of ischemia and symptoms for predicting long-term outcomes in diabetics. Zellweger et al. [53] recently evaluated 1430 consecutive diabetic patients, all of whom received rest ^{201}Tl/stress ^{99m}Tc-sestamibi myocardial perfusion SPECT (MPS), in order to assess this relationship. During the follow-up period (median of 2 years) with respect to risk and presenting symptoms, annual cardiac event (CE) rates (cardiac death or myocardial infarction) among patients with normal MPS findings were similar for patients with angina, asymptomatic patients, and patients with shortness of breath. Among patients with abnormal MPS results, however, patients with shortness of breath had significantly higher CE rates than patients with angina ($P = 0.008$) and asymptomatic patients ($P < 0.001$); the outcomes for asymptomatic patients and patients with angina were similar. (Adapted from Zellweger et al. [53].)

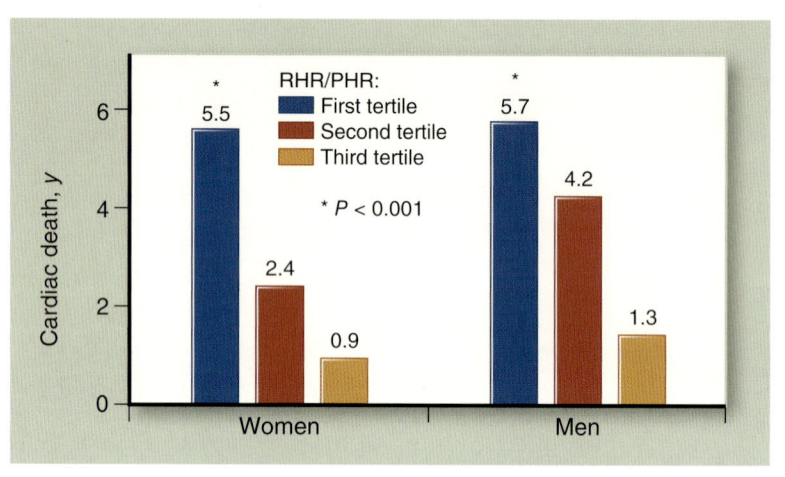

Figure 6-35. Prognostic impact of hemodynamic response to adenosine on patient survival. In many respects, the results of vasodilator stress myocardial perfusion SPECT (MPS) studies are more difficult to understand compared with those of exercise MPS in that there are a paucity of nonperfusion markers to consider. For example, although the positive predictive value of the electrocardiogram response is quite high, the negative value is not as good. Although symptoms often occur with vasodilator stress, their predictive value is very poor and is most often unrelated to coronary artery disease. Although "walking" vasodilator stress is performed, the exercise capacity is not maximal, hence not prognostically useful. Hence, it is potentially useful to identify additional putative markers of risk in patients undergoing vasodilator stress MPS.

To this end, Abidov et al. [54] recently identified both resting heart rate (RHR) and peak heart rate (PHR) as an important and powerful prognostic predictor of cardiac death in these patients. Both of these variables were both independent and incremental risk-adjusted predictors of cardiac death. Increasing values of PHR response to adenosine stress were strongly associated with improved survival, as were low RHRs. In both male and female patients, an increasing ratio of RHR to PHR was associated with increasing cardiac mortality rates. (Adapted from Abidov et al. [54].)

Prognostic Adenosine Score

Age (years)

+ % myocardium ischemic (%)

+ % myocardium fixed (%)

+ 10 (if dyspnea was presenting symptom)

− 20 (in patients undergoing walking adenosine)

+ 0.5 × (resting HR–peak HR)

+ 20 (if an abnormal rest ECG was present)

− % myocardium ischemic (if treated with early revascularization)

+ 10 (if treated with early revascularization)

A

Figure 6-36. Prognostic adenosine score. As discussed above, although the results of adenosine and exercise stress are equivalent in their clinical predictive value, the results of the former are often more challenging to apply to clinical management decisions in light of the relatively more limited data available from the test results (the absence of information on exercise tolerance and stress-induced symptoms, the altered accuracy of stress-induced electrocardiogram [ECG] changes). Prognostication is further obfuscated by the greater baseline risk of patients unable to undergo exercise stress, as pharmacologic stress patients are at greater baseline clinical risk, have more severe and frequent comorbidities, are more frequently older, diabetic, female, and with prior coronary artery disease. Also mentioned earlier, these higher risk factors associated with pharmacologic stress are also associated with increasing risk for any level of myocardioal perfusion SPECT (MPS) abnormality, further complicating the application of MPS results.

Optimizing the amount of prognostic information extracted from testing mandates incorporation of multiple, complementary data elements, and elimination of redundant data elements. This challenge is best addressed by a composite, validated clinical score, as exemplified by the Duke treadmill score. With this in mind, the Cedars-Sinai group has derived and validated a prognostic adenosine score in 5873 adenosine stress patients followed-up for 2.2 ± 1.1 years (94% complete follow-up, 387 cardiac deaths [6.6%]) [55]. Three distinct scores were published in this report: a simplified score (**A**), a more complex score including an ECG subscore (for a more robust risk estimate), and an additional score that includes a modifying factor for patients referred to "walking" adenosine studies. The relationship between the complex prognostic adenosine score and 2-year Kaplan-Meier survival free of cardiac death (CD) reveals that over the range of lower risk scores

Continued on the next page

Estimates of Patient Risk of Cardiac Death with Medical Therapy and Revascularization

Example: 80-year-old man with atypical angina

Normal rest ECG

Nonwalking adenosine

Resting HR 70, peak HR 80

SDS 24—% myocardium ischemic = 30%

SRS 0—% myocardium fixed = 0%

If treated with revascularization early after SPECT:

- 30 (% myocardium ischemic)

+ 10 (early revascularization)

Prognostic score: medical therapy: 105; early revascularization: 85

Estimated 2-year risk of CD:

No early revascularization: adenosine score = 105, CD = 9%

With early revascularization: adenosine score = 85, CD = 3%

C

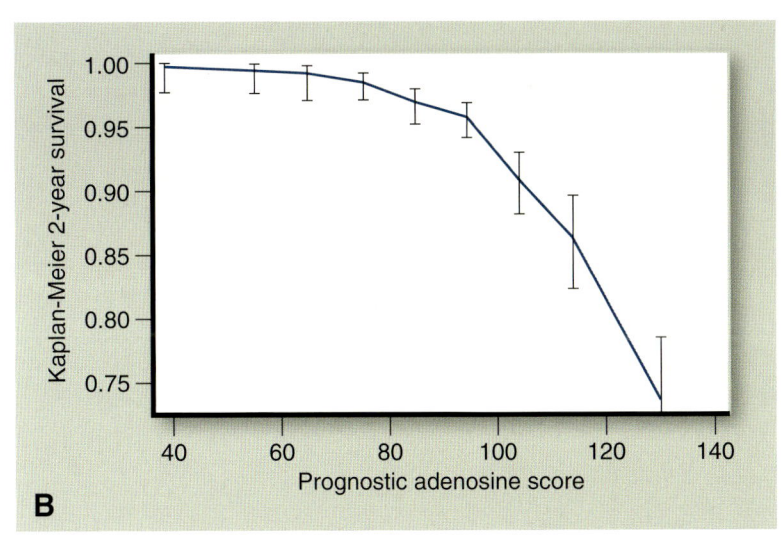

Figure 6-36. *(Continued)* (approximate score < 100) the confidence intervals are relatively narrow, permitting relatively more precise estimates of risk in lower risk patients (**B**). For values of the prognostic adenosine score greater than 100, the associated risk is sufficiently large that although the confidence intervals are wider, it is not as important. By calculating an individual patient's prognostic adenosine score (based on **A**), and determining the risk associated with the calculated score by use of **B**, estimates of patient risk of CD with medical therapy and revascularization can be determined (**C**). It is important to note that **C** also represents a new paradigm for noninvasive testing. Although the focus for many years has been on the estimation of patient risk, the determination of risk with two distinct therapeutic approaches also yields an estimate of patient benefit. Thus, rather than focus on the risk of adverse events, the focus can be shifted to the identification of the optimal management for a patient and the impact of therapeutic choices for different patients with different characteristics. This approach also teaches us the impact of different MPS data elements. While for many years the prognostic focus has been on summed stress scores, it is apparent that two patients with identical summed scores will have very different therapeutic recommendations if one patient has only reversible defects while the other has only fixed defects. HR—heart rate; SDS—summed difference score; SRS—summed rest score. (*Data from Hachamovitch et al.* [55].)

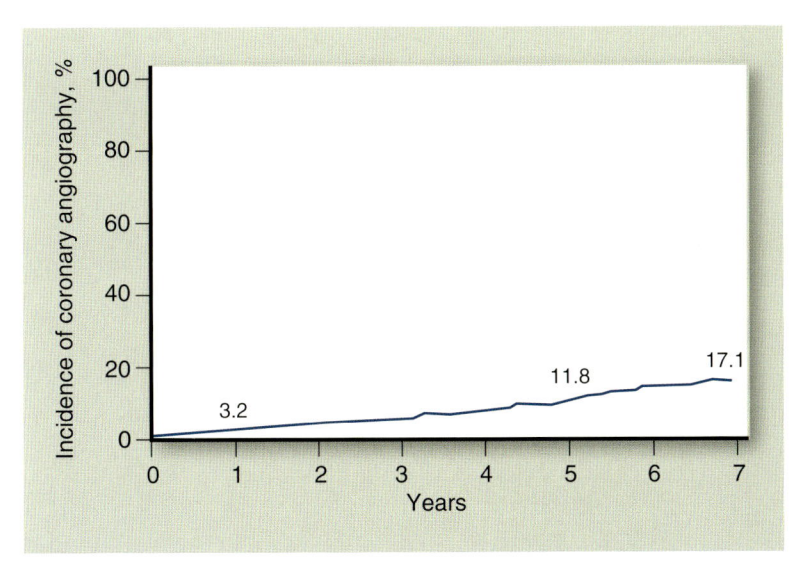

Figure 6-37. The cumulative incidence of coronary angiography in 4649 patients with an intermediate-risk Duke treadmill score and no stress myocardial perfusion defect. Note that the clinicians involved in the decision-making process seldom chose to perform cardiac catheterization in these patients. The findings of this study add strength to the concept that stress myocardial perfusion SPECT is highly effective in clinical decision making applied to the management of patients with intermediate-risk Duke treadmill scores. (*Adapted from Gibbons et al.* [42].)

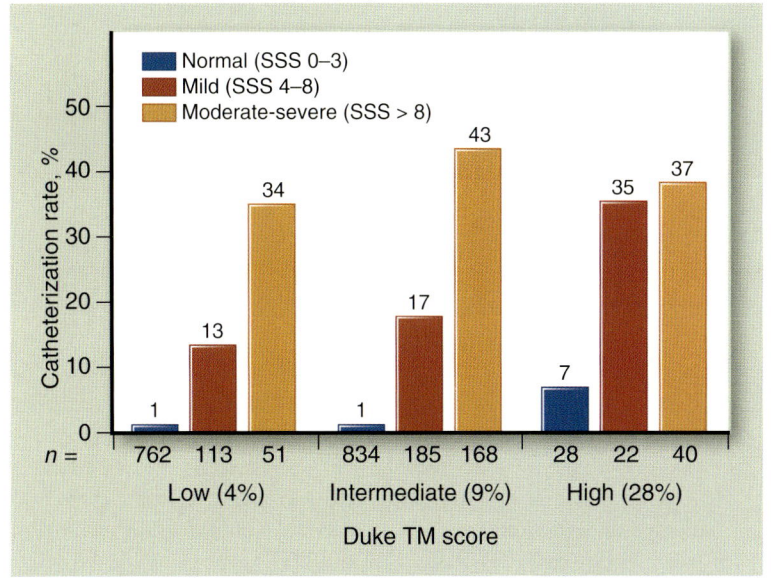

Figure 6-38. Catheterization rate as a function of summed stress score (SSS) and the Duke treadmill (TM) score. The catheterization rates are seen to follow the event rates in Figure 6-23. Note that in the patients in the intermediate Duke TM score group, only 1% who were found to have a normal myocardial perfusion SPECT study underwent subsequent early catheterization. Similarly, in patients in the high Duke TM score group, only 7% who were found to have a normal myocardial perfusion SPECT study underwent subsequent early catheterization. (*Adapted from Hachamovitch et al.* [22].)

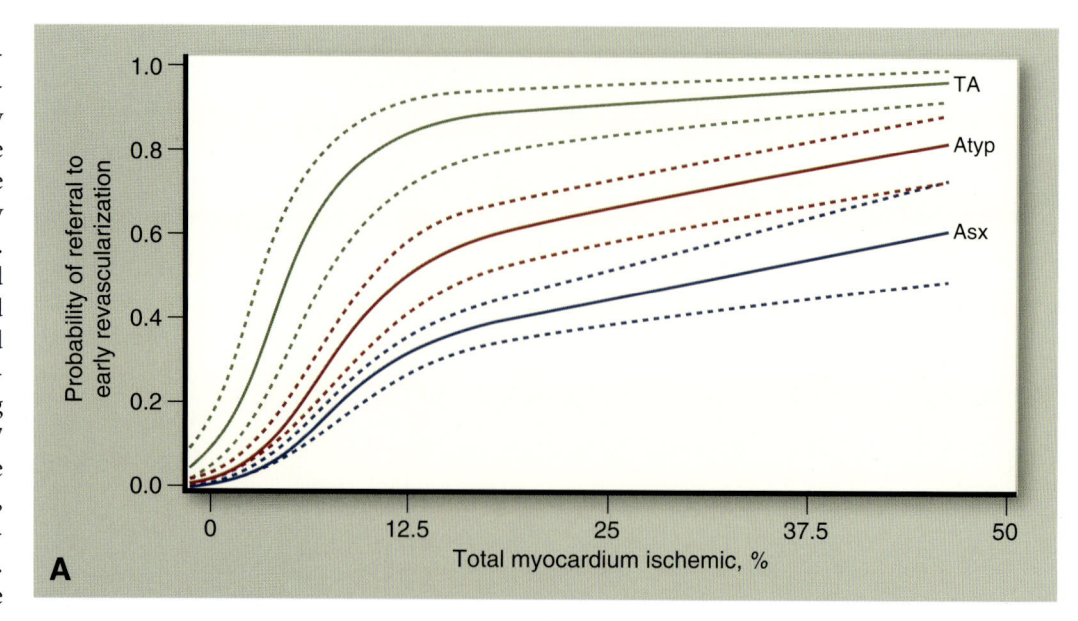

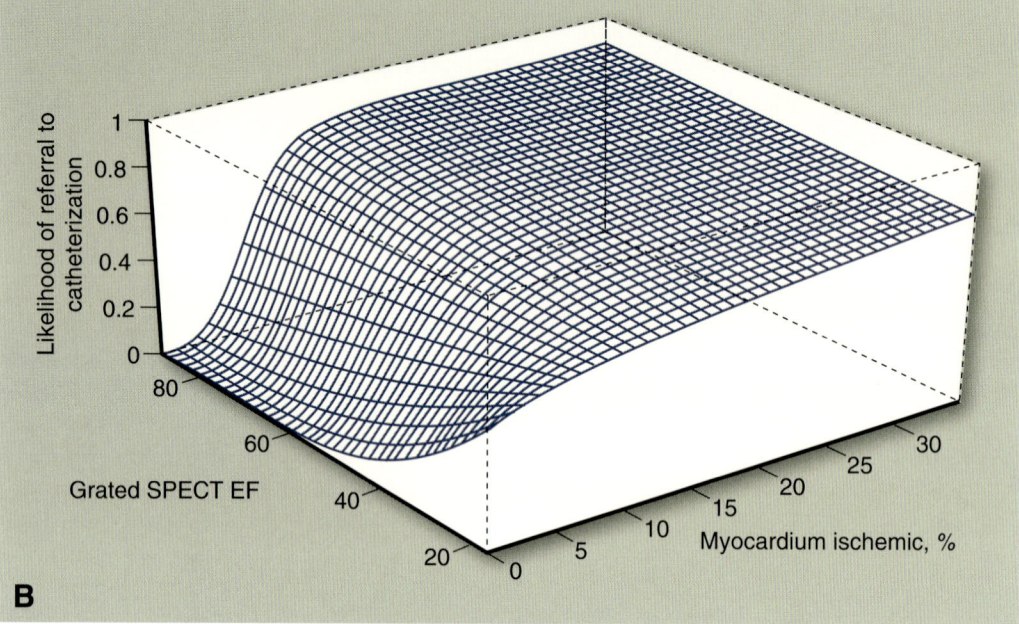

Figure 6-39. Drivers of referral to catheterization and revascularization after myocardial perfusion SPECT (MPS). It is currently assumed by many that physicians appropriately weigh the various patient characteristics available to the referring physician after the stress MPS study in formulating the final management decision. In 2003, Hachamovitch *et al.* [56] demonstrated that the amount of ischemia was strongly related to survival benefit with revascularization and at the same time contributed 83% of the information in a multivariable model predicting revascularization [51] based on data in 10,627 patients without prior coronary artery disease (CAD) referred to stress MPS (**A**). Importantly, the shape of this relationship also yields considerable insight into how doctors use MPS results. First, with increasing amounts of ischemia, there are increasing referral rates to revascularization. The ischemia-revascularization relationship, however, is highly nonlinear. With increasing ischemia in the range of no or mild ischemia (< 12.5% myocardium ischemic) there is a steep slope between ischemia and revascularization referral such that a small change in ischemia is associated with a large change in the likelihood of revascularization. At approximately 10% to 15% of the myocardium ischemic, this relationship plateaus, such that increasing amounts of ischemia are associated with relatively little increase in the rate of revascularization. Further, referring physicians did not act on the ischemia information alone, but other factors also influenced this referral decision. For example, for any level of ischemia, worsening presenting symptoms (asymptomatic [Asx], atypical symptoms [Atyp], or typical angina [TAP]) resulted in greater rates of referral.

Regarding ejection fraction (EF) (**B**), although revascularization yields the greatest survival benefit in patients with low EF and extensive CAD, whether post-MPS referral to catheterization and revascularization are proportional to patient risk as a function of EF and ischemia was examined only recently [56]. In a cohort of 3369 patients without prior myocardial infarction or revascularization who underwent exercise or adenosine stress MPS and were followed up for occurrence of early (< 60 days) post-SPECT revascularization, 445 patients were referred to catheterization (13.2%) and 254 to revascularization (7.5%) early after MPS. Logistic regression analysis was used to determine the association of clinical, historical stress, and MPS factors with referral to catheterization and revascularization in separate models. The likelihood of referral to catheterization increased with both increasing ischemia and decreasing EF. Referral rates to catheterization (**B**) increased with decreasing values of EF in the setting of no (< 5% myocardium ischemic) or mild to moderate amounts of ischemia (5%–15% myocardium ischemic), but this pattern was reversed in patients with severe ischemia (> 15% myocardium ischemic) wherein predicted referral rates to catheterization decreased with decreasing EF. Referral rates to revascularization increased markedly with increasing amounts of ischemia, plateauing beyond 15% myocardium ischemic, and demonstrated a mild decrease in referral rates with decreasing EF that was quantitatively not as significant as that found in the referral to catheterization model. Although referral to revascularization seemed to be in proportion to the anticipated risk in these patients, catheterization was the rate-limiting step in the evaluation of these patients and was significantly influenced by an EF-related referral bias in which clinicians may have been hesitant to consider revascularization in patients with low EF at the time of this study. This referral bias helps explain the findings from the Mayo Clinic that found that in a cohort of 77 patients with congestive heart failure, left ventricular EF less than 45%, and large reversible perfusion defects by SPECT, the 5-year revascularization rate was only 13% despite a 57.6% mortality rate over this same period of time. (*Adapted from* Hachamovitch *et al.* [56].)

Figure 6-40. Myocardial perfusion SPECT (MPS) results, post-MPS referral patterns to revascularization, and the subsequent post-test referral bias' obfuscation of post-MPS event rates. It has long been appreciated that the use of MPS data to dictate post-MPS management, as supported by the above, results in a high rate of catheterization in patients with abnormal MPS and a low rate of catheterization in patients with normal MPS, creating a partial verification bias associated with lowered specificity and increased sensitivity in studies assessing MPS test diagnostic accuracy. What is not generally appreciated, however, is that this same referral pattern to catheterization and revascularization that creates a diagnostic bias, also results in a prognostic bias (more specifically, a differential treatment selection bias) [57]. Since imaging results affect patient management, especially referral to revascularization, and revascularization affects risk, the association between test results and revascularization referral results in a lowering of observed patients' risk in proportion to their imaging results. Hence, as seen in Figures 6-15 and 6-30, risk is underestimated in patients with more abnormal MPS results, resulting in a flattening of the MPS result-risk relationship in proportion to intervention rates. A recent study examined the impact of revascularization on observed hard event (HE) rates in a cohort of patients with high pre-MPS likelihood of coronary artery disease [37]. Examining 240 patients treated medically and 204 patients treated with revascularization, this study found that the HE rate in patients referred to revascularization would have been nearly three times higher (11% vs 4.4%) if these patients would have been treated with medical therapy as opposed to revascularization. Thus, this study provides both evidence of this prognostic referral bias and a quantitative handle on its potential impact. (*Adapted from* Hachamovitch et al. [37].)

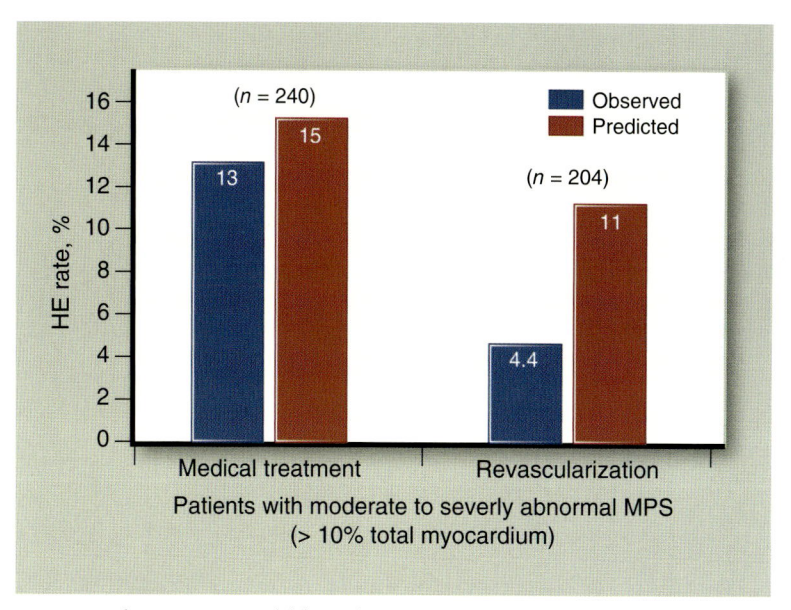

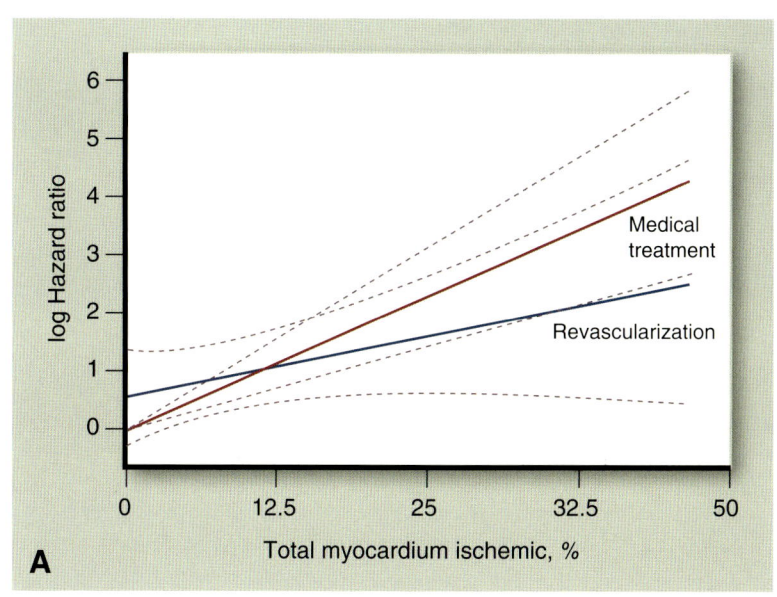

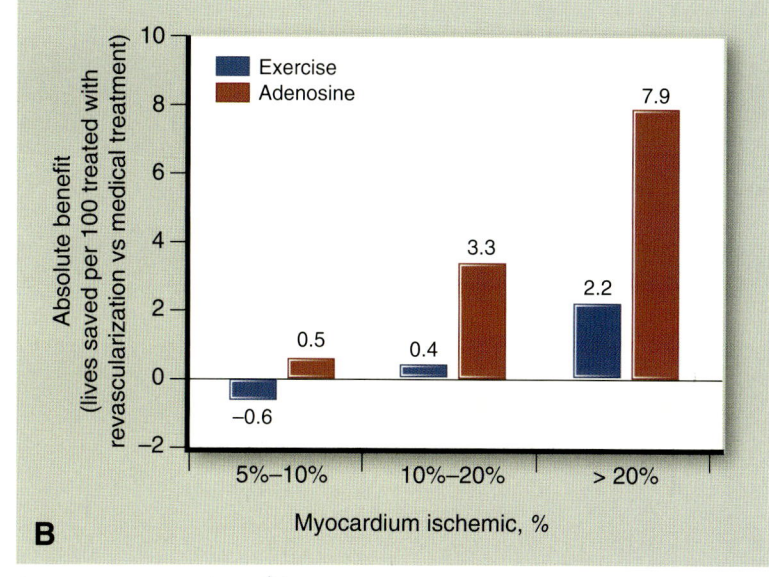

Figure 6-41. Using myocardial perfusion SPECT (MPS) for medical decision making: identification of optimal patient management. To date, almost all studies investigating the relationship of MPS results and patient risk have included only those patients who are treated medically (as patients treated with early revascularization are excluded or censored from these analyses since the decision to refer to early revascularization is usually based on the results of the MPS study), thus no prognostication can be extrapolated to patients treated with revascularization. In this context, an important study published in 2003 examined the relationship between the extent and severity of ischemia and the survival benefit associated with subsequent revascularization [47]. In this study, 10,627 patients without prior myocardial infarction or revascularization who underwent stress MPS and were followed up for a mean of 1.9 years (3.98% lost to follow-up). Over this time period, cardiac death occurred in 146 patients (1.4% mortality). The authors defined patient treatment on the basis of that received within 60 days post-MPS (revascularization [671 patients, 2.8% mortality] vs medical therapy [9956 patients, 1.3% mortality; $P = 0.0004$]). The authors used a risk-adjusted approach that included a propensity score to adjust for nonrandomization of treatment assignment, which was developed using logistic regression. This propensity score was used to adjust survival analyses.

Based on the Cox proportional hazards model most predictive of cardiac death ($\chi^2 = 539$, $P < 0.0001$), patients undergoing medical therapy as their initial treatment had superior survival to those patients referred to revascularization in the setting of no or mild ischemia. On the other hand, patients undergoing revascularization had an increasing survival benefit over patients undergoing medical therapy when moderate to severe ischemia (> 10% of the total myocardium ischemic) was detected by MPS (**A**).

Continued on the next page

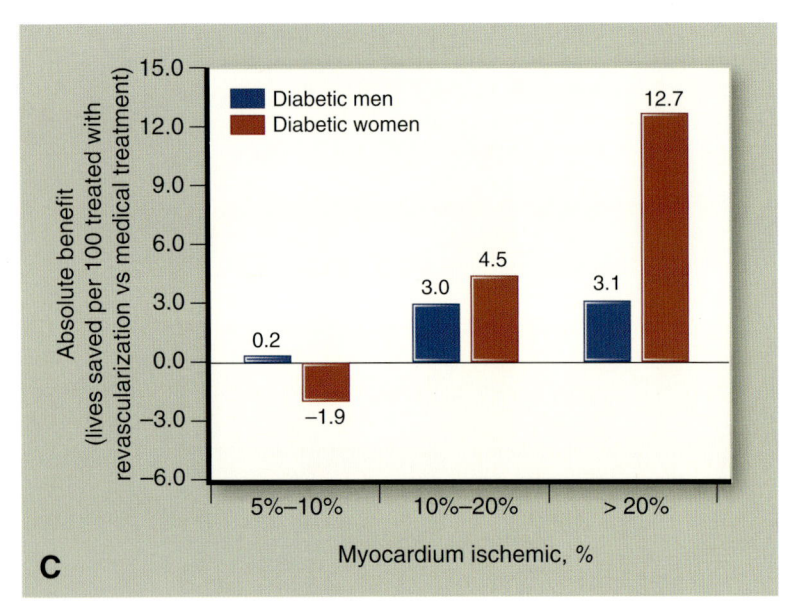

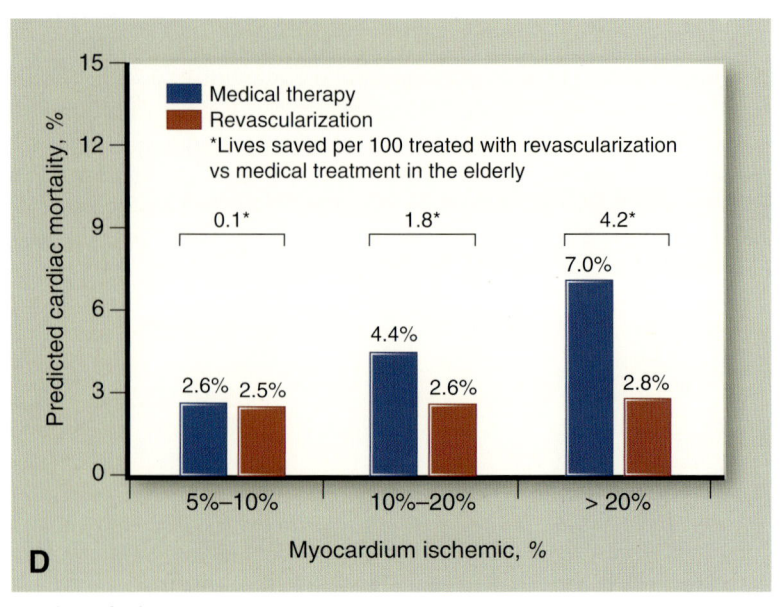

Figure 6-41. *(Continued)* While ischemia was the sole identifier of whether survival was enhanced with revascularization or medical therapy (relative benefit), the absolute benefit (*eg*, number of lives saved per 100 treated with different therapies) was impacted by baseline patient risk. Hence, the absolute benefit for revascularization over medical therapy was accentuated in the presence of greater clinical risk (patients undergoing pharmacologic stress, diabetic women, and elderly patients) (**B–D**) as well as in diabetics (not shown). (*Adapted from* Hachamovitch et al [47].)

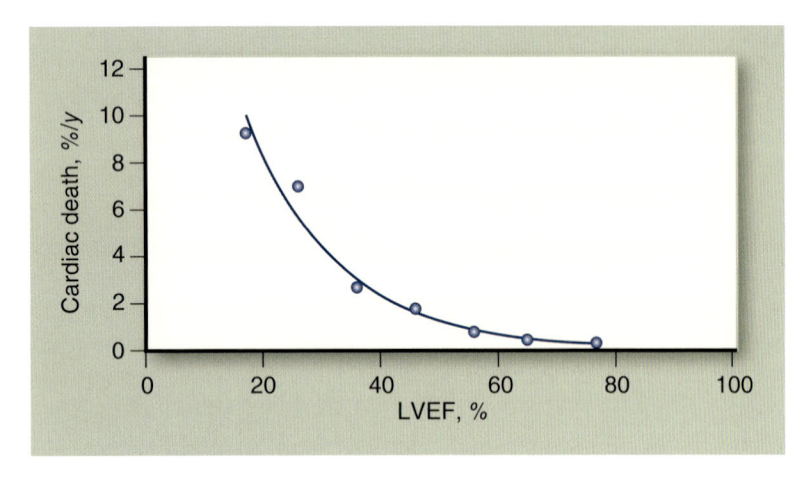

Figure 6-42. Relationship between left ventricular ejection fraction (LVEF) measured by gated SPECT and mortality rate and nonfatal myocardial infarction (MI). In 2686 consecutive patients undergoing stress ^{99m}Tc gated myocardial perfusion SPECT (MPS), there was a curvilinear inverse relationship between LVEF at rest by MPS, performed after stress, and cardiac death [27]. The LVEF was the strongest predictor of mortality in this group. The findings are similar to those reported for rest LVEF acquired with radionuclide angiography in patients after MI. (*Adapted from* Sharir et al. [27].)

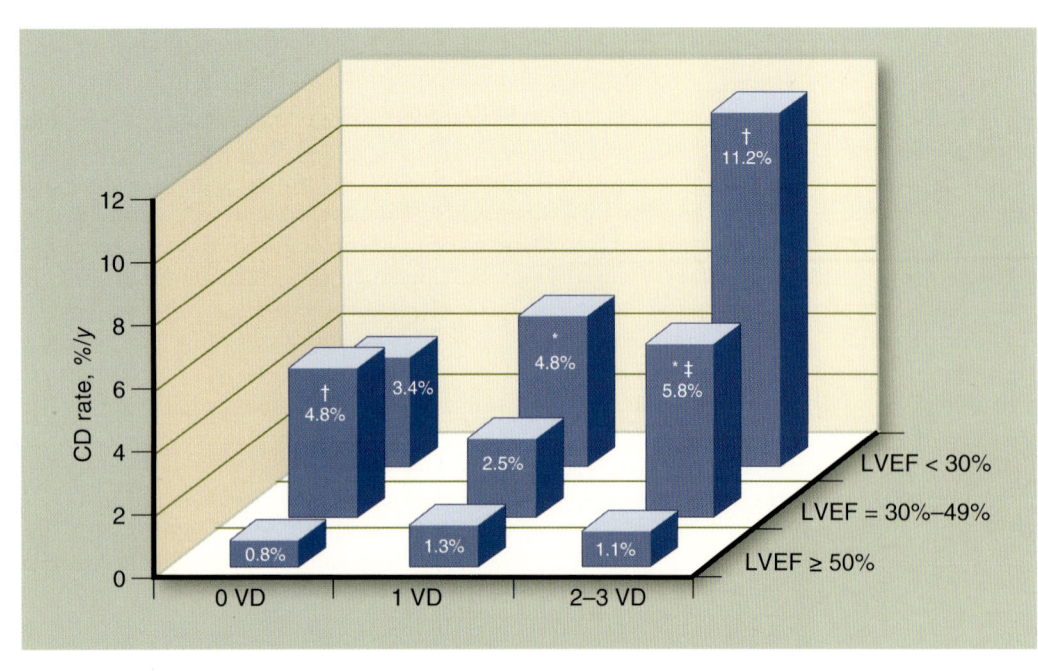

Figure 6-43. Added prognostic value of gated myocardial perfusion SPECT (MPS) left ventricular perfusion and function. An important early question that faced stress gated MPS was whether the data provided by the perfusion and function components of the test were additive or redundant. Travin *et al.* [28] reported on 3207 patients who underwent stress gated MPS and were followed up for hard events. Cox proportional hazards regression analysis revealed that the stress perfusion and gated ejection fraction components added incrementally to each other even after considering pre-MPS data. Annualized cardiac death (CD) rates were risk stratified by both perfusion and function data, with increasing risk as a function of both greater perfusion defects and decreasing ejection fraction. *$P < 0.05$ compared with EF $\geq$ 50%; †$P < 0.001$ compared with EF $\geq$ 50%; ‡$P < 0.05$ compared with 1 vessel disease (VD). LVEF—left ventricular ejection fraction. (*Adapted from* Travin et al. [28].)

160 Atlas of Nuclear Cardiology

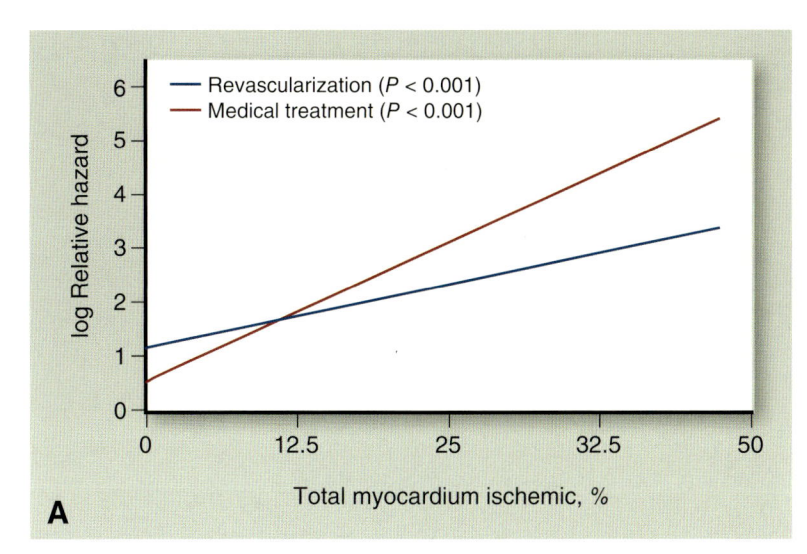

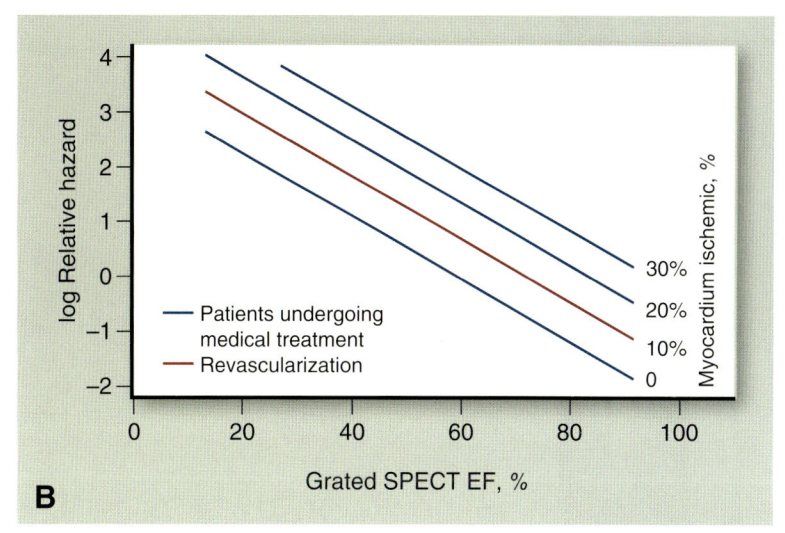

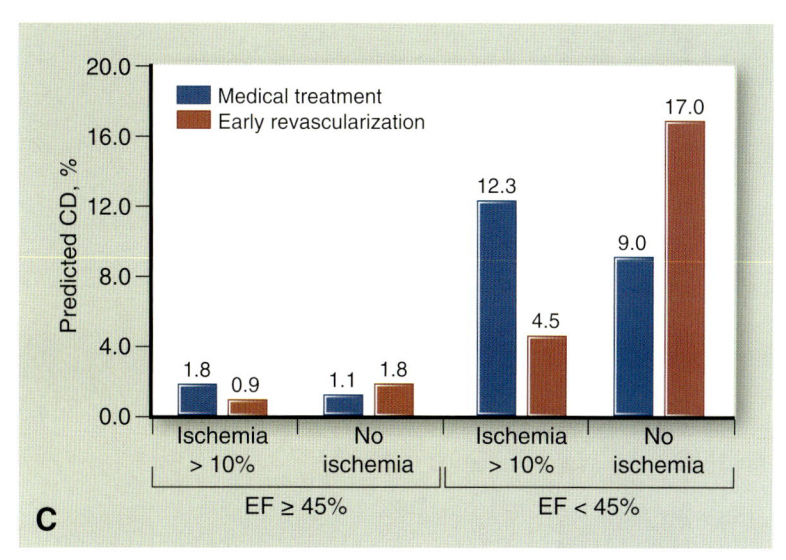

Figure 6-44. In the context of the results presented in Figure 6-40, specifically, the ability of myocardial perfusion SPECT (MPS)-determined ischemia to identify which patients may benefit from revascularization versus medical therapy, the role of gated ejection fraction (EF) in identifying patient benefit must also be assessed. In a study of 5366 consecutive patients without a history of prior revascularization followed up for 2.8 ± 1.2 years (during which 146 cardiac deaths occurred [2.7%, 1.0%/y]), the relative roles of ischemia and EF for the assessment of cardiac death (CD) risk and potential benefit with revascularization was examined [49]. A Cox proportional hazards survival model was used to adjust for differences in patients' baseline characteristics, and a propensity score to correct for nonrandomized patient referral to revascularization versus medical therapy. While this model identified EF to be by far the strongest predictor of CD, ischemia, but not EF, was found to have a significant interaction with therapy given. The latter indicates that the survival associated with any level of ischemia was dependent on the treatment given, and the survival associated with treatment dependent on the level of ischemia (*eg*, superior survival with medical therapy in the presence of little or no ischemia, enhanced survival with revascularization in the setting of increasing ischemia) (**A**).

Further, after adjusting for baseline differences, ischemia and EF added incrementally to each other with respect to the risk of CD, as the risk of CD increased with decreasing values of gated EF and the risk of CD at any level of EF increased with increasing amounts of ischemia (**B**). Interestingly, 10% myocardial ischemia appeared to identify patients who would have a survival benefit with revascularization across the spectrum of EF.

Thus, while simple measurement of EF alone defines patients at high risk, only ischemia appeared to identify a survival benefit with revascularization. These data illustrate the difference between risk assessment and prediction of benefit from revascularization. The added value of ischemia to EF was only present in medically treated patients, as the relationship between EF and ischemia in patients treated with revascularization is limited to a single line, as increasing levels of ischemia are not associated with increasing risk in the setting of revascularization. The relationship between ischemia and EF is further illustrated in **C**—absolute risk is greatest in the presence of lower EF (as evidenced by the higher CD rates on the *right* side of the figure). Irrespective of EF, in the absence of ischemia (no ischemia), the risk of CD is greater with early revascularization than medical therapy, while the converse is true in the presence of ischemia. Hence, although benefit is best predicted by ischemia, both risk and relative benefit is best predicted by the combination of EF and ischemia.

Risk Stratification and Patient Management 161

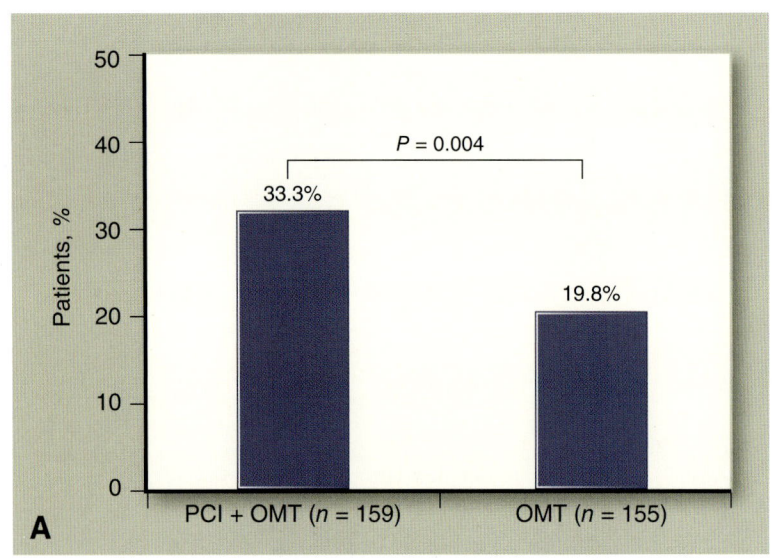

Figure 6-45. Clinical Outcomes Utilizing Revascularization and Aggressive Drug Evaluation (COURAGE) nuclear substudy. Shaw et al. [58] reported results of a substudy of the COURAGE trial. In this study of 314 patients in whom both pre- and 6- to 18-month postrandomization myocardial perfusion SPECT (MPS) was performed, patients assigned to percutaneous coronary intervention (PCI) and optimal medical therapy (OMT) demonstrated significantly greater ischemia reduction when compared with patients receiving OMT alone (PCI + OMT: 33% [n = 159]; OMT alone: 20% [n = 155]; P = 0.0004) (**A**). Importantly, the rate of subsequent cardiac events was strongly related to the amount of residual ischemia on MPS studies performed 6 to 18 months after randomization (**B**). MI—myocardial infarction. (*Adapted from* Shaw et al. [58].)

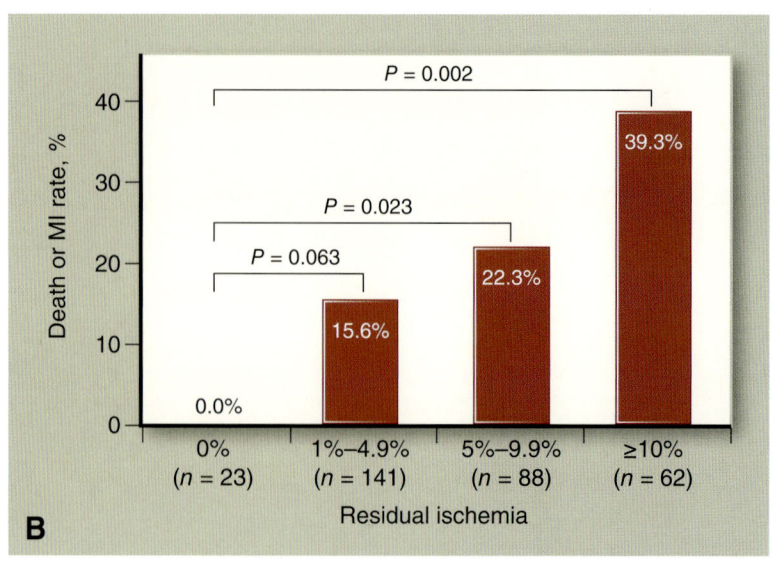

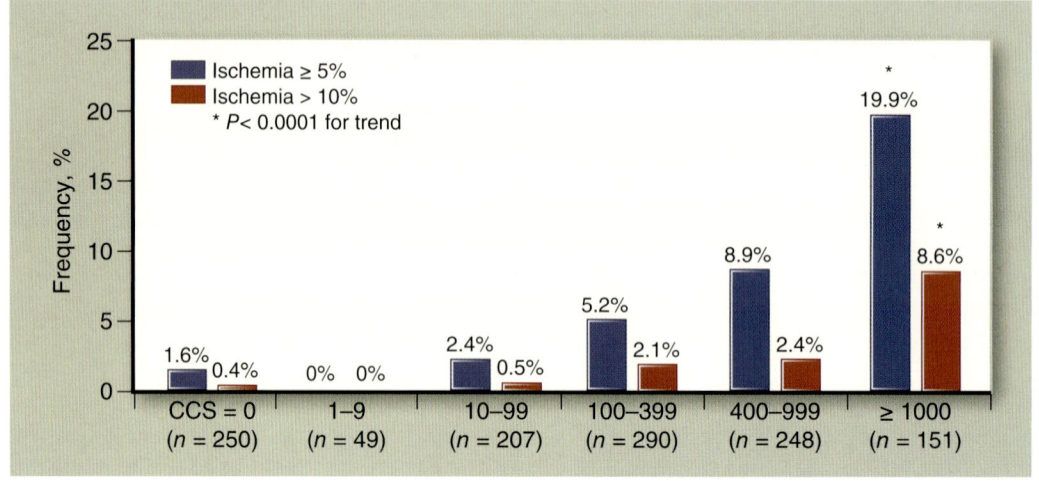

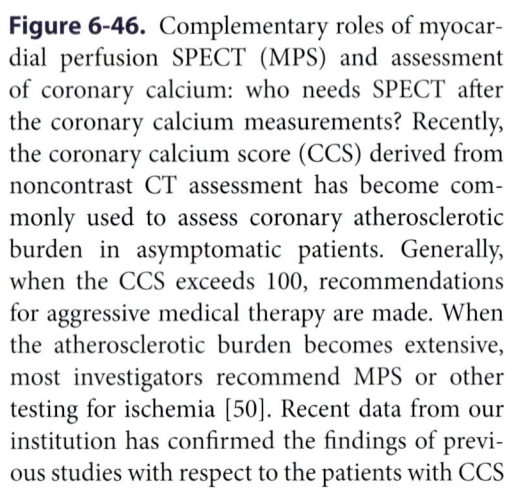

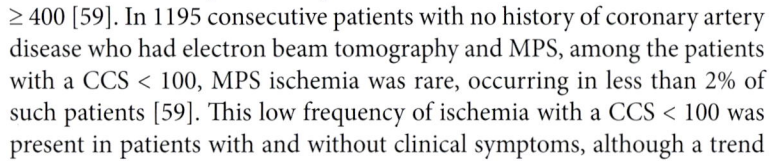

Figure 6-46. Complementary roles of myocardial perfusion SPECT (MPS) and assessment of coronary calcium: who needs SPECT after the coronary calcium measurements? Recently, the coronary calcium score (CCS) derived from noncontrast CT assessment has become commonly used to assess coronary atherosclerotic burden in asymptomatic patients. Generally, when the CCS exceeds 100, recommendations for aggressive medical therapy are made. When the atherosclerotic burden becomes extensive, most investigators recommend MPS or other testing for ischemia [50]. Recent data from our institution has confirmed the findings of previous studies with respect to the patients with CCS ≥ 400 [59]. In 1195 consecutive patients with no history of coronary artery disease who had electron beam tomography and MPS, among the patients with a CCS < 100, MPS ischemia was rare, occurring in less than 2% of such patients [59]. This low frequency of ischemia with a CCS < 100 was present in patients with and without clinical symptoms, although a trend toward more ischemia in symptomatic patients with scores 10 to 99 was observed. As the CCS increased in magnitude above 100, the frequency of myocardial ischemia on MPS increased progressively. Among patients with a CCS exceeding 1000, 20% manifested an ischemia by MPS. (*Adapted from* Berman et al. [59].)

162 Atlas of Nuclear Cardiology

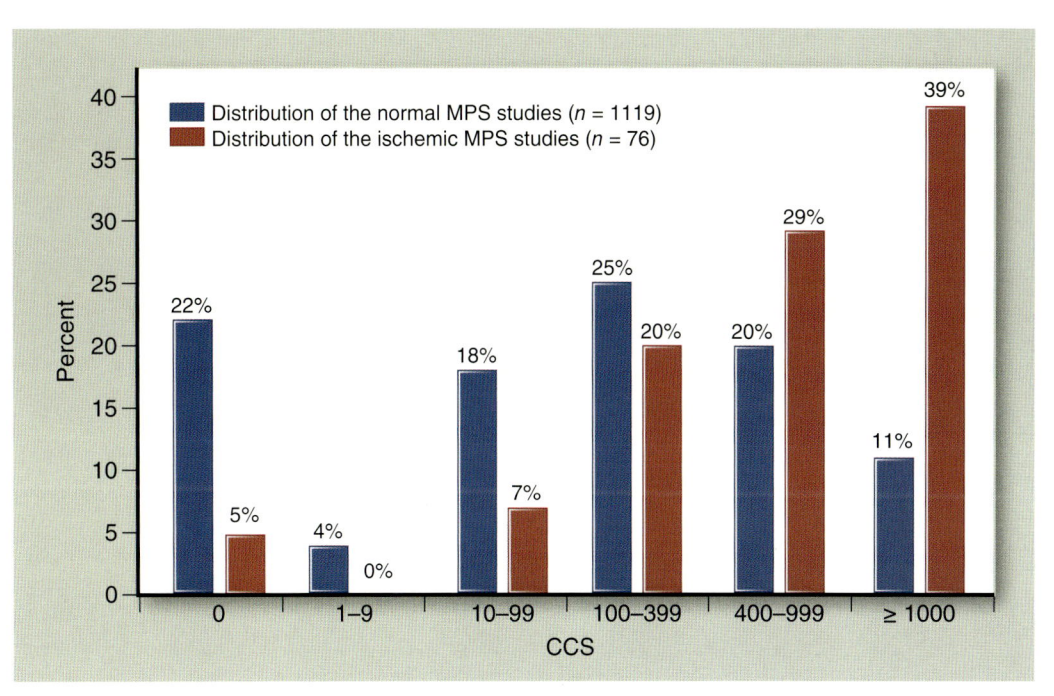

Figure 6-47. Complementary roles of myocardial perfusion SPECT (MPS) and assessment of coronary calcium: who needs coronary calcium measurement after SPECT? Of 1195 patients having both coronary calcium score (CCS) and SPECT studies in our institution, a large proportion had high enough CCS that there would be consensus that aggressive medical management is warranted: 56% had CCS > 100 and 31% had CCS > 400. While this frequency is inflated by a referral bias in which patients with high CCS were more likely to undergo MPS, these findings suggest that if testing begins with MPS in a given patient, further assessment of atherosclerotic burden by coronary calcium testing may be useful in assessment of the need for aggressive medical therapy and lifestyle recommendations in an attempt to prevent coronary events.

Clinical implications of Figures 6-45 through 6-47 can be summarized as follows: In asymptomatic patients, atherosclerosis imaging is more effective than imaging for ischemia, since it is better suited to defining subclinical disease in need of preventive treatment. Approximately 10% of asymptomatic patients undergoing atherosclerosis imaging will be defined as having sufficient subclinical disease so that ischemia testing is indicated. Patients who are able to exercise and are found to have extensive atherosclerosis but no ischemia by MPS appear to be at low risk for short- to intermediate-term cardiac events, thus not requiring coronary angiography. (*Adapted from* Berman *et al.* [59].)

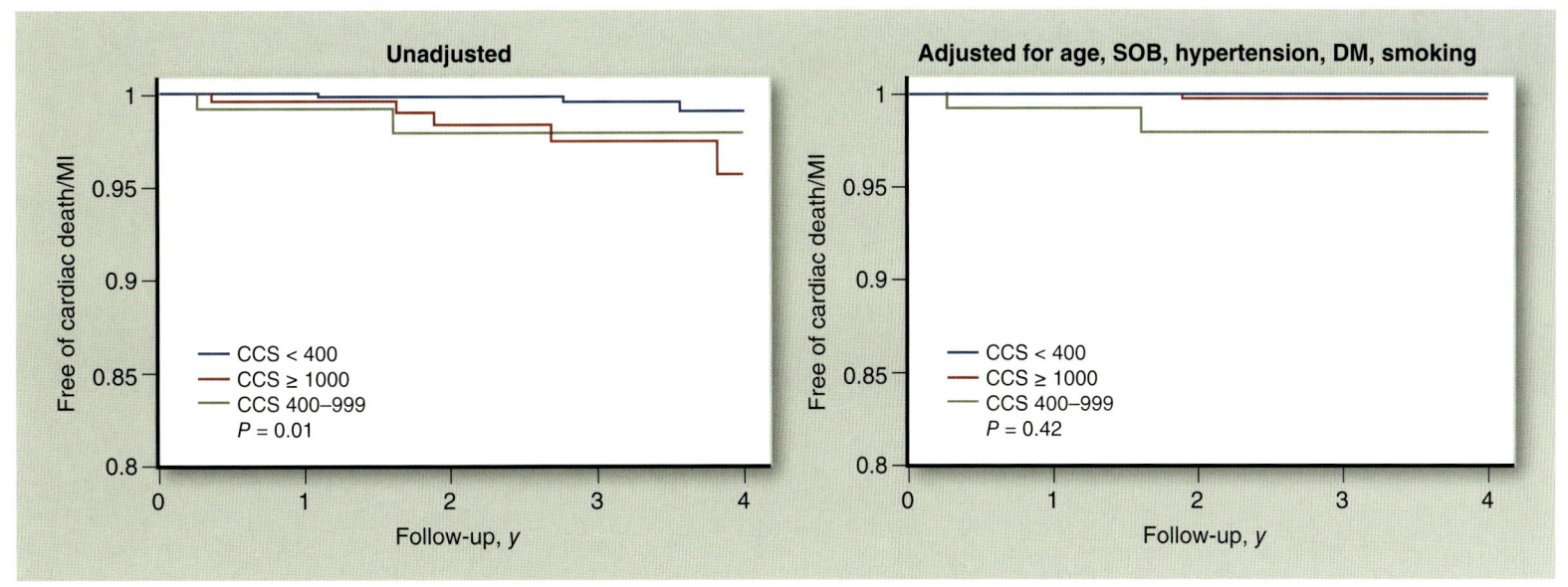

Figure 6-48. Prognosis of patients with high coronary calcium scores (CCS) and normal exercise myocardial perfusion SPECT (MPS). Until recently, there was no data upon which to justify the common practice of following medically, without coronary angiography, patients who have normal MPS associated with a very high CCS. A publication by Rozanski *et al.* [60] has provided data supporting this practice. The findings indicated that the 4-year cardiac event rate in patients without ischemia was equally low in patients with and without extensive coronary atherosclerosis (CCS > 1000). Given the known adverse prognostic implications of high CCS, these findings imply that in the absence of ischemia and with aggressive medical therapy, the adverse event rate in patients with coronary atherosclerosis is low in patients who are able to exercise. DM—diabetes mellitus; MI—myocardial infarction; SOB—shortness of breath. (*Adapted from* Rozanski *et al.* [60].)

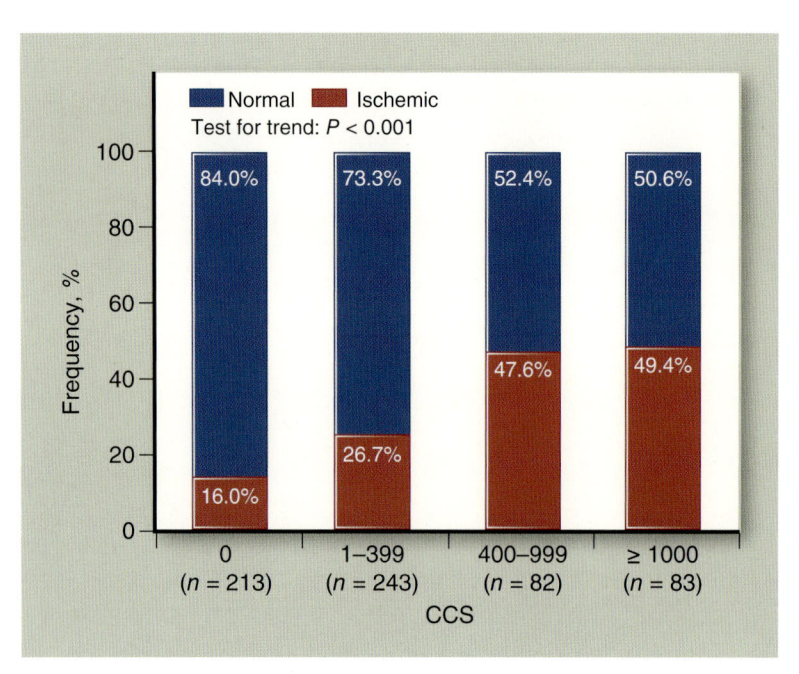

Figure 6-49. Relationship between PET-assessed ischemia and coronary calcium score (CCS). A more recent report of 695 symptomatic patients referred for adenosine stress PET who underwent CCS as part of routine image acquisition reported a 48.5% frequency of abnormal stress PET in patients with CCS ≥ 400, with an only slightly greater frequency (49.4%) of abnormal PET with a CCS ≥ 1000 [61]. Interestingly, 16% of patients with no measurable calcium had PET identified ischemia (negative predictive value 84%). The discrepancies in the reported frequencies of abnormal myocardial perfusion SPECT (MPS) in patients with high CCS appears to be largely explained by differences in the underlying patient risk. Recent subset analyses have supported this concept, indicating that the threshold of CCS warranting referral for MPS will vary further as a function of underlying patient risk. In this regard, the frequency of abnormal MPS for any level of CCS has been reported to be higher in patients with type 2 diabetes [62–64], patients with the metabolic syndrome [65], patients with a family history of premature coronary heart disease [63,64], and in patients with a high likelihood of coronary artery disease [64]. Although no validated threshold is currently recognized, in patient cohorts at greater risk for developing early atherosclerosis it has been suggested that a threshold CCS of ≥ 100 might be appropriate for these patients. (*Adapted from* Schenker et al. [61].)

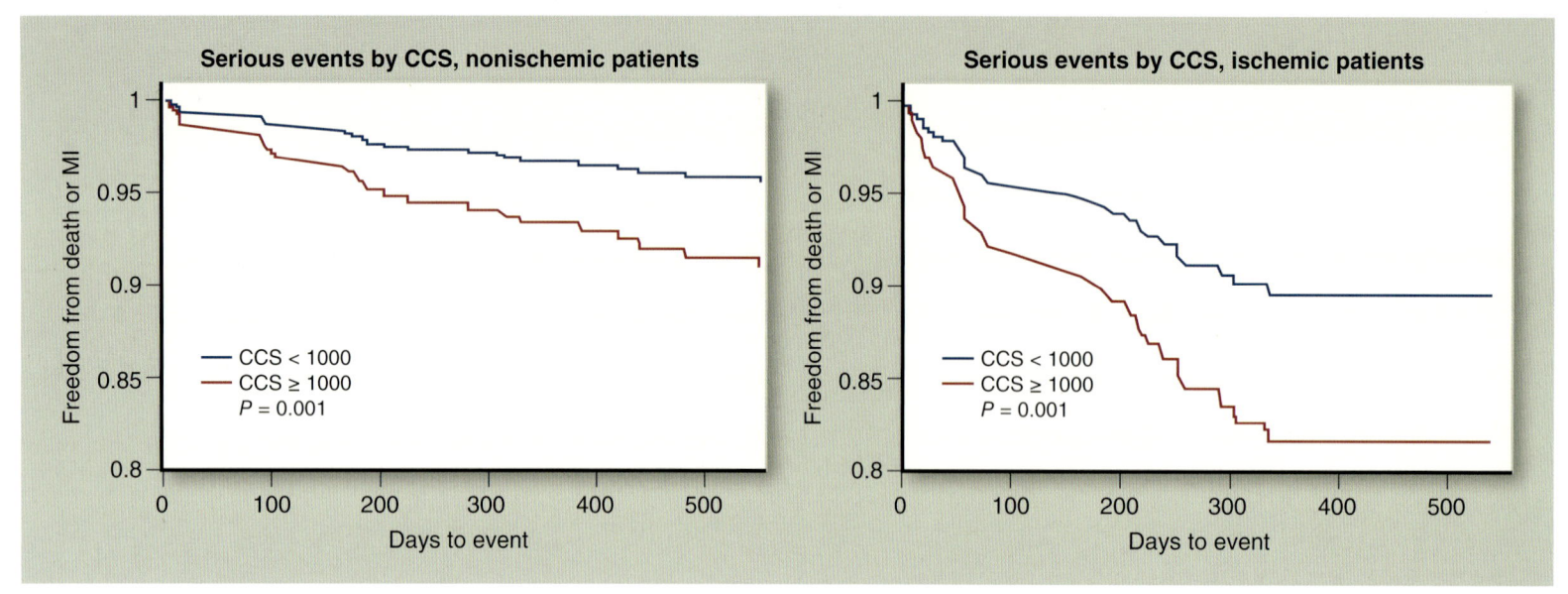

Figure 6-50. Prognosis of patients with high coronary calcium scores (CCS) and findings on PET with vasodilator stress. In contrast to the findings of Rozanski et al. [60] showing excellent prognosis in patients with high CCS and normal exercise myocardial perfusion SPECT (MPS), Schenker et al. [61] have shown that patients who have a nonischemic PET myocardial perfusion scan and have a CCS ≥ 1000 have a worse prognosis than those with a CCS < 1000 (*left*). These authors also demonstrated that when ischemia was seen on PET, those with a higher CCS also had a worse prognosis than those without extensive CCS (*right*). Multiple factors are likely to explain the difference between the prognostic implications of a very high CCS in patients with normal perfusion scans in these studies, with the most prominent being the pretest risk of the patients. In comparing the patients with normal perfusion scans in the two populations, those reported by Schenker et al. [61] had several features implying a "sicker" cohort as described above. The patients were referred for pharmacologic stress, older, more symptomatic, and had a higher pretest likelihood of coronary artery disease (CAD). The work of Schenker et al. [61] provides evidence that the measurement of the CCS adds to the prognostic information provided by myocardial perfusion imaging. MI—myocardial infarction. (*Adapted from* Schenker et al. [61].)

164 Atlas of Nuclear Cardiology

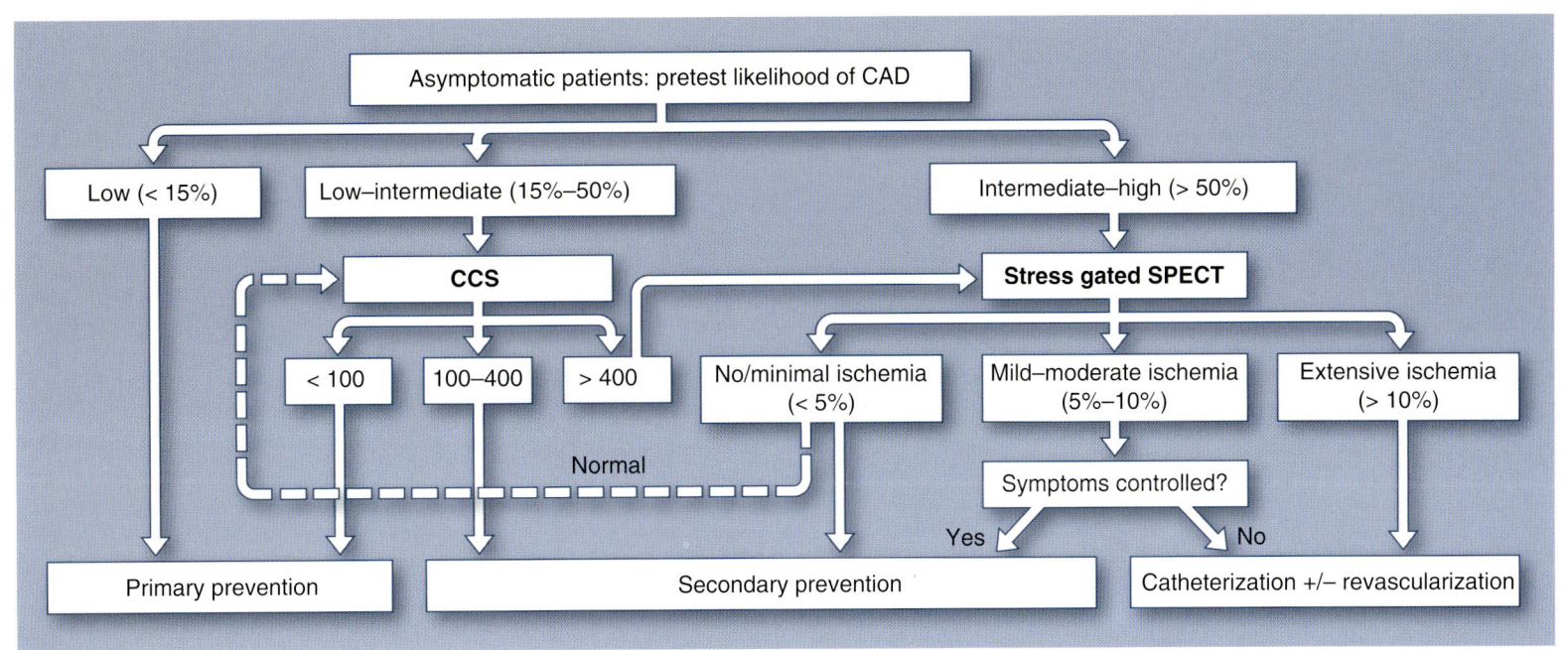

Figure 6-51. Conceptual approach to the use of CT coronary calcium measurements and nuclear testing in coronary artery disease (CAD) diagnosis and risk stratification in asymptomatic patients. First, the pretest likelihood of angiographically significant CAD is assessed as low (less than 10%), low-intermediate (10%–50%), high-intermediate (50%–85%), and high (> 85%) employing age, sex, risk factors, and symptoms. Patients with a low likelihood of CAD (in our experience < 15%) or low 10-year risk (< 10%) require only primary prevention guidelines regarding coronary risk factors (Adult Treatment Panel III) [16]. Patients with a low-intermediate likelihood of CAD (15%–50%), a group which by American College of Cardiology/American Heart Association guidelines might be selected for exercise testing, become excellent candidates for coronary calcium score (CCS) measurement in this approach. Since CCS provides a more sensitive, quantitative measurement of subclinical CAD in this population, we consider it more useful than the exercise electrocardiogram in selecting patients for aggressive medical management. Patients would then have the intensiveness of their medical therapy guided by the degree of CCS abnormality. Scores greater than 100 are regarded by many as the cutoff for recommending aggressive medical therapy with target low-density lipoprotein less than 70 and the target blood pressure would be 120/80 mm Hg [65]. Patients with scores ≥ 10 but < 100 might be considered as appropriate for aggressive medical therapy when CCS is 90th percentile or greater for age and gender [59], although the exact thresholds remain controversial. Regarding further testing, patients with CCS > 400 would be candidates for further testing with myocardial perfusion SPECT for purposes of risk/benefit assessment with respect to the possible need to consider revascularization. The exact cut-off above which patients should be referred for stress imaging is unclear; in the presence of symptoms, referral for nuclear testing might be appropriate with any abnormal score. In asymptomatic patients, the threshold for referral of 400 may be appropriate. In the CCS category of 100 to 400 it would not be cost effective to refer all patients for myocardial perfusion scanning; however, if tailoring this referral to the individual patient based on age, sex, and risk factors, selective referral for stress imaging might be appropriate. In this regard, a recent manuscript has shown that the category of 100 to 400 would deserve testing in diabetic patients [66], and preliminary data has suggested that this would be appropriate in patients with the metabolic syndrome [67].

In selected patients with normal or nearly normal nuclear scans, CCS might be appropriate in order to evaluate the extent of atherosclerosis and help guide medical management decisions [68], and to avoid missing extensive atherosclerosis simply because there is no regional stress-induced ischemia (*ie*, balanced reduction in flow). While CCS testing might not be needed in patients who are already following an aggressive medical management approach using secondary prevention guidelines, the CCS in this setting may help motivate patients to follow medical approaches to control CAD as well as to guide the intensity of medical management in settings in which the need for secondary prevention is not clear. (*Adapted from* Berman *et al.* [69].)

Acknowledgment

The authors gratefully acknowledge the valuable assistance of Xingping Kang, MD, in the preparation of this chapter.

References

1. Hasdai D, Gibbons RJ, Holmes DR Jr, et al.: Coronary endothelial dysfunction in humans is associated with myocardial perfusion defects. *Circulation* 1997, 96:3390–3395.

2. Ladenheim ML, Pollock BH, Rozanski A, et al.: Extent and severity of myocardial hypoperfusion as predictors of prognosis in patients with suspected coronary artery disease. *J Am Coll Cardiol* 1986, 7:464–471.

3. Garcia EV: Quantitative myocardial perfusion single-photon emission computed tomographic imaging: quo vadis? (Where do we go from here?). *J Nucl Cardiol* 1994, 1:83–93.

4. Sharir T, Germano G, Waechter PB, et al.: A new algorithm for the quantitation of myocardial perfusion SPECT. II: validation and diagnostic yield. J Nucl Med 2000, 41:720–727.

5. Germano G, Kavanagh P, Waechter P, et al.: A new algorithm for the quantitation of myocardial perfusion SPECT. I: technical principles and reproducibility. *J Nucl Med* 2000, 41:712–719.

6. Berman DS, Abidov A, Kang X, et al.: Prognostic validation of a 17-segment score derived from a 20-segment score for myocardial perfusion SPECT interpretation. *J Nucl Cardiol* 2004, 11:414–423.

7. Berman DS, Kiat H, Friedman JD, et al.: Separate acquisition rest thallium-201/stress technetium-99m sestamibi dual-isotope myocardial perfusion single-photon emission computed tomography: a clinical validation study. *J Am Coll Cardiol* 1993, 22:1455–1464.

8. Cerqueira MD, Weissman NJ, Dilsizian V, et al.: Standardized myocardial segmentation and nomenclature for tomographic imaging of the heart: a statement for healthcare professionals from the Cardiac Imaging Committee of the Council on Clinical Cardiology of the American Heart Association. *Circulation* 2002, 105:539–542.

9. Berman DS, Kang X, Gransar H, et al.: Quantitative assessment of myocardial perfusion abnormality on SPECT myocardial perfusion imaging is more reproducible than expert visual analysis. *J Nucl Cardiol* 2009, In press.

10. Slomka PJ, Nishina H, Berman DS, et al.: Automated quantification of myocardial perfusion SPECT using simplified normal limits. *J Nucl Cardiol* 2005, 12:66–77.

11. Mazzanti M, Germano G, Kiat H, et al.: Identification of severe and extensive coronary artery disease by automatic measurement of transient ischemic dilation of the left ventricle in dual-isotope myocardial perfusion SPECT. *J Am Coll Cardiol* 1996, 27:1612–1620.

12. Shaw LJ, Hachamovitch R, Berman DS, et al.: The economic consequences of available diagnostic and prognostic strategies for the evaluation of stable angina patients: an observational assessment of the value of precatheterization ischemia. *J Am Coll Cardiol* 1999, 33:661–669.

13. Matzer L, Kiat H, Van Train K, et al.: Quantitative severity of stress thallium-201 myocardial perfusion single-photon emission computed tomography defects in one-vessel coronary artery disease. *Am J Cardiol* 1993, 72:273–279.

14. Sharir T, Bacher-Stier C, Dhar S, et al.: Identification of severe and extensive coronary artery disease by postexercise regional wall motion abnormalities in Tc-99m sestamibi gated single-photon emission computed tomography. *Am J Cardiol* 2000, 86:1171–1175.

15. Borges-Neto S, Shaw LK, Tuttle RH: Incremental prognostic power of SPECT myocardial perfusion imaging in patients with know or suspected coronary artery disease. *Am J Cardiol* 2005, 95:182–188.

16. Berman DS, Hachamovitch R, Kiat H, et al.: Incremental value of prognostic testing in patients with known or suspected ischemic heart disease: a basis for optimal utilization of exercise technetium-99m sestamibi myocardial perfusion single-photon emission computed tomography. *J Am Coll Cardiol* 1995, 26:639–647 [published erratum appears in *J Am Coll Cardiol* 1996, 27:756].

17. Christian TF, Miller TD, Bailey KR, Gibbons RJ: Exercise tomographic thallium-201 imaging in patients with severe coronary artery disease and normal electrocardiograms. *Ann Intern Med* 1994, 121:825–832.

18. Hachamovitch R, Berman DS, Kiat H, et al.: Value of stress myocardial perfusion single photon emission computed tomography in patients with normal resting electrocardiograms: an evaluation of incremental prognostic value and cost-effectiveness. *Circulation* 2002, 105:823–829.

19. Klocke FJ, Baird MG, Lorell BH, et al.: ACC/AHA/ASNC guidelines for the clinical use of cardiac radionuclide imaging-executive summary. A report of the American College of Cardiology/American Heart Association Task Force on Practice Guidelines (ACC/AHA/ASNC committee to revise the 1995 guidelines for the clinical use of cardiac radionuclide imaging). *Circulation* 2003, 108:1404–1418.

20. Berman DS, Hachamovitch R, Shaw LJ, et al.: Nuclear cardiology. In *Hurst's The Heart*, edn 11. Edited by Fuster V, O'Rourke RA, Roberts R, et al. New York: McGraw-Hill Companies; 2004:563–597.

21. Ladenheim ML, Kotler TS, Pollock BH, et al.: Incremental prognostic power of clinical history, exercise electrocardiography and myocardial perfusion scintigraphy in suspected coronary artery disease. *Am J Cardiol* 1987, 59:270–277.

22. Hachamovitch R, Berman DS, Kiat H, et al.: Exercise myocardial perfusion SPECT in patients without known coronary artery disease: incremental prognostic value and use in risk stratification. *Circulation* 1996, 93:905–914.

23. Hachamovitch R, Berman DS, Shaw LJ, et al.: Incremental prognostic value of myocardial perfusion single photon emission computed tomography for the prediction of cardiac death: differential stratification for risk of cardiac death and myocardial infarction. *Circulation* 1998, 97:535–543.

24. Marwick TH, Shaw LJ, Lauer MS, et al.: The noninvasive prediction of cardiac mortality in men and women with known or suspected coronary artery disease. Economics of Noninvasive Diagnosis (END) Study Group. *Am J Med* 1999, 106:172–178.

25. Sharir T, Germano G, Kang X, et al.: Prognostic value of post-stress left ventricular volume and ejection fraction by gated myocardial perfusion single photon emission computed tomography in women: gender related differences in normal limits and outcome [abstract]. *Circulation* 2002, 106:II-523.

26. Zellweger MJ, Lewin HC, Lai S, et al.: When to stress patients after coronary artery bypass surgery? Risk stratification in patients early and late post-CABG using stress myocardial perfusion SPECT: implications of appropriate clinical strategies. *J Am Coll Cardiol* 2001, 37:144–152.

27. Sharir T, Germano G, Kang X, et al.: Prediction of myocardial infarction versus cardiac death by gated myocardial perfusion SPECT: risk stratification by the amount of stress-induced ischemia and the poststress ejection fraction. *J Nucl Med* 2001, 42:831–837.

28. Travin MI, Heller GV, Johnson LL, et al.: The prognostic value of ECG-gated SPECT imaging in patients undergoing stress Tc-99m sestamibi myocardial perfusion imaging. *J Nucl Cardiol* 2004, 11:253–262.

29. Thomas GS, Miyamoto MI, Morello AP, et al.: Technetium99m based myocardial perfusion imaging predicts clinical outcome in the community outpatient setting: The nuclear utility in the community ("nuc") study. *J Am Coll Cardiol* 2004, 43:213–223.

30. Heller GV, Herman SD, Travin MI, et al.: Independent prognostic value of intravenous dipyridamole with technetium-99m sestamibi tomographic imaging in predicting cardiac events and cardiac-related hospital admissions. *J Am Coll Cardiol* 1995, 26:1202–1208.

31. Kang X, Berman DS, Lewin HC, et al.: Incremental prognostic value of myocardial perfusion single photon emission computed tomography in patients with diabetes mellitus. *Am Heart J* 1999, 138(6 Pt 1):1025–1032.

32. Giri S, Shaw LJ, Murthy DR, et al.: Impact of diabetes on the risk stratification using stress single-photon emission computed tomography myocardial perfusion imaging in patients with symptoms suggestive of coronary artery disease. *Circulation* 2002, 105:32–40.

33. Vanzetto G, Ormezzano O, Fagret D, et al.: Long-term additive prognostic value of thallium-201 myocardial perfusion imaging over clinical and exercise stress test in low to intermediate risk patients : study in 1137 patients with 6-year follow-up. *Circulation* 1999, 100:1521–1527.

34. Diamond GA, Staniloff HM, Forrester JS, et al.: Computer-assisted diagnosis in the noninvasive evaluation of patients with suspected coronary artery disease. *J Am Coll Cardiol* 1983, 1(2 Pt 1):444–455.

35. Wackers FJ, Young LH, Inzucchi SE, et al.: Detection of silent myocardial ischemia in asymptomatic diabetic subjects: the DIAD study. *Diabetes Care* 2004, 27:1954–1961.

36. Sharir T, Berman DS, Lewin HC, et al.: Incremental prognostic value of rest-redistribution Tl-201 single-photon emission computed tomography. *Circulation* 1999, 100:1964–1970.

37. Hachamovitch R, Hayes SW, Friedman JD, et al.: Stress Myocardial Perfusion SPECT is Clinically Effective and Cost-effective in Risk-stratification of Patients with a High Likelihood of CAD but No Known CAD. *J Am Coll Cardiol* 2004, 43:200–208.

38. Stratmann HG, Tamesis BR, Younis LT, et al.: Prognostic value of dipyridamole technetium-99m sestamibi myocardial tomography in patients with stable chest pain who are unable to exercise. *Am J Cardiol* 1994, 73:647–652.

39. Gibbons RJ, Chatterjee K, Daley J, et al.: ACC/AHA/ACP-ASIM guidelines for the management of patients with chronic stable angina: a report of the American College of Cardiology/American Heart Association Task Force on Practice Guidelines (Committee on Management of Patients With Chronic Stable Angina). *J Am Coll Cardiol* 1999, 33:2092–2197.

40. Wagdy HM, Hodge D, Christian TF, et al.: Prognostic value of vasodilator myocardial perfusion imaging in patients with left bundle-branch block. *Circulation* 1998, 97:1563–1570.

41. Cottin Y, Rezaizadeh K, Touzery C, et al.: Long-term prognostic value of 201Tl single-photon emission computed tomographic myocardial perfusion imaging after coronary stenting. *Am Heart J* 2001, 141:999–1006.

42. Gibbons RJ, Hodge DO, Berman DS, et al.: Long-term outcome of patients with intermediate-risk exercise electrocardiograms who do not have myocardial perfusion defects on radionuclide imaging. *Circulation* 1999, 100:2140–2145.

43. Shaw L, Chaitman BR, Hilton TC, et al.: Prognostic value of dipyridamole thallium-201 imaging in elderly patients [comment]. *J Am Coll Cardiol* 1992, 19:1390–1398.

44. Calnon DA, McGrath PD, Doss AL, et al.: Prognostic value of dobutamine stress technetium-99m-sestamibi single-photon emission computed tomography myocardial perfusion imaging: stratification of a high-risk population [comment]. *J Am Coll Cardiol* 2001, 38:1511–1517.

45. Amanullah AM, Kiat H, Friedman JD, Berman DS: Adenosine technetium-99m sestamibi myocardial perfusion SPECT in women: diagnostic efficacy in detection of coronary artery disease. *J Am Coll Cardiol* 1996, 27:803–809.

46. Hachamovitch R, Hayes S, Friedman JD, et al.: Determinants of risk and its temporal variation in patients with normal stress myocardial perfusion scans: what is the warranty period of a normal scan? *J Am Coll Cardiol* 2003, 41:1329–1340.

47. Hachamovitch R, Hayes SW, Friedman JD, et al.: Comparison of the short-term survival benefit associated with revascularization compared with medical therapy in patients with no prior coronary artery disease undergoing stress myocardial perfusion single photon emission computed tomography. *Circulation* 2003, 107:2900–2907.

48. Berman DS, Kang X, Hayes SW, et al.: Adenosine myocardial perfusion single-photon emission computed tomography in women compared with men. Impact of diabetes mellitus on incremental prognostic value and effect on patient management. *J Am Coll Cardiol* 2003, 41:1125–1133.

49. Hachamovitch R, Rozanski A, Hayes SW, et al.: Predicting Therapeutic benefit from myocardial revascularization procedures: Are measurements of both resting left ventricular ejection fraction and stress-induced myocardial ischemia necessary? *J Nucl Cardiol* 2006, 13:768–778.

50. He ZX, Hedrick TD, Pratt CM, et al.: Severity of coronary artery calcification by electron beam computed tomography predicts silent myocardial ischemia. *Circulation* 2000, 101:244–251.

51. Iskander S, Iskandrian AE: Risk assessment using single-photon emission computed tomographic technetium-99m sestamibi imaging. *J Am Coll Cardiol* 1998, 32:57–62.

52. Abidov A, Hachamovitch R, Rozanski A, et al.: Prognostic implications of atrial fibrillation in patients undergoing myocardial perfusion single-photon emission computed tomography. *J Am Coll Cardiol* 2004, 44:1062–1070.

53. Zellweger MJ, Hachamovitch R, Kang X, et al.: Prognostic relevance of symptoms versus objective evidence of coronary artery disease in diabetic patients. *Euro Heart J* 2004, 25:543–550.

54. Abidov A, Hachamovitch R, Hayes SW, et al.: Prognostic impact of hemodynamic response to adenosine in patients older than age 55 years undergoing vasodilator stress myocardial perfusion study. *Circulation* 2003, 107:2894–2899.

55. Hachamovitch R, Hayes SW, Friedman JD, et al.: A prognostic score for prediction of cardiac mortality risk after adenosine stress myocardial perfusion scintigraphy. *J Am Coll Cardiol* 2005, 45:722–729.

56. Hachamovitch R, Friedman JD, Cohen I, et al.: Is there a referral bias against revascularization of patients with reduced LV ejection fraction? Influence of ejection fraction and inducible ischemia on post-SPECT management of patients without history of CAD. *J Am Coll Cardiol* 2003, 42:1286–1294.

57. Hachamovitch R, Di Carli MF: Methods and limitations of assessing new noninvasive tests: part I: Anatomy-based validation of noninvasive testing. *Circulation* 2008, 117:2684–2690.

58. Shaw LJ, Berman DS, Maron DJ, et al.: Optimal medical therapy with or without percutaneous coronary intervention to reduce ischemic burden: results from the Clinical Outcomes Utilizing Revascularization and Aggressive Drug Evaluation (COURAGE) trial nuclear substudy. *Circulation* 2008, 117:1283–1291.

59. Berman DS, Wong ND, Gransar H, et al.: Relationship between stress-induced myocardial ischemia and atherosclerosis measured by coronary calcium tomography. *J Am Coll Cardiol* 2004, 44:923–930.

60. Rozanski A, Gransar H, Wong ND, et al.: Clinical outcomes after both coronary calcium scanning and exercise myocardial perfusion scintigraphy. *J Am Coll Cardiol* 2007, 49:1352–1361.

61. Schenker MP, Dorbala S, Hong EC, et al.: Interrelation of coronary calcification, myocardial ischemia, and outcomes in patients with intermediate likelihood of coronary artery disease: a combined positron emission tomography/computed tomography study. *Circulation* 2008, 117:1693–1700.

62. Anand DV, Lim E, Hopkins D, et al.: Risk stratification in uncomplicated type 2 diabetes: prospective evaluation of the combined use of coronary artery calcium imaging and selective myocardial perfusion scintigraphy. *Eur Heart J* 2006, 27:713–721.

63. Blumenthal RS, Becker DM, Yanek LR, et al.: Comparison of coronary calcium and stress myocardial perfusion imaging in apparently healthy siblings of individuals with premature coronary artery disease. *Am J Cardiol* 2006, 97:328–333.

64. Rozanski A, Gransar H, Wong ND, et al.: Use of coronary calcium scanning for predicting inducible myocardial ischemia: Influence of patients' clinical presentation. *J Nucl Cardiol* 2007, 14:669–679.

65. Grundy SM, Cleeman JI, Merz CN, et al.: Implications of recent clinical trials for the National Cholesterol Education Program Adult Treatment Panel III guidelines. *Circulation* 2004, 110:227–239.

66. Anand DV, Lim E, Raval U, et al.: Prevalence of silent myocardial ischemia in asymptomatic individuals with subclinical atherosclerosis detected by electron beam tomography. *J Nucl Cardiol* 2004, 11:450–457.

67. Wong ND, Rozanski A, Gransar H, et al.: Metabolic syndrome and diabetes are associated with an increased likelihood of inducible myocardial ischemia among patients with subclinical atherosclerosis. *Diabetes Care* 2005, 28:1445–1450.

68. Berman DS, Hayes S, Friedman J, et al.: Normal myocardial perfusion SPECT does not imply the absence of significant atherosclerosis [abstract]. *Circulation* 2003, 108:IV-562.

69. Berman DS, Hachamovitch R, Shaw LJ, et al.: Roles of nuclear cardiology, cardiac computed tomography, and cardiac magnetic resonance: noninvasive risk stratification and a conceptual framework for the selection of noninvasive imaging tests in patients with known or suspected coronary artery disease. *J Nucl Med* 2006, 47:1107–1118.

The Role of Stress Myocardial Perfusion Imaging in Special Populations

Leslee J. Shaw and Jennifer H. Mieres

In decades past, the goal of observational research studies was to establish the prognostic value of myocardial perfusion single-photon emission CT (SPECT) and ventricular function measurements in generic cohorts of patients with known or suspected coronary disease. In more recent times, it has been observed that specific populations with unique needs and risks may limit the predictive value of prior prognostic models that were based on large but nondescript patient populations. In other words, any model that predicts major adverse clinical outcomes for laboratory populations (as a whole) may not be relevant to the subset of patients with unique but elevated cardiovascular risk. Such is the dilemma of defining the prognostic accuracy of SPECT imaging for special populations, including women, diabetic individuals, the elderly, obese patients, and ethnic minority cohorts, that are highlighted in this chapter. In the past few years, more recent data have unfolded that have identified very high-risk subsets for whom global predictive estimates may be less relevant. Physicians should take care to more closely align the abundance of evidence on risk stratification that matches the needs and specifications of their laboratory populations.

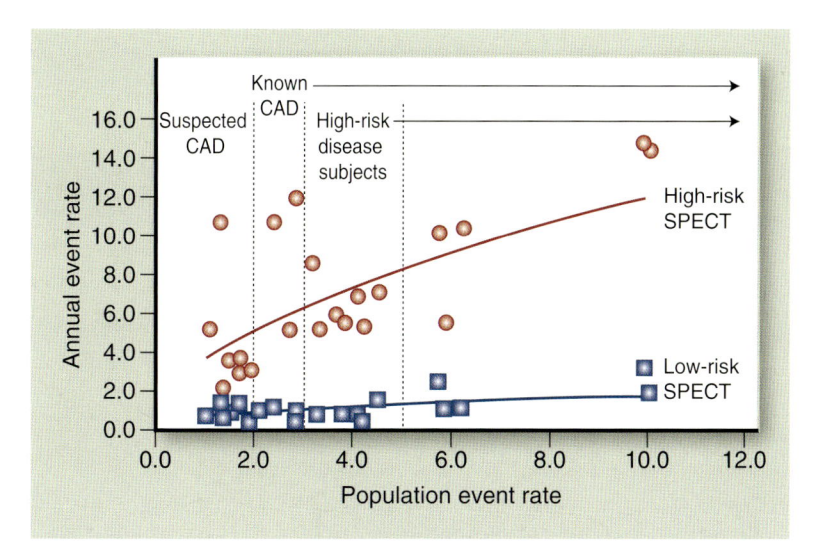

Figure 7-1. Risk stratification with single-photon emission CT (SPECT) imaging. A first step in applying the current evidence on risk stratification with SPECT imaging results to a given population is to understand what the baseline risk is for any given patient cohort [1]. Using this figure, one can visualize that risk stratification is effective for low- to high-risk SPECT results across a spectrum of population event rates. Although it is noted that the general risk for a suspected disease population is fewer than 2% per year for coronary heart disease death or nonfatal myocardial infarction [1,2], of this group, there are specific high-risk patient subsets, including diabetic individuals and the elderly, to name a few. Thus, this figure depicts generalities of risk that allow physicians to grasp the idea of risk stratification, even if it may not necessarily be applied to all patient cohorts [1].

Based on the application of risk stratification in this figure, women are unique in that a large proportion fall into the low-risk end of the spectrum. However, diabetic and elderly women and men, and probably those with the metabolic syndrome, form a very high-risk subset whose annual event risk is decidedly high. For African American and Hispanic patients with multiple risk factors, the risk of events is also elevated when compared with white, non-Hispanic patients. With regard to minority patient populations, physicians should take care to also consider nonclinical factors that may elevate a patient's risk, including delays in health care seeking and treatment, the absence of a regular source of care, and other financial hurdles that may render patients at greater risk on presentation to a SPECT imaging laboratory. CAD—coronary artery disease. (*Adapted from* Shaw and Iskandrian [1].)

Figure 7-2. High-risk coronary heart disease (CHD) (equivalent) populations. Over time, there has been growing support for the definition of *high risk* that now includes the cohort with established coronary disease as well as those whose event risk is equivalent to that of patients with obstructive coronary disease. The table delineates the segments of the population that may be considered as risk-equivalent cohorts.

The notion of defining patient cohorts who are CHD risk equivalents was initially introduced by the National Cholesterol Education Panel Adult Treatment Program III when it delineated diabetic patients as being risk equivalent, with an ensuing event rate over 10 years of 20% or higher [2]. In addition, the table details a number of high-risk patient subsets by categories, including those for patients with extracardiac atherosclerosis and those who have clustered risk factors. There are also subsets of patients who, by their extensive comorbidity, have an elevated risk, including the elderly, those with chronic kidney disease, and—a characteristic notable for any stress-testing laboratory—those who are functionally impaired. Functional impairment is a risk factor that is becoming more and more common with the epidemic of obesity and diabetes in the United States. For a single-photon emission CT laboratory, this potentially encumbers up to half of a referral population. Functional impairment is a surrogate marker for an aggregation of risk factors that act to limit a patient's abilities to perform maximal exercise. This is perhaps the most overlooked risk factor in a patient's clinical history. Thus, physicians should take care to discern a patient's physical work capacity and to decide on the use of pharmacologic stress in patients who have limited exercise abilities. CABS—coronary artery bypass surgery; CVD—cardiovascular disease; FRS—Framingham risk score; PCI—percutaneous coronary intervention.

High-Risk Coronary Heart Disease (Equivalent) Populations*

Known ischemic heart disease
  Stable coronary artery disease
  Post-MI/acute coronary syndrome
  Post-PCI/CABS
Known vascular disease
  Preoperative screening for noncardiac surgery
  Peripheral artery disease/CVD
CHD risk equivalent
  Diabetic patients
Degree of comorbidity
  Elderly
  Pharmacologic stress
  Functionally impaired
  Chronic kidney disease
Clustering of risk factors
  Metabolic syndrome
  Intermediate FRS and coronary calcium score
  High C-reactive protein

*Includes cohorts whose cardiac event risk is equivalent to the population with existing ischemic heart disease (ie, 10-year risk of cardiac death or nonfatal MI of 20% or greater).

Figure 7-3. Growth in the number of elderly patients. Estimates from the Centers for Disease Control and Prevention have noted that at or around the turn of the century, there was a notable change in the number of elderly patients [3]. Specifically, the growth slope has increased steadily over the past 50 years but tended toward a sharp ascent at the start of the 21st century. Following the observations of the past few years, projections through the year 2050 reveal that the number of the elderly in the United States will only continue to grow. Many experts posit that this growing elderly population will place further encumbrances on our health care system. However, it is clear that the need for chronic disease services will escalate dramatically, which is particularly relevant for a single-photon emission CT (SPECT) imaging laboratory. With the growing number of elderly patients having a greater prevalence of coronary disease, the requirements for diagnostic testing are also expected to expand. Thus, one would expect SPECT growth rates to emulate the growth in the elderly, diabetic, and obese populations.

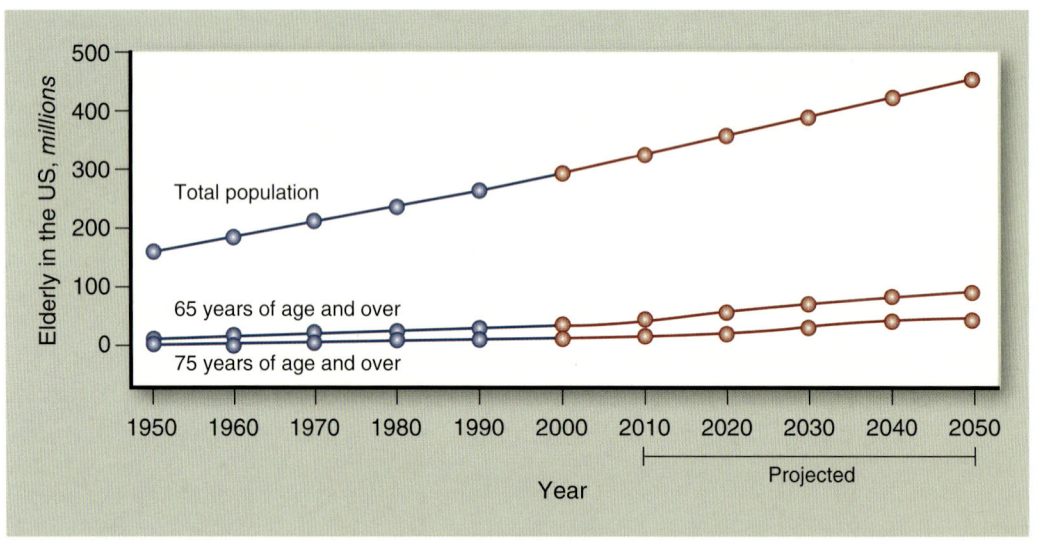

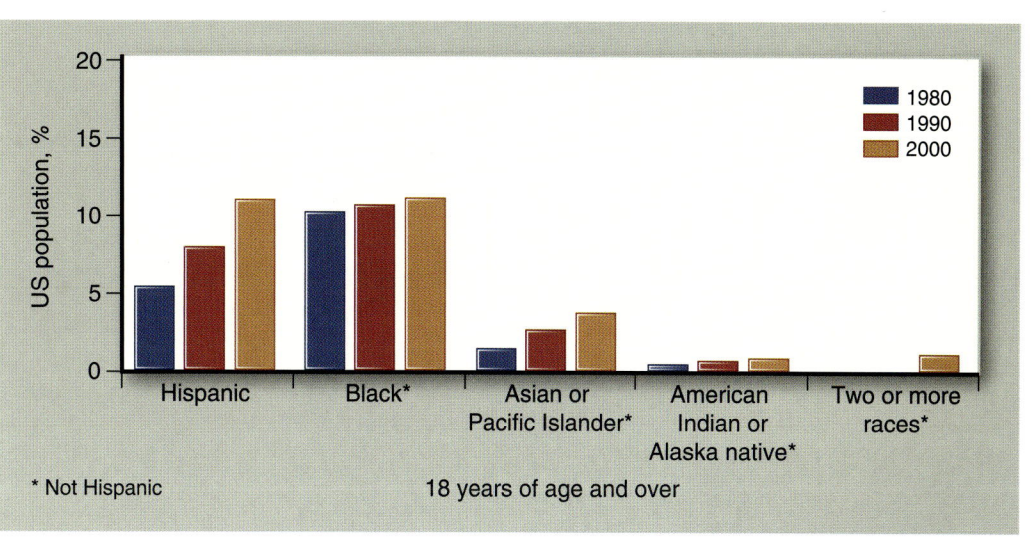

Figure 7-4. Diversity in the US population. Another population trend that has notable implications for the need for cardiovascular services, particularly cardiac imaging laboratories, is the ever-increasing diversity in the US population [3]. The influx of a greater percentage of Hispanic patients with high rates of obesity and risks associated with hyperlipidemia brings unique challenges to current cardiovascular medical practice. Furthermore, African American patients with multiple risk factors at much younger ages and less prevalent obstructive coronary disease bring additional challenges to diagnostic testing. Only recently has prognostic evidence been available to guide decision making in these two cohorts of patients. It is hoped that additional evidence of specific challenges in ethnic minority populations regarding the metabolic syndrome and/or diabetes will further aid in the development of guidelines targeted to the special needs of these patients.

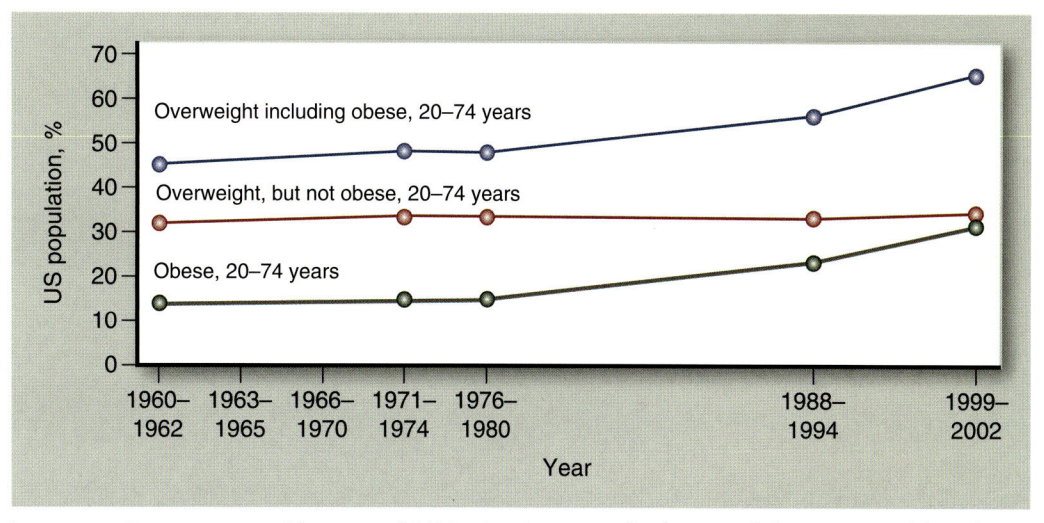

Figure 7-5. Prevalence of obesity. Over the past several decades, the prevalence of obesity has skyrocketed. Concomitant with the rising prevalence of obesity, a similar trend has been noted for diabetes [3]. For the obese patient, hypertension, poor eating habits, and functional disability are common. Thus, we would also expect to see a similar trend in the rate of the metabolic syndrome. For the single-photon emission CT (SPECT) imaging laboratory, the growing prevalence of obese patients presents unique challenges. First, any imaging laboratory can expect a greater percentage of their population to be obese. Second, obese patients are difficult to image and due to poor functional capacity, they more often require pharmacologic stress. Breast attenuation problems will pose a problem for obese women and men. Positron emission tomography imaging may also provide unique advantages for the obese patient, although this has yet to be established. Third, because of the frequent clustering of risk factors in obese patients, physicians are frequently referring them at younger ages and, as such, expected likelihood of risk predictions must not only consider comorbidities but importantly the age of the patient. Although not specified, the time duration of excess weight will also be important. Therefore, for a patient who gains weight later in life, a higher body mass index may be less relevant than it is for the patient who has been obese his or her entire life. Finally, many obese patients will be referred for a preoperative evaluation (eg, bariatric surgery) that may require unique imaging challenges and near-term risk predictions.

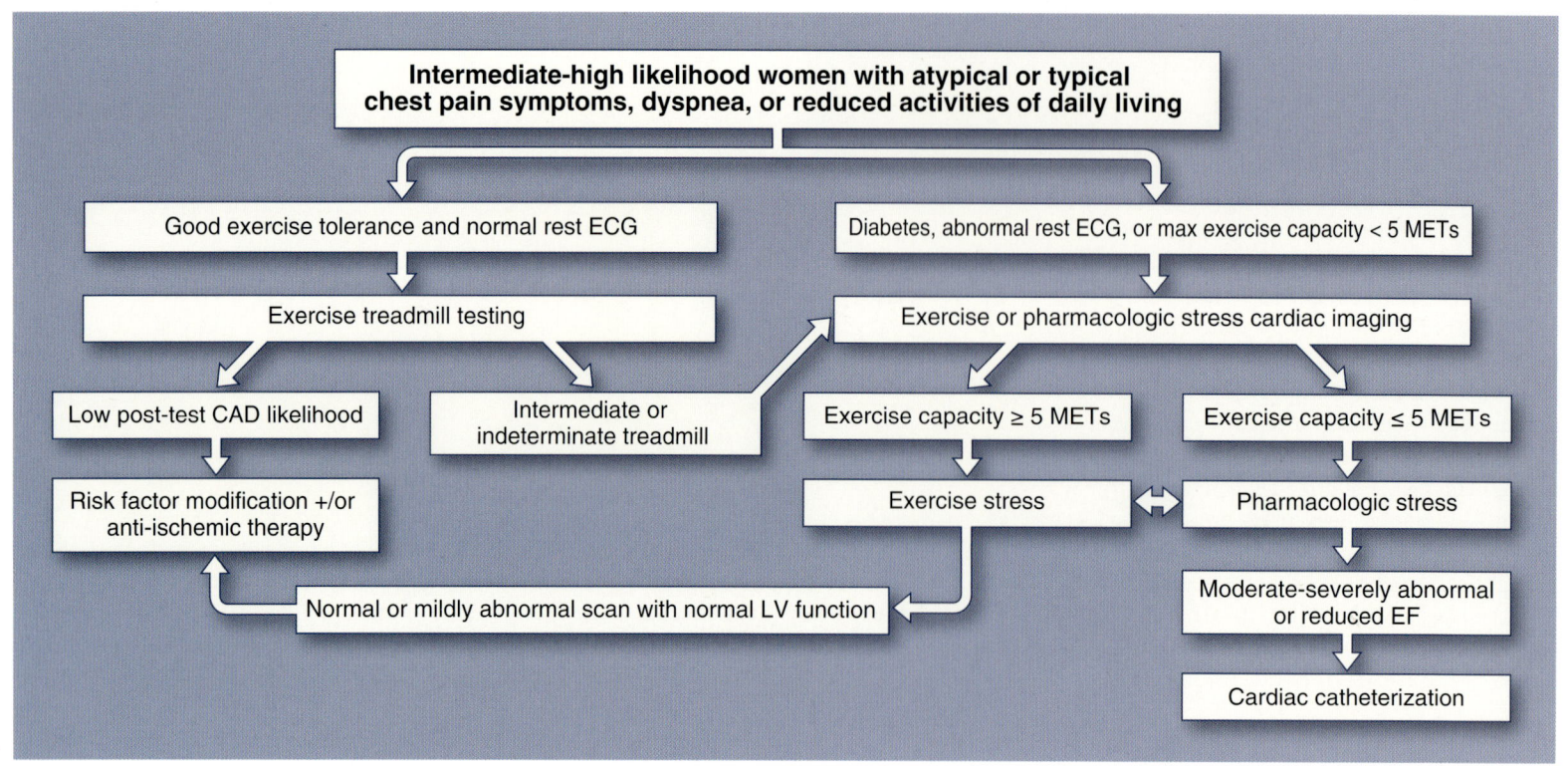

Figure 7-6. Predictive value of cardiac imaging in women. As early as a decade ago, our knowledge base of the predictive value of common cardiac imaging modalities in women was inadequate. As a result, much historical data were filled with problems and noted frequent limitations for female patients. However, our evidence base is now so robust that the American Heart Association (AHA) and American Society of Nuclear Cardiology have assimilated evidence into clinical guidelines [4,5]. From the 2005 AHA guidelines, a clinical algorithm was put forth as a guide to discerning optimal female candidates for stress testing [4]. Several notable changes to this algorithm stand in controvert to the existing stress-testing guidelines from the American College of Cardiology (ACC)/AHA [6]. First, the authors used a wider berth of descriptors for female symptomatology and highlighted the importance of functional capacity. In fact, declining abilities in performing activities of daily living should be considered an important landmark for female patients presenting with angina or equivalents, such as excessive dyspnea. This broader inclusion of symptoms is important because women present more often with atypical or nonexertional chest pain symptoms.

An additional point that is not noted in this figure is that because of a greater frequency in atypical presentation, physicians rely more often on imaging results to guide management decisions. Thus, in practice, single-photon emission CT (SPECT) imaging is frequently being used as a first-line test, although this is not supported by ACC/AHA guidelines [6]. This is in large part due to the numerous problems with the exercise electrocardiogram (ECG), which can result in diagnostic sensitivity and specificity measures in the range of 65% to 70% [4]. Reasons for the diminished accuracy include lower ECG voltage, sex hormones, and, most importantly, a failure to achieve maximal stress. For all women who undergo initial exercise testing in which the results are indeterminate or intermediate, sequential SPECT imaging is recommended. Use of the Duke treadmill score (defined as exercise time: 4 × chest pain index [0 = no chest pain, 1 = non-limiting chest pain, 2 = exercise-limiting chest pain] and 5 × ST segment deviation [+ or – used in absolute terms]) may help to define an intermediate patient who may benefit from sequential SPECT imaging [7].

Based on the AHA guidelines for cardiac imaging in women, only women with resting ST-T wave changes, functional disability, established coronary disease, or diabetes are recommended to undergo initial cardiac imaging [4]. Diabetic women are one of the highest-risk cohorts referred to any SPECT imaging laboratory. Of this group, those requiring insulin to manage their diabetes are at even greater risk. Another group that should also be considered at elevated risk and perhaps in the future may also have recommendations for direct cardiac imaging includes women with the metabolic syndrome. CAD—coronary artery disease; EF—ejection fraction; LV—left ventricular; METs—metabolic equivalents. (*Adapted from* Mieres *et al.* [4].)

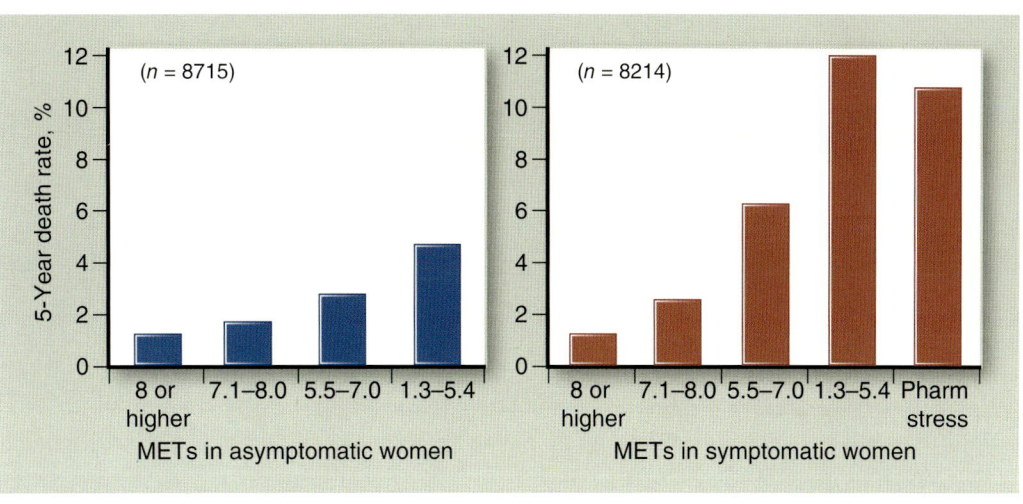

Figure 7-7. Functional disability in women. Concomitant functional disability with chest pain is common in women and may occur in half of symptomatic females [8]. Women not achieving 4.7 metabolic equivalents (METs) or higher should be considered at high risk and frequently will have inadequate heart rate response and a reduced likelihood of provocative ischemia, and may benefit from referral to pharmacologic stress imaging. Women who achieve submaximal exercise are often left with diagnostic uncertainty, leading to greater rates of anxiety and depression with regard to the etiology of their symptoms [9]. Upcoming data will suggest that the use of preexercise testing questionnaires, such as the Duke Activity Status Index, will aid in test selection and referral of women to pharmacologic or exercise stress. Importantly, guideline data do support the use of pharmacologic stress testing in patients unable to achieve 5 METs. However, physicians often initially try exercise testing to garner insight into the patient's physical work abilities. In the future, the application of physical functioning questionnaires that focus on activities of daily living and recreational activities may be sufficient evidence on which to guide test use and decision making. Pharmacologic stress (pharm stress) = women referred for adenosine or dipyridamole single-photon emission CT or dobutamine stress echocardiography. (*Adapted from* Shaw et al. [8].)

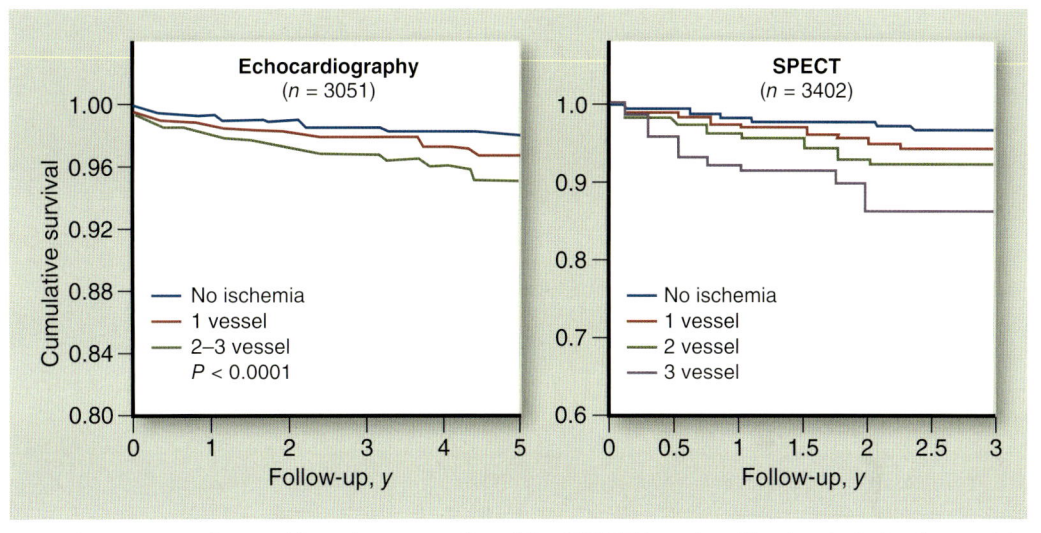

Figure 7-8. Prognostic accuracy of exercise echocardiography and single-photon emission CT (SPECT) in women. Several large, observational series of women have reported a high degree of prognostic accuracy for both exercise echocardiography and SPECT imaging. In the Economics of Noninvasive Diagnosis (END) study of 3402 women with chest pain, risk stratification was gender neutral; *ie*, there was no difference in the prognostic accuracy of SPECT imaging in women versus men. A woman with no inducible ischemia had a 99% cardiac survival at 3 years, a rate similar to that of the enrolled men with chest pain [10]. Survival decrementally worsened such that women with multivessel ischemia had 3% to 5% annual death rates ($P < 0.0001$). It appears that women who are referred to exercise echocardiography are lower risk (as can be seen in the figure [note: different y-axis scales]) [11], and higher-risk patients are referred for SPECT imaging. Yet, despite being lower risk, effective risk stratification is possible with exercise echocardiography in women, as noted by a recent report in 3051 women.

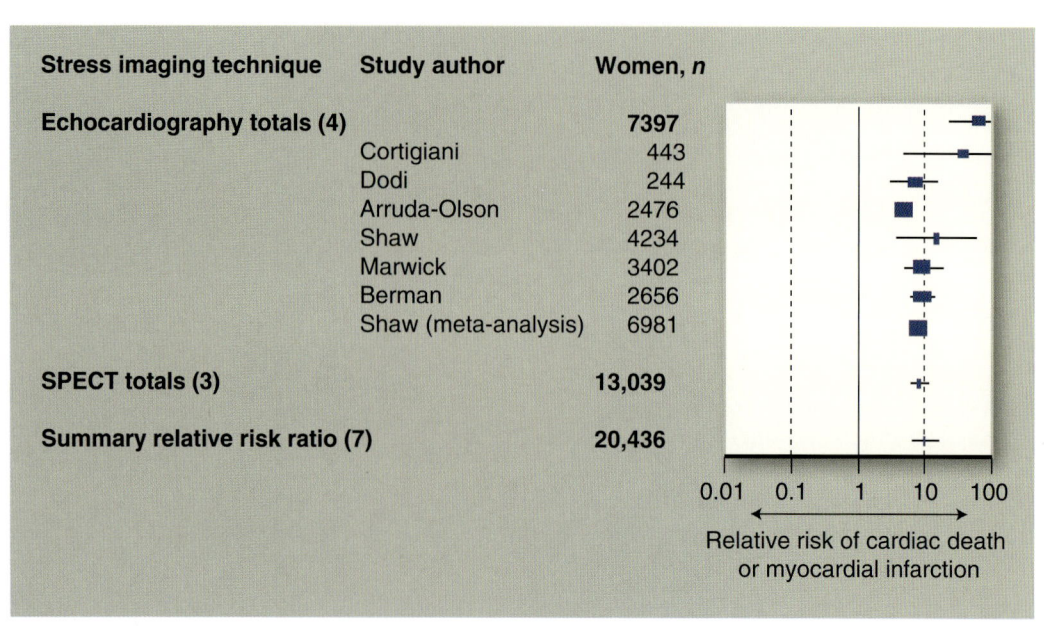

Figure 7-9. Accuracy of echocardiography and single-photon emission CT (SPECT) in predicting cardiac death or myocardial infarction. When accumulating the evidence on the predictive accuracy of a normal- and high-risk perfusion scan in women, one can expect annual rates of cardiac death or nonfatal myocardial infarction to range from 0.7% to 6.3%, respectively [4,10,12]. These results, when synthesized into a meta-analysis including more than 20,000 women, reveal a high degree of accuracy for both echocardiography and SPECT imaging [11]. Although these two modalities often compete in the research arena, the good news for women is that they both work very well for risk stratification and, as such, local expertise should guide their application. It appears from the literature that optimal allocation of testing would allow for the use of exercise echocardiography in lower-risk women and SPECT imaging in higher-risk women, for whom precise delineation of defect extent and severity is crucial to effective decision making. When one examines the extent of vascular territory involvement with reduced stress perfusion, cardiac survival can range from 99% to approximately 85% for those with no ischemia to three vascular territories

Stress imaging technique	Study author	Women, n
Echocardiography totals (4)		7397
	Cortigiani	443
	Dodi	244
	Arruda-Olson	2476
	Shaw	4234
	Marwick	3402
	Berman	2656
	Shaw (meta-analysis)	6981
SPECT totals (3)		13,039
Summary relative risk ratio (7)		20,436

Relative risk of cardiac death or myocardial infarction

[10]. By comparison, including the extent and severity of perfusion abnormalities, low-risk, mildly abnormal, moderately abnormal, and severely abnormal SPECT results have annual cardiac death rates, proportionally, of 0.8%, 1.6%, 2.8%, and 6.1%, respectively, for nondiabetic women [12]. (*Adapted from* Shaw *et al.* [11].)

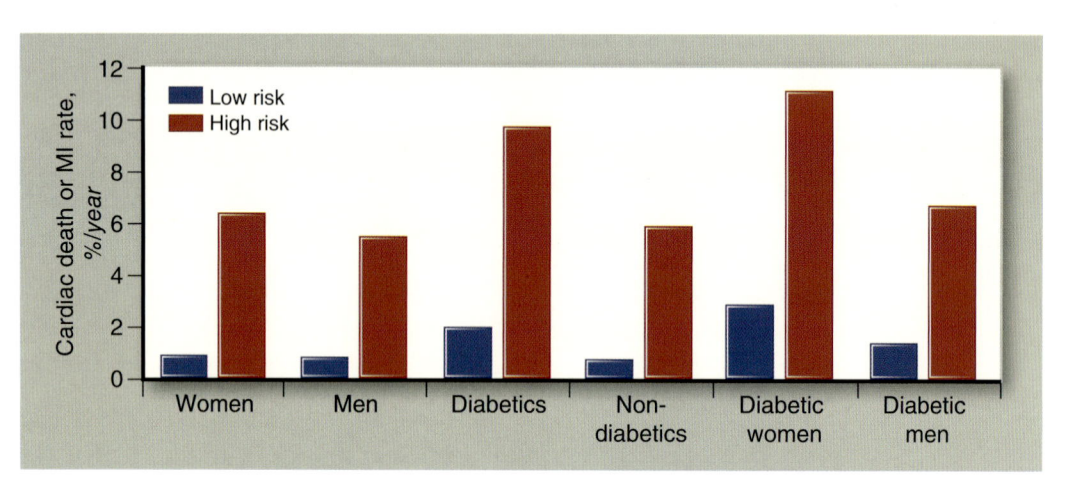

Figure 7-10. Diabetes and rate of cardiac death or myocardial infarction (MI). Risk is decidedly higher for diabetic women than nondiabetic women and men [12]. As stated earlier, for all the cohorts of patients referred for single-photon emission CT imaging, diabetic women are one of the highest-risk groups. In general, the overall event rates for diabetic women are approximately 50% higher than those for nondiabetic women [4]. (*Adapted from* Shaw and Iskandrian [1].)

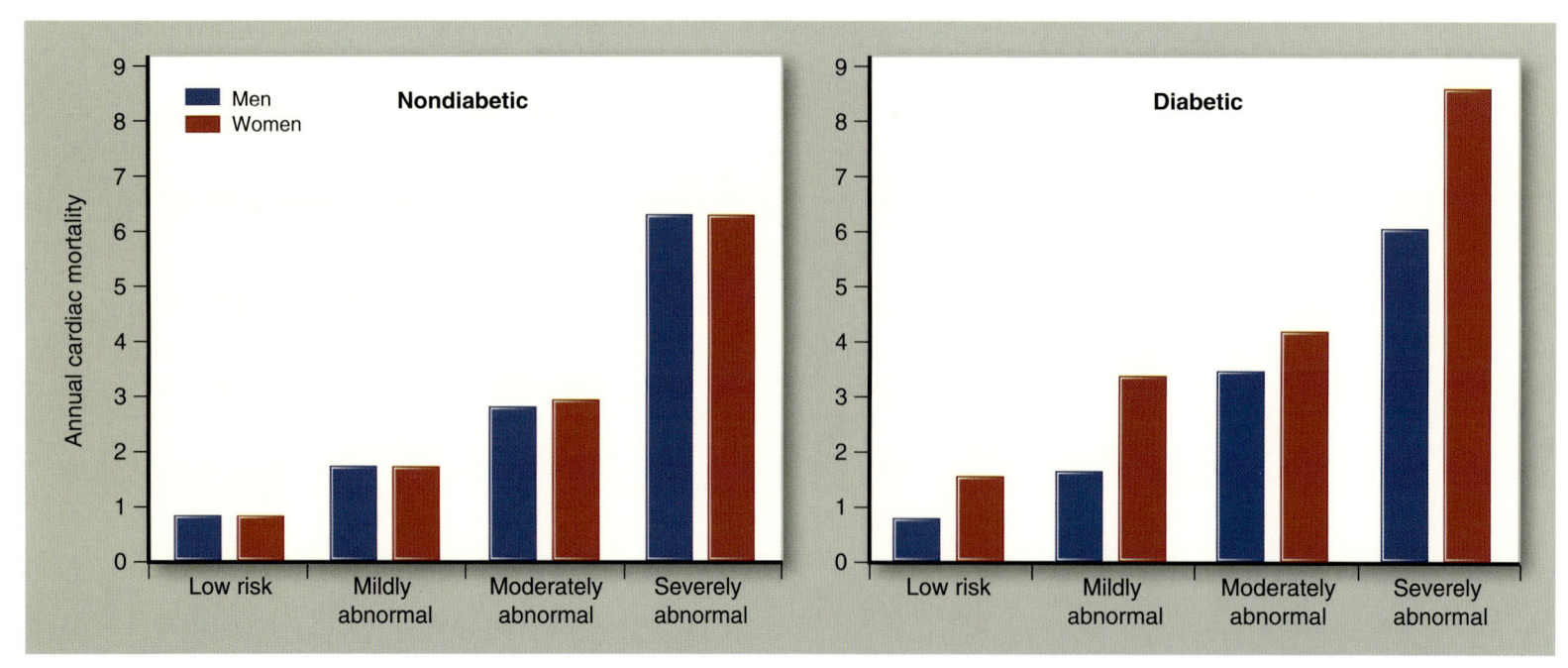

Figure 7-11. The annual cardiac mortality rates for 6173 diabetic and nondiabetic women and men by adenosine single-photon emission CT (SPECT) imaging [12]. In a report on diabetic women, yearly death rates ranged from 1.5% to 8.5% for normal to severely abnormal SPECT imaging results [12]. Thus, effective risk stratification is possible for women, including very high-risk diabetic patients [1]. Of note, normal stress perfusion results are associated with a low annual cardiac death or myocardial infarction rate.

Continued on the next page

174 Atlas of Nuclear Cardiology

Figure 7-11. *(Continued)* For women with severely abnormal studies, the rate of "hard" cardiac events is elevated approximately nine- to 10-fold [11]. In the example shown here, women have a higher rate of annual major adverse cardiac events, in large part because of their older age and more frequent comorbidity. However, there are subsets of younger women with more nonanginal symptoms who are at very low risk. This is the major challenge in evaluating women with suspected myocardial ischemia, *ie*, ferreting out from the diverse group of women those who are truly at risk. Furthermore, of those at risk, there are subsets of women whose risk is decidedly higher than that of their male counterparts. Diabetic women and those with functional disability are examples of high-risk women. From this figure, women with severely abnormal SPECT studies, including multivessel ischemia or high-risk summed stress score, should be considered candidates for aggressive anti-ischemic therapy and coronary angiography [4]. If a physician is able to exclude any possibility of breast artifact, even in the setting of nonobstructive coronary disease, recent evidence is supportive of treatment toward ameliorating a woman's ischemic burden. *(Adapted from* Berman et al. [12].*)*

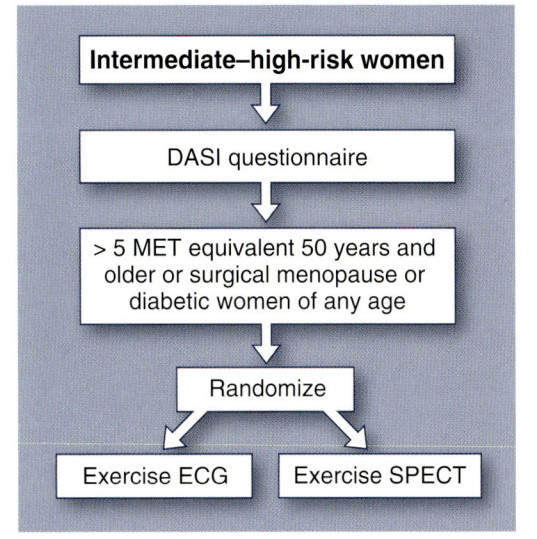

Figure 7-12. What Is the Optimal Method for Ischemia Evaluation in Women? (WOMEN) study. The WOMEN study is an exciting randomized trial that could have significant ramifications for diagnostic testing in female patients with suspected myocardial ischemia. This trial is randomizing 824 women to receive an exercise electrocardiogram (ECG) or a single-photon emission CT (SPECT) study as their initial diagnostic test. The primary aim of this study is to discern the negative predictive value of the exercise ECG as compared with SPECT in this diagnostic cohort of women. Secondary aims of quality of life and cost are also being explored. Although current practice is using a SPECT-driven strategy, current guidelines lack the evidence to make definitive changes supporting a greater utilization and indications for cardiac imaging. Thus, the WOMEN study will be pivotal in supporting the use of SPECT imaging in all intermediate-risk women with stable chest pain symptoms. DASI—Duke Activity Status Index (a 12-item quality-of-life measure estimating activities of daily living); MET—metabolic equivalent.

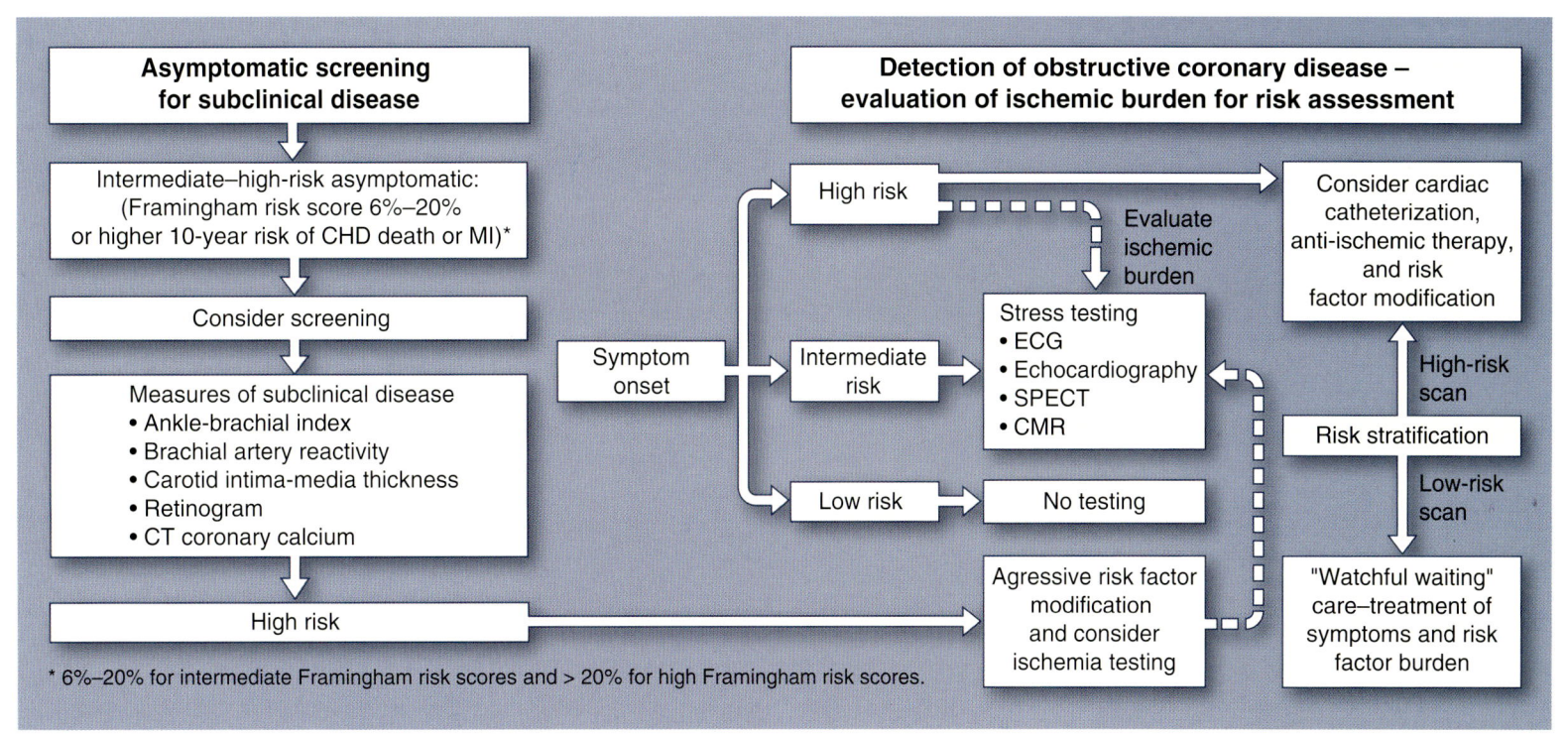

Figure 7-13. Strategy for identification of high-risk asymptomatic and symptomatic women. As more evidence unfolds regarding optimal female candidates for noninvasive testing, there is an unfolding paradigm that includes a diverse strategy for the identification of high-risk asymptomatic and symptomatic women [13]. What is key from this testing paradigm is that risk assessment is the driving force for interpretation of test results, in large part because of the reduced prevalence of obstructive coronary disease in women. In fact, a disconnect exists between a woman's predicted risk and her obstructive coronary disease burden. For the latter case, the extent and severity of ischemia are better tracking mechanisms for a woman's risk of adverse cardiac events. Using this paradigm, intermediate-risk (based on the Framingham risk score) asymptomatic women are candidates for some type of subclinical disease testing including measures of endothelial function (*eg*, brachial artery reactivity testing) or atherosclerotic disease burden (*eg*, coronary calcium screening). Women with high-risk calcium scores, for example, should then be referred for additional ischemia testing based on the current evidence [14].

Continued on the next page

Figure 7-13. *(Continued)* For the symptomatic woman, risk stratification after a stress test is an effective means on which to guide the intensity of posttest management. Low-risk women do not require additional testing, whereas those with high-risk stress test results should be considered candidates for cardiac catheterization. Evidence of ischemia should not be considered a benign finding and treatment should be oriented toward resolution of stress-induced findings with aggressive anti-ischemic therapies. CHD—coronary heart disease; CMR—cardiovascular magnetic resonance (imaging); ECG—electrocardiogram; MI—myocardial infarction; SPECT—single-photon emission CT. (*Adapted from* Shaw et al. [13].)

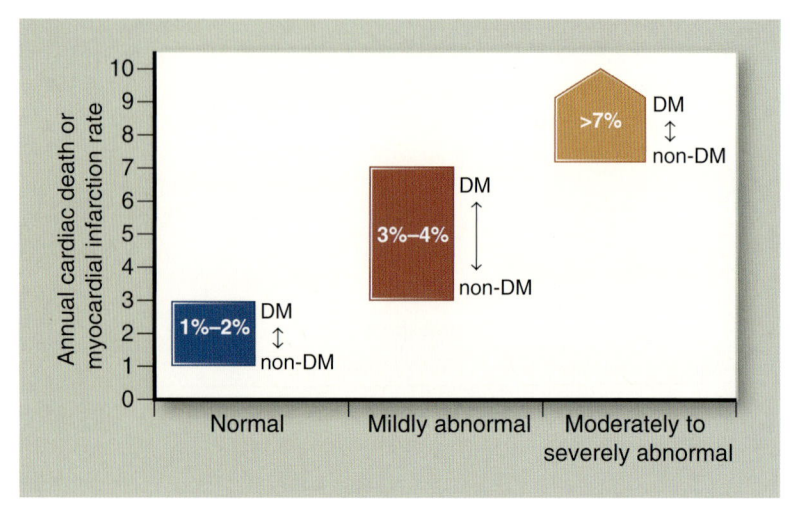

Figure 7-14. Cardiac event rates in diabetic versus nondiabetic patients. Diabetic patients have a life expectancy that is estimated to be approximately one decade less than that of their nondiabetic counterparts, and for our purposes, their ensuing risk associated with any single-photon emission CT (SPECT) abnormality will be exacerbated. The benefit of screening diabetic patients is that because of the frequent occurrence of neuropathy, silent ischemia and infarction are more prevalent. Thus, an imaging strategy, such as that utilizing SPECT, is valuable to discern the extent and severity of provocative ischemia. Because microvascular and macrovascular complications occur at the onset of hyperglycemia, on initial diagnosis, some assessment of cardiac risk should be performed. In a meta-analysis, annual cardiac death or myocardial infarction rates were 1.9% for diabetic patients and 0.6% for nondiabetic patients with a normal stress perfusion scan [1]. For a severely abnormal SPECT study, the annual rates increased to 5.8% for nondiabetic patients and were as high as 9.6% for patients with diabetes. These results reveal that diabetic patients have a higher than expected cardiac event rate when compared with nondiabetic patients [15]. So for the nuclear cardiologist, one could expect that concurrent with their higher baseline risk, all predicted event rates will be elevated and adjusted accordingly for diabetic patients. As noted in the report by Kang et al. [15], we can expect that any risk associated with a given severity of SPECT abnormalities is higher for diabetic than nondiabetic individuals. This statement is probably also true for patients with the metabolic syndrome, particularly those with four or five risk factors for the metabolic syndrome (defined as insulin resistance [with or without glucose intolerance], reduced high-density lipoprotein cholesterol, increased triglycerides, hypertension, and abdominal obesity). DM—diabetes mellitus. (*Adapted from* Kang et al. [15].)

Figure 7-15. Adenosine stress single-photon emission CT (SPECT) and cardiac mortality in patients with diabetes. A recent report using adenosine stress SPECT may be more generalizable to the diabetic patient who is functionally impaired as a result of obesity or peripheral arterial disease [12]. In this analysis, insulin-dependent diabetic patients were at very high risk, with death rates that were approximately twofold higher in the setting of an abnormal SPECT study as compared with non–insulin-dependent diabetic or nondiabetic patients. In this report, nearly one in 10 insulin-dependent diabetic patients with abnormal SPECT findings died annually, a rate twice that of non–insulin-dependent diabetic or nondiabetic patients. (*Adapted from* Berman et al. [12].)

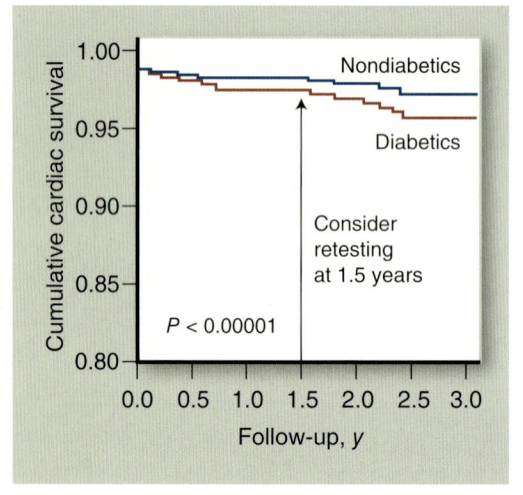

Figure 7-16. Clinical worsening in diabetic patients. Because of the more frequent aggressive disease process in individuals with diabetes, progression can be expected to occur earlier and at a more rapid rate when compared with nondiabetic patients. Thus, for the diabetic patient presenting with symptoms suspected of myocardial ischemia but with normal stress single-photon emission CT findings, consideration should be given to retesting at or around 1.5 years of follow-up. In the survival curve shown in the figure, there is a drastic decrease in survival between 1 to 2 years of follow-up, thereby demonstrating a trend toward an increase in the rate of cardiac death at that time. (*Adapted from* Giri et al. [16].)

176 Atlas of Nuclear Cardiology

Figure 7-17. Risk stratification in pharmacologic versus exercise stress testing. It is expected that by 2030, nearly 20% of the US population will be 65 years of age or older [3]. As elderly patients have more frequent chronic diseases, including coronary artery disease, prevalence rates approach one in three patients for those older than 70 years. Comorbid conditions are also prevalent, including hypertension, vascular diseases, and osteoarthritis [3]. Elderly patients also have frequent physical disability, with estimates from the Centers for Disease Control and Prevention reporting that from one to three of 10 elderly individuals require assistance or are unable to perform activities of daily living including self-care and household cleaning [3]. For a single-photon emission CT (SPECT) imaging laboratory, this would translate into an estimated physical work capacity of less than 4 metabolic equivalents (METs) and an increased need for the use of pharmacologic stress imaging [3,6]. Experientially, we have observed the representation of patients referred to pharmacologic stress grow from approximately 20% to 40% of any laboratory's patient population.

Physiologically, peak maximal oxygen consumption values decline with age. Based on a 2005 report, the average peak MET value for patients older than 74 years is less than 5 METs [17]. Thus, one can envision that the vast majority of elderly patients would require the use of pharmacologic stress SPECT. Consequent to this, it is essential to note whether risk stratification is equally accurate for exercise and pharmacologic stress. Results from a meta-analysis showed a similarly marked separation in expected cardiac event rates for patients undergoing exercise and pharmacologic stress; ie, the death or myocardial infarction (MI) rates were low for patients with normal stress perfusion SPECT results and increased dramatically for those with abnormal stress myocardial perfusion findings. However, as the degree of comorbidity drives the expected event rate and pharmacologic stress patients are frequently encumbered with multiple chronic conditions, there is a necessary escalation in expected event rates for low-risk to severely abnormal findings. As can be seen from a meta-analysis, low-risk pharmacologic stress SPECT is associated with an annual rate of cardiac death or nonfatal myocardial infarction of approximately 1.2%, as compared with 0.7% for exercise stress with normal perfusion [1]. A similarly greater event rate is noted for pharmacologic versus exercise stress in patients with abnormal myocardial perfusion results.

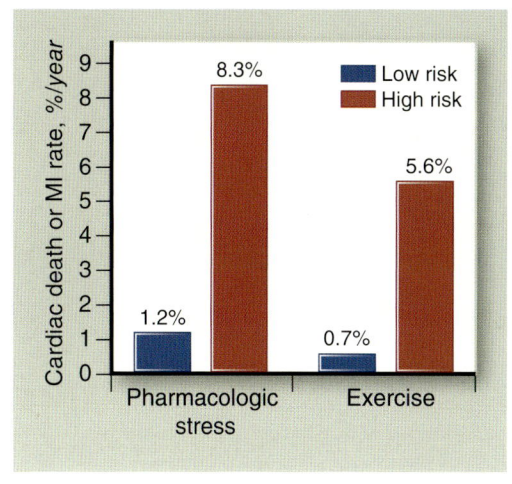

Diagnostic Accuracy of Stress Myocardial Perfusion SPECT Compared with Exercise ECG in Women With Type 2 Diabetes

Modality (n = 104)	Sensitivity, %	Specificity, %
Stress myocardial perfusion SPECT	94	97
Exercise ECG	49	61

A

Prognosis by Pharmacologic Stress Myocardial Perfusion PET in Obese Patients

PET results	Cardiac death	Acute MI	Combined events
Normal (n = 89)	0.0%	0.0%	0.0%
Abnormal (n = 45)	11.1%	4.4%	15.6%
P value	< 0.001	0.025	< 0.001

B

Figure 7-18. A, Diagnostic accuracy of dipyridamole stress myocardial perfusion single-photon emission CT (SPECT) as compared with exercise electrocardiography in asymptomatic type 2 diabetic women [18]. **B,** Prognosis by pharmacologic stress myocardial perfusion positron emission tomography (PET) in obese patients [19]. MI—myocardial infarction.

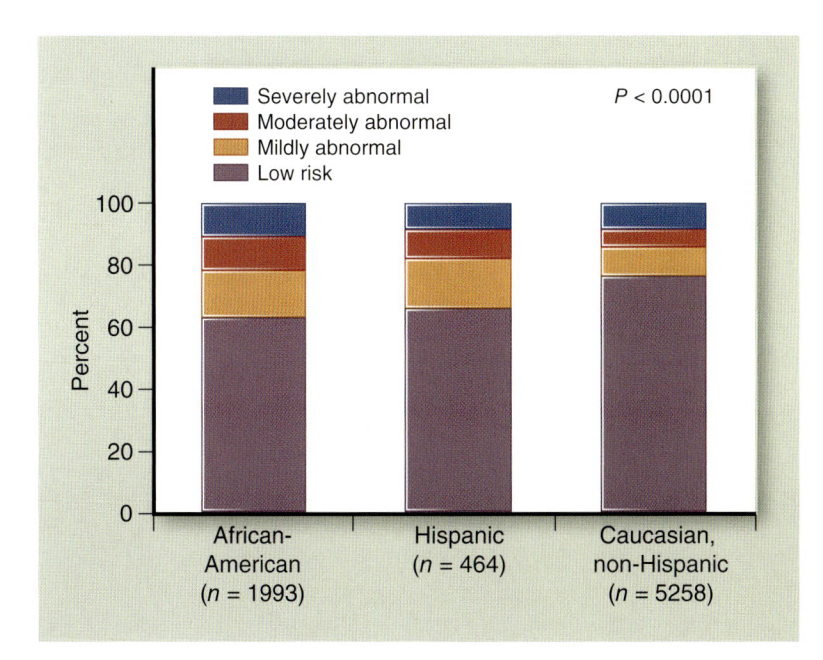

Figure 7-19. Prevalence of cardiovascular diseases according to ethnicity. Epidemiologic evidence is supportive of substantial variability in the prevalence of cardiovascular diseases in diverse ethnic populations [20]. Although it appears that the etiology for ethnic differences is multifaceted, there is supportive evidence that there are true phenotypic differences across racial and ethnic subsets of the population. This variability may be seen in the frequency, clustering of multiple risk factors, and treatment effectiveness in Hispanic populations with hypertriglyceridemia. African American and Asian Indian patients have some of the highest rates of atherosclerotic disease [19]. Yet, for African American patients, higher coronary disease mortality occurs in the setting of more frequent risk factors at a younger age and with less obstructive coronary disease [20]. This uncoupling between risk factor burden and coronary disease extent suggests that other factors may play a prominent role in risk assessment and, for our discussion, the role of single-photon emission CT imaging. This figure from a report published by the Myoview Multicenter Registry reveals that African American and Hispanic patients have a substantially higher rate of stress perfusion abnormalities (using the summed stress score risk groupings) [20].

Continued on the next page

Figure 7-19. *(Continued)* This finding was provocative to those familiar with laboratory datasets, as these ethnic minority cohorts are largely younger. Greater rates of provocative ischemia in the setting of nonobstructive coronary disease point to a greater role of microvascular or endothelial dysfunction as a prominent factor affecting outcome in certain minority patient populations [21].

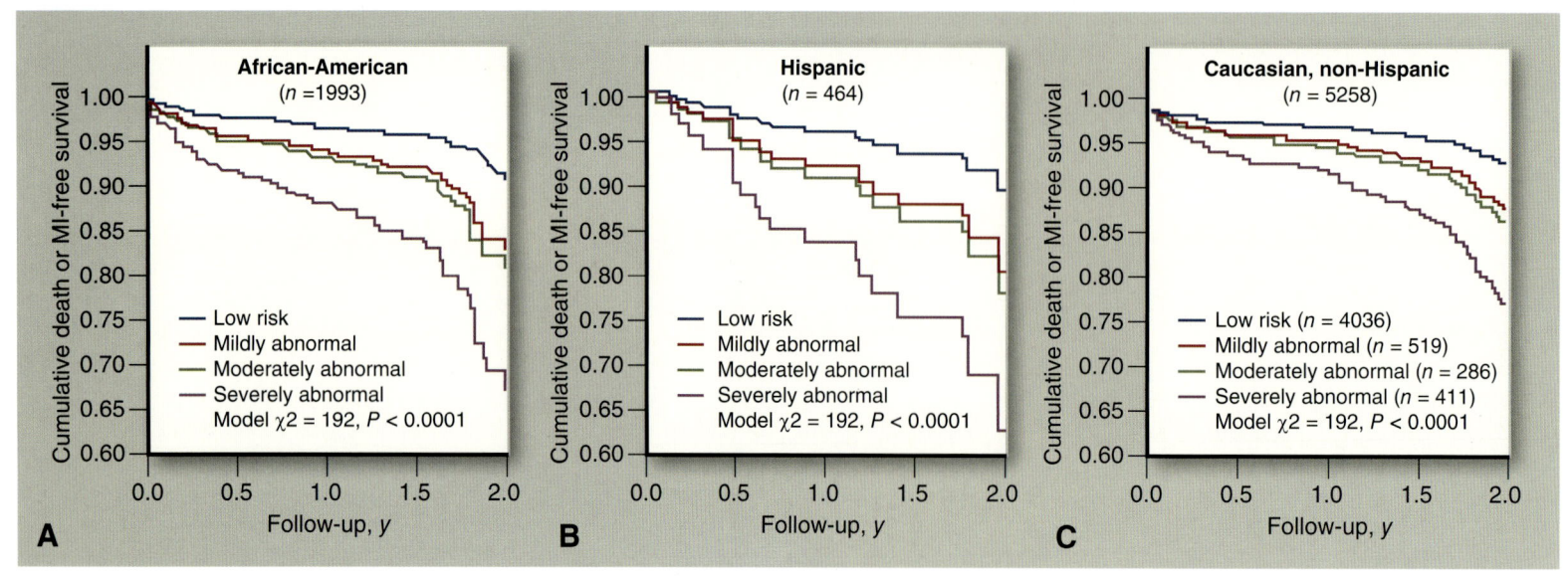

Figure 7-20. Event-free survival in African American and Hispanic patients versus white non-Hispanic patients. An examination of the dramatic differences in event-free survival for African American (**A**) and Hispanic patients (**B**) as compared with white non-Hispanic patients (**C**) reveals several notable phenomena [20]. This was the first study to find that in sufficiently large populations, effective risk stratification is possible using the 20-segment model summed stress score risk groupings in ethnic minority cohorts. Additionally, because of greater comorbidity, African American and Hispanic patients have decidedly higher rates of cardiac death or nonfatal myocardial infarction (MI) when compared with their white non-Hispanic counterparts. Thus, similar to our findings in diabetic patients, one must realize that comorbidity or the underlying hazard (or risk) in the population will drive the expected event rates. Therefore, for higher-risk patient subsets, although one may stratify risk from low to high, the event rates will be higher in minority populations because of more frequent risk factors and greater comorbidity burden. The effective risk stratification is notable given the evidence of less-prevalent obstructive coronary disease and is supportive of a greater role for physiologic or flow abnormalities in risk assessment for ethnic minority patients, particularly black and Hispanic patients. A low event rate in 4629 Asian patients with normal stress myocardial perfusion single-photon emission CT findings was recently reported, with annual cardiac event rates of approximately 0.7% [22].

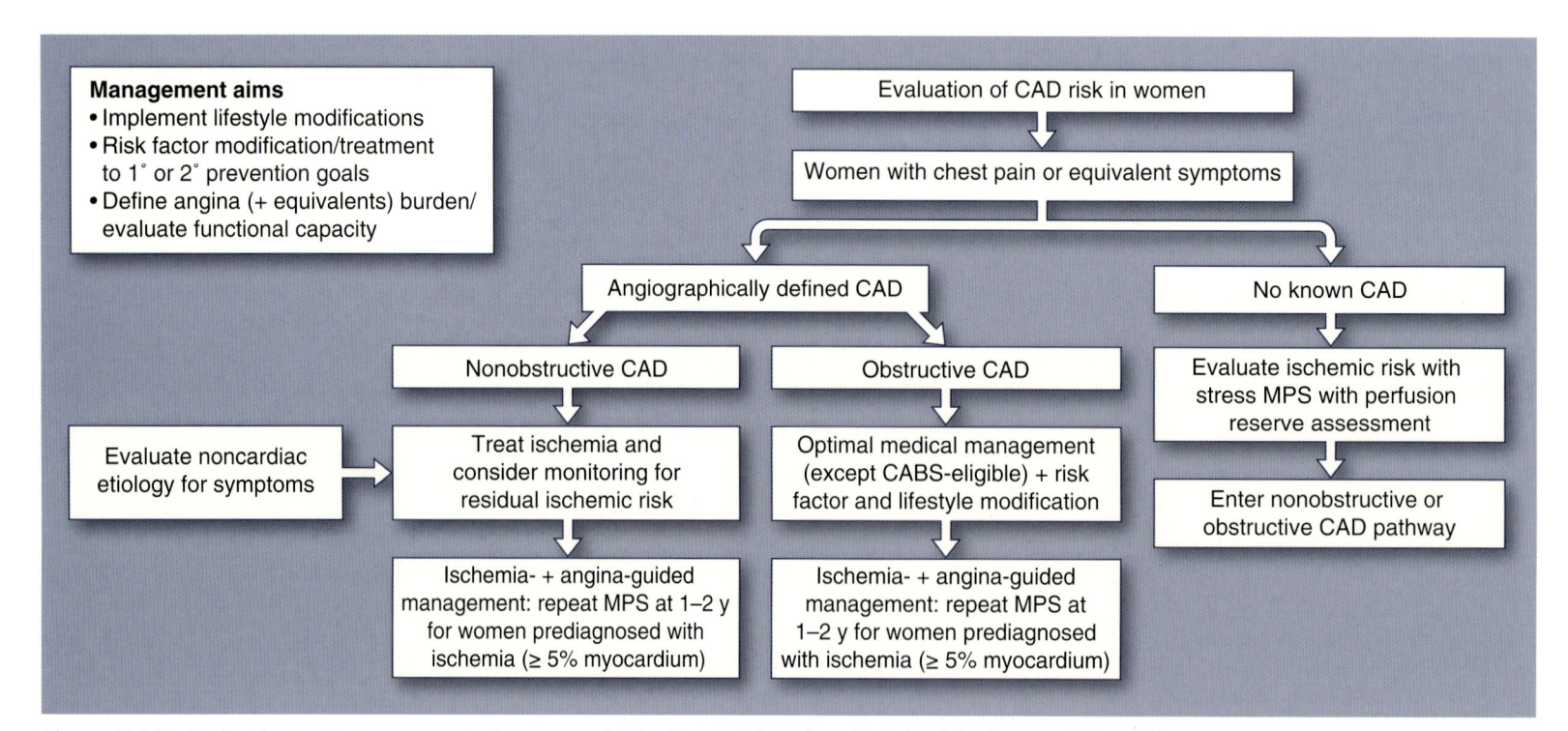

Figure 7-21. Evaluation and management of women at high risk or with suspected myocardial ischemia. Although this figure describes the care of symptomatic women, it may also be applied to the special populations described in this chapter. Using this management strategy, treatment is guided for two primary goals: optimal risk factor control/lifestyle modifications as well as resolution of ischemic symptoms.

Continued on the next page

Figure 7-21. *(Continued)* Using this strategy, as recently reported in the Clinical Outcomes Using Revascularization and Aggressive Drug Evaluation (COURAGE) trial, optimal medical therapy (OMT) becomes the default strategy for all patients with chronic stable angina [23], with the exception of patients eligible for coronary artery bypass surgery (CABS). A critical element to this management strategy is that a reevaluation of ischemic risk be considered after approximately 1 year following OMT, especially for those with persistent chest pain. It should be noted that the repeat scan is performed with the patient on medical therapy so as to evaluate the efficacy of therapy in ameliorating ischemia. At that time, patients with significant residual ischemia in the setting of obstructive coronary artery disease (CAD) should be considered for revascularization. For patients with nonobstructive CAD, consideration of noncardiac etiology for symptoms should be primary, followed by a management strategy that is guided by the presence and severity of inducible ischemia and treatment responsiveness to antianginal therapies [24].

References

1. Shaw LJ, Iskandrian AE: Prognostic value of gated myocardial perfusion SPECT. *J Nucl Cardiol* 2004, 11:171–185.

2. Expert Panel on Detection, Evaluation, and Treatment of High Blood Cholesterol in Adults: Executive Summary of the Third Report of the National Cholesterol Education Program (NCEP) Expert Panel on Detection, Evaluation, and Treatment of High Blood Cholesterol in Adults (Adult Treatment Panel III). *JAMA* 2001, 285:2486–2497.

3. National Center for Health Statistics: Health, United States 1999: health and aging chartbook. Available at http://www.cdc.gov/nchs/data/hus/hus99cht.pdf. Accessed April 25, 2005.

4. Mieres JH, Shaw LJ, Arai A, et al.: Role of noninvasive testing in the clinical evaluation of women with suspected coronary artery disease: consensus statement from the Cardiac Imaging Committee, Council on Clinical Cardiology, and the Cardiovascular Imaging and Intervention Committee, Council on Cardiovascular Radiology and Intervention, American Heart Association. *Circulation* 2005, 111:682–696.

5. Mieres JH, Shaw LJ, Hendel RC, et al.; Writing Group on Perfusion Imaging in Women: American Society of Nuclear Cardiology consensus statement: Task Force on Women and Coronary Artery Disease—the role of myocardial perfusion imaging in the clinical evaluation of coronary artery disease in women. *J Nucl Cardiol* 2003, 10:95–101.

6. Gibbons RJ, Balady GJ, Bricker JT, et al.; American College of Cardiology/American Heart Association Task Force on Practice Guidelines. Committee to Update the 1997 Exercise Testing Guidelines: ACC/AHA 2002 guideline update for exercise testing: summary article. A report of the American College of Cardiology/American Heart Association Task Force on Practice Guidelines (Committee to Update the 1997 Exercise Testing Guidelines). *J Am Coll Cardiol* 2002, 40:1531–1540.

7. Alexander KP, Shaw LJ, Shaw LK, et al.: Value of exercise treadmill testing in women. *J Am Coll Cardiol* 1998, 32:1657–1664.

8. Shaw LJ, Olson MB, Kip K, et al.: The value of estimated functional capacity in estimating outcome: results from the NHLBI-sponsored Women's Ischemia Syndrome Evaluation (WISE) study. *J Am Coll Cardiol* 2006, 47:S36–S43.

9. Olson MB, Kelsey SF, Matthews K, et al.: Symptoms, myocardial ischaemia, and quality of life in women: results from the NHLBI-sponsored WISE study. *Eur Heart J* 2003, 24:1506–1514.

10. Marwick TH, Shaw LJ, Lauer MS, et al.: The noninvasive prediction of cardiac mortality in men and women with known or suspected coronary artery disease. Economics of Noninvasive Diagnosis (END) Study Group. *Am J Med* 1999, 106:172–178.

11. Shaw LJ, Vasey C, Sawada S, et al.: Impact of gender on risk stratification by exercise and dobutamine stress echocardiography: long-term mortality in 4234 women and 6898 men. *Eur Heart J* 2005, 26:447–456.

12. Berman DS, Kang X, Hayes SW, et al.: Adenosine myocardial perfusion single-photon emission computed tomography in women compared with men. Impact of diabetes mellitus on incremental prognostic value and effect on patient management. *J Am Coll Cardiol* 2003, 41:1125–1133.

13. Shaw LJ, Bairey Merz CN, Pepine CJ, et al.; WISE Investigators: Insights from the NHLBI-sponsored Women's Ischemia Syndrome Evaluation (WISE) study. Part I: gender differences in traditional and novel risk factors, symptom evaluation, and gender-optimized diagnostic strategies. *J Am Coll Cardiol* 2006, 47:S4–S20.

14. Computed tomographic imaging within nuclear cardiology. *J Nucl Cardiol* 2005, 12:131–142.

15. Kang X, Berman DS, Lewin HC, et al.: Incremental prognostic value of myocardial perfusion single photon emission computed tomography in patients with diabetes mellitus. *Am Heart J* 1999, 138:1025–1032.

16. Giri S, Shaw LJ, Murthy DR, et al.: Impact of diabetes on the risk stratification using stress single photon emission computed tomography myocardial perfusion imaging in patients with symptoms suggestive of coronary artery disease. *Circulation* 2002, 105:32–40.

17. Gulati M, Black HR, Shaw LJ, et al.: The prognostic value of a nomogram for exercise capacity in women. *N Engl J Med* 2005, 353:468–475.

18. Smanio PE, Carvalho AC, Tebexreni AS, et al.: Coronary artery disease in asymptomatic type-2 diabetic women. A comparative study between exercise test, cardiopulmonary exercise test, and dipyridamole myocardial perfusion scintigraphy in the identification of ischemia. *Arq Bras Cardiol* 2007, 89:263–269, 290–297.

19. Yoshinaga K, Chow BJ, Williams K, et al.: What is the prognostic value of myocardial perfusion imaging using rubidium-82 positron emission tomography? *J Am Coll Cardiol* 2006, 48:1029–1039.

20. Shaw LJ, Hendel RC, Cerqueira M, et al.: Ethnic differences in the prognostic value of stress technetium-99m tetrofosmin gated single photon emission computed tomography myocardial perfusion imaging. *J Am Coll Cardiol* 2005, 45:1494–1504.

21. Bairey Merz CN, Shaw LJ, Reis SE, et al.; WISE Investigators: Insights from the NHLBI-sponsored Women's Ischemia Syndrome Evaluation (WISE) study. Part II: gender differences in presentation, diagnosis, and outcome with regard to gender-based pathophysiology of atherosclerosis and macrovascular and microvascular coronary disease. *J Am Coll Cardiol* 2006, 47:S21–S29.

22. Matsuo S, Nakajima K, Horie M, et al.; J-ACCESS Investigators: Prognostic value of normal stress myocardial perfusion imaging in Japanese population. *Circ J* 2008, 72:611–617.

23. Shaw LJ, Berman DS, Maron DJ, et al.; COURAGE Investigators: Optimal medical therapy with or without percutaneous coronary intervention to reduce ischemic burden: results from the Clinical Outcomes Utilizing Revascularization and Aggressive Drug Evaluation (COURAGE) trial nuclear substudy. *Circulation* 2008, 117:1283–1291.

24. Peix A, García EJ, Valiente J, et al.: Ischemia in women with angina and normal coronary angiograms. *Coron Artery Dis* 2007, 18:361–366.

Imaging Cardiac Metabolism

Heinrich Taegtmeyer and Vasken Dilsizian

Cardiac metabolism is the process that converts energy providing fuels to ATP. ATP is largely used to maintain myocardial contraction and to regulate the membrane pumps and movements of ions in and out of the cell. For a given physiologic environment, the heart consumes the most efficient metabolic fuel. In the normally oxygenated heart, fatty acids account for the majority of ATP production with glucose making only a small contribution to the ATP production, unless there is an insulin surge. During an acute increase in work load, for example, inotropic stimulation, the heart immediately mobilizes its metabolic reserve contained in glycogen (transient increase in glycogen oxidation) and meets the needs for additional energy from the oxidation of carbohydrate substrates (glucose and lactate). When the oxygen supply is decreased, the heart helps protect itself from an oxygen-lacking fate of infarction by switching its energy source to glycolysis, down-regulating mitochondrial oxidative metabolism, and reducing contractile function.

The interrelationship between mechanical function, myocardial perfusion, metabolic, and energy consuming processes within the heart is complex. A metabolic switch from fatty acids to glucose seems pivotal in preserving myocardial viability and likely represents the earliest adaptive response to myocardial ischemia. Perhaps the most dramatic clinical application for metabolic switch from fatty acid utilization to glycolysis is in myocardial hibernation. Hibernating myocardium represents dysfunctional but viable myocardium most likely the result of extensive cellular reprogramming due to repetitive episodes of chronic ischemia. While the true mechanism for viability remodeling in hibernation is likely to be much more complex, it is thought to be related, in part, to the increased glycogen content and myocardial ATP levels in such cells, simulating the fetal heart. Because glucose transport and phosphorylation is readily tracked by the uptake and retention of [^{18}F]-2-deoxy, 2-fluoroglucose, hibernating myocardium is readily detected by enhanced glucose uptake in the same regions by external detectors, such as PET.

Recent clinical studies have also shown the potential utility of metabolic adaptation in the emergency department as well as for detection of coronary artery disease in the form of "ischemic memory." Ischemic memory represents prolonged but reversible metabolic recovery after transient myocardial ischemia, also known as "metabolic stunning." Other disease entities where metabolic imaging by nuclear techniques can play an important role include identification of microvascular disease and subendocardial ischemia in symptomatic women with nonobstructive coronary artery disease, diabetic heart disease, and left ventricular remodeling in hypertrophy and congestive heart failure. There has been dramatic increase in the prevalence of left ventricular remodeling in hypertophy and heart failure in recent years. Emerging evidence suggests a role of altered metabolism in the progression of both left ventricular hypertrophy and remodeling. Some of the clinical evidence includes 1) variable prognosis in patients with similar left ventricular mass in hypertrophy, 2) loss of metabolic flexibility, which may portend worse prognosis in patients with heart failure, and 3) development of modulators for medical treatment in heart failure, such as fatty acid oxidation inhibitors (ranolazine) and insulin sensitizers.

Metabolic adaptation represents one of the earliest responses to myocardial ischemia, left ventricular remodeling, and diabetic and uremic heart disease. Recognizing key intracellular signals that link energy substrate metabolism with gene expression may allow the discovery of more specific molecular targets for imaging, diagnosis, and treatment of cardiovascular disease.

Single Photon and Positron-emitting Radiotracers

SPECT Radiotracers

^{123}I-BMIPP	13 hour half-life, cyclotron-produced

PET Radiotracers

^{11}C-palmitate	20 minute half-life; cyclotron-produced
^{11}C-acetate	20 minute half-life; cyclotron-produced
^{18}F-fluorodeoxyglucose	110 minute half-life; cyclotron-produced

Figure 8-1. Single photon and positron-emitting metabolic radiotracers. By labeling various compounds of physiologic interest, valuable insights into biochemical pathways and tissue metabolism can be obtained in functional and dysfunctional myocardium. Current Food and Drug Administration–approved and Centers for Medicare & Medicaid Services–reimbursable PET myocardial metabolic radiotracer is limited to ^{18}F-fluorodeoxyglucose (FDG). FDG is a glucose analogue that is used clinically to image myocardial glucose utilization with PET. ^{11}C-palmitate is a PET radiolabeled straight-chain fatty acid, and β-methyl p-[^{123}I]-iodophenyl-pentadecanoic acid (^{123}I-BMIPP) is a SPECT radiolabeled branched-chain fatty acid. Both radiotracers interrogate myocardial fatty acid metabolism in vivo. Uptake and clearance of ^{11}C-palmitate from the myocyte occurs quite rapidly via β-oxidation, while the methyl chain in ^{123}I-BMIPP results in metabolic trapping of the radiotracer in the myocyte. ^{11}C-acetate is a PET radiolabeled short-chain acid that is ideal for in vivo assessment of myocardial oxidative metabolism.

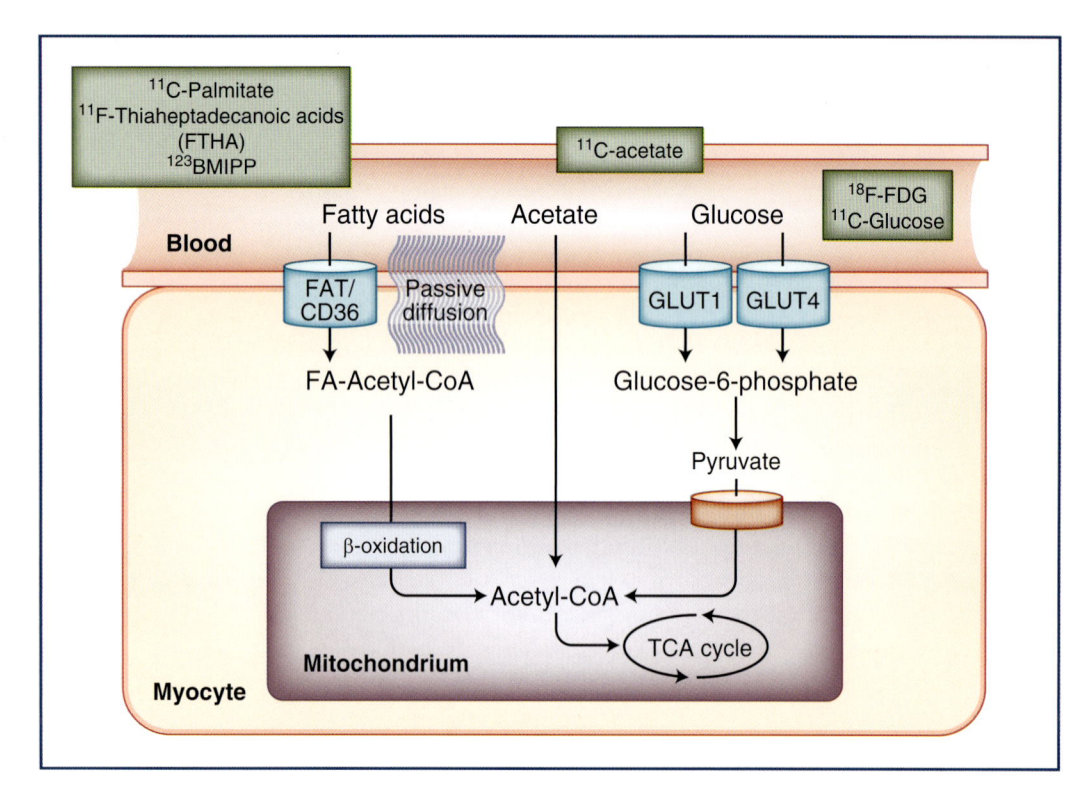

Figure 8-2. Imaging cardiac metabolism. Fatty acid, glucose, and oxidative metabolism assessment with various SPECT and PET radiotracers are shown. Free fatty acids account for the majority of ATP production when the heart is in a normal, fasting state. Following uptake of the radiotracers by active transport or diffusion, fatty acids are converted by β-oxidation into acetyl-coenzyme A (CoA). Under anaerobic or non-fasting conditions, energy production shifts to glucose metabolism. Conversion of glucose via glucose-6-phosphate and pyruvate provides the source of acetyl-CoA. Oxidative metabolism also provides an important contribution to cardiac metabolism. In mitochondria, ATP production occurs via the tricarboxylic acid (TCA) cycle. BMIPP—β-methyl p-[^{123}I]-iodophenyl-pentadecanoic acid; FA—fatty acid; FAT/CD36—fatty acid translocase; FDG—fluorodeoxyglucose; THA—thiaheptadecanoic acid; GLUT1 and GLUT4—glucose transporters 1 and 4.

Metabolic Signals in Normal and Diseased Heart: New Opportunities for Molecular Imaging

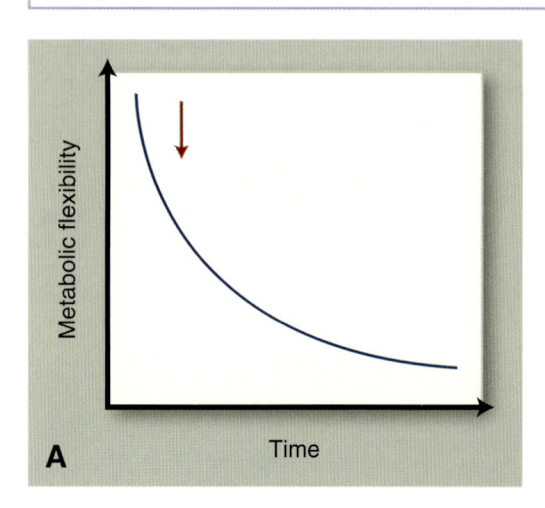

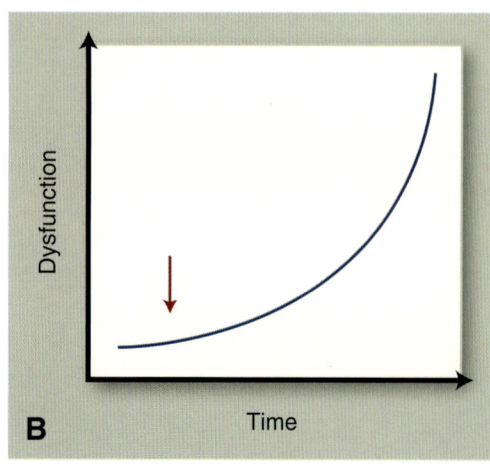

Figure 8-3. A refined understanding of metabolic regulation may result in the early diagnosis of myocardial ischemia and heart failure. The hyperbolic curves illustrate a hypothetical time course of the rapid loss of metabolic flexibility antedating contractile dysfunction in the path of metabolic and functional remodeling of the stressed heart. The loss of metabolic flexibility (**A**, *arrow*) and changes in gene expression likely precede the onset of severe contractile dysfunction (**B**, *arrow*) [1]. The concept depicted in this figure is supported by the observation that transcriptional changes of enzymes and proteins of energy substrate metabolism antedate any contractile dysfunction in hearts from diabetic animals [2]. (*Adapted from* Taegtmeyer et al. [1].)

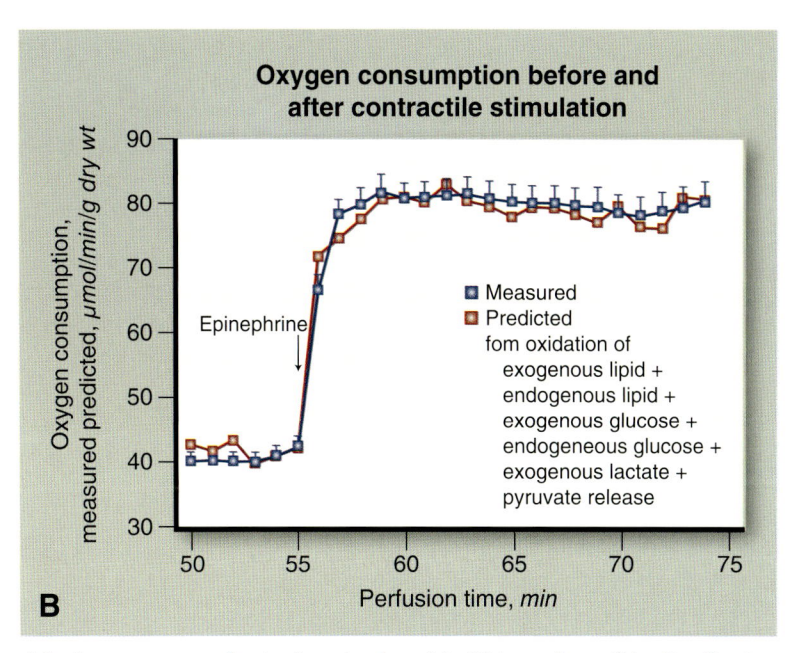

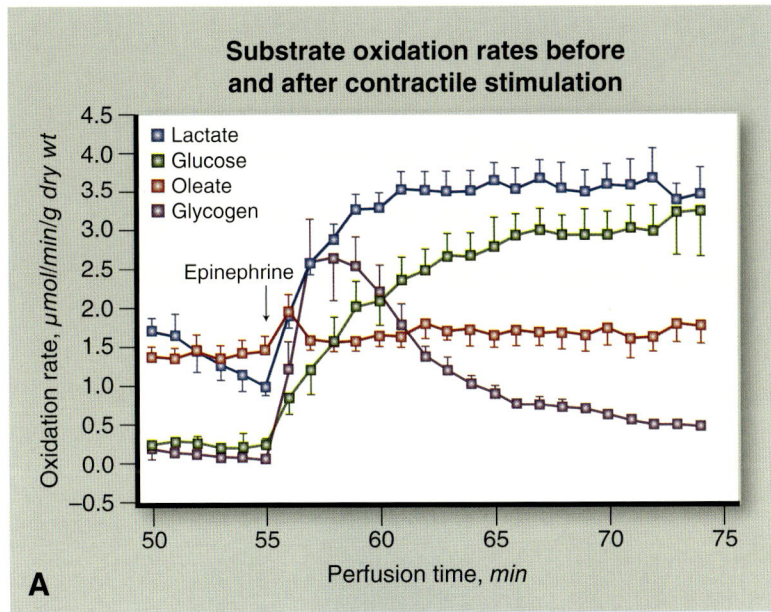

Figure 8-4. **A** and **B**, Major energy substrate oxidation rates before and after contractile stimulation. Fuel selection during acute transition from low to high workload (1 μM epinephrine and afterload increase by 40%) of isolated working rat heart is shown. When the workload is acutely increased, glycogen and, to a lesser extent, lactate are important energy substrates for the aerobic heart (**A**). With more prolonged adrenergic stimulation, nonesterified fatty acids and lactate are the major respiratory substrates for the heart, which is in keeping with the in vivo observations in the exercising state. When all relevant exogenous and endogenous substrates are examined, the increase in carbohydrate oxidation upon adrenergic stimulation is shown to be selective. Although exogenous fatty acid oxidation is not significantly changed, total β-oxidation was increased by 40%, and the increase was associated with a decrease in the level of malonyl-coenzyme A (CoA). Carbohydrate oxidation is increased selectively because total β-oxidation, regulated mostly by malonyl-CoA levels in the cytosol, is independent of the activity of pyruvate dehydrogenase complex in the mitochondria. Using values of the distribution between oxidation and release of lactate or pyruvate during adrenergic stimulation, the calculated effective value of ATP synthesized/O_2 consumed ratio (not to be confused with the ATP/O_2 ratio calculated for complete oxidation) is 5.4 for glucose and 5.7 for glycogen, which is higher than those calculated for oleate (5.0) and lactate (4.8). The higher ATP yield with glycogen during periods of high energy demand provides a potential explanation for why the heart adopts the strategy of preferential increase in carbohydrate oxidation to deal with increased energy demand. **B**, Measured and predicted values for oxygen consumption. Predicted rates are based on the sum of the measured rates of oxygen of every major substrate (glucose, glycogen, lactate, oleate, triglycerides, and release of pyruvate). The close agreement between measured and predicted MVO_2 validates the assumption of uniform isotopic dilution, and that every major oxidizable substrate was quantitatively accounted for in the heart. (*Adapted from* Goodwin et al. [3].)

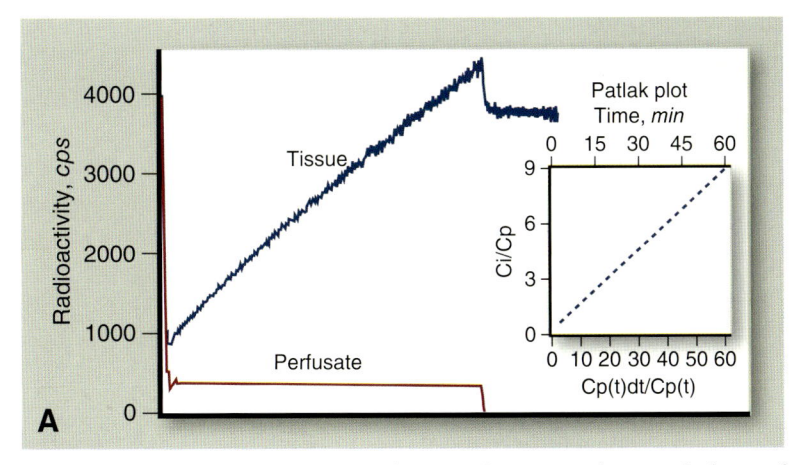

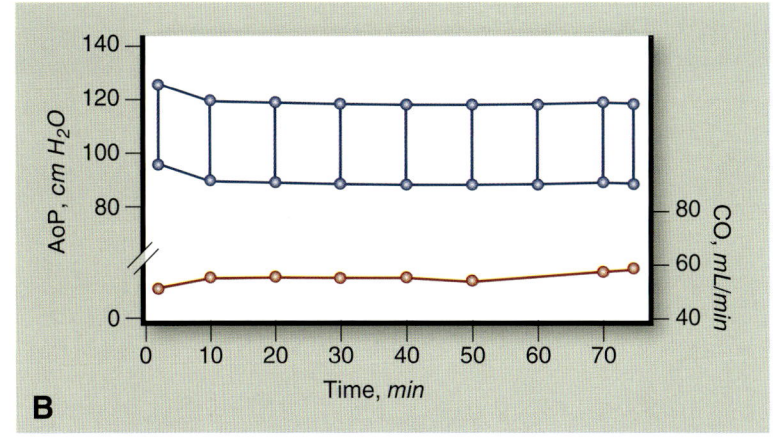

Figure 8-5. Direct evidence that the initial steps in the metabolism of fluorodeoxyglucose (FDG) are the same as for glucose and that FDG is retained by the tissue in proportion to the rate of glucose utilization. The underlying premise of FDG PET imaging is that FDG behaves similarly to the tracee, glucose, with respect to facilitated transport across the sarcolemma and subsequent intracellular phosphorylation by hexokinase. Time-activity curves obtained in an isolated working rat heart (afterload = 100 cm H_2O, preload = 15 cm H_2O) with Krebs-Henseleit saline containing glucose (10 mM) and FDG (350 uCi/200 mL perfusate) for the first 60 minutes is shown. After an initial phase of tracer equilibrium (**A**), myocardial uptake of FDG was linear (*top curve*), whereas tracer activity in the perfusate remained constant (*bottom curve*). Graphical analysis of the myocardial and perfusate FDG concentrations acquired between 5 and 60 minutes by Patlak analysis (*inset* in **A**) showed a stable and linear plot from 20 to 60 minutes. Aortic pressures and cardiac output were also stable throughout the experiment (**B**). At 60 minutes, when the perfusion medium was changed to buffer containing no tracer, radioactivity in the tissue fell abruptly and then remained stable for the duration of the washout period. The above phenomena suggest clearance of the radiotracer from the heart chambers and the vascular and extracellular spaces and metabolic trapping of FDG. Tissue accumulation of FDG decreased with a reduction in work load and with the addition of competing substrates. Insulin caused a significant increase in FDG accumulation in hearts from fasted but not from fed animals. These data confirm the utility of FDG to assess myocardial glucose metabolism in the clinical setting by showing that tissue uptake and retention of the tracer in the isolated working rat heart responds to physiologic interventions in the same way as glucose. (*Adapted from* Nguyen et al. [4].)

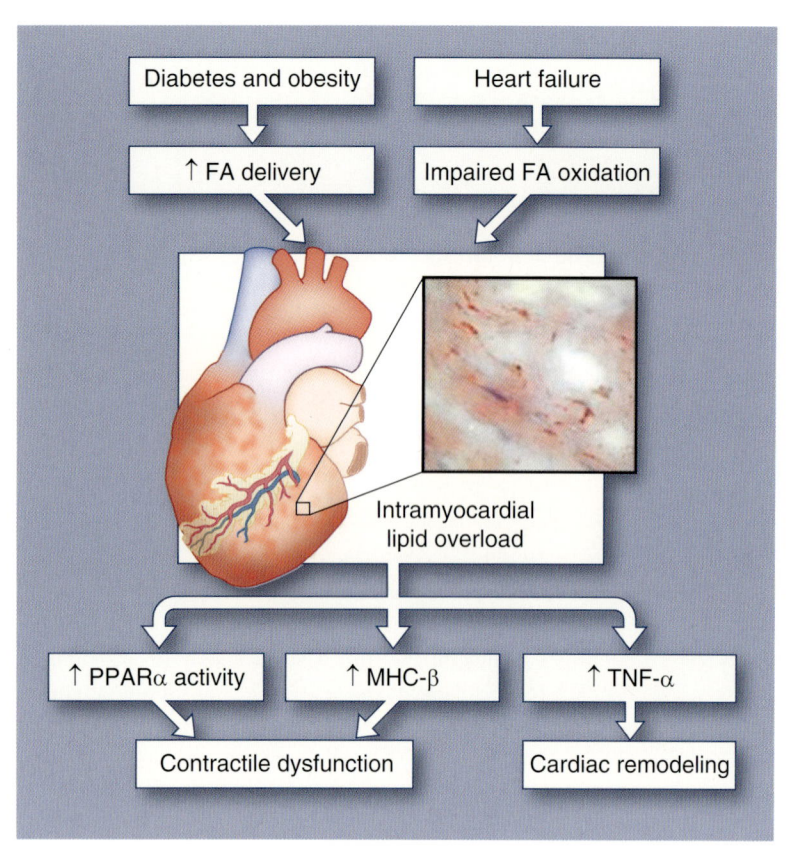

Figure 8-6. Left ventricular dysfunction in patients with diabetes and/or obesity or heart failure may be association with altered metabolism independent of the presence of underlying coronary artery disease. For example, patients with similar glycemic control (HgA1c) can have dramatically different rates of left ventricular dysfunction. Both increased fatty acid (FA) delivery (eg, diabetes, obesity) and impaired FA oxidation (eg, heart failure) result in severe intramyocardial triglyceride accumulation. Triglycerides are the "canary in the coal mine" for a host of other lipotoxic intermediates, including oxygen-derived free radicals, diacylglycerol, and ceramide. Oil-red-O stain of triglycerides is shown in failing heart muscle. MHC-β—myosin heavy chain–β; PPARα—peroxisome proliferation–activated receptor α; TNF-β—tumor necrosis factor–α. (*Adapted from* Sharma *et al.* [5].)

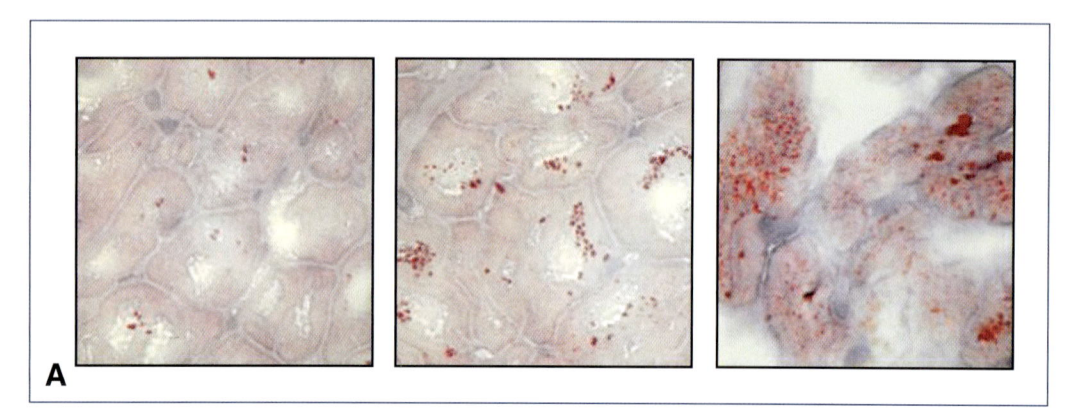

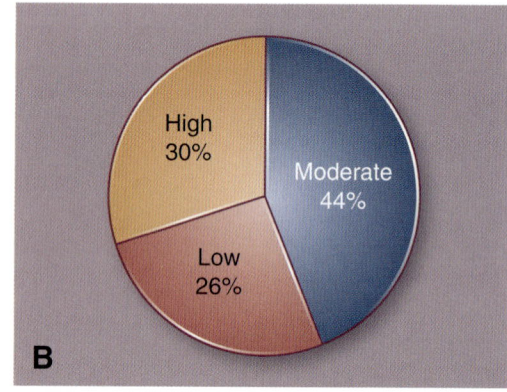

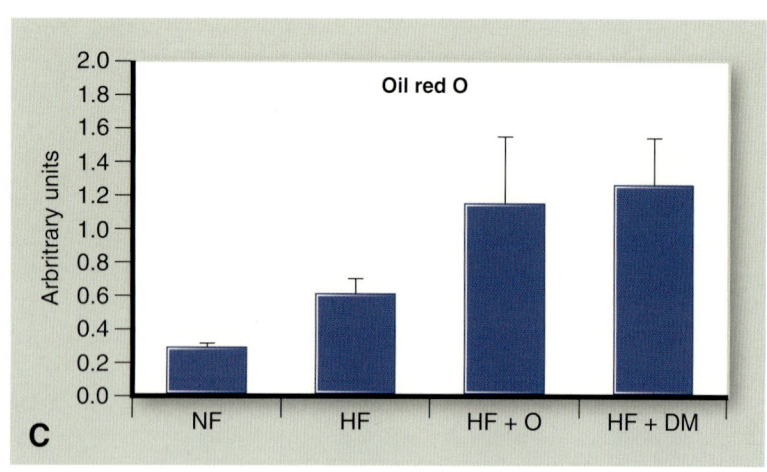

Figure 8-7. Intramyocardial triglyceride overload and changes in gene expression are associated with contractile left ventricular dysfunction in patients with nonischemic heart failure. Low, intermediate, and high intramyocardial lipid accumulation can be appreciated histologically in heart tissue samples from these patients (**A**). In a study of 27 nonischemic failing hearts, high amounts of intramyocardial lipid overload was present in 30% of hearts (**B**). The highest levels of lipid staining were observed in failing hearts of patients with coexisting diabetes or obesity (body mass index > 30) (**C**). Intramyocardial lipid deposition was associated with an upregulation of peroxisome proliferation–activated receptor (PPAR) α–regulated genes, myosin heavy chain–β, and tumor necrosis factor–α. Intramyocardial lipid overload is a relatively common finding in nonischemic heart failure and is associated with a distinct gene expression profile that is similar to an animal model of lipotoxicity and cardiac dysfunction. Metabolic imaging may play an important role for detection of subclinical disease early in the process of left ventricular dysfunction and/or remodeling. Early identification may be more amenable to medical therapy, such as PPAR agents, insulin, and fish oil analogues, and in prevention. DM—diabetes mellitus; HF—heart failure; NF—nonfailing; O—obesity. (*Adapted from* Sharma *et al.* [5].)

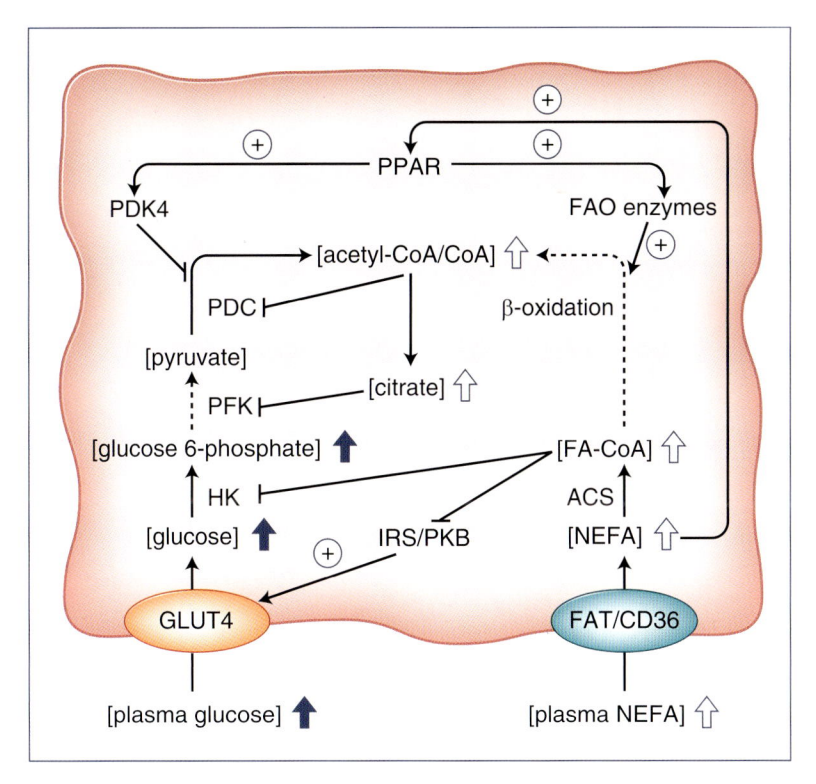

Figure 8-8. Mechanisms of fatty acid (FA) inhibition on glucose utilization by the heart. During diabetes, both plasma glucose and plasma nonesterified FA (NEFA) levels are elevated. The latter results in increased intracellular levels of FAs and their fatty acetyl-coenzyme A (FA-CoA) derivatives. FA-CoAs inhibit insulin-mediated glucose transport by inhibiting insulin receptor substrates (IRS) and protein kinase B (PKB). FA-CoAs can directly inhibit hexokinase (HK). Increased β-oxidation (due to increased substrate availability and increased gene expression of FA oxidation [FAO] enzymes via peroxisome proliferation–activated receptor [PPAR] activation) results in an increase in the mitochondrial acetyl-CoA/CoA ratio. The combined effects of increased PDK4 expression (induced through FA activation of PPAR) and increased acetyl-CoA/CoA ratio severely inhibit the pyruvate dehydrogenase complex (PDC). In addition, the increased acetyl-CoA/CoA ratio promotes citrate efflux from the mitochondrion into the cytosol, where it is able to inhibit phosphofructokinase (PFK). Despite decreased insulin-mediated glucose transport, glucose uptake by the diabetic heart is comparable to the normal heart because of the hyperglycemia. Glycolytic intermediates therefore accumulate in the cardiomyocyte. (*Adapted from* Taegtmeyer *et al.* [6].)

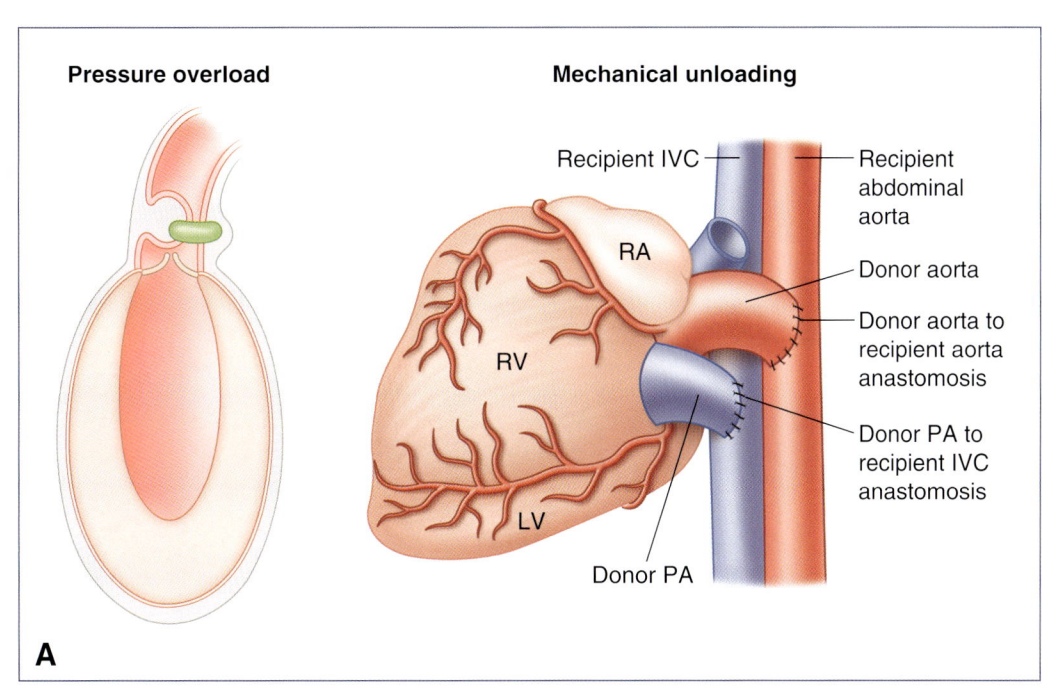

Figure 8-9. Metabolic processes are transcriptionally regulated in response to chronic changes in the work load of the heart. The change in cardiac mass by both pressure overload and ventricular unloading is a mechanism of adaptation accompanied by the re-expression of fetal genes (**A**). However, cardiac hypertrophy, if not treated, evolves to an uncompensated state of heart failure, whereas the process of atrophy induced by ventricular unloading rapidly stabilizes and shows no further progression thereafter. Therefore, unloading the failing heart reduces cardiac mass by a self-limited process and limits energy expenditure by preserving the expression of fetal isoforms of proteins regulating myocardial energetics. These mechanisms can explain the clinical improvement of patients with heart failure after treatment by a left ventricular assist device (LVAD). Unloading the heart with a LVAD is now used in clinical practice for patients with advanced heart failure awaiting heart transplantation, and mechanical unloading may improve cardiac function to an extent that makes transplantation no longer necessary. Such improvement results from a better contractile performance of the myocytes after LVAD therapy, indicating that mechanical unloading in vivo affects the expression of genes coding for contractile proteins and/or metabolic enzymes. These clinical results prompted investigators to assess the molecular response of the heart to unloading [7].

Continued on the next page

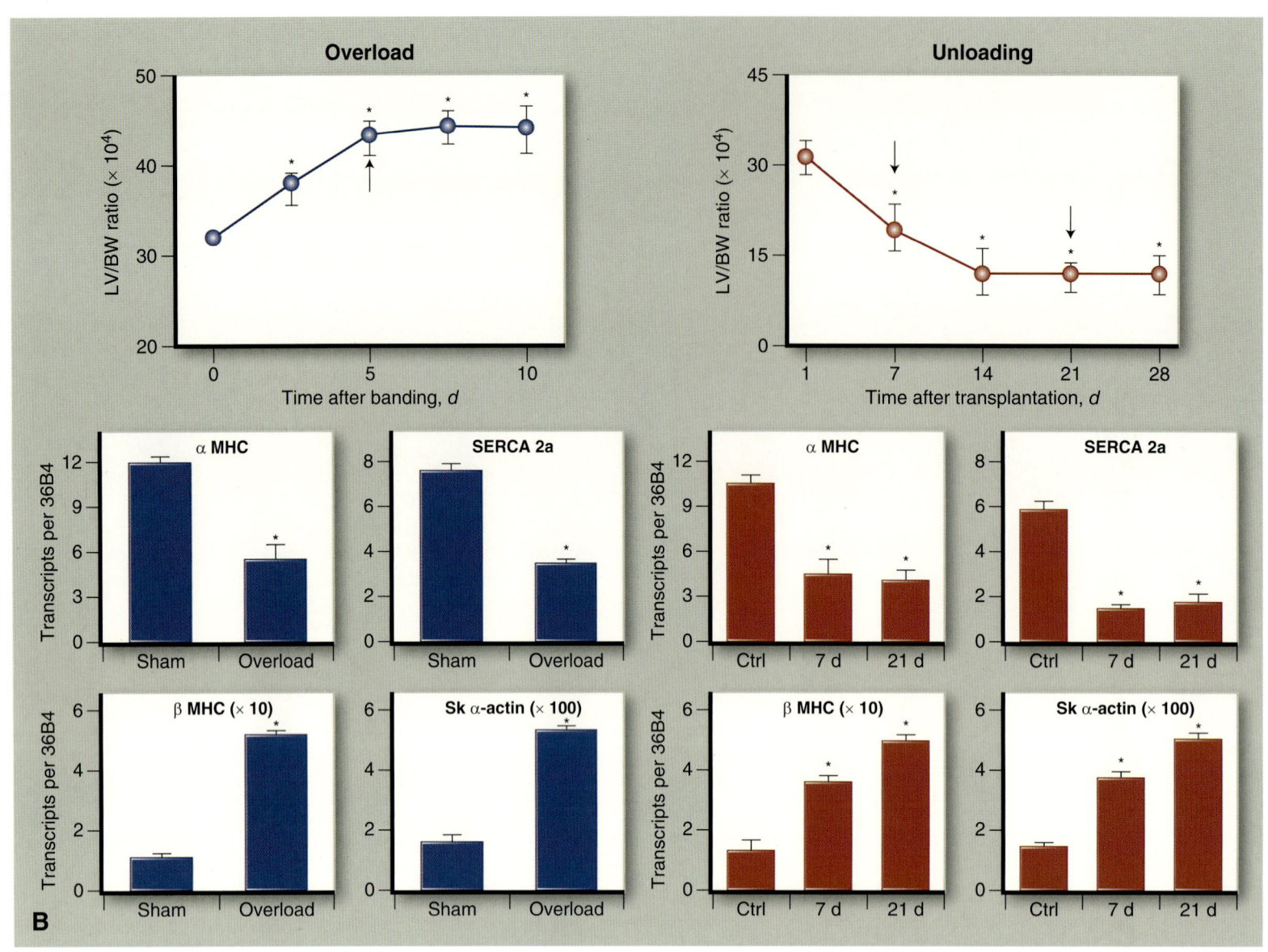

Figure 8-9. *(Continued)* The t*op two panels* of **B** show the changes in left ventricular mass (LV/BW ratio) in response to pressure overload and unloading. The *lower panels* show the expression of α myosin heavy chain (α MHC), β MHC, SERCA 2a, and SK α-actin in 1) hypertrophied hearts compared with hearts from sham-operated rats, and 2) unloaded hearts compared with control hearts up to 28 days after transplantation. Data are reported as the number of mRNA transcripts per number of 36B4 molecules (constitutive housekeeping gene product). Both conditions induced a re-expression of growth factors and proto-oncogenes, and a downregulation of the "adult" isoforms, but not of the "fetal" isoforms, of proteins regulating myocardial energetics. Therefore, opposite changes in cardiac workload in vivo induce similar patterns of gene response. Reactivation of fetal genes may underlie the functional improvement of an unloaded failing heart. Ctrl—control. (*Adapted from* Depre *et al.* [7].)

186 Atlas of Nuclear Cardiology

Figure 8-10. Peroxisome proliferation–activated receptor α (PPARα) activation of target metabolic genes. PPARα, a transcription factor that modulates fatty acid metabolism, regulates substrate preference in the heart. Although in acute ischemia there is a switch in substrate preference from fatty acids to glucose, metabolic gene expression in repetitive ischemia is not well described. In a mouse model of ischemic cardiomyopathy, the role of metabolic gene expression induced by repetitive ischemia/reperfusion was assessed [8]. In response to repetitive ischemia, there was a reversible downregulation of the genes that modulate fatty acid metabolism and myosin heavy chain isoforms in the heart. Overexpression of extracellular superoxide dismutase, an endogenous antioxidant enzyme, in hearts exposed to repetitive ischemia failed to cause the decrease in metabolic and myosin isoform gene expression. When fatty acid metabolism—in hearts exposed to repetitive ischemia—was pharmacologically reactivated, there was worsened contractile function, microinfarctions, and triglyceride accumulation within cardiomyocytes. These findings suggest that downregulation of fatty acid metabolic gene expression in the hibernating myocardium is an adaptive mechanism. Furthermore, modulation of myocardial metabolism may provide a pharmacologic target for cardiac protection in repetitive ischemia. In another experimental model of insulin resistance and type 2 diabetes, changing the metabolic profile, reducing myocardial lipid accumulation, and promoting the down-regulation of PPARα-regulated genes, PPARγ activation led to an increased capacity of the myocardium to oxidize glucose and to a tighter coupling of oxidative metabolism [9]. Perhaps phenotypic characterization of genetic variables, such as PPAR, may play an important role in the future for drug development and individualized medicine. (*Adapted from* Dewald *et al.* [8].)

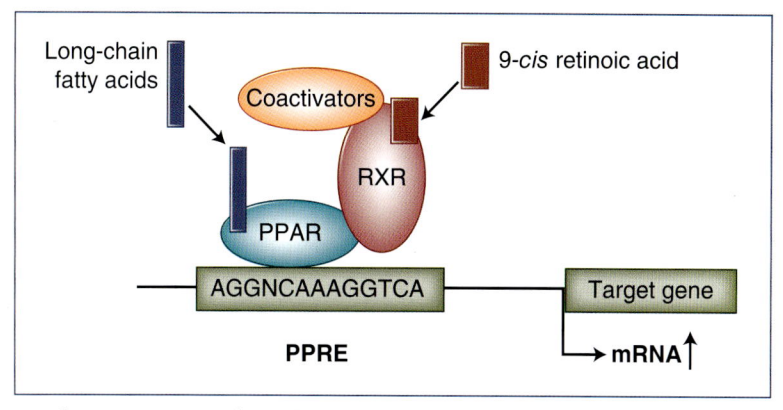

Clinical Application of Myocardial Metabolism: PET and SPECT Techniques

PET Techniques: ^{11}C-palmitate

Image acquisition to start at 15–20 mCi bolus injection of the tracer and to continue 40–60 min

Initial uptake and distribution in the myocardium is determined primarily by regional blood flow

In the cytosol, ^{11}C-palmitate is esterified to ^{11}C-acyl-CoA, which is mediated by thiokinase, an energy-dependent reaction, resulting in trapping of the tracer in the myocardium

Thereafter, ^{11}C-acyl-CoA either enters the endogenous lipid pool as ^{11}C glycerides and ^{11}C phospholipids or moves via the carnitine shuttle to the mitochondria, where rapid degradation by ß-oxidation results in the generation of carbon dioxide

A

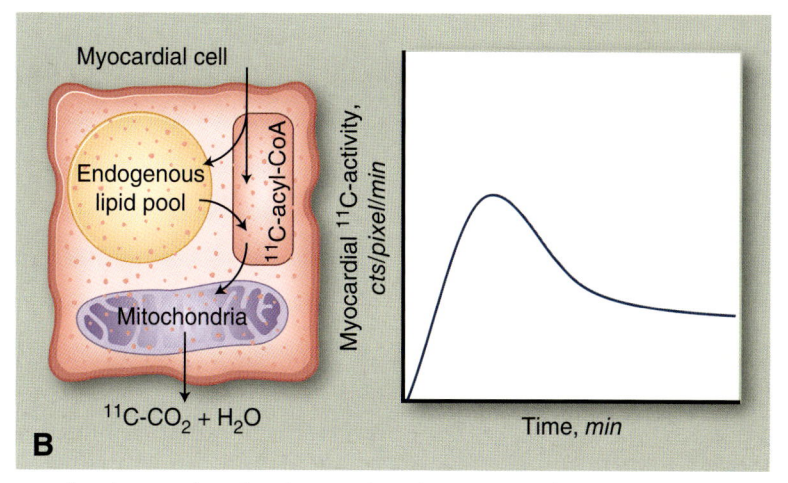

B

Figure 8-11. PET techniques: ^{11}C-palmitate. **A,** The principle of using a metabolic tracer for myocardial imaging is based on the concept that viable myocytes in hypoperfused and dysfunctional regions are metabolically active, while scarred or fibrotic tissue is metabolically inactive. Under fasting and aerobic conditions, long-chain fatty acids are the preferred fuel in the heart because they supply 65% to 70% of the energy for the working heart, and approximately 15% to 20% of the total energy supply comes from glucose. As such, early studies focused on the characterization of myocardial kinetics of the long-chain fatty acid, ^{11}C-palmitate, using PET. Uptake of ^{11}C-palmitate in the myocardium is dependent on regional perfusion, diffusion across the sarcolemmal membrane, transporter protein, and acceptance in the cytosol by binding to CoA. In normally perfused myocardium, the extraction fraction of ^{11}C-palmitate is 40%. The transporter protein of long-chain fatty acids across myocardial cells has a molecular weight of 40 kD; within the myocyte fatty acids are bound to storage protein with a molecular weight of 12 kD. Once in the cell, metabolic activation of ^{11}C-palmitate occurs by binding to coenzyme A. Depending on demand, about 80% of the extracted ^{11}C-palmitate is activated for transport from the lipid pool into the mitochondria (via the carnitine shuttle) for breakdown by β-oxidation. β-Oxidation results in the generation of carbon dioxide, which appears in the venous effluent of the coronary circulation in less than a minute after ^{11}C-acyl-CoA transfer into the mitochondria.

B, External measurement by dynamic PET imaging allows the observation of tracer inflow, peak accumulation, and release of the tracer within a particular region of interest in the myocardium. Fatty acid imaging with radioiodine-labeled fatty acid analogues such as β-methyliodopentadecanoic acid is also possible using SPECT. (**B,** *adapted from* Feinendegen [10].)

SPECT Techniques: ¹²³I-BMIPP

¹²³I-BMIPP is a methyl branched-chain fatty acid, which is trapped in myocardial cells with limited catabolism

Uptake of BMIPP from the plasma into myocytes occurs via CD36 transporter protein present on the sacrolemmal membrane

Once in the cell, BMIPP will either back-diffuse to the plasma, accumulate in the lipid pool, or undergo limited alpha- and beta-oxidation; enzymatic conversion of BMIPP to BMIPP-CoA or triacylglycerol in the myocyte is ATP dependent and is an irreversible step

Thus, uptake of BMIPP in the myocardium most likely reflects activation of fatty acids of CoA, and indirectly, of cellular ATP production resulting from fatty acid metabolism

A

B

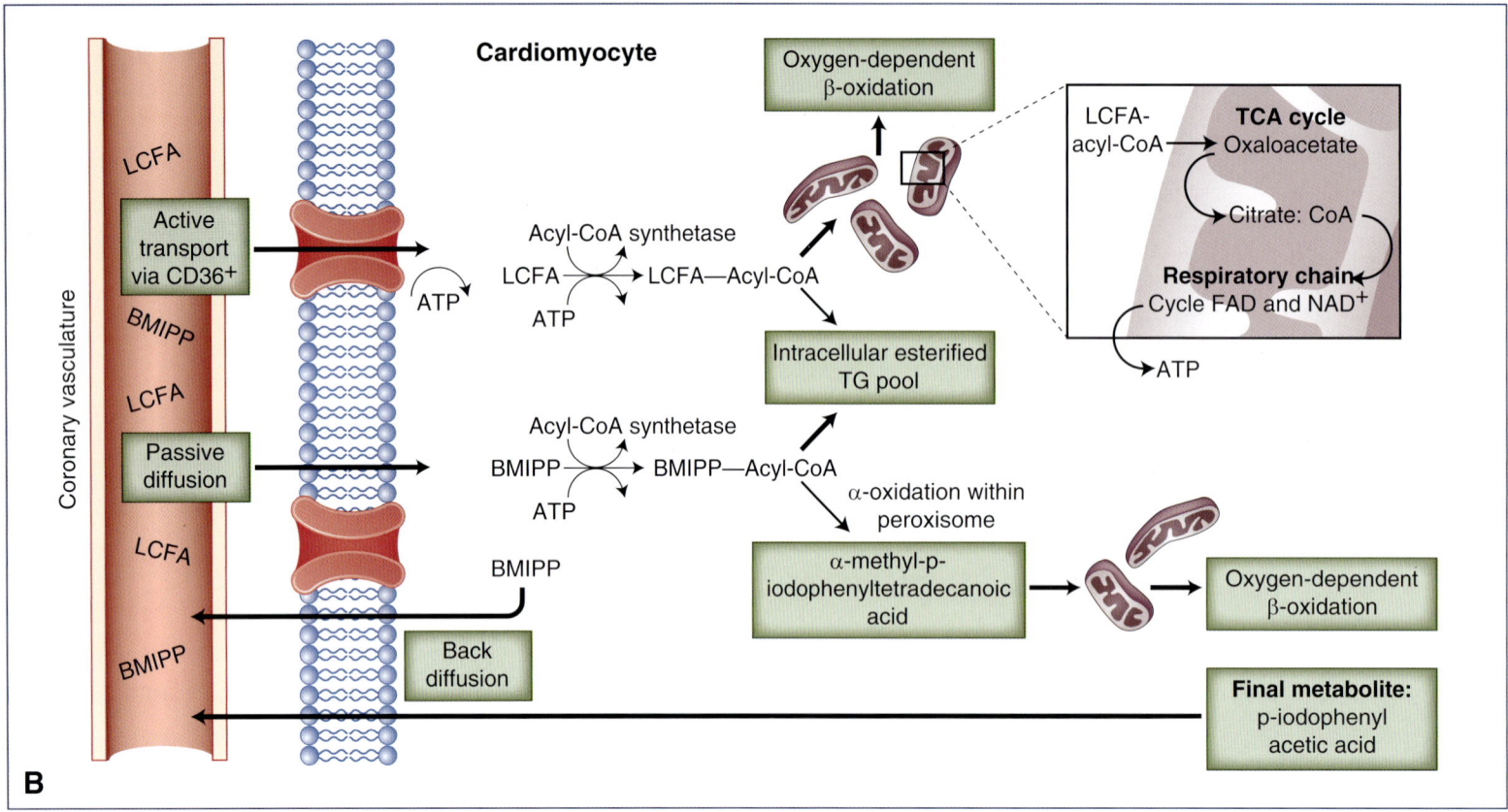

Figure 8-12. A, SPECT techniques: β-methyl-p-[¹²³I]-iodophenyl-pentadecanoic acid (¹²³I-BMIPP). Alterations in myocardial fatty acid metabolism were first evaluated noninvasively in humans using the positron-emitting radiotracer 11C-palmitate, which requires an on-site cyclotron and a PET camera. Because most nuclear cardiology laboratories are equipped with SPECT cameras, investigators subsequently focused their attention on developing gamma-emitting fatty acid tracers. In contrast to palmitate, BMIPP is an iodine-labeled, methyl branched-chain fatty acid that is predominantly trapped in myocardial cells with limited catabolism. Uptake of BMIPP from the plasma into myocytes occurs via CD36 transporter protein present on the sarcolemmal membrane. Once in the cell, BMIPP will either back-diffuse to the plasma, accumulate in the lipid pool, or undergo limited alpha- and beta-oxidation. Enzymatic conversion of BMIPP to BMIPP-CoA or triacylglycerol in the myocyte is ATP dependent and is an irreversible step. Such conversion prevents back-diffusion of BMIPP to the plasma and facilitates its cellular retention. The prolonged retention of BMIPP in the myocardium combined with rapid clearance from the blood and diminished uptake in the liver and lung results in excellent visualization and imaging of the myocardium by SPECT techniques. Thus, BMIPP provides a means of measuring myocardial fatty acid utilization in vivo. In the setting of myocardial ischemia, reduction in ATP production secondary to diminished fatty acid metabolism is mirrored by decreased myocardial BMIPP uptake. Although BMIPP is approved for clinical use in Japan, it has not yet received approval by the US Food and Drug Administration. **B,** Major metabolic pathways and regulatory steps of BMIPP in the myocyte. Under normoxic conditions, the myocardium preferentially oxidizes long-chain fatty acids (LCFAs) to generate ATP. Fatty acids enter the endothelial cell via diffusion or active transport through integral CD36⁺ membrane-bound proteins. The ATP-dependent activation of fatty acids by acyl-coenzyme A (CoA) synthetase involves its transformation to acyl-CoA moieties, which can then undergo β-oxidation in the mitochondria. The majority of LCFA-acyl-CoA derivatives are metabolized via β-oxidation, whereas the remainder of the acyl-CoA and acyl moieties is incorporated into the intracellular esterified triglyceride (TG) pool. BMIPP, however, is not initially metabolized by β-oxidation because the methyl substitution precludes the formation of the keto-acyl-CoA intermediate. BMIPP must first undergo an obligatory initial α-oxidation conversion step in the cytosol or primarily the peroxisome, to α-methyl-p-iodopheny-tetradecanoic acid (AMIPT). AMIPT is metabolized by rounds of β-oxidation in the mitochondria to the end product, 2-(p-[¹²³I]-iodophenyl) acetic acid, which does not accumulate intracellularly. BMIPP appears to be primarily activated (esterified-CoA) in the cytosol and incorporated into triglyceride storage products into the endogenous lipid pool (70%). BMIPP if not activated can undergo early washout back into the bloodstream. TCA—tricarboxylic acid cycle. *(Adapted from* Messina et al. [11]*.)*

188 Atlas of Nuclear Cardiology

Figure 8-13. PET techniques: ^{11}C-acetate. **A**, ^{11}C-acetate is a short-chain acid that is avidly extracted by the myocardium with a first-pass extraction of 63% at blood flows of 1 mL/g/min and is metabolized predominantly by mitochondrial oxidative metabolism. Once in the cytosol, the tracer is converted to acetyl-CoA by acetyl CoA synthase, and is oxidized by the tricarboxylic acid cycle in the mitochondria to ^{11}C-carbon dioxide and water. Thus, the washout rate of ^{11}C-acetate from myocardium is directly related to oxidative tricarboxylic acid cycle flux. Given the close link between tricarboxylic acid cycle and oxidative phosphorylation, the myocardial turnover and clearance of ^{11}C-acetate in the form of ^{11}C-carbon dioxide may reflect overall oxidative metabolism and provide insight into the mitochondrial function of viable myocardium. Alternative metabolic pathways of ^{11}C-acetate include incorporation into amino acids, ketones, and fatty acids by de novo synthesis or chain elongation. However, these latter pathways are thought to be modest and unlikely to compromise estimation of regional myocardial oxygen consumption per minute.

B, Myocardial ^{11}C-acetate tissue time-activity curve demonstrating biexponential clearance of the tracer from myocardium. Monoexponential fitting of the early portion of the clearance phase yields the slope k_{mono}, while biexponential least-square fitting of the clearance phase yields k_1 and k_2 slopes. The rapid phase of clearance (k_1) represents oxidation of extracted ^{11}C-acetate by the mitochondria to ^{11}C-carbon dioxide, and the slower phase of clearance (k_2) represents incorporation of ^{11}C-acetate into amino acids and other alternate metabolic pathways. In patients with recent myocardial infarction and chronic stable angina, preservation of myocardial oxidative metabolism is shown to predict functional recovery after revascularization [12,13]. When clearance rates of ^{11}C-acetate are within 2 standard deviations of the normal mean, the positive predictive accuracy for recovery of function after revascularization is 84% in patients with recent myocardial infarction and 79% in patients with chronic stable angina. Conversely, when clearance rates of ^{11}C-acetate are more than 2 standard deviations below the normal mean, the negative predictive values are 70% in patients with recent myocardial infarction and 83% in patients with chronic stable angina. (**B**, adapted from Schelbert [14].)

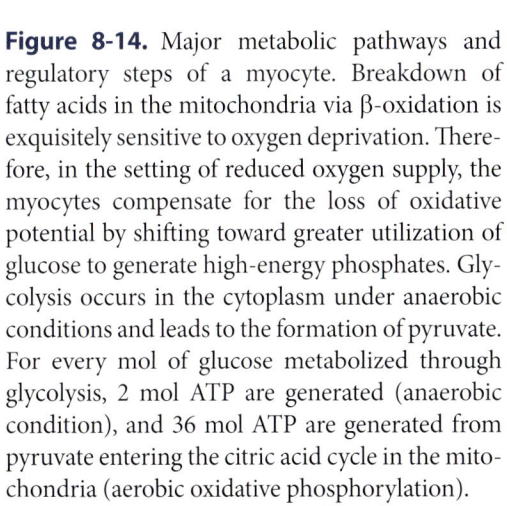

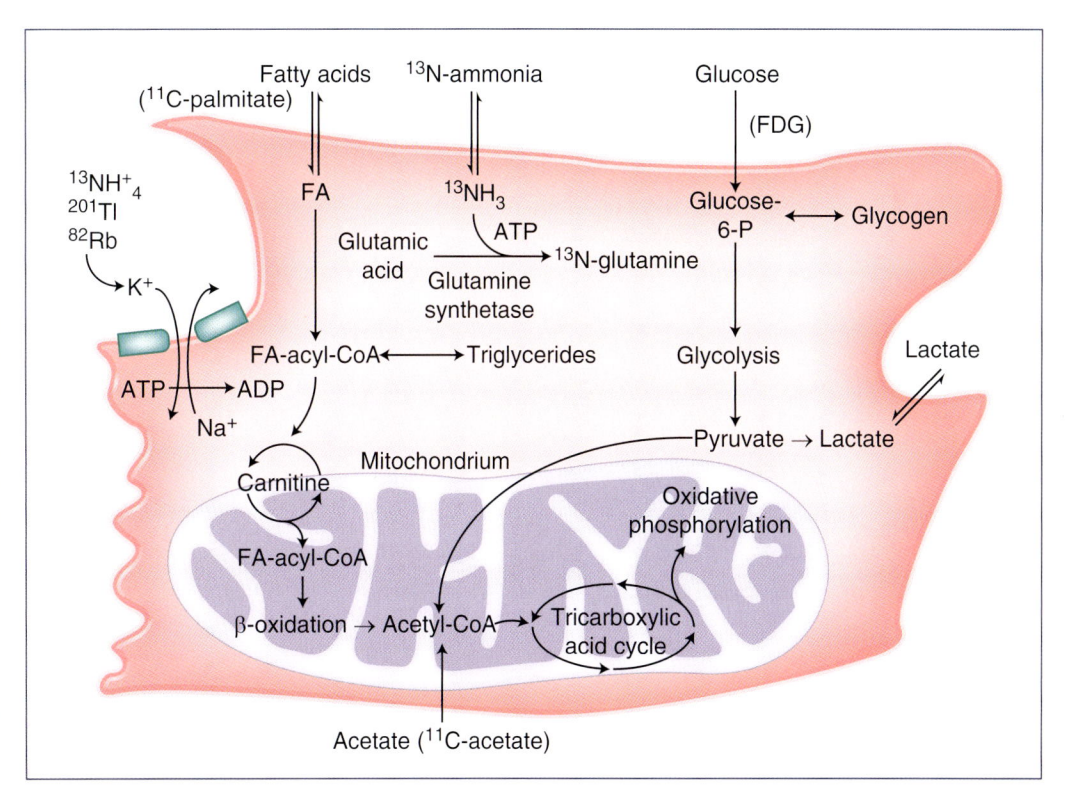

PET Techniques: ^{11}C-acetate

Initial tracer uptake provides an indirect estimate of regional myocardial blood flow

In the cytosol, ^{11}C-acetate is converted directly to ^{11}C-acetyl-CoA and is oxidized by the tricarboxylic acid cycle in the mitochondria to ^{11}C-carbon dioxide and water

Because the washout rate of ^{11}C-acetate from myocardium is directly related to oxidative tricarboxylic acid cycle flux, it is an ideal indicator of myocardial oxidative metabolism

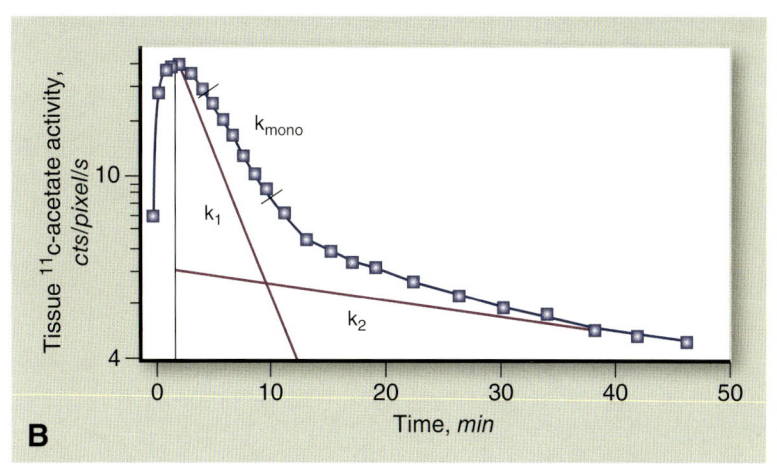

Figure 8-14. Major metabolic pathways and regulatory steps of a myocyte. Breakdown of fatty acids in the mitochondria via β-oxidation is exquisitely sensitive to oxygen deprivation. Therefore, in the setting of reduced oxygen supply, the myocytes compensate for the loss of oxidative potential by shifting toward greater utilization of glucose to generate high-energy phosphates. Glycolysis occurs in the cytoplasm under anaerobic conditions and leads to the formation of pyruvate. For every mol of glucose metabolized through glycolysis, 2 mol ATP are generated (anaerobic condition), and 36 mol ATP are generated from pyruvate entering the citric acid cycle in the mitochondria (aerobic oxidative phosphorylation).

Continued on the next page

Figure 8-14. *(Continued)* Because glycolysis can generate ATP under anaerobic conditions, glycolysis becomes an attractive alternate metabolic pathway for ATP generation in hypoperfused myocardium with a limited supply of oxygen. Although the amount of energy produced by glycolysis may be adequate to maintain myocyte viability and preserve the electrochemical gradient across the cell membrane, it may not be sufficient to sustain contractile function. In hibernation, the adaptive response of the myocardium in the setting of prolonged resting hypoperfusion (reduced oxygen supply) is a reduction in myocardial contractile function (reduced oxygen demand), thereby preserving myocardial viability in the absence of clinically evident ischemia. FDG—[^{18}F]-fluorodeoxyglucose. (*Adapted from* Dilsizian [15].)

Figure 8-15. PET techniques: [^{18}F]-fluorodeoxyglucose (FDG). FDG is a glucose analogue used to image myocardial glucose utilization with PET. Following intravenous injection of 5 to 10 mCi FDG, FDG rapidly exchanges across the capillary and cellular membranes and is phosphorylated by hexokinase to FDG-6-phosphate. Once phosphorylated, FDG is not metabolized further in the glycolytic pathway, fructose-pentose shunt, or glycogen synthesis. Because the dephosphorylation rate of FDG is slow, essentially it becomes trapped in the myocardium, allowing adequate time to image regional glucose uptake by PET or SPECT. In the fasting and aerobic conditions, fatty acids are the preferred source of myocardial energy production, with glucose accounting for some 15% to 20% of the total energy supply. However, in the fed state, plasma insulin levels increase, glucose metabolism is stimulated, and tissue lipolysis is inhibited, resulting in reduced fatty acid delivery to the myocardium. The combined effects of insulin on these processes and the increased arterial glucose concentration associated with fed state result in preferred glucose utilization by the myocardium.

PET Techniques: FDG

- Glucose analogue that competes with glucose for hexokinase
- Phosphorylated by hexokinase to FDG-6-phosphate
- Trapped within myocytes
  - Impermeable to the sarcolemma
  - Poor substrate for further metabolism
  - Slow dephosphorylation
- Myocardial uptake is influenced by metabolic and hormonal milieu

Figure 8-16. Standardization schemes for optimizing [^{18}F]-fluorodeoxyglucose (FDG) image quality. Diagnostic quality of FDG imaging is critically dependent on a number of factors, such as hormonal milieu, substrate availability, and regional blood flow. This becomes particularly evident when studying patients with clinical or subclinical diabetes. Most clinical studies are performed after 50 to 75 g glucose loading with oral dextrose approximately 1 to 2 hours before the FDG injection. Although 90% of FDG images are of adequate-to-excellent diagnostic quality in nondiabetic patients, the quality of FDG images after glucose loading is less certain in patients with clinical or subclinical diabetes mellitus. Because the increase in plasma insulin levels after glucose loading may be attenuated in patients with diabetes mellitus, tissue lipolysis is not inhibited, and free fatty acid levels in the plasma remain high. Acquiring good quality FDG images in diabetics may be challenging. Standardization schemes used to optimize FDG image quality include intravenous insulin injections after glucose loading, hyperinsulinemic-euglycemic clamping, and use of nicotinic acid derivative.

Standardization Schemes for Optimizing FDG Image Quality

Intravenous Bolus of Regular Insulin

- Most common and clinically feasible approach
- Regular insulin is administered according to plasma glucose level and predetermined sliding scale
- Plasma glucose level is assessed every 15 minutes with administration of additional boluses of insulin, if necessary
- FDG dose is injected once the plasma glucose level is below 140 mg/dL

Hyperinsulinemic-Euglycemic Clamping

- Insulin and glucose are infused simultaneously to achieve a stable plasma insulin level of 100 to 120 IU/L and a normal plasma glucose level
- The rate of glucose infusion (20% dextrose solution with potassium chloride) is adjusted intermittently based on measured glucose levels
- Although it provides excellent image quality, the technique is rather tedious and impractical for routine clinical studies

Use of Nicotinic Acid Derivative

- Approximately 2 hours before the FDG dose injection, a single dose of nicotinic acid derivative is given orally followed by glucose loading
- FDG image quality is shown comparable to that obtained after the clamp technique in the same patient population

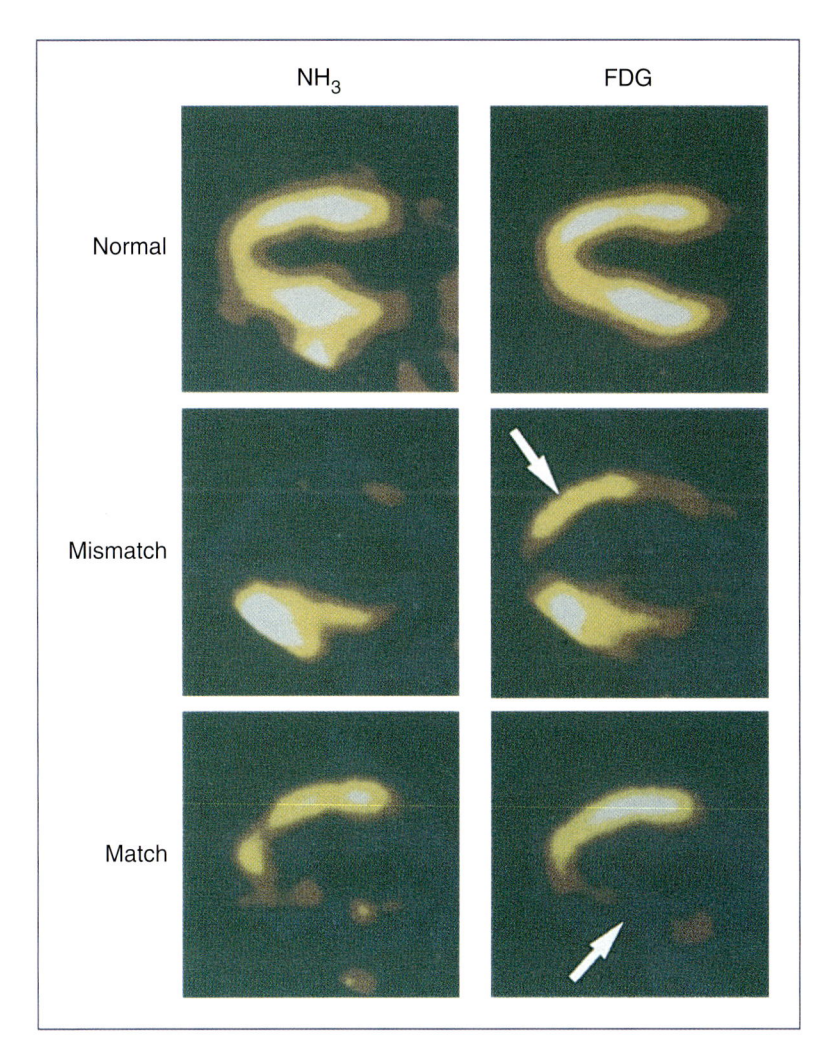

Figure 8-17. Patterns of normal, mismatch, and match under glucose-loading. Preserved or increased myocardial glucose utilization in the setting of prolonged hypoperfusion at rest is termed a *mismatch pattern*. On the NH$_3$ images, there is severely reduced blood flow in the anterior and lateral regions that have preserved metabolism on the [^{18}F]-fluorodeoxyglucose (FDG) images (*arrow*) consistent with myocardial viability. Reduced or absent myocardial glucose utilization in hypoperfused myocardial regions is termed a *match pattern*. On the NH$_3$ images, there is severely reduced blood flow in the inferior region that has absent myocardial metabolism on the FDG images (*arrow*) consistent with scarred myocardium. The application of such PET patterns in patients with chronic ischemic left ventricular dysfunction confers high positive and negative predictive accuracies for recovery of regional function after revascularization, with an overall accuracy between 80% and 90% [16]. However, clinically meaningful increases in global left ventricular function after revascularization are best attained if the extent of hibernating and stunned myocardium is 17% to 25% of the left ventricular mass or more [17]. (*Courtesy of* Dr. James Arrighi.)

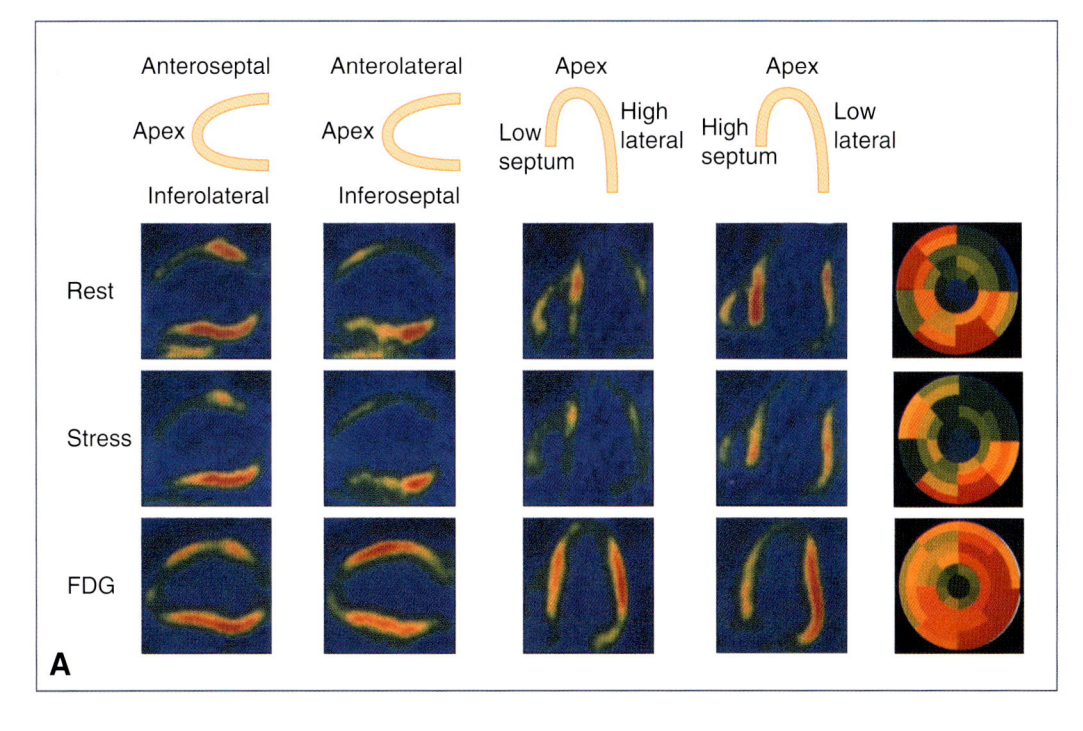

Figure 8-18. Examples of PET mismatch and match patterns. Increased [^{18}F]-fluorodeoxyglucose (FDG) uptake in asynergic myocardial regions with reduced blood flow at rest (mismatch pattern) has become a scintigraphic marker of hibernation. **A,** A patient with severely dilated left ventricle, diffuse hypokinesis, and apical dyskinesis (left ventricular ejection fraction [LVEF], 12%) had severe triple vessel disease. Coronary angiogram revealed 100% occlusion of the proximal left anterior descending (LAD) coronary artery, D1, and D2; subtotal occlusion of the proximal right coronary artery (RCA; and 90% OM1 occlusion. In this patient, four long-axis slices (two horizontal long-axis and two vertical long-axis images) encompassing the entire left ventricle along with corresponding bull's-eye images for rest and stress ^{13}N-ammonia and FDG uptake are shown.

Continued on the next page

Imaging Cardiac Metabolism

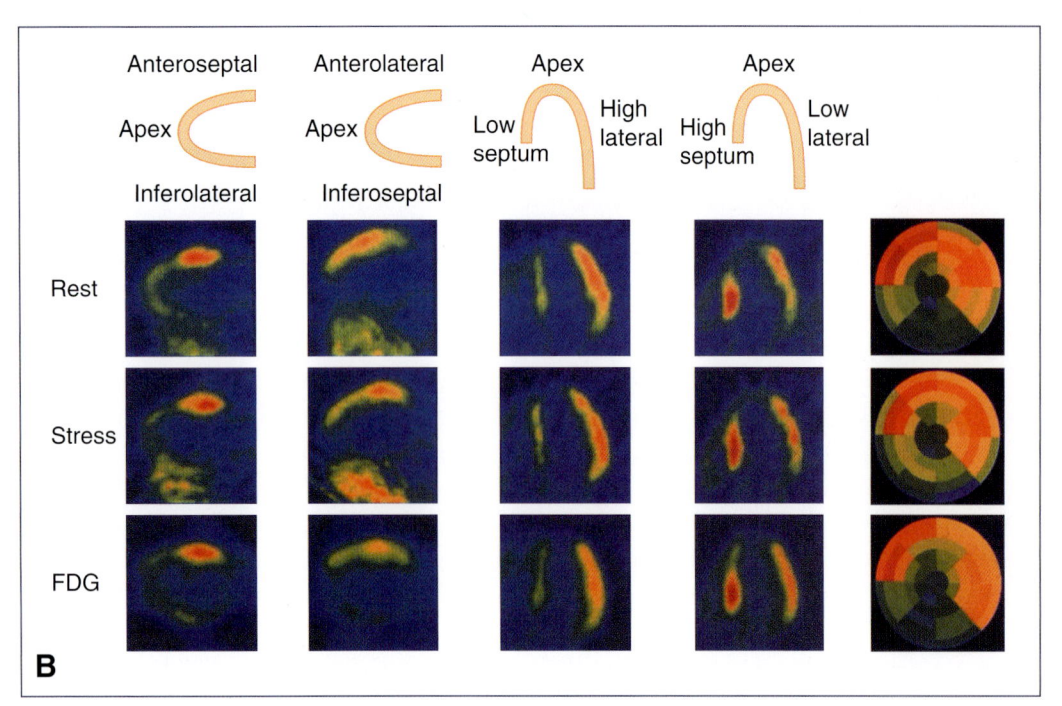

Figure 8-18. *(Continued)* Rest ^{13}N-ammonia images show irreversible defects in the apical and anterolateral regions with partial reversibility in the anterior and inferoseptal regions. Stress ^{13}N-ammonia images show markedly decreased perfusion in the apical, anterior, anterolateral, and inferoseptal regions. However, FDG images acquired under glucose-loaded conditions show preserved or increased glucose utilization in all abnormally perfused myocardial regions at rest, the scintigraphic hallmark of hibernation. In patients with chronic ischemic left ventricular dysfunction, rest and stress myocardial perfusion images alone may significantly underestimate the presence and extent of hibernating but viable myocardium. **B,** Decreased or absent FDG uptake in asynergic myocardial regions with reduced blood flow at rest (match pattern) represents scarred myocardium. A patient with previous coronary bypass surgery presented with significantly dilated left ventricle, apical dyskinesis, septal and inferior akinesis (LVEF, 36%), and congestive heart failure. Coronary angiogram revealed severe native disease of all three vessels, patent left and right internal mammary grafts to the LAD and RCA, critical stenoses of the OM1 vein graft, and a patent OM2 vein graft. In this patient, rest and stress ^{13}N-ammonia images show irreversible defects in the inferior, apical, and inferoseptal regions. FDG images acquired under glucose-loaded conditions show absence of glucose utilization in all abnormally perfused myocardial regions at rest. Such asynergic myocardial regions demonstrating matched reduction in perfusion and metabolism represent scarred myocardium and are unlikely to recover function after revascularization.

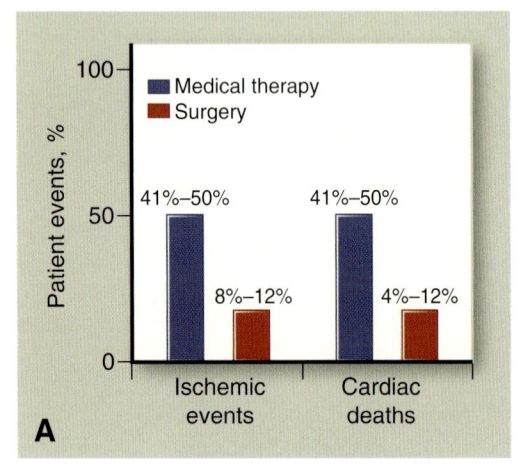

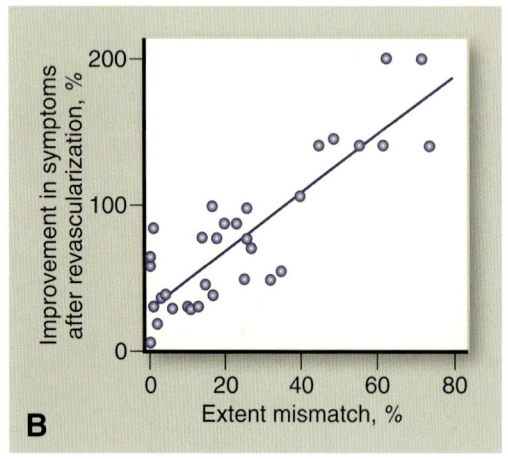

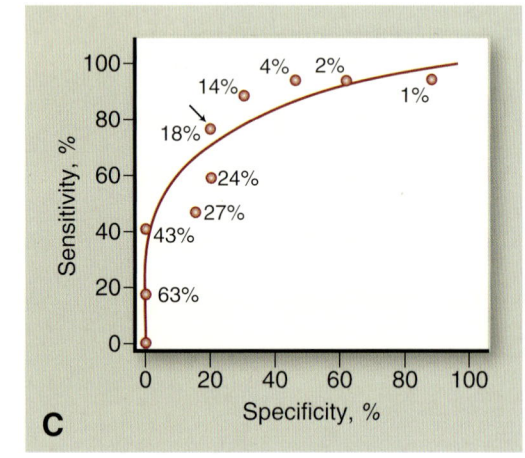

Figure 8-19. PET mismatch and prognosis. The prognostic significance of perfusion-metabolism mismatch pattern in ischemic cardiomyopathy has been shown in a number of nonrandomized, retrospective studies with PET [18,19]. **A,** Patients with perfusion-metabolism mismatch pattern who were treated surgically had lower ischemic event rates and fewer deaths when compared with those treated with medical therapy. In contrast, patients with perfusion-metabolism match pattern displayed no such difference in outcomes between surgical and medical management. Moreover, the patients with myocardial viability (mismatch pattern) who underwent revascularization manifested a significant improvement in heart failure symptoms and exercise tolerance [20,21]. **B,** The relation between the anatomic extent of perfusion:metabolism PET mismatch pattern (expressed as percent of the left ventricle) and the change in functional status after revascularization (expressed as percent improvement from baseline) is shown. The scatterplot shows that the greatest improvement in heart failure symptoms occurs in patients with the largest mismatch defects on quantitative analysis of PET images. **C,** Receiver-operating characteristic curve for different anatomic extent of perfusion-metabolism mismatch to predict a change (at least one grade) in functional status after revascularization is shown. When the extent of PET mismatch involves 18% or more of the left ventricular mass, the sensitivity for predicting a change in functional status after revascularization is 76% and the specificity is 78% (area under the fitted curve = 0.82). (**A,** *adapted from* Eitzman *et al.* [18] and DiCarli *et al.* [19]; **B** and **C,** *adapted from* DiCarli *et al.* [20].)

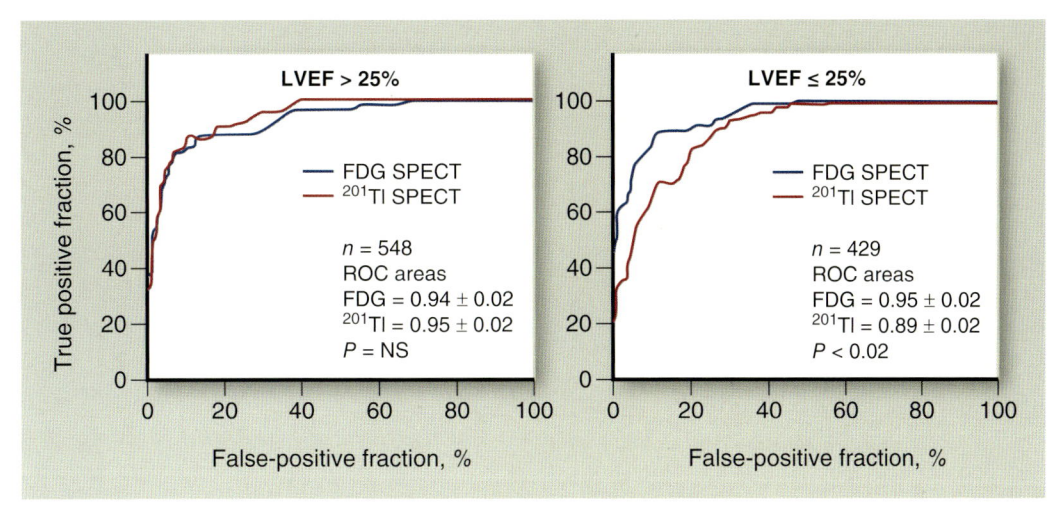

Figure 8-20. In patients with chronic coronary artery disease, differences between high-energy collimator SPECT and PET technologies and [^{18}F]-fluorodeoxyglucose (FDG) and ^{201}Tl tracers are examined for their ability to differentiate viable from nonviable myocardium. Plots of receiver-operating characteristic (ROC) curves for ^{201}Tl and FDG SPECT to predict myocardial viability as defined by 60% FDG PET threshold value for patients with left ventricular ejection fraction (LVEF) above 25% (*left*) and for patients with LVEF 25% or less (*right*) are shown. Area under the ROC curve for FDG SPECT and ^{201}Tl SPECT are displayed for each panel. ^{201}Tl tends to underestimate myocardial viability in patients with LVEF 25% or less, but not in patients with LVEF above 25%. Of the severe asynergic regions, 73% of discordant regions between ^{201}Tl and FDG PET were located in the inferior segment, compared with only 27% of regions with concordance between ^{201}Tl and FDG PET ($P < 0.001$). (*Adapted from* Srinivasan *et al.* [22]).

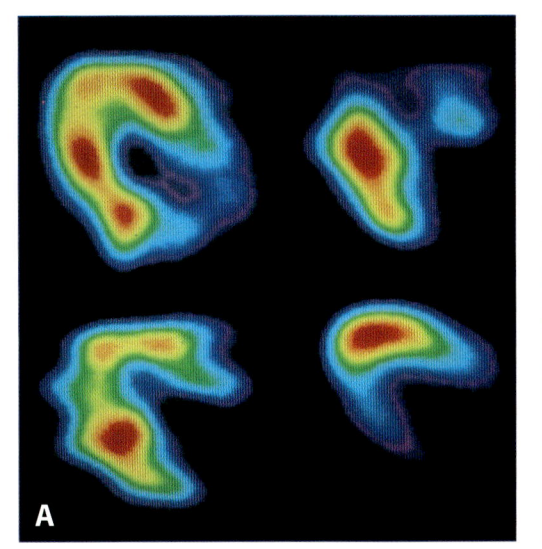

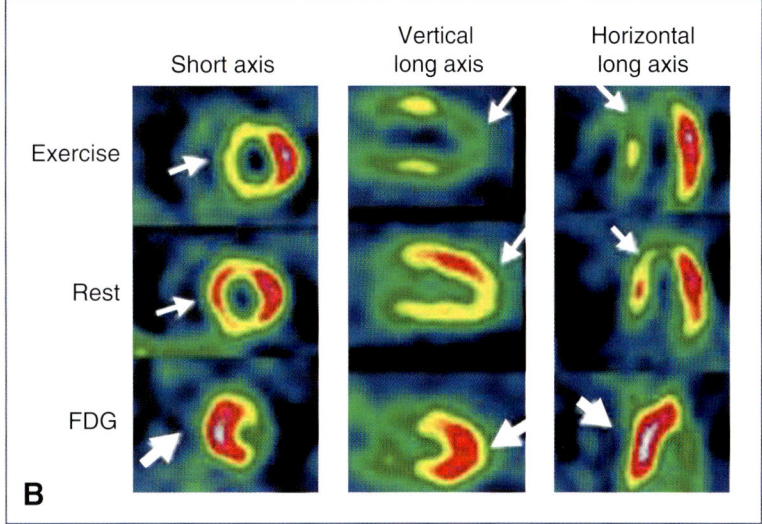

Figure 8-21. Metabolic alterations in postischemic myocardium in patients with angina. Physical exercise is probably the most common precipitating factor responsible for myocardial ischemia in patients with coronary artery disease, manifested as angina and, most importantly, left ventricular dysfunction. Although recovery of such stress-induced left ventricular dysfunction is thought to occur within minutes after the termination of exercise, persistent contractile dysfunction has been observed in some patients up to 90 minutes after the termination of exercise, which has been attributed to stunned myocardium. **A,** Transaxial rubidium-82 (^{82}Rb) PET images reflecting myocardial blood flow at rest, during exercise, and after exercise are shown along with [^{18}F]-fluorodeoxyglucose (FDG) images after exercise. At rest (*top left*), the distribution of myocardial blood flow is homogeneous in all myocardial regions. During exercise (*top right*), there are extensive blood flow abnormalities in the apical and anteroseptal regions that improve on the postexercise images (*bottom left*) and are comparable to the ^{82}Rb rest image (*top left*). FDG was injected 8 minutes after the termination of exercise. The FDG image recorded 60 minutes after tracer injection (*bottom right*) shows metabolic alterations in the previously ischemic regions.

B, Simultaneous myocardial perfusion and metabolism imaging after dual intravenous injection of ^{99m}Tc-sestamibi and FDG at peak exercise. Dual isotope simultaneous acquisition was carried out 40 to 60 minutes after the exercise study was completed. Rest ^{99m}Tc-sestamibi imaging was carried out separately. In this patient with angina and no prior myocardial infarction, there is evidence for extensive reversible perfusion defect in the anterior, septal, and apical regions. The coronary angiogram showed 90% stenosis of the left anterior descending and 60% stenosis of the left circumflex coronary arteries. The corresponding FDG image shows intense uptake in the regions with reversible sestamibi defects reflecting the metabolic correlate of exercise-induced myocardial ischemia. (**A,** *from* Camici *et al.* [23]; with permission; **B,** adapted from He *et al.* [24].)

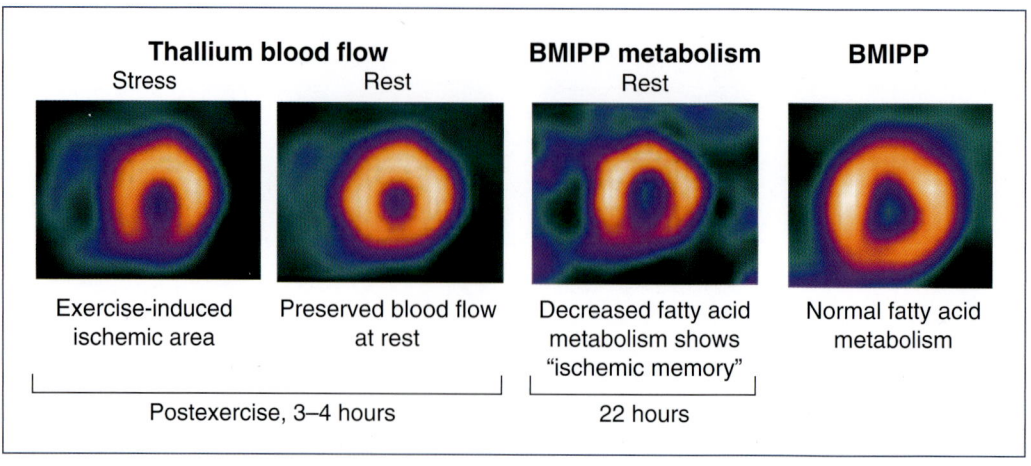

Figure 8-22. SPECT showing delayed recovery of regional fatty acid metabolism after transient exercise-induced ischemia, termed *ischemic memory*. Representative stress and rest reinjection short-axis thallium tomograms demonstrate a reversible inferior defect consistent with exercise-induced myocardial ischemia. A β-methyl-p-[^{123}I]-iodophenyl-pentadecanoic acid (BMIPP)-labeled CT injected and acquired at rest 22 hours after exercise-induced ischemia shows persistent metabolic abnormality in the inferior region despite complete recovery of regional perfusion at rest, as evidenced by thallium reinjection image. The tomogram on the *far right* shows retention of BMIPP in the heart of a normal adult for comparison. (*Adapted from* Taegtmeyer and Dilsizian [25] and Dilsizian *et al.* [26].)

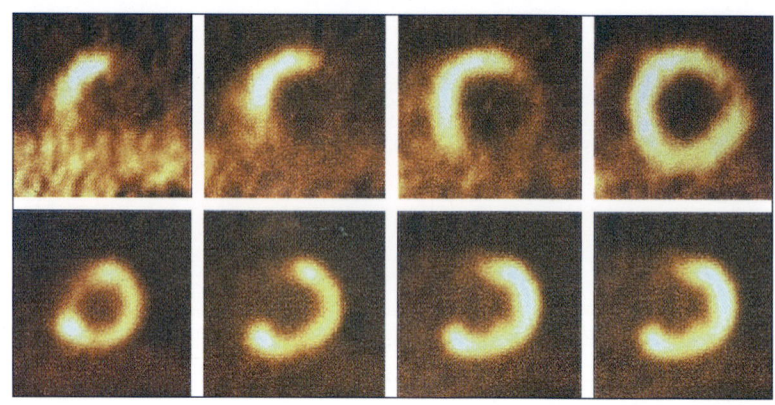

Figure 8-23. PETs demonstrating perfusion–metabolism mismatch (reduced blood flow with preserved or enhanced [^{18}F]-fluorodeoxyglucose [FDG] uptake) in a patient with chronic ischemic left ventricular dysfunction and heart failure symptoms. The principle of using a metabolic tracer, such as FDG, is based on the concept that viable myocytes in hypoperfused and dysfunctional regions are metabolically active, while scarred or fibrotic tissue is metabolically inactive. Although fatty acids are the primary source of myocardial energy production in the fasting state, in the setting of reduced oxygen supply (a consequence of hypoperfusion at rest), the myocytes compensate for the loss of oxidative potential by shifting toward greater glucose utilization to generate high-energy phosphates. Thus, in chronic ischemia, aerobic metabolism is slowed while the anaerobic metabolism is accelerated, a reversal of the well-known Pasteur effect [27]. Such increased FDG uptake (anaerobic metabolism) in asynergic myocardial regions with reduced blood flow at rest has become a scintigraphic marker of hibernation. *Top row*, Short-axis [^{13}N]-ammonia scans demonstrate large lateral and inferior perfusion defects at rest. *Bottom row*, The corresponding FDG images acquired under fasting conditions demonstrate that FDG metabolic activity is preserved in the lateral and inferior regions (mismatch pattern). On the other hand, the lack of FDG metabolic activity in the anterior and septal regions reflects the utilization of fatty acid rather than glucose as the primary fuel in such normally perfused myocardial regions.

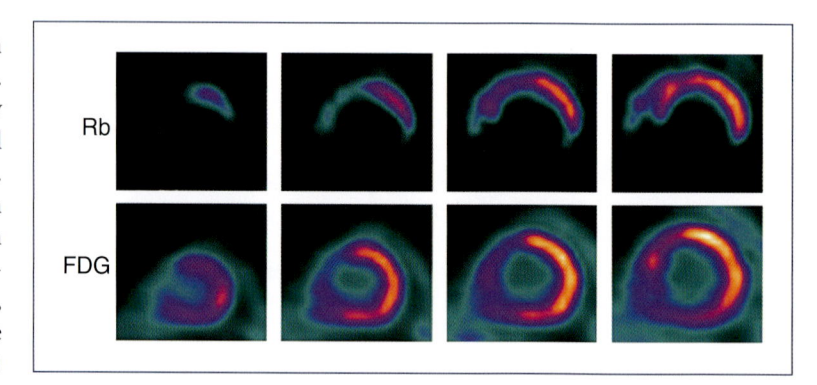

Figure 8-24. PET scan showing perfusion–metabolism mismatch in hibernating heart tissue as an example of preserved cardiometabolic reserve. *Top*, Rubidium (Rb)-82-labeled PET in short-axis view shows markedly decreased perfusion defects in the apical, inferior, inferolateral, and septal regions of the left ventricle at rest, which extends from distal to basal slices. *Bottom*, Images acquired under glucose-loaded conditions, labeled with [^{18}F]-fluorodeoxyglucose (FDG), show perfusion–metabolism mismatch pattern (the scintigraphic hallmark of hibernation) in all abnormally perfused myocardial regions at rest. An exception is the anteroseptal region, which demonstrates matched perfusion–metabolism pattern (compatible with scarred myocardium). (*Adapted from* Taegtmeyer and Dilsizian [25].)

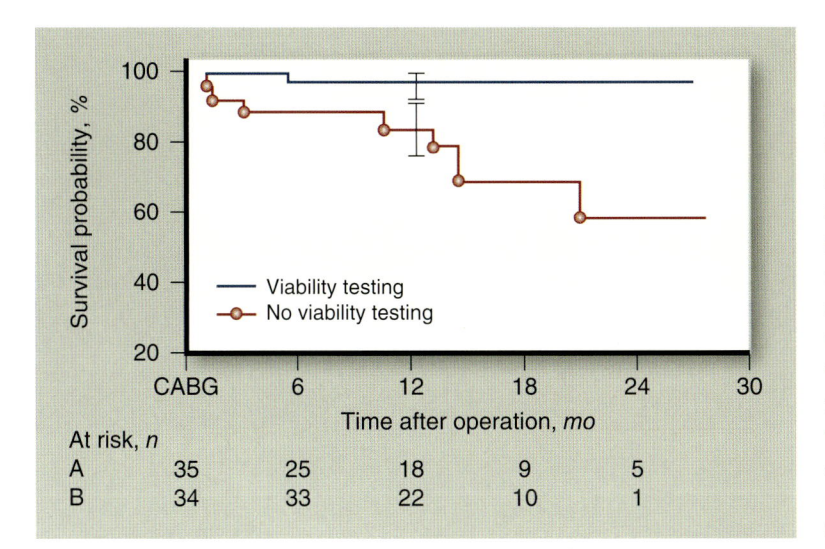

Figure 8-25. Myocardial viability testing prior to surgical revascularization. Determination of myocardial viability evaluation in patients with coronary artery disease and severe left ventricular dysfunction before referral to coronary artery revascularization affects clinical outcome with respect to both in-hospital mortality and 1-year survival rate. In this retrospective study, the perioperative and postoperative event-free survival rate was significantly lower in patients who were referred to revascularization on the basis of clinical presentation and angiographic data but without viability testing (group A) compared with those who were selected according to the extent of viable tissue determined by PET (group B) in addition to clinical presentation and angiographic data. There were four in-hospital deaths (11.4%) in group A and none in group B ($P = 0.04$). Moreover, after 12 months, the survival rate was 79% in group A and 97% in group B ($P = 0.01$). (*Adapted from* Haas *et al.* [21].)

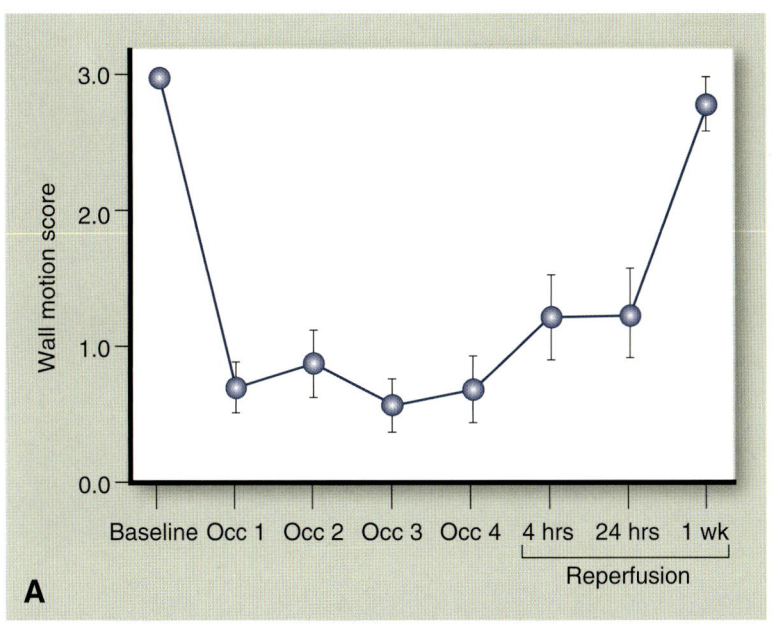

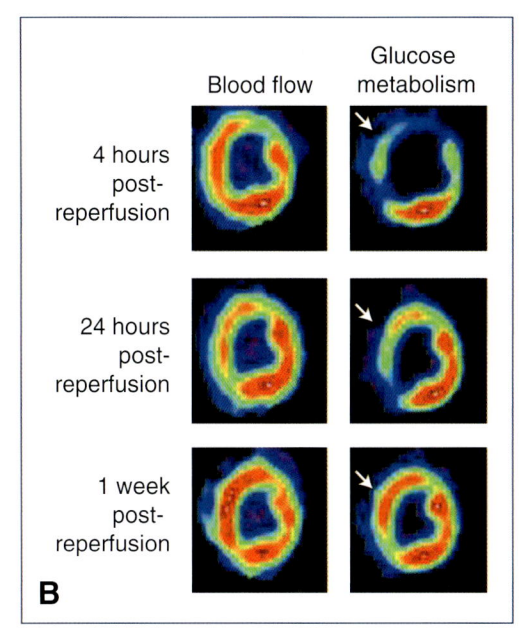

Figure 8-26. Alterations in contractile function, regional blood flow, and glucose metabolism in myocardial stunning. **A,** Anesthesized dogs were subjected to four sequential 5-minute intervals of balloon left anterior descending coronary artery occlusion (Occ), each separated by 5 minutes of reperfusion. Regional blood flow, metabolism, and function were evaluated 4 hours, 24 hours, and 1 week after reperfusion. Regional wall motion was severely depressed in the anterior and anteroseptal regions after the four cycles of ischemia, remained impaired 24 hours after reperfusion, and normalized 1 week later consistent with myocardial stunning. **B,** Representative mid short-axis PET images of [^{13}N]-ammonia (blood flow) and fluorodeoxyglucose (glucose metabolism) obtained 4 hours, 24 hours, and 1 week after reperfusion. In images obtained 4 hours after reperfusion, regional myocardial blood flow is near normal in the anterior and anteroseptal region, whereas glucose utilization is severely reduced (*arrow*). In images obtained 24 hours after reperfusion, regional myocardial blood flow remains near normal with evidence of partial recovery in glucose utilization in the anterior and anteroseptal regions (*arrow*). In images obtained 1 week after reperfusion, there is complete recovery of glucose utilization in the regions of stunned myocardium that appear homogeneous with remote myocardial regions (*arrow*). These findings suggest that in repetitive myocardial stunning, a unique metabolic adaptation occurs (abnormal glucose utilization despite restoration of regional blood flow) that is different from the adaptation typically described in clinical and experimental models of myocardial hibernation (preserved or enhanced glucose utilization in a region with decreased regional blood flow). (*Adapted from* DiCarli *et al.* [28].)

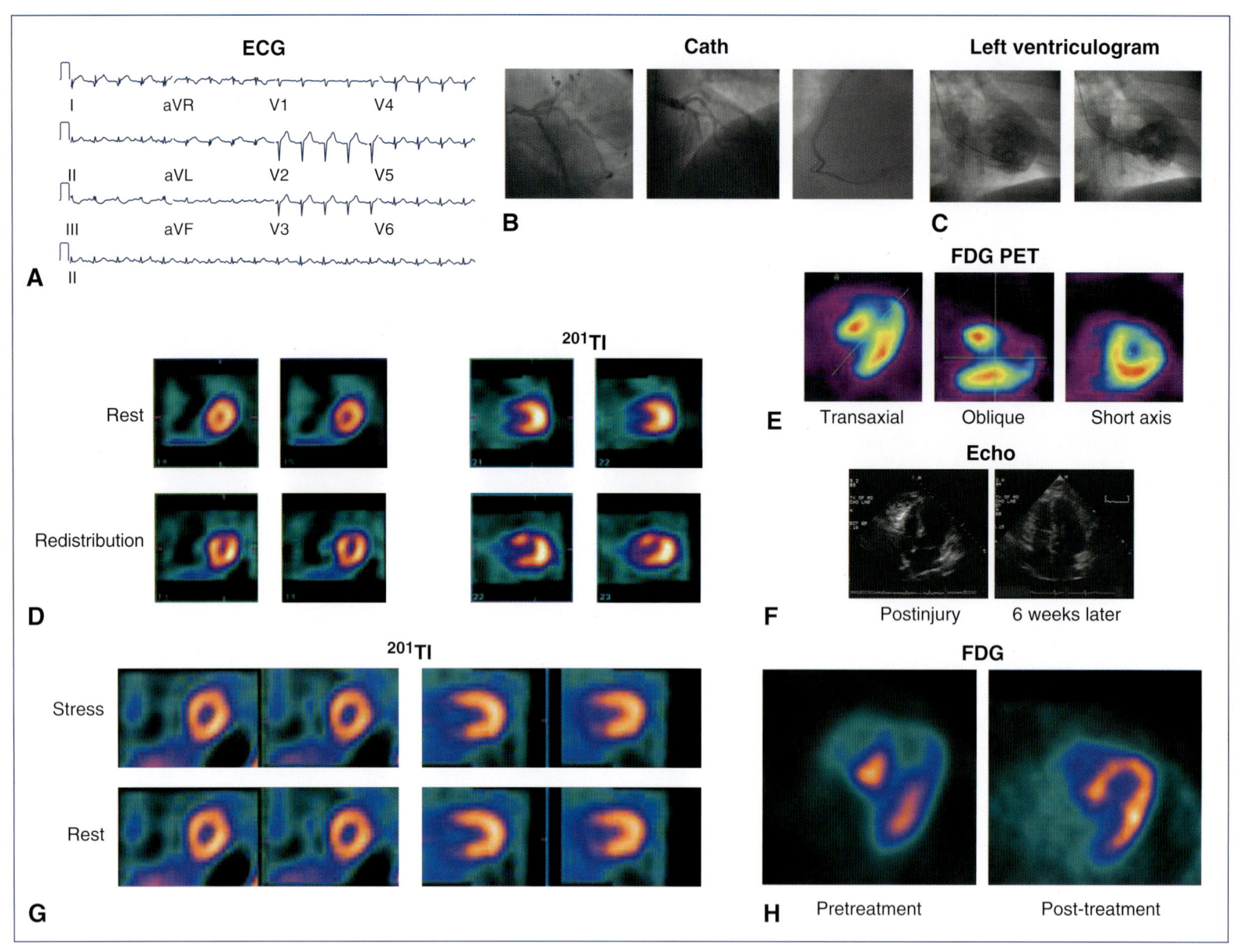

Figure 8-27. Scintigraphic pattern of stunned myocardium. A patient with end-stage liver disease and family history of coronary artery disease presents to the emergency department with 1 hour of new onset chest pain. The electrocardiogram (ECG) pattern is consistent with acute ST segment elevation myocardial infarction (**A**). The coronary angiogram shows normal appearing, insignificant coronary artery disease (**B**). The left ventriculogram shows extensive left ventricular apical, anterior, and anterolateral akinesis with a calculated ejection fraction of 30% (**C**, *left panel* diastole, *right panel* systole). The patient had a mild rise in cardiac enzymes (troponin = 1.5, serum creatine kinase = 76, MB = 5, %MB = 6.6) indicative of myocardial injury. Rest-redistribution ^{201}Tl SPECT images acquired within 1 week after the onset of chest pain show normal perfusion at rest (*top row*) with evidence for rapid ^{201}Tl washout in the anterior region on ^{201}Tl redistribution images (*bottom row*) consistent with reverse redistribution (**D**). Fluorodeoxyglucose (FDG) PET images acquired within days after the thallium study show severely impaired glucose utilization in the anterior and apical regions (**E**). These scintigraphic findings (abnormal glucose utilization or retention of ^{201}Tl on redistribution images despite normal regional blood flow on rest ^{201}Tl) are compatible with stunned myocardium. Repeat echocardiography (**F**), myocardial perfusion SPECT (**G**), and FDG PET (**H**) studies approximately 6 weeks after the acute ischemic injury show complete resolution of the extensive left ventricular apical akinesis (**F**) with homogeneous and normal glucose utilization in all myocardial regions (**H**) and no evidence of myocardial ischemia (**G**).

Similar presentation of transient left ventricular apical ballooning by echocardiography, termed Tako-tsubo, has been observed in critically ill patients being admitted to the medical intensive care unit for noncardiac medical disorders. Elevated serum creatine kinase has been described in up to 50% of patients with ventricular apical ballooning with a subset of these patients also exhibiting ECG evidence of Q-wave and/or ST segment displacement. Although possible triggering factors have been suggested in the literature, the underlying pathophysiology for the left ventricular dysfunction and apical ballooning has not been elucidated. The transient nature of the apical dysfunction in a subset of patients could be attributed to transient ischemic injury and myocardial stunning. (*Courtesy of* Mark Kelemen and Vasken Dilsizian.)

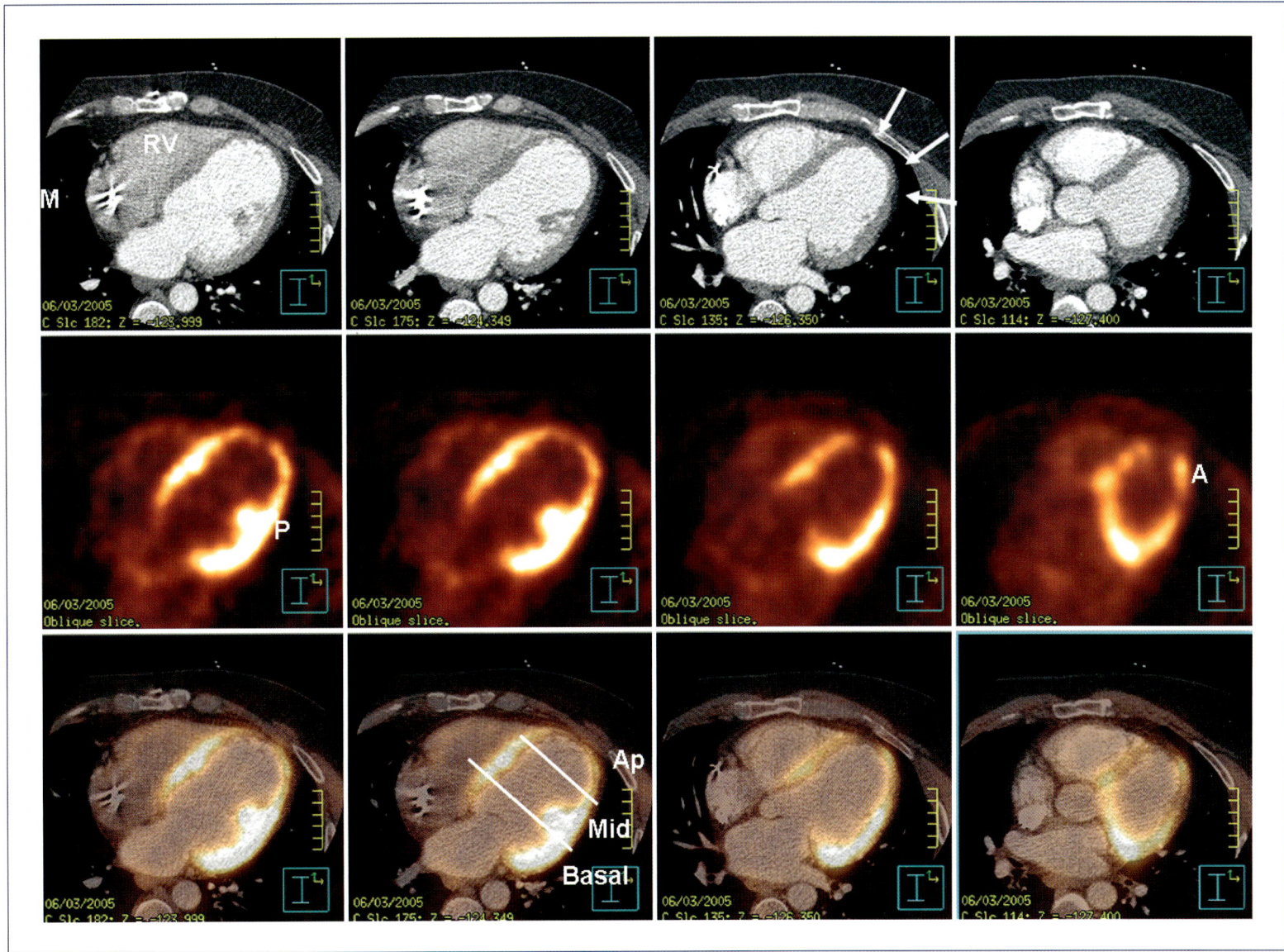

Figure 8-28. PET-guided ventricular tachycardia (VT) ablation therapy. Myocardial scar usually acts as the substrate for reentrant VT and is present in the majority of patients with ischemic and nonischemic cardiomyopathy. During reentrant VT an electrical wave front enters and traverses the myocardial scar via a network of such electrically conducting channels. After exiting the scar, it depolarizes the rest of the ventricle and returns to the original entry site, repeating the cycle. This concept of entry sites, slowly conducting channels, and exit sites has been successfully validated in post–myocardial infarction patients during clinical electrophysiologic studies.

The current "gold standard" of defining myocardial scar is based on endocardial bipolar voltage recordings using a 3D mapping system with a roving mapping catheter. Accordingly, regions with greater than 1.5 mV are classified as normal myocardium, 0.5 to 1.5 mV as abnormal myocardium, and less than 0.5 mV as scarred myocardium. Of significant interest for electrophysiologists is the ability of PET to define myocardial scar. Different from delayed-enhanced MRI and CT, which provide a morphologic substrate assessment, PET allows a metabolic characterization of the myocardial scar and its border zone. In addition, PET can be safely performed in patients with an implanted cardiac defibrillator or renal insufficiency.

Current software developments are aiming at exporting this detailed 3D imaging information into the actual ablation procedure and provide anatomic guidance for patients with recurrent episodes of VT. In a recent study of patients undergoing VT ablation, a good correlation was found between PET-derived metabolic scar maps and endocardial voltage (r = 0.89, $P < 0.05$). Scar size, location, and border zone accurately predicted high-resolution voltage map findings (r = 0.87, $P < 0.05$). Moreover, PET/CT maps correctly predicted nontransmural epicardial scar that was confirmed with epicardial mapping despite normal endocardial map [29].

Fusion of [^{18}F]-fluorodeoxyglucose (FDG) PET and CT images. Contrast-enhanced CT demonstrates all cardiac chambers (right ventricle [RV] and left ventricle [LV]) and metal artifact of implantable cardioverter defibrillator lead (M) in the right atrium. Significant wall thinning (*arrows*) noted in apical and lateral LV wall consistent with myocardial infarction (*top*). Matching decrease in signal intensity in apical and lateral wall segments observed in PET images. Preserved metabolism of papillary muscle (P) seen. Note areas of preserved metabolic activity (A) within lateral wall, which appears uniformly thinned by CT images (*middle*). PET images are fused with corresponding CT datasets to allow visualization of metabolic and anatomic datasets. LV wall is divided in apical (Ap), mid, and basal section for conventional 17-segment analysis (*bottom*). (Adapted from Dickfield et al. [29].)

Figure 8-29. Metabolic alterations in renal failure. **A,** The concurrent pathogenic factors contributing to the development of uremic cardiomyopathy and altered metabolism with declining kidney function in chronic kidney disease (CKD) is shown. While myocardial infarction and ischemic heart disease account for the significant portion of patients with heart failure and left ventricular remodeling, several sequelae of renal failure that accrue with loss of renal function can also contribute to left ventricular remodeling, termed *uremic cardiomyopathy*. The United States Renal Data System has reported near-equivalent rates of myocardial infarction and cardiac death in dialysis patients and an approximately 10-fold higher rate of heart failure in the same population [30]. The common occurrence of heart failure in the dialysis population is thought to be related to left ventricular hypertrophy (LVH) that occurs frequently in patients with CKD. Although hypertension is common among patients with kidney disease, several investigators have suggested that elevated blood pressure becomes increasingly volume-dependent with a concomitant increase in arterial stiffening, activation of neurohormones, and endothelial dysfunction as renal function declines. Individuals with CKD, therefore, are faced with both pressure- and volume-overload states contributing to the development of left ventricular remodeling and heart failure. The cardiomyopathy typical of CKD and the associated uremia is thought to lead to a myocyte–capillary mismatch, with a diminished vascular supply relative to the number and volume of functioning myocytes [31]. The oxygen-poor milieu will lead to diffuse myocardial ischemia with an anticipated decline in aerobic myocardial fatty acid utilization and a shift to anaerobic metabolism, with increased uptake of glucose as the principal energy providing substrate [32,33]. The shift from a predominance of aerobic (fatty acid) to anaerobic (glucose) metabolism appears to account for a significant portion of the excessive cardiovascular morbidity and mortality observed across all stages of kidney disease.

In a prospective study of 130 asymptomatic end-stage renal disease (ESRD) patients undergoing hemodialysis (**B**), the prevalence of coronary artery disease was assessed by performing dual isotope thallium and β-methyl-p-[^{123}I]-iodophenyl-pentadecanoic acid (BMIPP) SPECT at rest followed by coronary angiography [34].

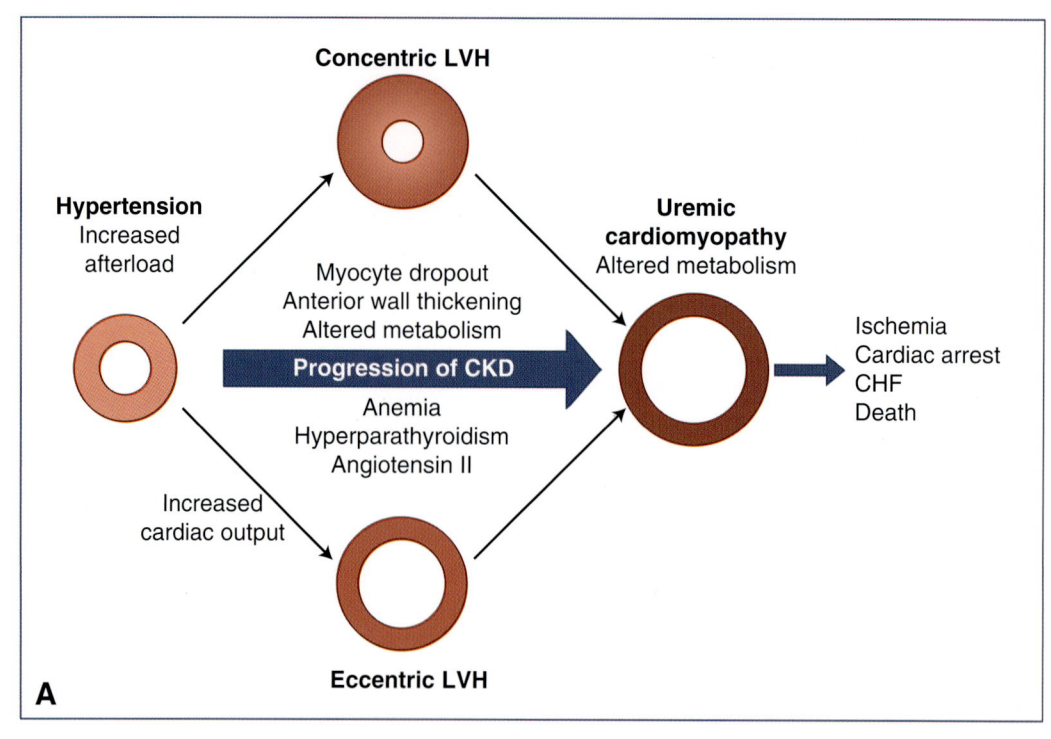

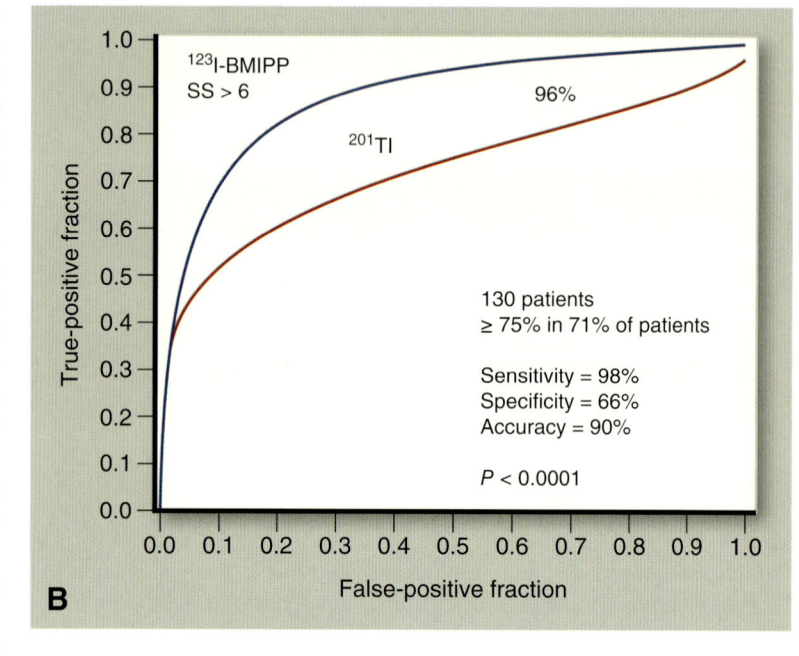

Continued on the next page

198 Atlas of Nuclear Cardiology

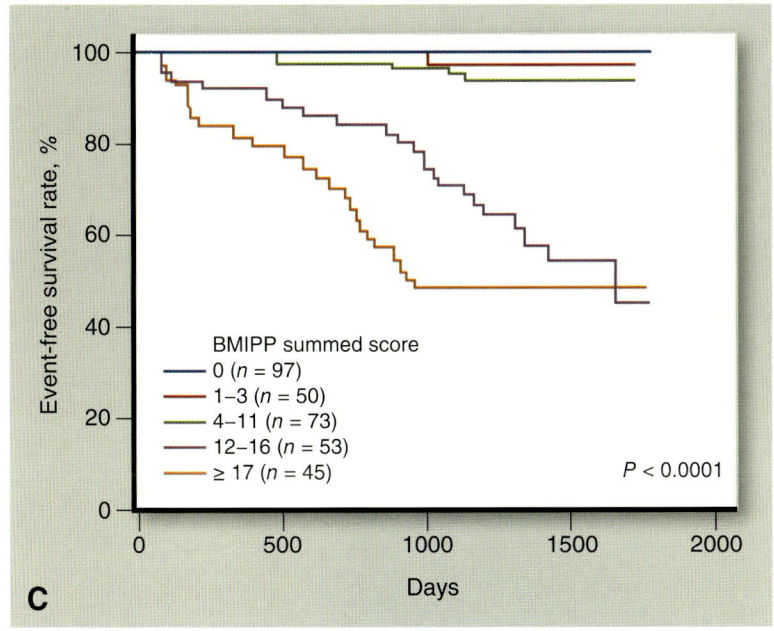

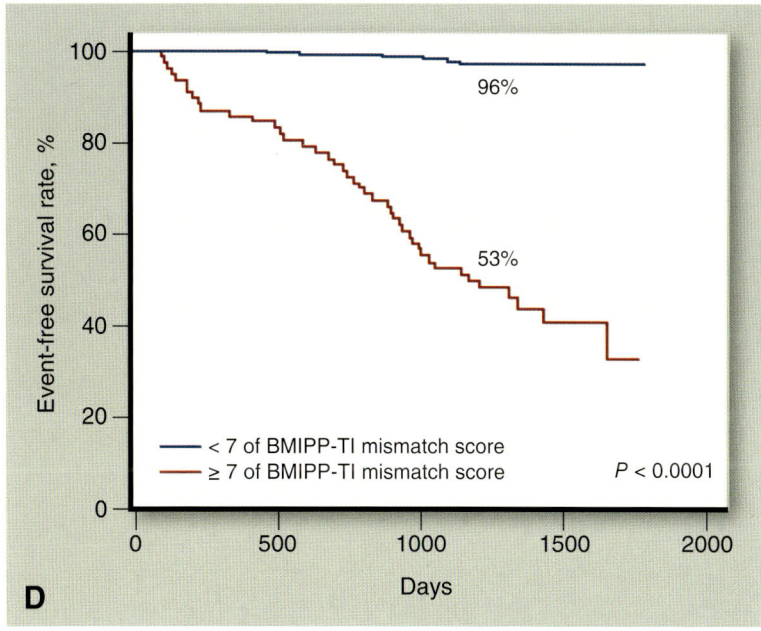

Figure 8-29. *(Continued)* Significant coronary artery luminal narrowing (> 75%) was present in 71.5% (93 of 130) of ESRD patients with an additional five patients exhibiting coronary vasospasm. When reduced myocardial metabolism with BMIPP (summed score of 6 or more) was used to define an abnormal scan, the sensitivity, specificity, and accuracy for detecting coronary artery disease with rest BMIPP SPECT was 98%, 66%, and 90%, respectively [34]. In a subsequent publication by the same investigators, the prognostic significance of reduced myocardial metabolism with BMIPP in conjunction with perfusion abnormalities assessed with thallium in ESRD patients was examined [32]. Among 318 prospectively enrolled asymptomatic hemodialysis patients without prior myocardial infarction, 50 (16%) died of cardiac events during a mean follow-up period of 3.6 + 1.0 years. Kaplan-Meier survival estimates showed 61% event-free survival at 3 years among patients with summed BMIPP score of 12 or more, and 98% in patients with a summed BMIPP score of below 12, with graded relationship between survival and severity of summed BMIPP score (**C**). When BMIPP uptake (metabolism) was assessed in relation to regional thallium uptake (perfusion), indicating myocardial ischemia, the sensitivity and specificity of metabolism–perfusion mismatch for predicting cardiac death was 86% and 88%, respectively. Kaplan-Meier survival estimates showed 53% event-free survival at 3 years among patients with a BMIPP–thallium mismatch score of 7 or more, and 96% in patients with a BMIPP–thallium mismatch score of below 7 (**D**). These findings support the assertion that altered cardiac metabolism (indicating silent myocardial ischemia) is highly prevalent in ESRD patients and can identify the subgroup of patients who are at high risk for cardiac death. The shift from a predominance of aerobic (fatty acid) to anaerobic (glucose) metabolism appears to account for a significant portion of the excessive cardiovascular morbidity and mortality observed across all stages of kidney disease. CHF—congestive heart failure. (**A**, *adapted from* Dilsizian and Fink [35]; **B**, *adapted from* Nishimura et al. [34]; **C**, **D**, *adapted from* Nishimura et al. [32].)

References

1. Taegtmeyer H, Golfman L, Sharma S, et al.: Linking gene expression to function: metabolic flexibility in the normal and diseased heart. *Ann NY Acad Sci* 2004, 1015:202–213.

2. Depre C, Young ME, Ying J, et al.: Streptozotocin-induced changes in cardiac gene expression in the absence of severe contractile dysfunction. *J Mol Cell Cardiol* 2000, 32:985–996.

3. Goodwin GW, Taylor CS, Taegtmeyer H: Regulation of energy metabolism of the heart during acute increase in heart work. *J Biol Chem* 1998, 273:29530–29539.

4. Nguyen VT, Mossberg KA, Tewson TJ, et al.: Temporal analysis of myocardial glucose metabolism by 2-[18F]fluoro-2-deoxy-D-glucose. *Am J Physiol* 1990, 259: H1022–H1031.

5. Sharma S, Adrogue JV, Golfman L, et al.: Intramyocardial lipid accumulation in the failing human heart resembles the lipotoxic rat heart. *FASEB J* 2004,18:1692–1700.

6. Taegtmeyer H, McNulty P, Young ME: Adaptation and maladaptation of the heart in diabetes: part I: general concepts. *Circulation* 2002, 105:1727–1733.

7. Depre C, Shipley GL, Chen W, et al.: Unloaded heart in vivo replicates fetal gene expression of cardiac hypertrophy. *Nat Med* 1998 4:1269–1275.

8. Dewald O, Sharma S, Adrogue J, et al.: Downregulation of peroxisome proliferator-activated receptor-alpha gene expression in a mouse model of ischemic cardiomyopathy is dependent on reactive oxygen species and prevents lipotoxicity. *Circulation* 2005 112:407–415.

9. Golfman LS, Wilson CR, Sharma S, et al: Activation of PPARgamma enhances myocardial glucose oxidation and improves contractile function in isolated working hearts of ZDF rats. *Am J Physiol Endocrinol Metab* 2005, 289:E328–E336.

10. Feinendegen LE: Myocardial imaging of lipid metabolism with labeled fatty acids. In *Myocardial Viability: A Clinical and Scientific Treatise*. Edited by Dilsizian V. Armonk, New York: Futura; 2000:349–389.

11. Messina SA, Aras O, Dilsizian V: Delayed recovery of fatty acid metabolism after transient myocardial ischemia: a potential imaging target for "ischemic memory." *Curr Cardiol Rep* 2007, 9:159–165.

12. Gropler RJ, Siegel BA, Sampathkumaran K, et al.: Dependence of recovery of contractile function on maintenance of oxidative metabolism after myocardial infarction. *J Am Coll Cardiol* 1992, 19:989–997.

13. Gropler RJ, Geltman EM, Sampathkumaran K, et al.: Functional recovery after coronary revascularization for chronic coronary artery disease is dependent on maintenance of oxidative metabolism. *J Am Coll Cardiol* 1992, 20:569–577.

14. Schelbert HR: Principles of positron emission tomography. In *Marcus Cardiac Imaging: A Companion to Braunwald's Heart Disease*, edn 2. Edited by Skorton DJ, Schelbert HR, Wolf GL, Brundage BH. Philadelphia: WB Saunders; 1996:1063–1092.

15. Dilsizian V: Perspectives on the study of human myocardium: viability. In *Myocardial Viability: A Clinical and Scientific Treatise*. Edited by Dilsizian V. Armonk, New York: Futura; 2000:3–22.

16. Tillisch JH, Brunken R, Marshall R, *et al.*: Reversibility of cardiac wall-motion abnormalities predicted by positron tomography. *N Engl J Med* 1986, 314:884–888.

17. Dilsizian V, Arrighi JA: Myocardial viability in chronic coronary artery disease: perfusion, metabolism and contractile reserve. In *Cardiac Nuclear Medicine*, edn 3. Edited by Gerson MC. New York: McGraw-Hill; 1996:143–191.

18. Eitzman D, Al-Aouar Z, Kanter HL, *et al.*: Clinical outcome of patients with advanced coronary artery disease after viability studies with positron emission tomography. *J Am Coll Cardiol* 1992, 20:559–565.

19. DiCarli MF, Davidson M, Little R, *et al.*: Value of metabolic imaging with positron emission tomography for evaluating prognosis in patients with coronary artery disease and left ventricular dysfunction. *Am J Cardiol* 1994, 73:527–533.

20. DiCarli MF, Asgarzadie F, Schelbert HR, *et al.*: Quantitative relation between myocardial viability and improvement in heart failure symptoms after revascularization in patients with ischemic cardiomyopathy. *Circulation* 1995, 92:3436–3444.

21. Haas F, Haehnel CJ, Picker W, *et al.*: Preoperative positron emission tomography viability assessment and perioperative and postoperative risk in patients with advanced ischemic heart disease. *J Am Coll Cardiol* 1997, 30:1693–1700.

22. Srinivasan G, Kitsiou AN, Bacharach SL, *et al.*: ^{18}F-fluorodeoxyglucose single photon emission computed tomography: Can it replace PET and thallium SPECT for the assessment of myocardial viability? *Circulation* 1998, 97:843–850.

23. Camici P, Araujo LI, Spinks T, *et al.*: Increased uptake of 18F-fluorodeoxyglucose in postischemic myocardium of patients with exercise-induced angina. *Circulation* 1986, 74:81–88.

24. He ZX, Shi RF, Wu YJ, *et al.*: Direct imaging of exercise-induced myocardial ischemia with fluorine-18-labeled deoxyglucose and Tc-99m-sestamibi in coronary artery disease. *Circulation* 2003, 108:1208–1213.

25. Taegtmeyer H, Dilsizian V: Imaging myocardial metabolism and ischemic memory. *Nat Clin Pract Cardiol* 2008, 5:S42–S48.

26. Dilsizian V, Bateman TM, Bergmann SR, *et al.*: Metabolic imaging with beta-methyl-para-[^{123}I]-iodophenyl-pentadecanoic acid (BMIPP) identifies ischemic memory following demand ischemia. *Circulation* 2005, 112:2169–2174.

27. Krebs H: The Pasteur effect and the relation between respiration and fermentation. *Essays Biochem* 1972, 8:1–34.

28. DiCarli MF, Prceevski P, Singh TP, *et al.*: Myocardial blood flow, function, and metabolism in repetitive stunning. *J Nucl Med* 2000, 41:1227–1234.

29. Dickfeld T, Lei P, Dilsizian V, *et al.*: Integration of three-dimensional scar maps for ventricular tachycardia ablation with positron emission tomography-computed tomography. *J Am Coll Cardiol Imag* 2008; 1:73-82.

30. United States Renal Data System: USRDS 2006 annual data report: *Atlas of End-Stage Renal Disease in the US*. Bethesda: National Institutes of Health, National Institutes of Diabetes and Digestive and Kidney Diseases; 2006.

31. Tyralla K, Amann K: Morphology of the heart and arteries in renal failure. *Kidney Int* 2003, 63:S80–S83.

32. Nishimura M, Tsukamoto K, Hasebe N, *et al.*: Prediction of cardiac death in hemodialysis patients by myocardial fatty acid imaging. *J Am Coll Cardiol* 2008, 51:139–145.

33. Lodge MA: Evidence for inverse relationship between myocardial glucose utilization with PET and severity of renal dysfunction. *J Nucl Med* 2007, 48 [abstract]:108P.

34. Nishimura M, Hashimoto T, Kobayashi H, *et al.*: Myocardial scintigraphy using a fatty acid analogue detects coronary artery disease in hemodialysis patients. *Kidney Int* 2004, 66:811–819.

35. Dilsizian V and Fink J: Deleterious effect of altered myocardial fatty acid metabolism in kidney disease. *J Am Coll Cardiol* 2008, 51:146–148.

Nuclear Investigation in Heart Failure and Myocardial Viability

9

Vasken Dilsizian and Jagat Narula

Heart failure (HF) is evolving as an enormous cardiovascular health problem worldwide. In the United States alone, 5 million patients suffer from symptomatic disease, and more than half a million patients are newly diagnosed with HF every year. There are at least 1 million hospitalizations that result in 6.5 million hospital days and nearly 300,000 deaths each year. The total inpatient and outpatient costs for HF are approximately $35 billion. It has been increasingly realized that a much larger number of subjects may harbor asymptomatic ventricular dysfunction, and an enormous number may suffer from diseases that render them susceptible to development of HF. It is therefore important that clinicians are able to predict evolution and progression of the disease so that appropriate preventive measures are undertaken. For this purpose, various novel strategies are being developed for the identification of neurohumoral alterations that form the basis of ventricular remodeling

The objective of myocardial viability assessment in HF is to identify prospectively patients with potentially reversible left ventricular dysfunction in whom prognosis may be favorably altered with coronary artery revascularization. The concept that impaired left ventricular function may be reversible after revascularization is now well established. Pathophysiologic paradigms have emerged that describe the relationship between myocardial perfusion and ventricular function pertaining to myocardial stunning and hibernation. In these paradigms, myocardial function is depressed but myocytes remain viable, and therefore left ventricular dysfunction may be completely reversible. Parallel advances in the mechanisms underlying altered myocardial states and development of new radiotracers in nuclear cardiology have resulted in breakthroughs that contribute importantly to differentiating viable from nonviable myocardium in dysfunctional regions.

In this chapter, clinical experience of recent years, histomorphologic and structural changes in cardiomyopathy, left ventricular remodeling, and nuclear techniques that are most useful in clinical practice are presented.

Heart Failure: Pathogenetic Basis of Radionuclide Imaging

Figure 9-1. Priorities in imaging of heart failure (HF). Concerned with the enormity of the problem and enthused by the success of containment of the coronary disease epidemic, the American College of Cardiology–American Heart Association (ACC-AHA) proposed reclassification of HF in four stages [1]. These guidelines have emphasized the evolution and progression of the disease so that preventive measures can be enacted. *Stage A* identifies the patient who is at high risk for developing HF but has no structural disorder of the heart and is referred to as pre-HF. *Stage B* refers to a patient with a structural disorder of the heart who has never developed symptoms of HF. *Stage C* denotes the patient with past or current symptoms of HF associated with underlying structural heart disease. Finally, *Stage D* designates the patient who has advanced disease and requires specialized treatment strategies such as mechanical circulatory support, continuous inotropic infusions, cardiac transplantation, or hospice care. Only the latter two stages qualify for the traditional clinical diagnosis of HF. This classification recognizes that there are established risk factors and structural prerequisites for the development of HF and the process of ventricular remodeling determines the progression. It also recognizes that the therapeutic interventions performed even before the appearance of left ventricular dysfunction or symptoms can reduce the morbidity and mortality of HF. This classification system is intended to complement the widely used New York Heart Association (NYHA) classification, which primarily defines the severity of symptoms in patients who would correspond to stages B through D. Whereas the NYHA functional classification may change frequently over time, the ACC-AHA classification objectively identifies patients in the course of their disease and recommends treatments that are appropriate at each stage. As patients advance from one stage to the next, progression of the disease can be slowed or contained, but patients are expected to continue to receive the appropriate therapy for the highest stage achieved. Although patients may improve symptomatically to revert to a lower NYHA class, they may not return to earlier ACC-AHA stages. To fulfill the expectations of this classification, it may be necessary that an imager identify the subset of patients who are likely to remodel and determine the potential rate of remodeling. It may also be important to identify more established patients who are more likely to show reverse remodeling [2].

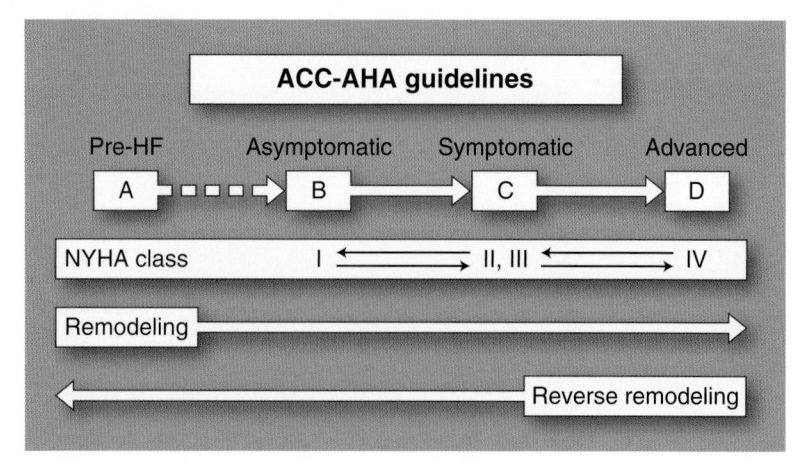

Development of Imaging Strategies for Prevention of Heart Failure

It is well established that myocardial neurohumoral upregulation contributes to ventricular remodeling and development of heart failure (HF) after myocardial infarction (MI). In particular, myocardial overexpression of the renin-angiotensin cascade is associated with interstitial fibrosis and ventricular dysfunction. Transgenic mice with deficient angiotensin II type 1 receptor expression exhibit minimal geometric and structural remodeling following MI, and show lesser upregulation of fetal genes, transforming growth factor-β1, and collagen deposition in comparison with the wild-type animals.

Clinical use of angiotensin-converting enzyme inhibitors and angiotensin receptor blockers in MI retards ventricular remodeling, delays development of HF, reduces rehospitalization for worsening HF, and improves survival. Because myocardial neurohumoral upregulation is associated with ventricular remodeling, we hypothesized that a novel diagnostic strategy targeted at detecting the extent of neurohumoral upregulation in the myocardium would allow identification of patients at risk of developing HF. In addition, such a strategy should allow optimization of pharmacologic therapy in HF patients.

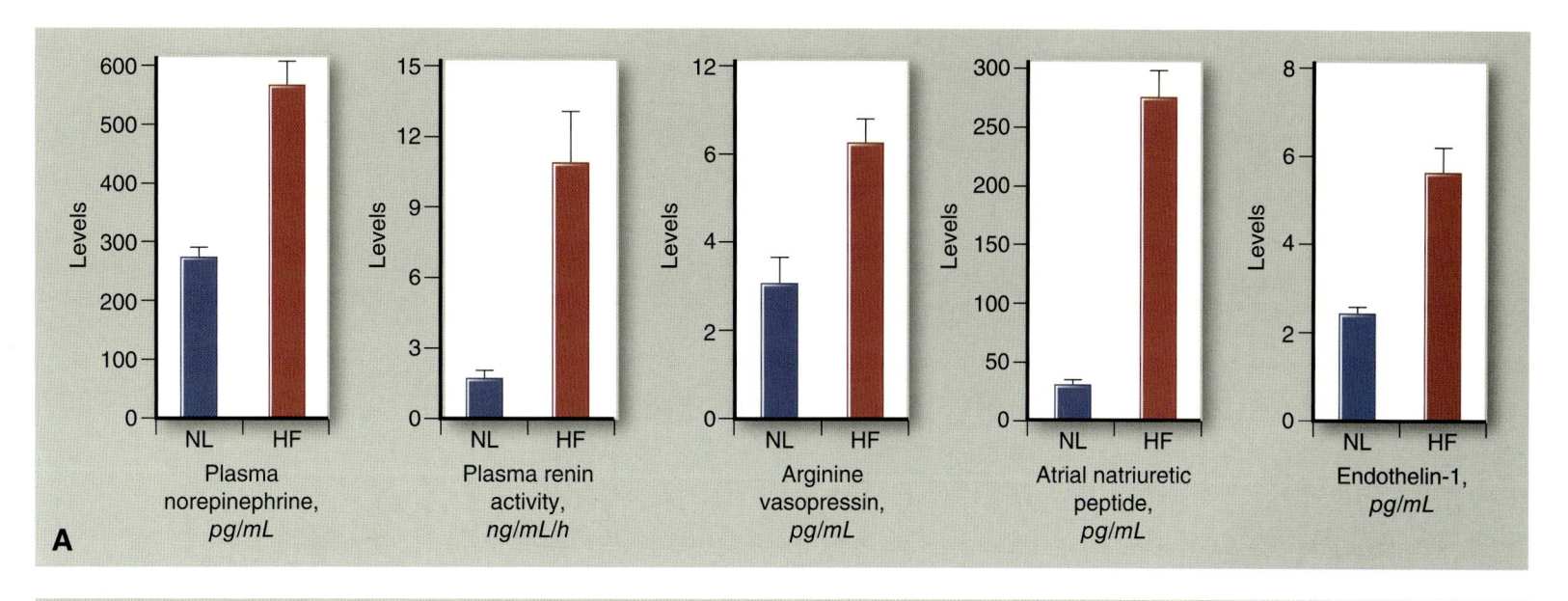

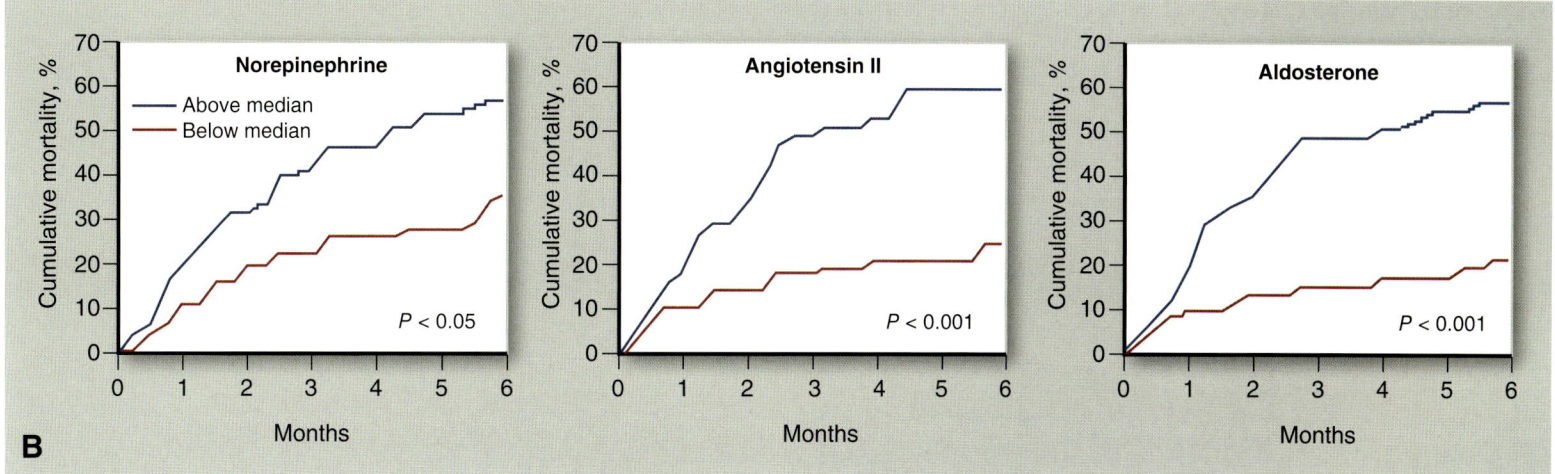

Figure 9-2. Neurohumoral upregulation in heart failure (HF). The process of remodeling or progression of HF is closely associated with widespread derangement of circulating neurohormones, the most notable being the activation of the sympathetic nervous system and the renin-angiotensin-aldosterone system. The increase in these neurohormones may constitute a part of the disease spectrum, represent a pathogenetic basis, or occur as a compensatory phenomenon. Neurohumoral upregulation over prolonged periods leads to progressive left ventricular remodeling and dysfunction. Other neurohormones that are elevated in HF include the vasoconstrictors vasopressin and endothelin, the vasodilators like natriuretic peptides, and the inflammatory cytokines like tumor necrosis factor-α (**A**). The degree of neurohormonal activation measured in the circulation is proportional to the severity of HF and demonstrates prognostic importance. As observed in the Cooperative North Scandinavian Enalapril Survival Study (CONSENSUS) (**B**) [3], the baseline neurohormone levels of norepinephrine, angiotensin II, and aldosterone were strong markers of subsequent mortality. Similar data are available from a number of other studies and for other neurohormones. NL—normal. (*Adapted from* Swedberg et al. [3].)

Nuclear Investigation in Heart Failure and Myocardial Viability 203

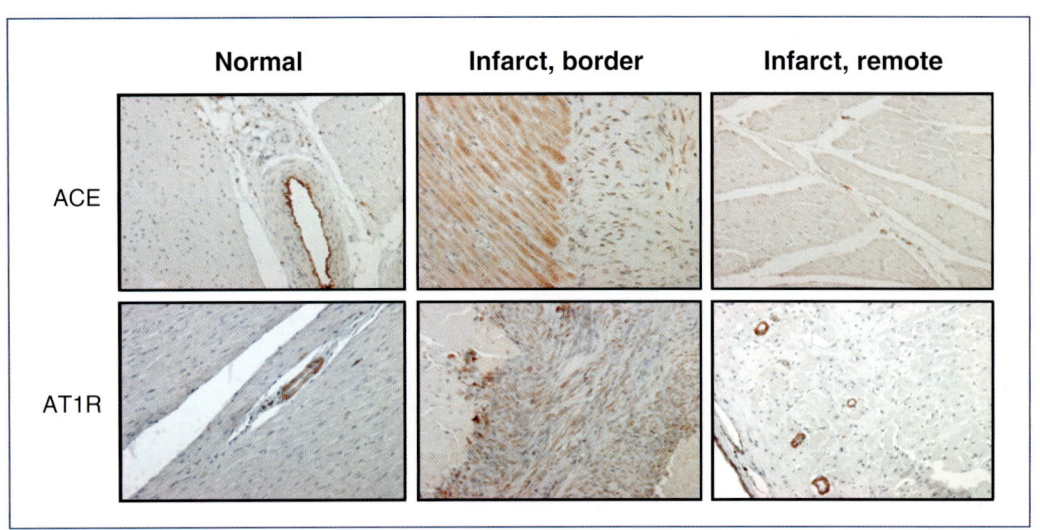

Figure 9-3. Myocardial neurohumoral upregulation after myocardial infarction. More so than the circulating levels, parallel upregulation of neurohumoral activity at the myocardial level is mechanistically more important. The increase in the hormonal system may reflect in the coronary sinus efflux. The converting enzyme and angiotensin upregulation is seen in myocytes, whereas receptors for angiotensin are preferentially expressed on the interstitial myofibrolasts. Shown here is upregulation of angiotensin-converting enzyme (ACE), angiotensin, and angiotensin II type 1 receptor (AT1R) in failing myocardium. Immunolabeled micrographs of ACE and AT1R from a normal and failing ovine heart showed altered distribution of ACE and AT1R in the infarct and peri-infarct zones of the myocardium. In the normal sheep myocardium (*top* and *bottom left*), ACE was confined to the vascular endothelium and AT1R was exclusively localized to vascular smooth muscle cells. In the failing sheep myocardium, there was upregulation of ACE in the cardiomyocytes in the infarct border zone (*top middle*) and myofibroblasts in the infarct center (*top right*). On the other hand, AT1R was normally observed in the vascular medial layer (*bottom middle*) and was significantly upregulated in myofibroblasts in the infarcted region (*bottom right*). (*Adapted from* Shirani *et al.* [4].)

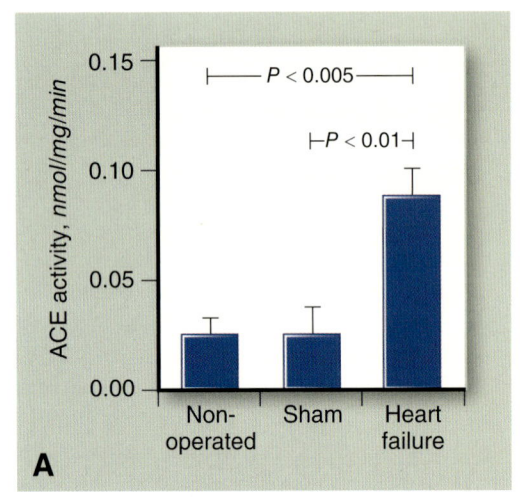

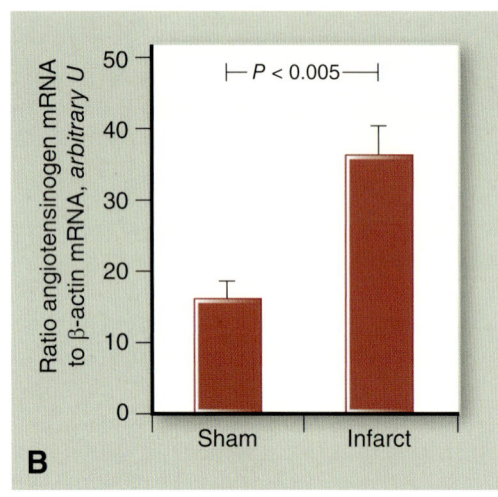

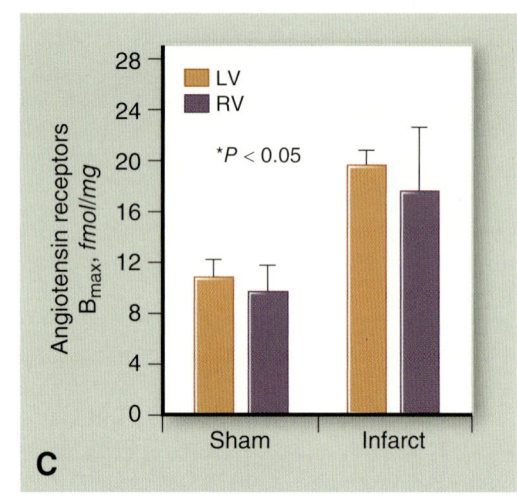

Figure 9-4. Upregulation of the tissue renin-angiotensin system in the noninfarcted myocardium after myocardial infarction. There is increasing evidence that in heart failure activation of the tissue renin-angiotensin system is associated with increased expression of several components of the pathway, including antiotensin-converting enzyme (ACE), angiotensinogen, and angiotensin II type I receptors. These data show a significant increase in ACE activity (**A**), the level of angiotensinogen mRNA (**B**), and the density of angiotensin II receptors (**C**). Although serum renin-angiotensin activity often returns to relatively normal levels in well-compensated heart failure, tissue renin-angiotensin activity may remain elevated in the myocardium and contribute to the progression of myocardial remodeling. LV—left ventricle; RV—right ventricle. (*Adapted from* Hirsch *et al.* [5]; Lindpaintner *et al.* [6]; and Meggs *et al.* [7].)

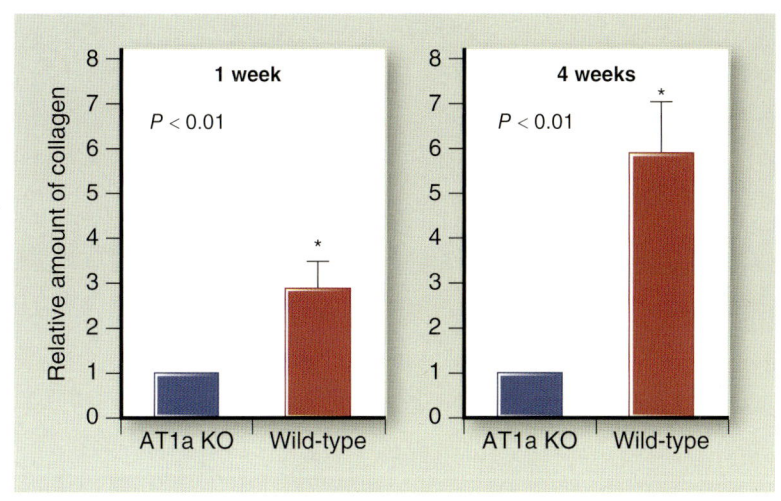

Figure 9-5. The role of myocardial renin-angiotensin system in reactive fibrosis and remodeling in noninfarcted myocardium. The extent of interstitial fibrosis and perivascular fibrosis is shown in angiotensin II type 1a (AT1a) receptor knockout (KO) mice and wild-type mice at 1 and 4 weeks after large acute myocardial infarction. At 4 weeks after infarction, control mice showed more marked left ventricular remodeling and fibrosis than did the AT1a KO mice. In addition, the cumulative 4-week mortality rate for the AT1a KO mice was reduced from 22.7% to 5.9% compared with controls, despite similar initial infarct size. These findings indicate that AT1a receptors play a pivotal role in the progression of left ventricular remodeling after myocardial infarction. (*From* Harada *et al.* [8]; with permission.)

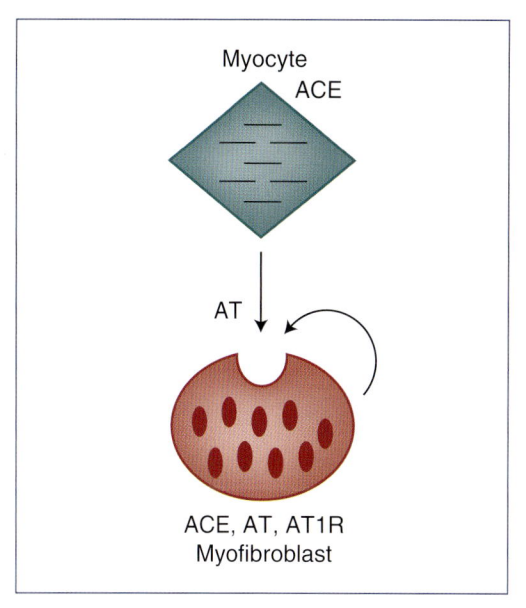

Figure 9-6. Predicting likelihood of ventricular remodeling. It is proposed that continuous growth stimulation of myofibriblasts may lead to collagen formation, interstitial fibrosis, and remodeling. As such, the assessment of angiotensin-converting enzyme (ACE) overexpression in myocytes or AT1R upregulation on myofibroblasts will allow prediction and likelihood of myofibroblast proliferation, rate of remodeling, and development of heart failure.

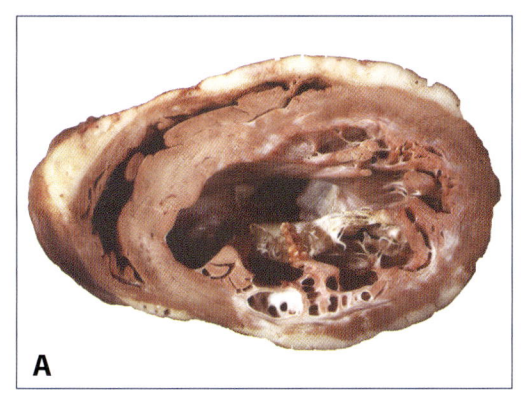

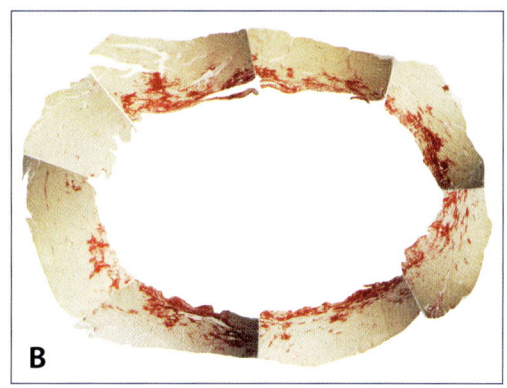

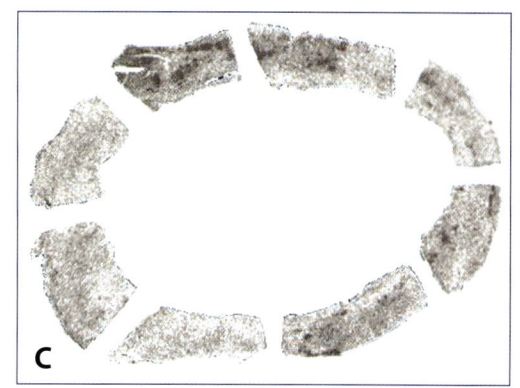

Figure 9-7. Targeting of angiotensin-converting enzyme (ACE) overexpression. Five radiolabeled ACE inhibitors have been employed for imaging: an iodotyrosyl derivative of the ACE inhibitor lisinopril ([^{125}I]351A), [^{18}F]-captopril, [^{18}F]-fluorobenzoyl-lisinopril, [^{11}C]-zofenoprilat, and [^{99m}Tc]-lisinopril. All of these radiotracers have been shown to bind specifically to the active site of ACE with the binding density correlating closely with literature values for enzyme activity. In an ex vivo study of explanted hearts of patients with ischemic cardiomyopathy, [^{18}F]-fluorobenzoyl-lisinopril was shown to specifically bind to tissue (myocardial) ACE with the highest activity in regions adjacent to infarcted myocardium [9]. Specific ACE binding was about twice as great as the nonspecific binding, and ACE binding in peri-infarct segments was about 1.3 fold greater than binding in remote, noninfarct segments. Gross pathology of a mid-ventricular slice (**A**) with corresponding contiguous mid-ventricular slices stained with Picrosirius red stain (for assessment of collagen deposition) (**B**) and [^{18}F]-fluorobenzyl-linsinopril autoradiographic images (**C**) are shown. [^{18}F]-fluorobenzoyl-lisinopril binding to ACE is nonuniform in infarct, peri-infarct and remote, noninfarct segments. Increased [^{18}F]-fluorobenzoyl-lisinopril binding can be seen in the segments adjacent to the collagen replacement. (*Adapted from* Dilsizian *et al.* [9].)

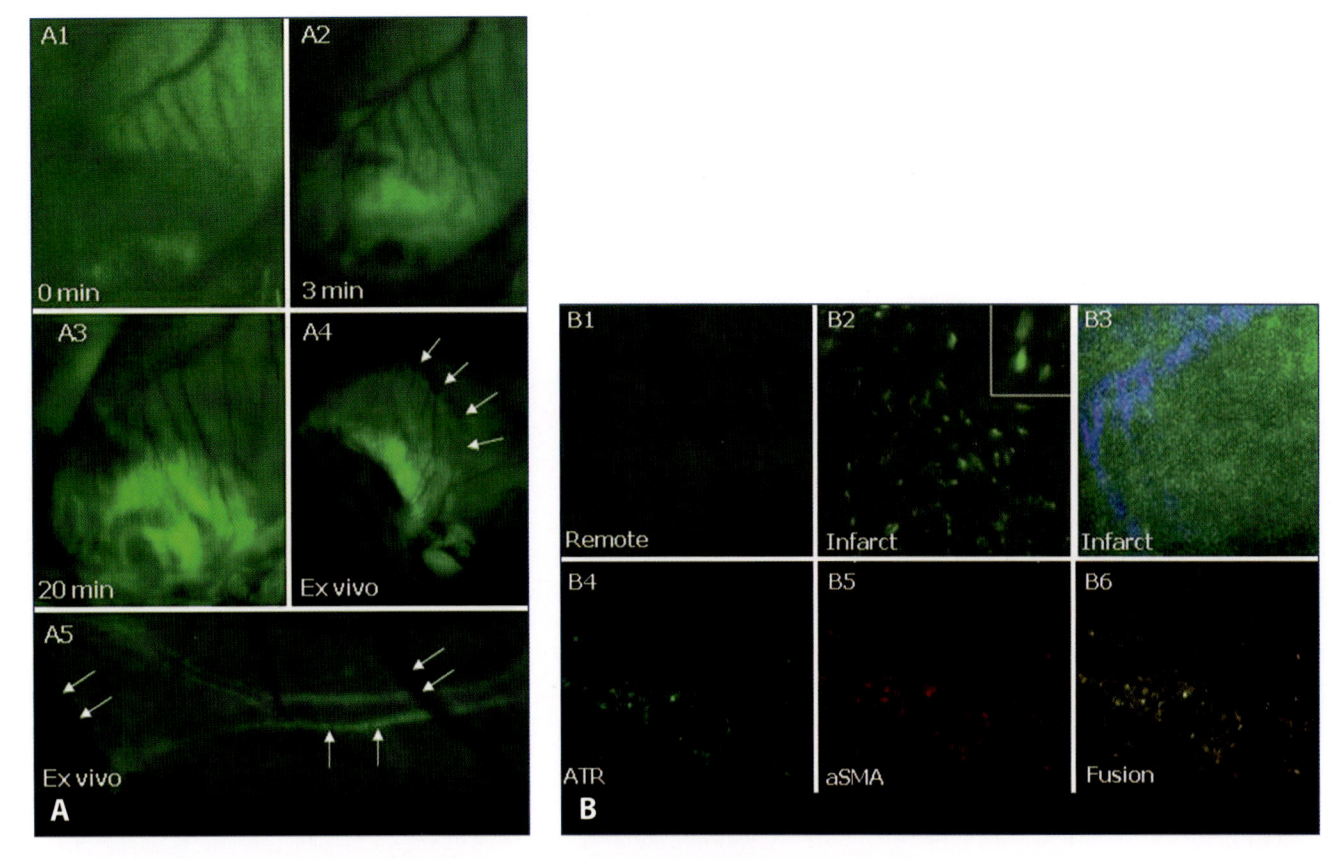

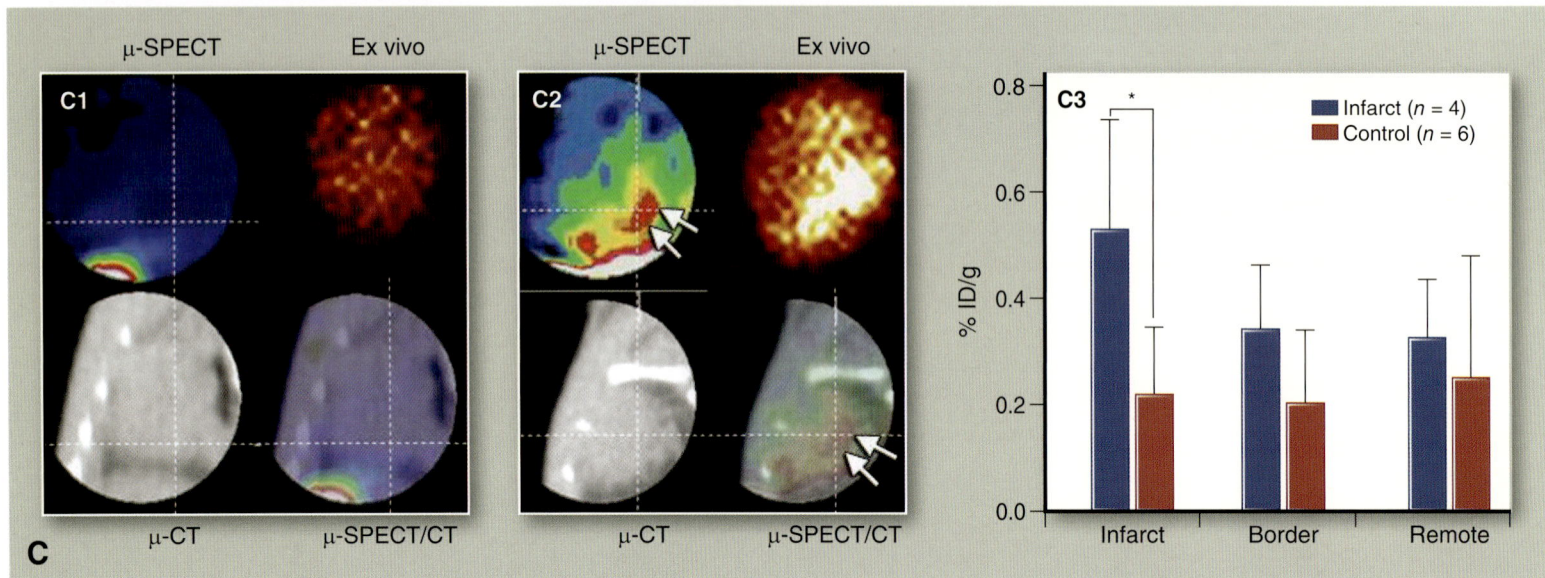

Figure 9-8. Imaging of angiotensin receptors on the myofibroblasts. To evaluate the feasibility of noninvasive imaging of angiotensin II (AT) receptor upregulation in a mouse model of post–myocardial infarction (MI) heart failure (HF), AT receptor imaging was performed at various time points after permanent coronary artery ligation, or in controls using a fluoresceinated angiotensin peptide analog (APA) or losartan. **A,** The intravital microscopy images show a 3-week old MI in the murine heart failure model from baseline (*A1*), and 3 minutes (*A2*), and at 20 minutes (*A3*) after administration of green fluorescent APA, demonstrating gradual increase of the fluorescent APA in infarcted region. Fluorescent uptake was maximum at 20 minutes after intravenous APA injection. The ex vivo image (*A4*) demonstrates APA uptake in the border zone (*arrows*), as thinned out infarct zone has collapsed and is therefore not visible. *Panel A5* shows APA uptake in smooth muscle cell layer of a small coronary artery (*vertical arrows*) as well as minimal uptake in thinner veins (*diagonal arrows*). **B,** Upon confocal microscopic characterization, the remote zone (*B1*) demonstrates no APA uptake in interstitium or cardiomyocytes. The cells of nonmyocytic origin demonstrate fluorescent APA uptake in the infarct zone (*B2*), with an enlarged image of myofibroblast uptake (*inset*). These cells in the infarct region (*B4, green*) also stained positively for smooth muscle actin (SMA) (*B5, red*), showing colocalization (*B6, yellow*), indicating AT receptor expression on myofibroblasts. Two-photon microscopy demonstrated fluorescent APA intracellularly within the myofibroblast (*B3, green*), with collagen surrounding the myofibroblast using second harmonic generation imaging (*B3, blue*). **C,** For noninvasive radionuclide imaging, the μ-SPECT and μ-CT images are performed; a control mouse after ^{99m}Tc-losartan administration shows no uptake in the heart (*C1*) in the in vivo and ex vivo images. There is only some liver uptake on the *bottom left* of the SPECT image. In the 3-week post-MI animal, significant radiolabeled losartan uptake is observed in the anterolateral wall (*C2, arrows*). The infarct uptake on the in vivo image is confirmed in the ex vivo image. The histogram (*C3*) demonstrates significantly (*asterisk*) higher uptake in the infarcted region (0.524 ± 0.212 % ID [injected dose]/g) as compared with control noninfarcted animals (0.215 ± 0.129 % ID/g; $P \leq 0.05$). (*Adapted from Verjans et al.* [10].)

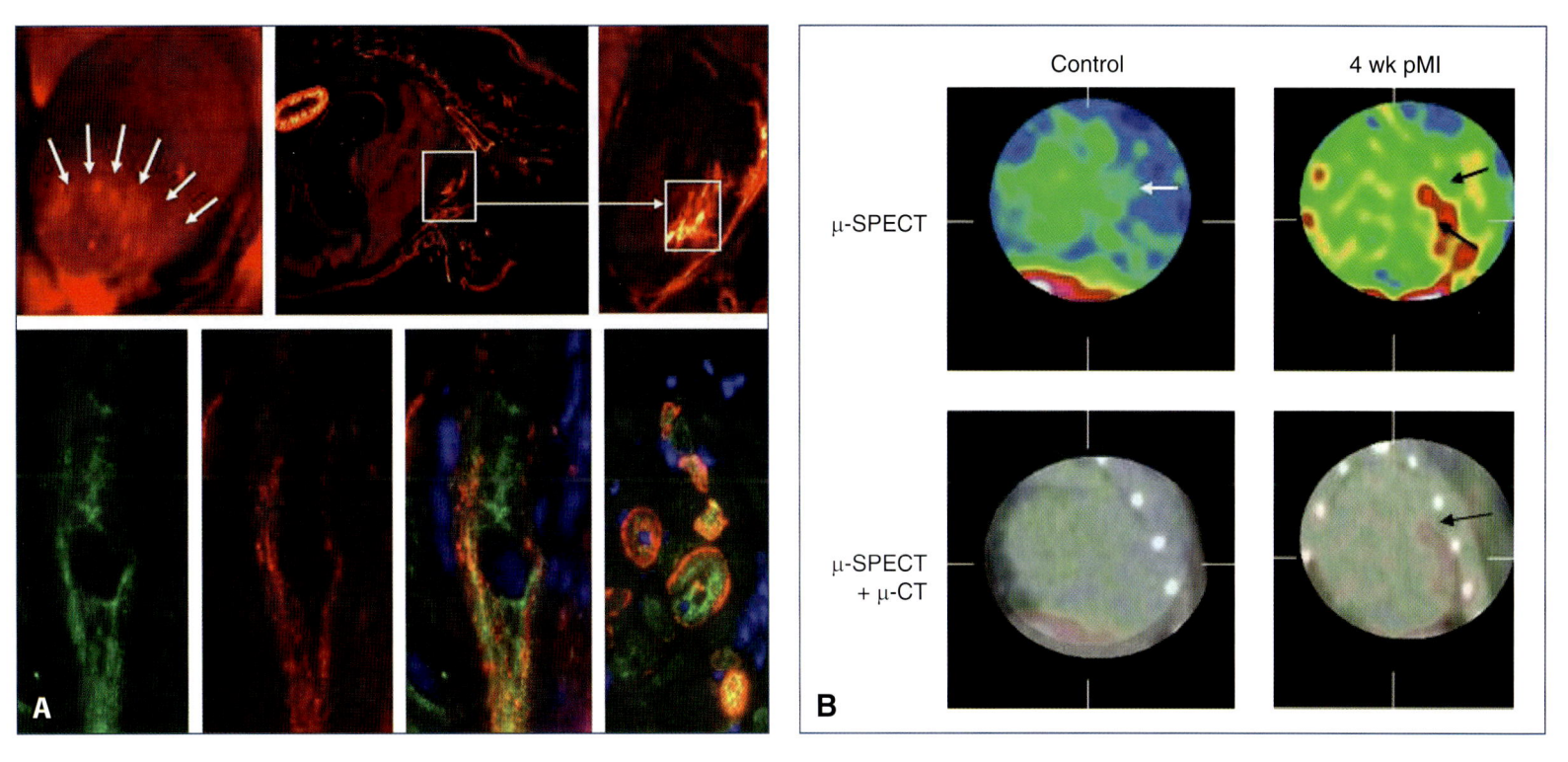

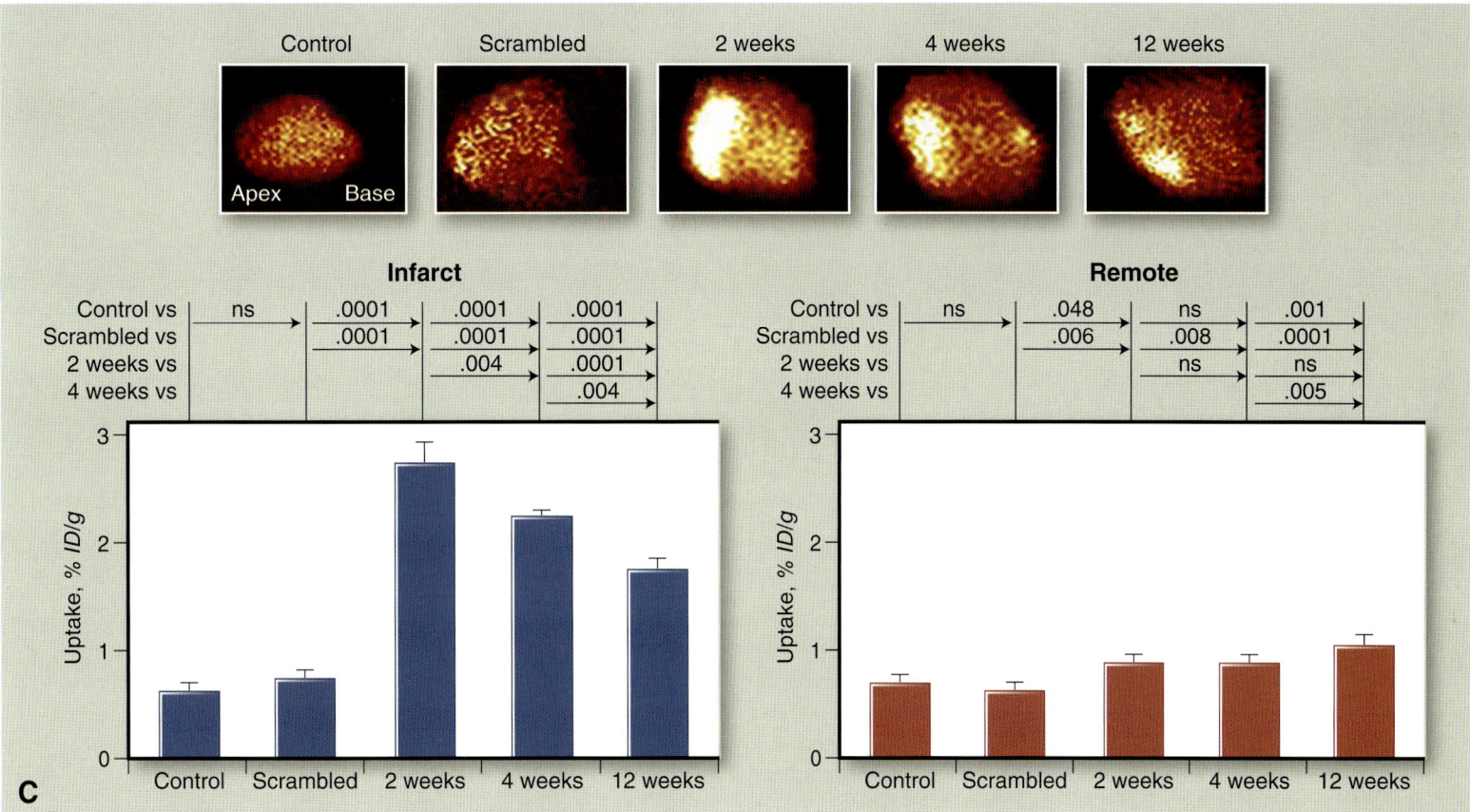

Figure 9-9. Imaging of integrin expression on myofibroblasts. Collagen production and fibrosis in the myocardium are associated with myofibroblastic proliferation. Besides up-regulation of angiotensin receptors, myofibroblasts demonstrate integrin moieties. The RGD peptide (containing the arginine-glycine-aspartate motif) that binds to integrins such as αvβ3 has been used to identify neovascularization in post-infarct animal models. Since integrin αvβ3 is associated with the supermature focal adhesion molecules on the cell membrane of myofibroblasts, we hypothesized that appropriately labeled RGD probes should identify myofibroblasts in post–infarct myocardium. For the experiment shown here, Cy5.5-RGD imaging peptide (CRIP) labeled with ^{99m}Tc was used in a murine model of post–myocardial infarction (MI) ventricular dysfunction. Scrambled CRIP(sCRIP) was used for tracer control.

Continued on the next page

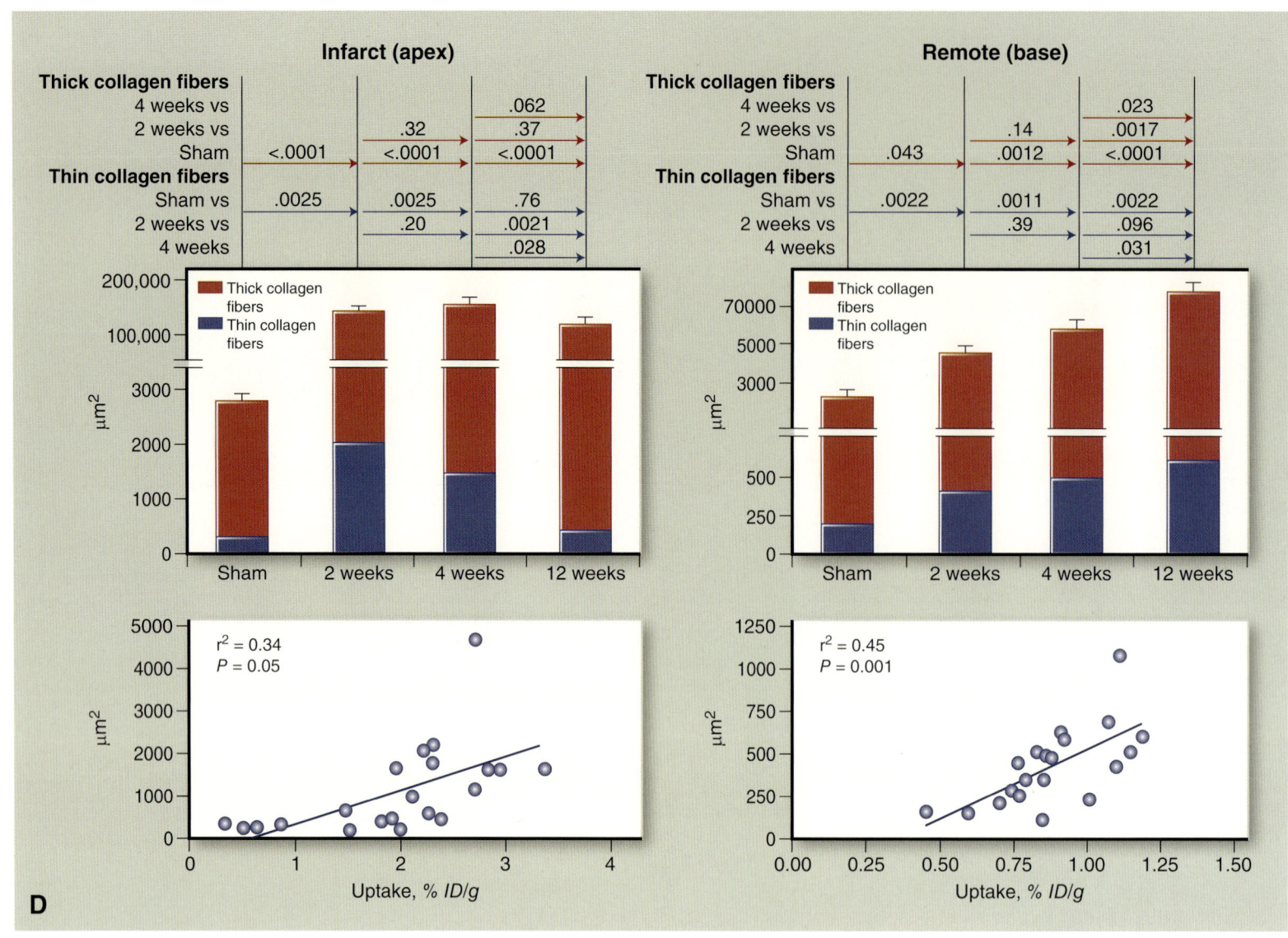

Figure 9-9. *(Continued)* Probe targeting was evaluated 3.5 hours after intravenous administration of CRIP in 2-week post-MI animals. **A,** Localization of the Cy5.5 fluorescence (*red*) was clearly observed in the infarct and peri-infarct zones in vivo (*top left, arrows*). A 30-μ whole mouse slice demonstrates myocardial uptake of the probe (*top middle, square*); intense uptake is seen in the kidney, which serves as the route of excretion. Magnification (*top right*) of the area enclosed by the box in the top middle panel demonstrates fluorescent probe localization in the subendocardium. For further characterization of the probe targets (*bottom panels*), we correlated the uptake of intravenously administered CRIP in 2-week post-MI animals (*red*) with concurrent staining of the sections by anti-alpha smooth muscle actin antibody (*green*); colocalization is shown by overlay (*bottom, second from right*). The localization of CRIP was observed in spindle-shaped myofibroblasts in the infarct area. CRIP colocalization is seen in transversely sectioned myofibroblasts (*bottom right*).

B, In vivo μ-SPECT and μ-SPECT/μ-CT fusion images in frontal projection are shown in unmanipulated control and 4-week post-MI animals 3.5 hours after radiolabeled CRIP administration. No uptake of ^{99m}Tc-labeled CRIP is observed in the unmanipulated animal (control). On the other hand, intense anterior uptake is seen in the infarcted mouse (4 wk pMI). The cardiac localization is confirmed in the μ-CT fusion image.

C, Ex vivo images of the heart are presented (*top*). Control heart with CRIP probe and 4-week post-MI heart with sCRIP show no radiotracer uptake. On the other hand, intense CRIP uptake is seen in the 2-week post-MI animal. The uptake in the infarcted area was highest in mice 2 weeks after MI, followed by 4 and 12 weeks. Quantitative Tc-CRIP uptake (*bottom*) in the infarct (apex) and remote (base) areas is presented as the percent injected dose (ID)/g uptake. The infarct area shows the highest uptake in mice 2 weeks after MI, followed by 4 and 12 weeks after MI. On the other hand, the uptake in the remote areas shows trends toward higher uptake from 2 to 12 weeks after MI. Quantitative data confirmed the findings of ex vivo images. Data are presented as mean ± standard error of the mean.

D, The total collagen content in the infarcted area remains similar with the passage of time; however, it increases significantly in the remote region (*top*). Characterization of the collagen fibers by polarization reveals that the thin or new collagen fibers decreased in the infarct region (suggestive of cessation of collagen production and maturation of the collagen fibers) and increased substantially in the remote area (suggesting ongoing production of the new collagen with increasing total collagen content). The prevalence of new collagen fibers paralleled the CRIP uptake and demonstrated a significant direct correlation, both in infarct and remote zones (*bottom*). (*Adapted from* Borne et al. [11].)

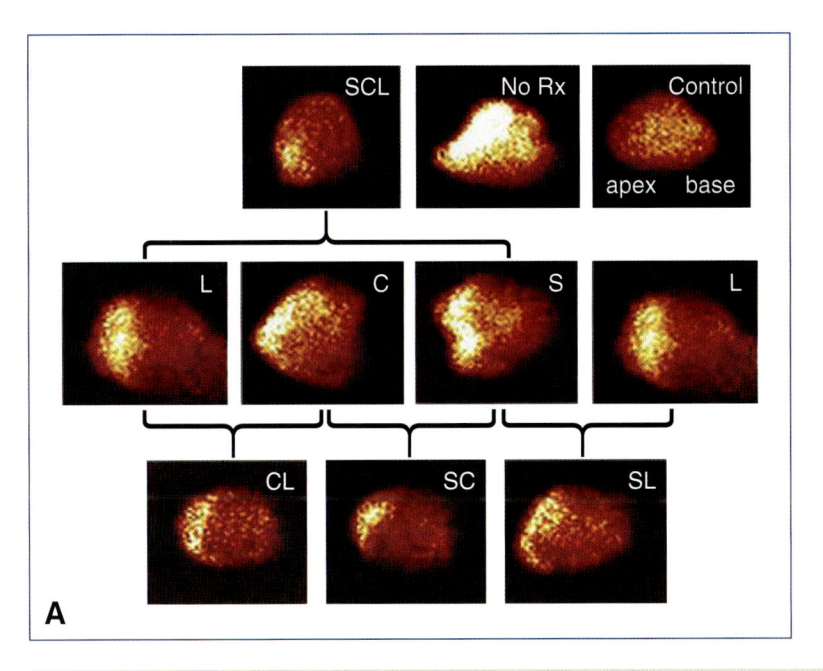

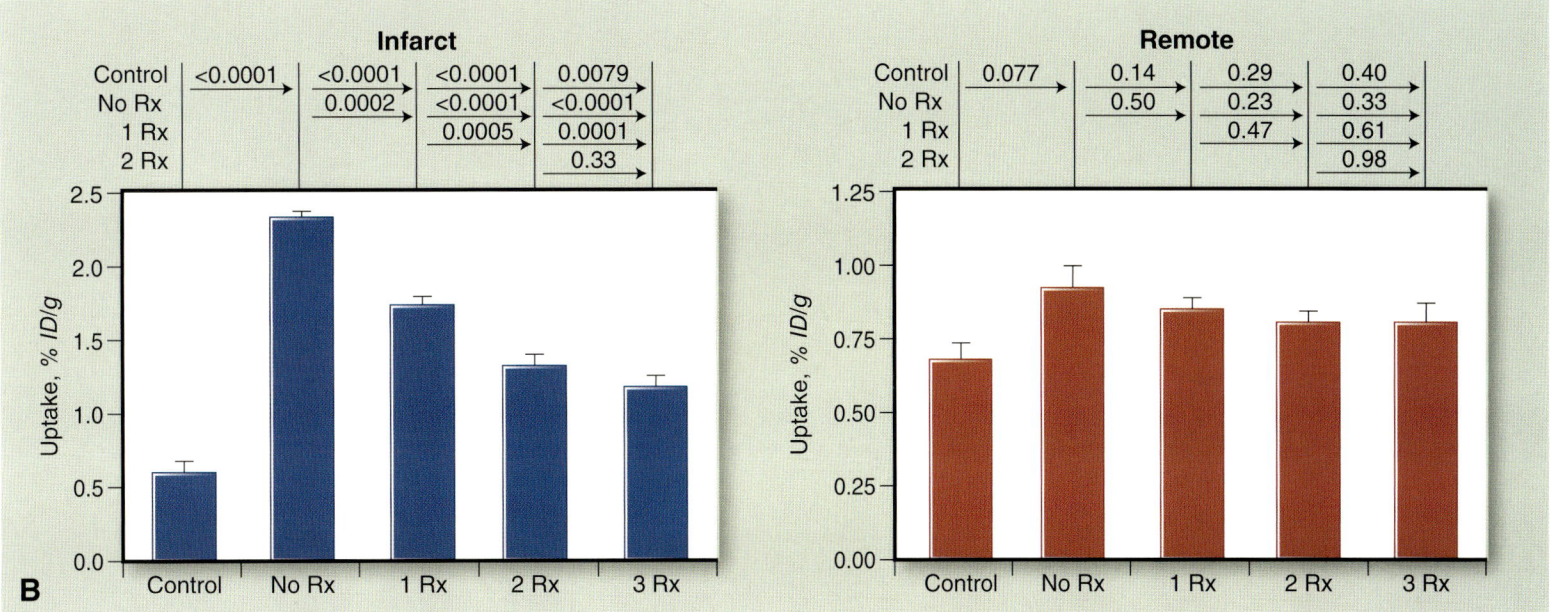

Figure 9-10. Efficacy of neurohumoral antagonists in prevention of remodeling. **A,** Disease control (unmanipulated) heart with Cy5.5-RGD imaging peptide (CRIP) probe shows no radiotracer uptake in ex vivo image of the heart. However, intense Tc-CRIP uptake is found in 4-week untreated (no Rx) post–myocardial infarction animals (*upper panel, right*). The uptake in the infarcted area is reduced after neurohumoral treatment with solitary agents and combination therapy (*middle* and *lower panels*) (losartan [L], captopril [C], spironolactone [S]). Losartan images are displayed twice (*middle panel*) for the convenience of comparison.

B, Quantitative CRIP uptake in the infarct (apex) (*left*) and remote (base) (*right*) areas. The % injected dose (ID)/g uptake in the infarct area is greatest in untreated mice, followed by treatment with one (1 Rx), two (2 Rx), and three (3 Rx) agents, respectively. Quantitative data confirmed the findings of ex vivo images. Data are presented as mean ± SEM.

Continued on the next page

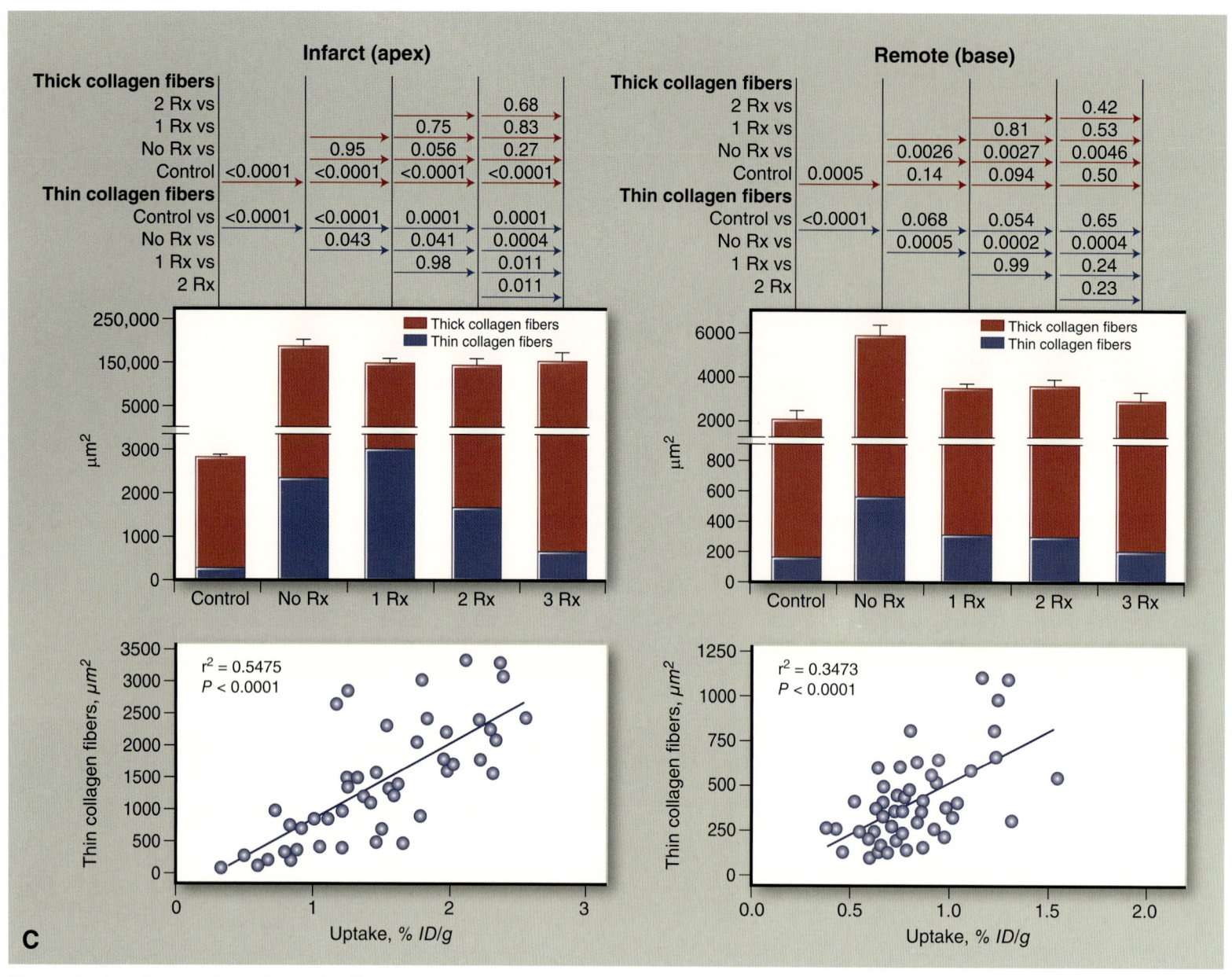

Figure 9-10. *(Continued)* **C,** The total collagen content does not change substantially with treatment in the infarcted zone, but does so in the remote areas (*top*). Further characterization of the collagen fibers by polarization reveals that the thin or new collagen fibers decreased both in the infarct and remote regions after treatment. This indicates cessation of new collagen production and maturation of the collagen fibers after treatment. The prevalence of new collagen fibers parallels the CRIP uptake and demonstrates a significant direct correlation, both in infarct and remote regions (*bottom*). (*Adapted from* Borne et al. [12].)

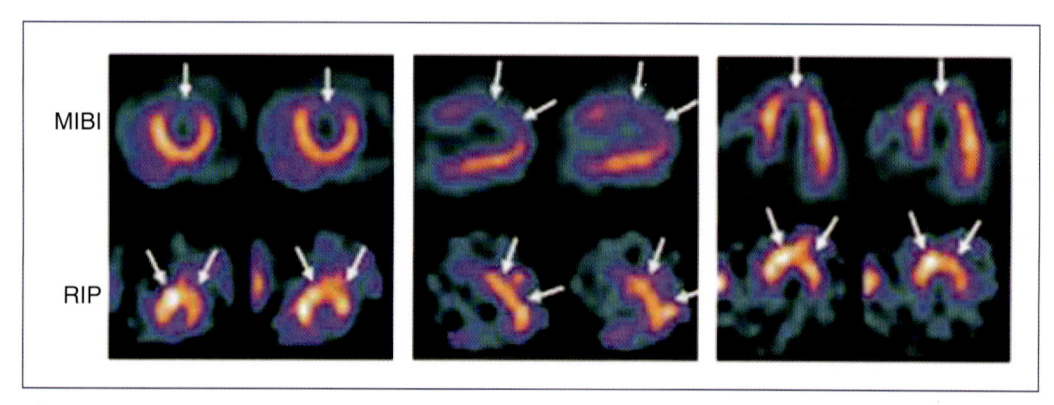

Figure 9-11. Noninvasive SPECT imaging of αvβ3 upregulation in a patient 3 weeks after myocardial infarction (MI). In a clinical study, ^{99m}Tc-labeled RGD imaging peptide (RIP) in 10 patients at 3 weeks after MI demonstrated the feasibility of targeted imaging of interstitial alterations. After intravenous injection of the radiotracer, imaging was performed, and uptake was seen in transverse (*top*), vertical long axis (*middle*) and horizontal long axis (*bottom*) views reflecting active remodeling regions. These images corresponded with the baseline MIBI perfusion defects (*arrows*). The area of radiotracer uptake was generally greater than the perfusion deficit. The RGD imaging peptide uptake extends beyond perfusion deficit (*arrows*) in this set of images. One-year follow-up MRI studies confirmed that the extent of fibrosis colocalized with earlier radiotracer uptake in patients. (*Adapted from* Verjans et al. [13].)

210 Atlas of Nuclear Cardiology

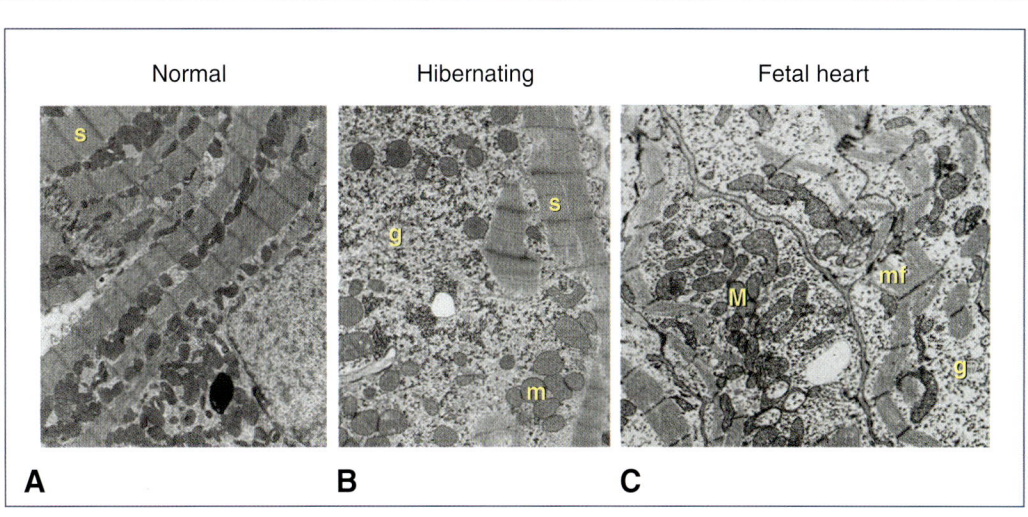

Development of Strategies for Identification of Viable Myocardium and Reversibility in Ischemic Cardiomyopathy

Figure 9-12. Structural correlates of myocardial viability in normal (**A**), hibernating (**B**), and 30-week gestation fetal heart (**C**). Irrespective of the inciting stimulus of decrease in regional blood flow, the myocardium undergoes metabolic, structural, and functional remodeling in response to myocardial ischemia, termed *programmed cell survival* [14]. When compared with the normal myocardium (**A**), electron micrograph of the hibernating myocardium (**B**) shows depletion of sarcomeres (s) (present only at the cell periphery) and contractile filament material (mf), accumulation and storage of glycogen (g), and the appearance of numerous small mitochondria (m). Because some of these structural changes of altered myocytes resemble those of embryonic cells (**C**), such changes have been attributed to a dedifferentiation process. Moreover, altered myocytes have been shown to re-express contractile proteins that are specific to the fetal heart, such as the alpha-smooth muscle cell actin. Beyond structural similarities on electron micrograph, hibernating myocardium resembles the fetal heart by its preferential metabolism of glucose and the presence of large amounts of glycogen in the cardiomyocytes. Recent literature on programmed cell survival and apoptosis provide support of a direct link between metabolic pathways and cellular adaptation or maladaptation [15]. It has been proposed, therefore, that perhaps metabolic reprogramming of the ischemic myocardium initiates and sustains the functional and structural remodeling of hibernating myocardium (scale bar = 1.0 μm). (*Adapted from* Depre and Taegmeyer [15] and Kim *et al.* [16].)

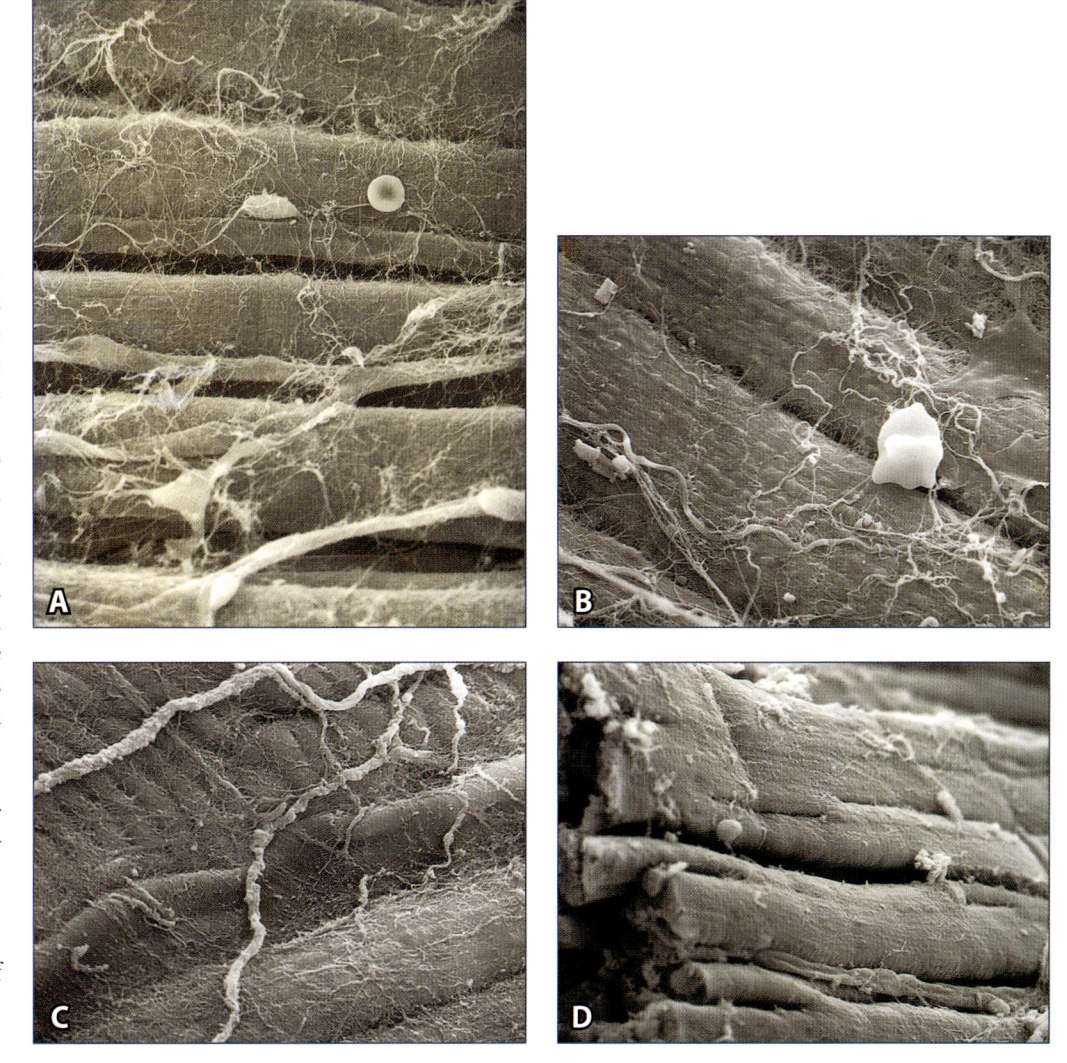

Figure 9-13. Scanning electron micrographs from normal tissue, a nonischemic region, and stunned myocardial regions. **A**, Normal tissue shows the usual dense and florid collagen weave enveloping the individual myocytes. There are abundant collagen struts that interconnect myocyte to myocyte and myocyte to capillary. The collagen struts are also connected to collagen weave (× 3000). **B**, In the nonischemic myocardial region, collagen cables are smooth and continuous, branch off into smaller cables, and connect with the underlying collagen weave on the surface of the myocyte (× 5700). **C**, In the stunned myocardial region, the collagen cables are characterized by a rough, irregular, notched appearance. The collagen weave is generally matted with a beaded and granular appearance, suggestive of degeneration (× 9000). **D**, In another example of stunned myocardium, the normally ubiquitous myocyte to myocyte struts are minimal to absent, with nodular or nublike structures likely indicative of broken collagen struts. In addition, there is almost complete absence of the perimysial weave (× 2100). (*Courtesy of* Calvin Eng; *from* Zhao *et al.* [17].)

Nuclear Investigation in Heart Failure and Myocardial Viability

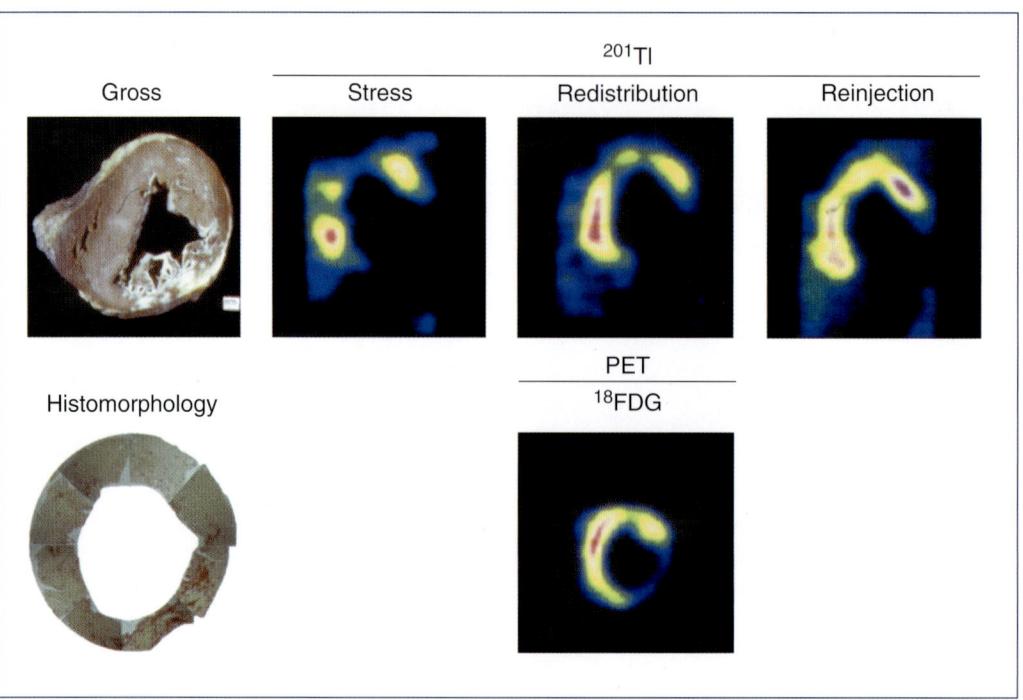

Figure 9-14. Disparity between left ventricular contractile dysfunction and the extent of myocardial injury assessed by thallium scintigraphy. Correlation between gross pathology, histomorphology, and ^{201}Tl and [^{18}F]-fluorodeoxyglucose (FDG) PET studies from a patient with stable chronic ischemic heart disease and severe left ventricular dysfunction who underwent orthotopic cardiac transplantation is demonstrated. Gross pathology and histomorphology of a midventricular slice is shown (*left*) with corresponding thallium and FDG PET images (*right*). On the thallium study, there are extensive abnormalities in the anterior, septal, and inferolateral regions during stress. On the redistribution image, there is partial reversibility of the anterior region, complete reversibility of the septum, and irreversible defect in the inferolateral region. After ^{201}Tl reinjection, there is complete reversibility of the septal and anterior regions with persistent irreversible defect in the inferolateral region. The corresponding FDG PET image shows preserved metabolic activity and hence viability in all regions except for the inferolateral region. On gross pathology, there is white fibrotic myocardium in the inferolateral region, and histomorphologic analysis shows a significant amount of red-stained collagen intermixed within normal tissue. Because structural changes in hibernating myocardium are chronic in nature and have developed over a prolonged period, some regions viable by scintigraphic or echocardiographic techniques may be irreversible despite successful revascularization. (*Courtesy of* Jamshid Shirani.)

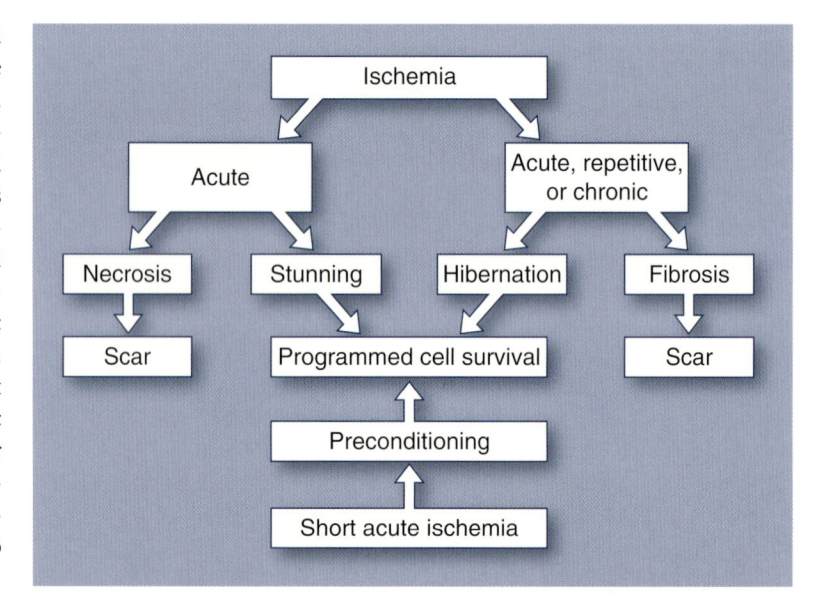

Figure 9-15. Imbalance between oxygen supply, usually due to reduced myocardial perfusion, and oxygen demand, determined primarily by the rate and force of myocardial contraction, is termed *ischemic myocardium*. If the oxygen supply-demand imbalance is transient (*ie*, triggered by exertion), it represents reversible ischemia. On the other hand, if regional oxygen supply-demand imbalance is prolonged, high-energy phosphates will be depleted, regional contractile function will progressively deteriorate, and cell membrane rupture with cell death will follow (myocardial necrosis and fibrosis). The phenomena of stunning, hibernation, and ischemic preconditioning represent different mechanisms of acute and chronic adaptation to a temporary or sustained reduction in coronary blood flow. Such modulated responses to ischemia are regulated to preserve sufficient energy to protect the structural and functional integrity of the cardiac myocyte. In contrast to programmed cell death, or apoptosis, Taegtmeyer [18] has coined the term *programmed cell survival* to describe the commonality between myocardial stunning, hibernation, and ischemic preconditioning independent from their disparate myocardial responses to acute and chronic ischemia. (*Adapted from* Taegtmeyer [18].)

Figure 9-16. Requirements for cellular viability. To date, the most common definition of myocardial viability has been the temporal improvement in contractile function of a dysfunctional region after restoration of blood flow. Requirements for cellular viability include sufficient myocardial blood flow, intact sarcolemmal membrane function, and preserved metabolic activity. Myocardial blood flow has to be adequate to deliver substrate to the myocyte to be used in the metabolic process, as well as to remove the end products of the metabolic process. If regional blood flow is severely reduced or absent, then the metabolites and end products will accumulate, causing inhibition of the enzymes of the metabolic pathway, depletion of high-energy phosphates, cell membrane disruption, and cell death. Thus, at either extreme of the range of blood flow, myocardial perfusion tracers provide information regarding myocardial viability. However, in regions in which the reduction in blood flow is of intermediate severity, perfusion information alone may be insufficient to determine viability, and additional pieces of data such as metabolic indexes would be necessary. Intact sarcolemmal membrane function to maintain electrochemical gradients across the cell membrane is a requirement for myocyte viability. Because cell membrane integrity is highly dependent on preserved intracellular metabolic activity to generate high-energy phosphates, tracers that reflect sarcolemmal cation flux as well as perfusion, such as ^{201}Tl and ^{82}Rb, should parallel the viability information provided by markers of metabolic activity, *eg*, [^{18}F]-fluorodeoxyglucose. Thus, in the setting of reduced regional blood flow and function, techniques that assess intact cellular sarcolemmal function or metabolic processes provide unique insight into the presence or absence of myocardial viability.

Requirements for Cellular Viability

- Adequate myocardial blood flow
- Sarcolemmal membrane integrity
- Preserved metabolic activity

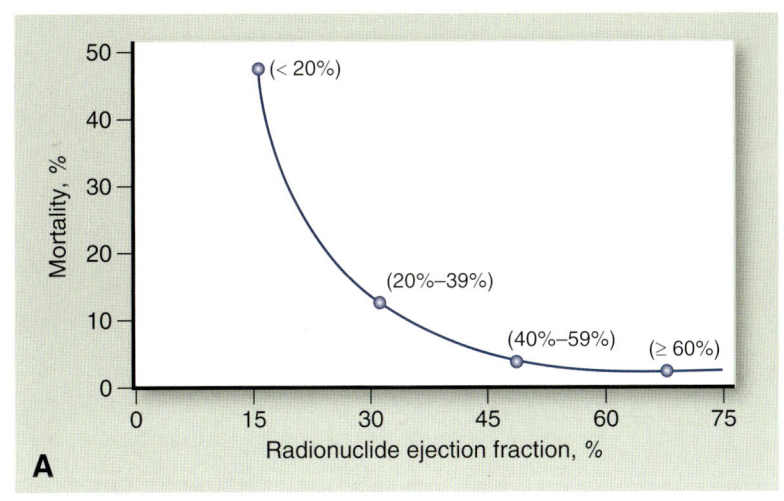

Figure 9-17. Left ventricular ejection fraction (LVEF). LVEF is a major determinant of survival in patients with acute and chronic coronary artery disease. **A,** In patients with acute myocardial infarction, the Multicenter Postinfarction Trial showed a curvilinear relationship between mortality rates in the first year after myocardial infarction and predischarge LVEF. This relationship has been demonstrated conclusively in virtually every study assessing patient outcome after myocardial infarction. It is apparent from the curve that attempts to risk-stratify patients with preserved left ventricular function ($\geq 50\%$) further will be problematic, because this cohort will have few cardiac-related deaths during the subsequent year after infarction. On the other hand, among patients with moderate-to-severe left ventricular dysfunction, further risk stratification is both feasible and clinically relevant. **B,** In chronic stable coronary artery disease, the cumulative 4-year survival of the medically treated Coronary Artery Surgery Study registry patients based on LVEF at rest is shown. Patients with normal ($> 50\%$) or mildly reduced (35%–49%) left ventricular function have an excellent 4-year survival on medical therapy (92% and 83%, respectively). On the other hand, patients with moderate to severely reduced ($< 34\%$) left ventricular function have a significantly lower 4-year survival (58%) when treated with medical therapy alone. (*Adapted from* [19] and Mock *et al.* [20].)

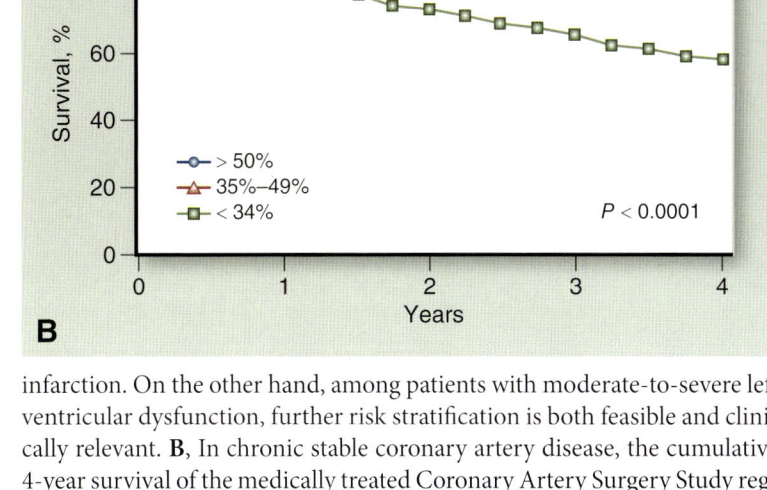

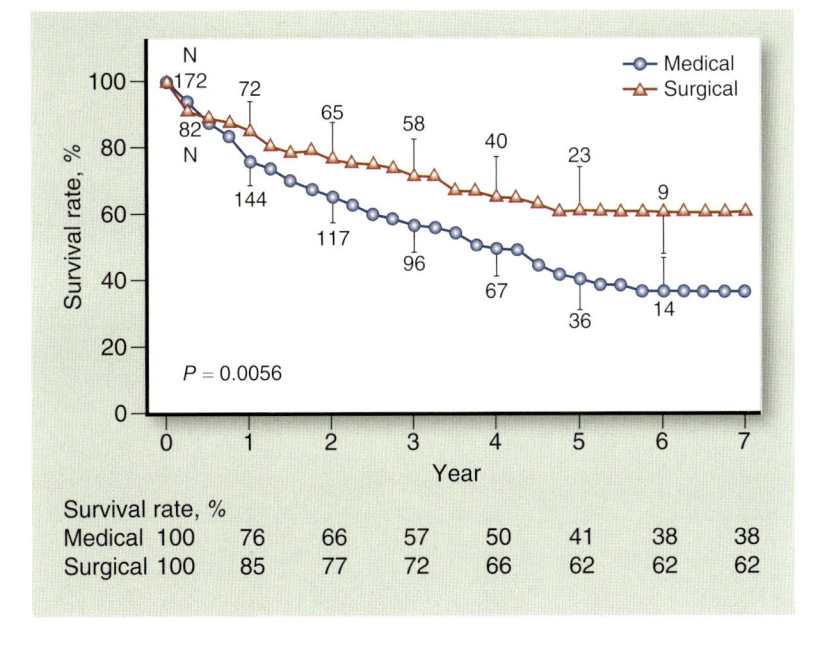

Figure 9-18. Life-table cumulative survival for surgically and medically treated Coronary Artery Surgery Study registry patients with severely reduced left ventricular ejection fraction (LVEF). Short- and long-term surgical survival benefits are greatest in patients with the most severe left ventricular dysfunction. Among the patients with LVEF of 25% or lower, the 5-year survival rate is 62% with surgical treatment and 41% with medical treatment. The 1- and 2-year survival rates of surgically treated patients is 85% and 77%, in contrast to 76% and 66% in the medically treated patients, respectively. Myocardial reperfusion via revascularization ameliorates ischemic injury, recruits hibernating regions, and prevents future infarction. However, the operative risk of coronary artery bypass surgery is increased in this patient population, which explains the reluctance of cardiac surgeons to operate on these patients without evidence of myocardial viability. With increased surgical expertise and improved intraoperative myocardial preservation techniques, combined with accurate prospective assessment of myocardial viability, surgical mortality rates have decreased substantially since the 1980s. (*Adapted from* Alderman *et al.* [21].)

Nuclear Investigation in Heart Failure and Myocardial Viability

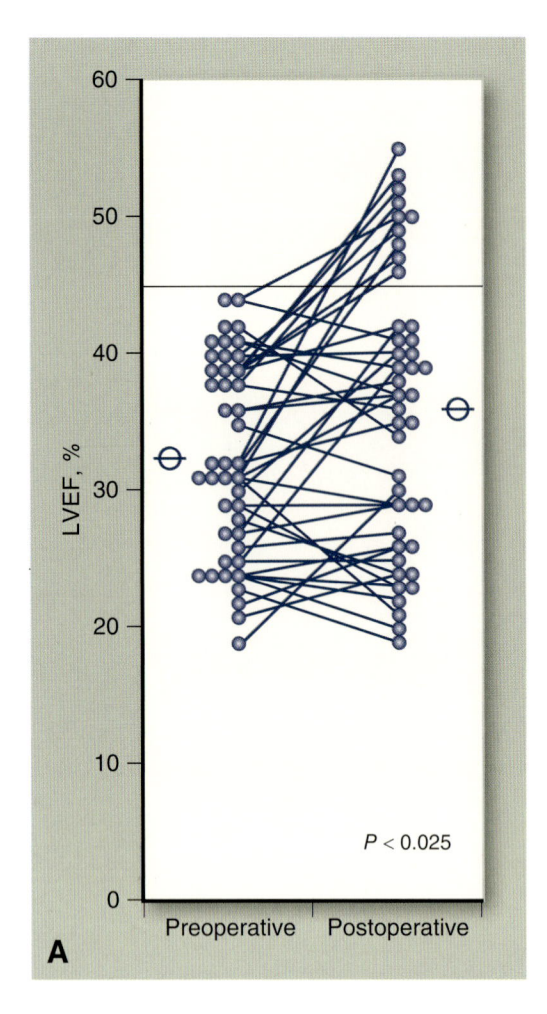

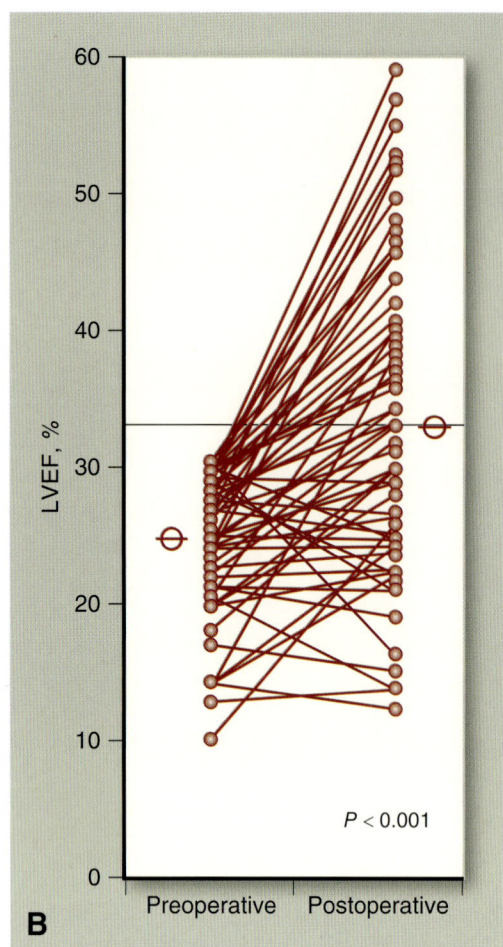

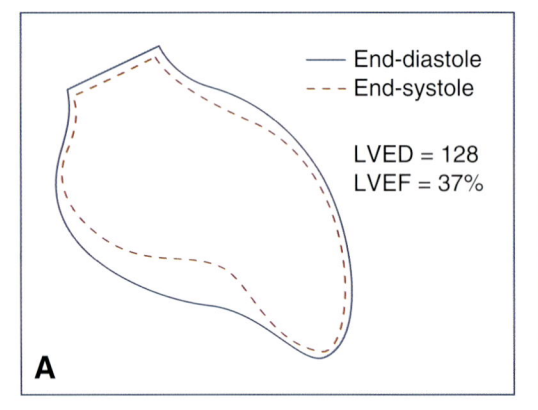

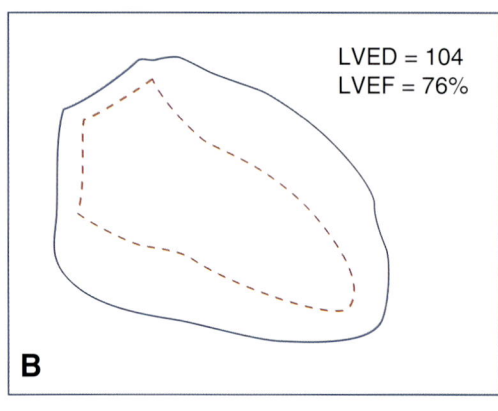

Figure 9-19. Change in left ventricular ejection fraction (LVEF) at rest before (preoperative) and after (postoperative) coronary artery bypass surgery. In patients with moderate (**A**) and severe (**B**) left ventricular dysfunction, successful coronary artery revascularization resulted in improved left ventricular function at rest in approximately one third of patients. Thus, the conventional wisdom that impaired left ventricular function at rest is an irreversible process has been challenged by such observations. Substantial data now exist to indicate that under certain conditions, when viable myocytes are subjected to hypoperfusion or transient periods of ischemia, prolonged alterations in regional and global left ventricular function may occur and this dysfunction may be completely reversible. (*Adapted from* Bonow and Dilsizian [22] and Elefteriades *et al.* [23].)

Figure 9-20. Hibernating myocardium. Recovery of regional and global left ventricular function at rest following revascularization is shown in a patient with totally occluded left anterior descending coronary artery and left ventricular dysfunction. End-diastolic and end-systolic silhouettes of the left ventricle from the right anterior oblique contrast ventriculography before (**A**) and 8 months after (**B**) coronary artery bypass surgery are shown. Preoperatively, the anteroapical region is akinetic, associated with a left ventricular ejection fraction (LVEF) of 37% at rest. Postoperatively, the anteroapical regional contraction is normal and the LVEF at rest has nearly doubled to 76%. LVED—left ventricular end-diastolic volume. (*Adapted from* Rahimtoola [24].)

214 Atlas of Nuclear Cardiology

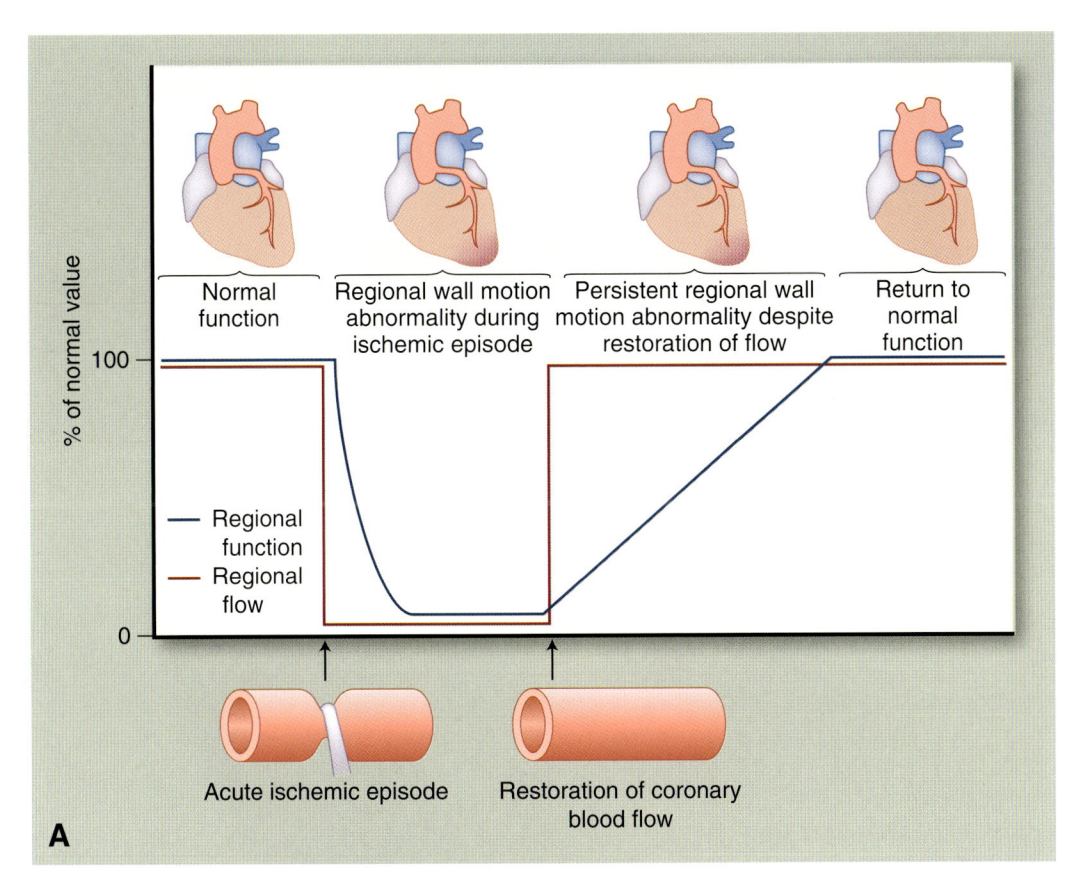

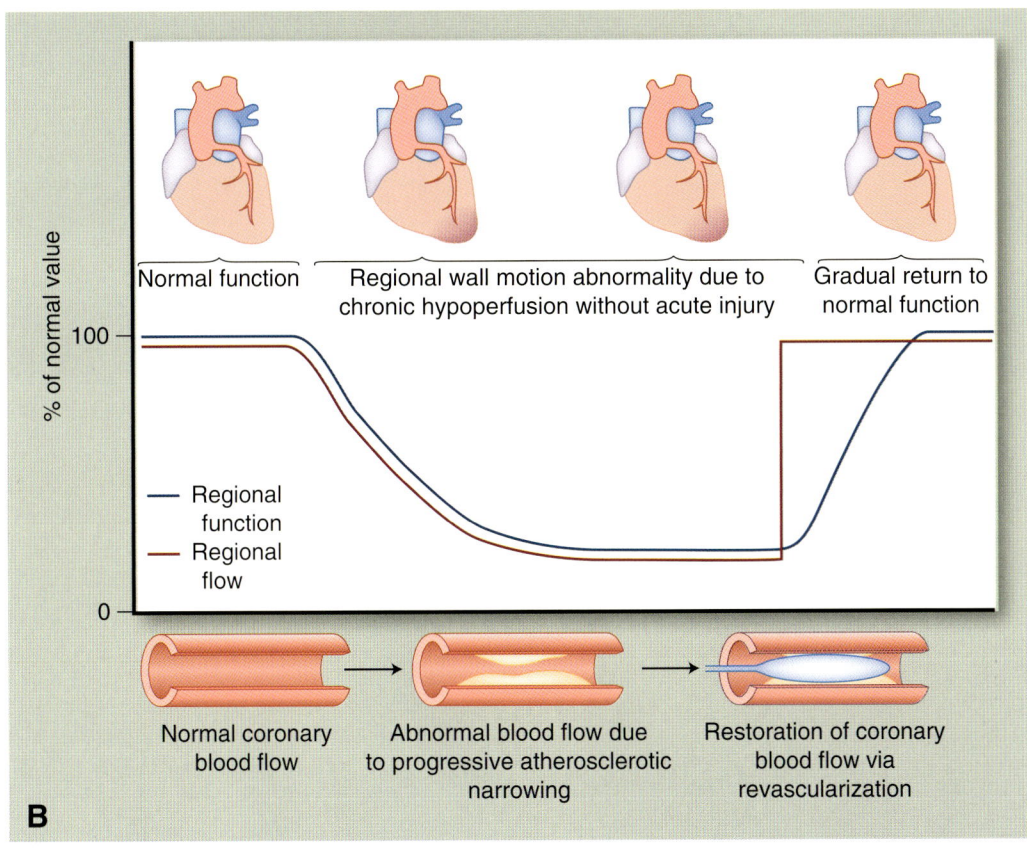

Figure 9-21. Pathophysiologic paradigms concerning the relationship between myocardial perfusion and left ventricular function in stunned and hibernating myocardium. **A,** Stunned myocardium refers to the state of delayed recovery of regional left ventricular dysfunction after a transient period of ischemia that has been followed by reperfusion [25]. The ischemic episodes that ultimately lead to myocardial stunning can be single or multiple, brief or prolonged, but never severe enough to result in myocardial necrosis. **B,** Hibernating myocardium refers to an adaptive rather than injurious response of the myocardium, in which viable but dysfunctional myocardium arises from prolonged myocardial hypoperfusion at rest in the absence of clinically evident ischemia [24]. In stunning, interventions aimed at decreasing the frequency, severity, or duration of ischemic episodes would result in improved contractile function. In hibernation, interventions that favorably alter the supply/demand relationship of the myocardium, either improvement in blood flow or reduction in demand, would be expected to improve contractile function. It is very likely, however, that in patients with chronic coronary artery disease, the adaptive responses of hibernation and injurious responses of stunning coexist.

Nuclear Investigation in Heart Failure and Myocardial Viability

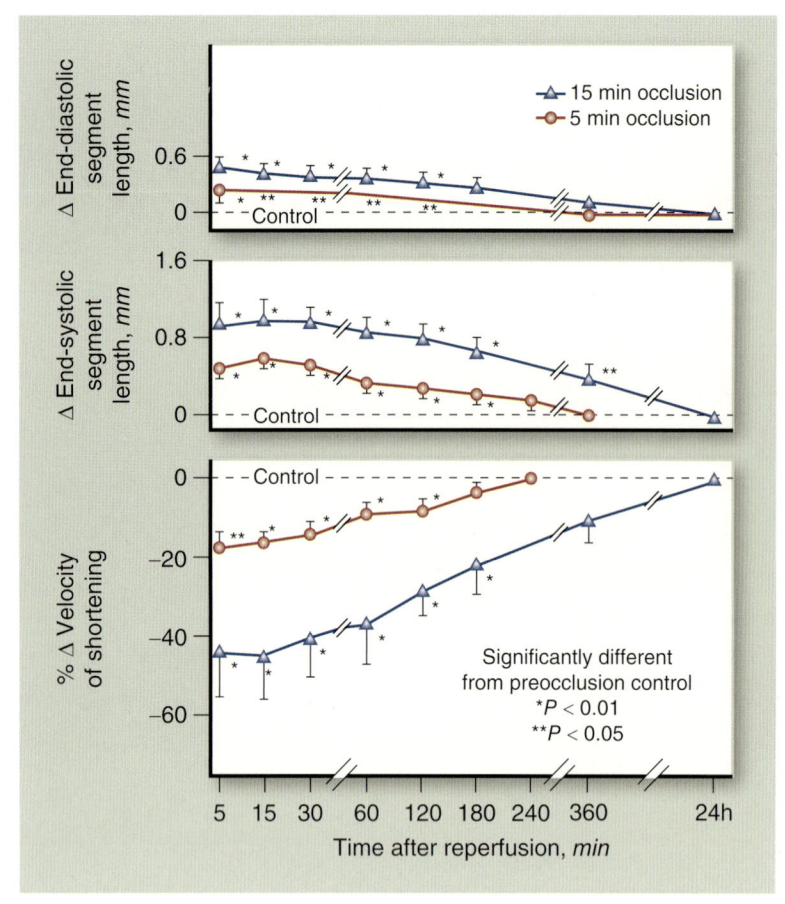

Figure 9-22. Experimental evidence for stunned myocardium. Conscious dogs were subjected to 5 or 15 minutes of coronary artery occlusion followed by reperfusion. Recovery times for end-diastolic and end-systolic segment length and velocity of shortening are shown after 5-minute (*circles*) and 15-minute (*triangles*) occlusions. Recovery times from 5 minutes to 24 hours after reperfusion are also shown. During the occlusion phase, regional systolic thickening was absent in the ischemic zone, and the electrocardiogram showed ST segment elevation. During the reperfusion phase, ST segments returned to baseline within 1 minute, and reactive hyperemia was observed within the ischemic zone. Systolic thickening, however, remained depressed for more than 3 hours after the 5-minute coronary occlusion and for more than 6 hours after the 15-minute occlusion. (*Adapted from* Heyndrickx *et al.* [26].)

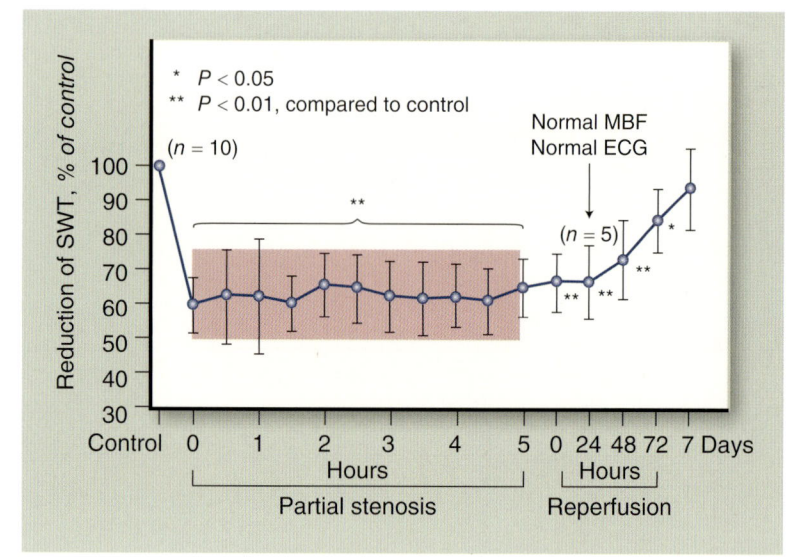

Figure 9-23. Experimental model for short-term hibernation demonstrating balanced reduction of myocardial function and myocardial blood flow (MBF) (contraction-perfusion match). Changes in systolic wall thickening (SWT) in the ischemic area during 5-hour partial coronary artery occlusion and after reperfusion are plotted as a percent of control at frequent intervals to indicate the sustained nature of the regional dysfunction. Data points are ± 1 SD, which is within the limits of a 25% to 50% decrease in function (*shaded area*). After reperfusion, regional dysfunction initially remained depressed but showed late recovery. At 24 hours after reperfusion, five of the 10 dogs had dysrhythmia. Thus, only the data obtained from the remaining five dogs were analyzed. The findings in this canine model indicate that prolonged moderate regional dysfunction caused by nontransmural ischemia during partial stenosis can be sustained for 5 hours. Furthermore, after reperfusion, there is complete recovery of regional and global contractile function within a period of 7 days. ECG—electrocardiogram. (*Adapted from* Matsuzaki *et al.* [27].)

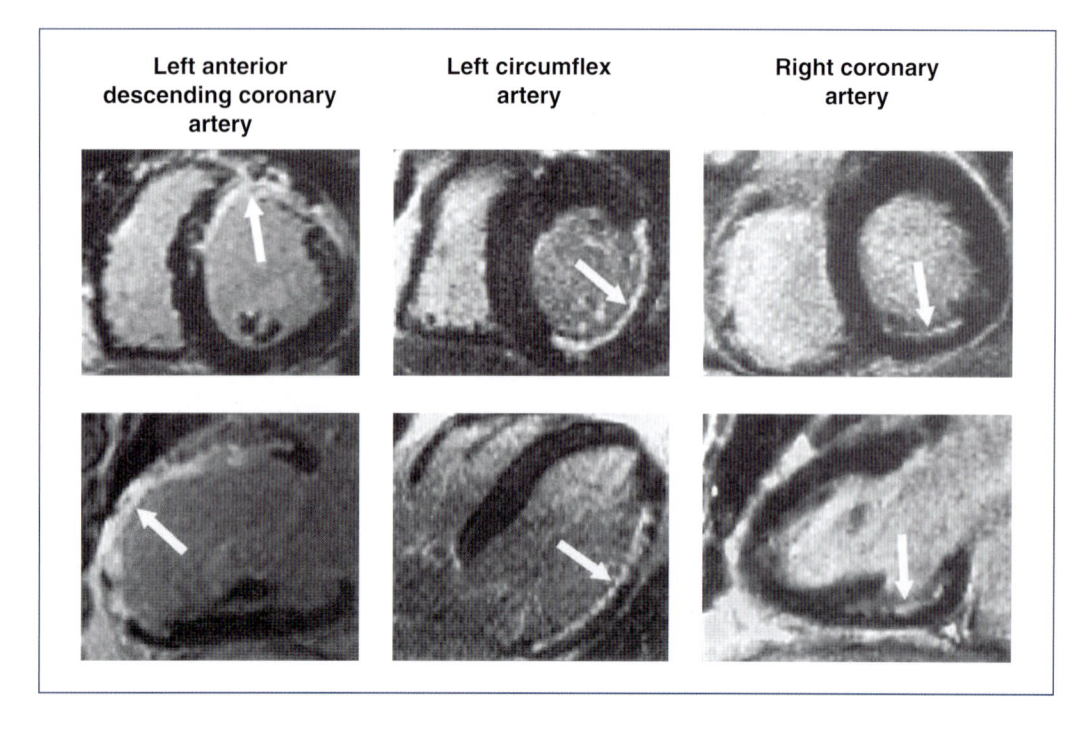

Figure 9-24. Contrast-enhanced images obtained by MRI in chronic left ventricular dysfunction. The earliest observation of signal-intensity changes in infarcted myocardium with contrast-enhanced cardiac magnetic resonance (CMR) dates back to 1993. While studying myocardial perfusion patterns in patients with acute and chronic myocardial infarction, increased signal intensity (greater T1 shortening after contrast) was observed in the infarcted, nonviable myocardium (approximately 10 minutes after bolus injection of the contrast), and was subsequently termed *delayed hyperenhancement*. Reversibly injured myocardium did not exhibit increased contrast concentration or enhancement.

Continued on the next page

Figure 9-24. *(Continued)* Several procedural and technologic improvements since 1993 have allowed CMR to take a more preeminent clinical role for the assessment of scarred myocardium in recent years. The current technique involves rapid infusion of a gadolinium chelate followed by a high resolution cardiac-gated T1-weighted pulse sequence 5 to 30 minutes thereafter. If imaging is performed too early (< 5 minutes after contrast infusion) or too late (> 30 minutes after contrast infusion), it may result in under- or overestimation of infarct size. A potential mechanism for the late gadolinium enhancement may relate to cellular degradation in the infarct region of the myocardium, increase in tissue permeability in the region, and consequent increase in the distribution volume of the extravascular space. When combined with slow washout characteristic of gadolinium chelates from infarcted myocardium, the net result is delayed contrast-enhanced T1-weighted images that appear bright in the infarcted tissue. Because the contrast used is primarily an extracellular, interstitial agent, it has been hypothesized that it is the increased volume of distribution of the contrast molecules within the infracted imaging voxel that is responsible for the greater shortening of the T1 relaxation time. The accuracy of this technique has been validated by comparison with histopathology [28], nuclear techniques [29], as well as recovery of function (or lack thereof) after revascularization [30].

Late gadolinium-enhanced images are shown in a short-axis view *(upper panels)* and a long-axis view *(lower panels)* in three patients. Hyperenhancement is present *(arrows)* in various coronary perfusion territories—the left anterior descending coronary artery, the left circumflex artery, and the right coronary artery—with a range of transmural involvement. *(Adapted from Kim et al. [30].)*

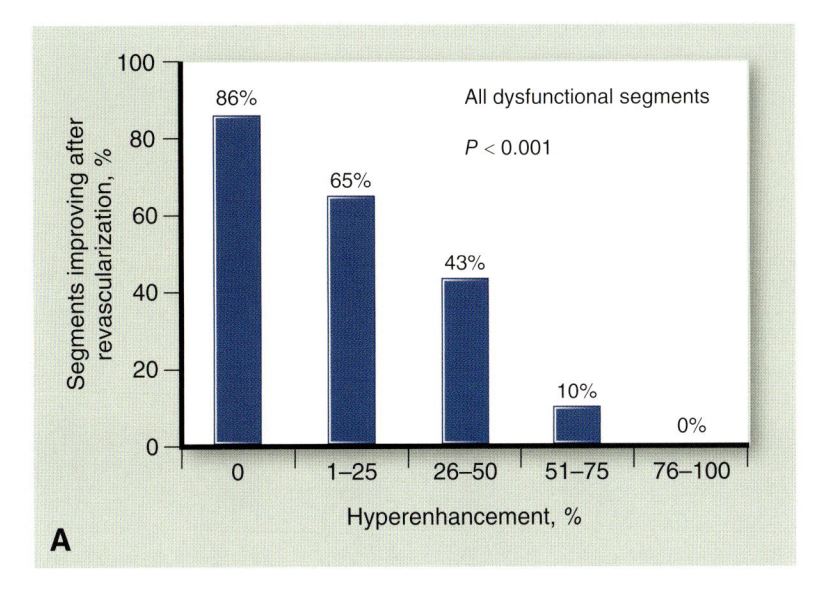

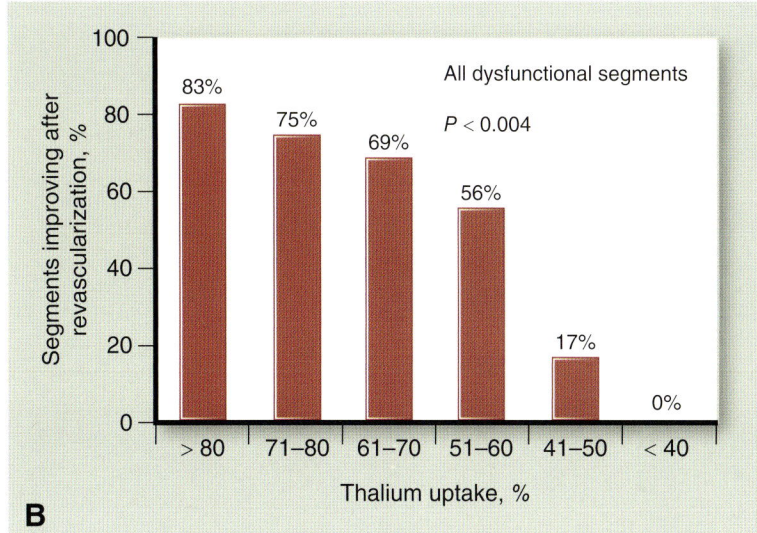

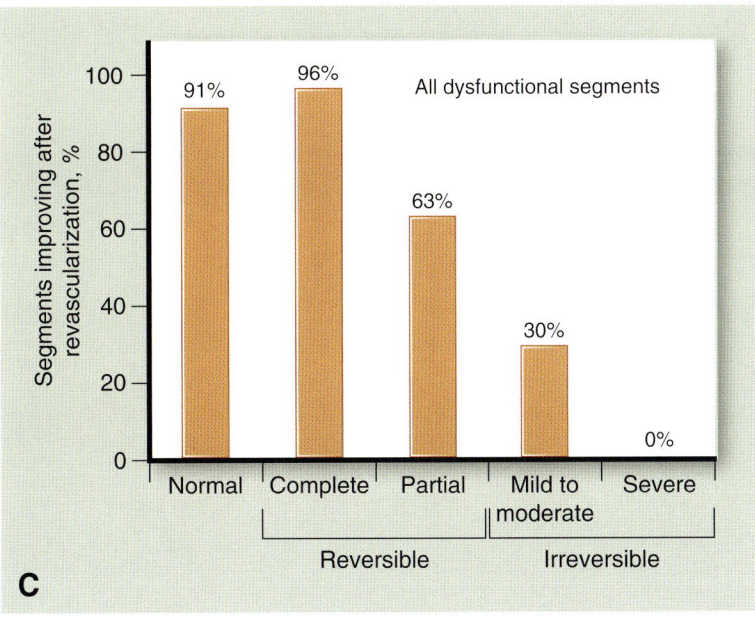

Figure 9-25. The ratio of viable to scarred myocardium dictates recovery of function after revascularization. Relationship between recovery of function after revascularization with contrast-enhanced cardiac magnetic resonance (CMR) (**A**) [30] and two thallium protocols optimized for viability detection: 1) rest-redistribution (**B**) [31] and 2) stress-redistribution-reinjection (**C**) [32] imaging are shown. The rest-redistribution protocol assesses myocardial viability alone while the stress-redistribution-reinjection protocol assesses myocardial ischemia and viability. When taking into consideration regions with reversible defects (ischemia) and success of revascularization (reexamining regional perfusion or vessel patency after revascularization) stress-redistribution-reinjection thallium imaging yields excellent positive and negative predictive accuracy for recovery of function after revascularization [32,33]. Irrespective of the imaging modality applied, the data suggest that recovery of function after revascularization is a continuum and is coupled to the ratio of viable to scarred myocardium within dysfunctional myocardial segments. The extent of infarct size on CMR or percent thallium defect on SPECT correlated with decreasing likelihood of functional recovery after revascularization.

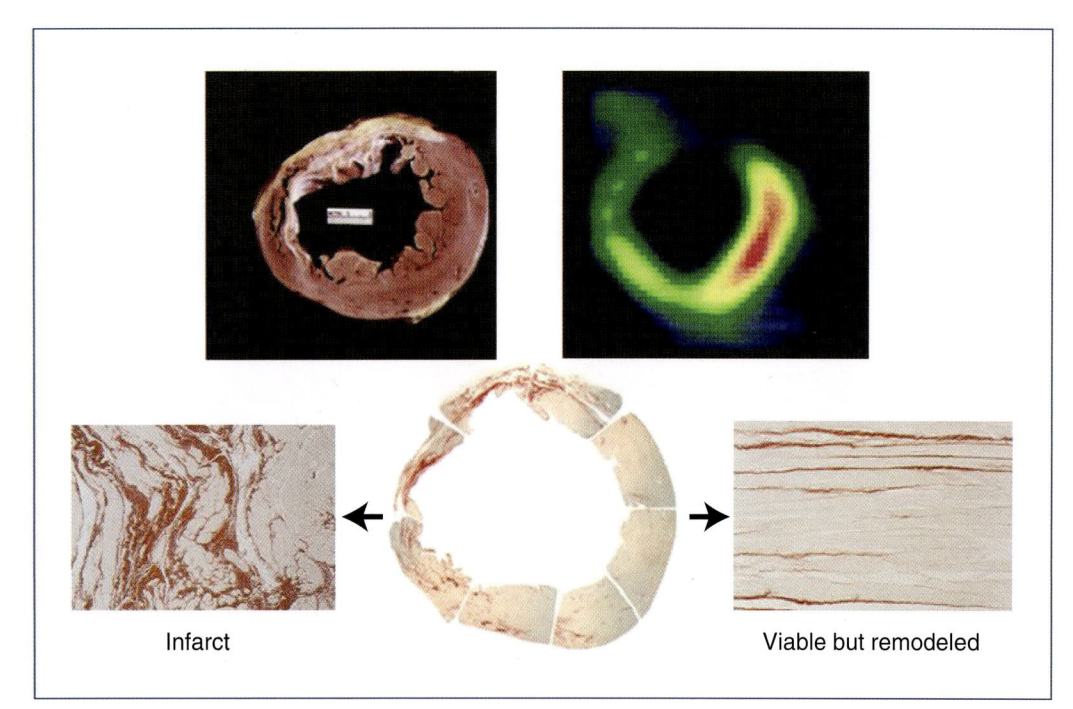

Figure 9-26. Left ventricular (LV) remodeling. An advantage of thallium SPECT protocols over delayed enhancement cardiac magnetic resonance is in providing additional insight into potential mechanisms of the underlying cause of regional and global LV dysfunction. Regional LV dysfunction could be attributed to scarred, hibernating, stunned, or remodeled myocardium. Having two or three sets of images with thallium SPECT, one can tease out three scintigraphic patterns that can differentiate between the three pathophysiologic conditions of scarred, hibernating, or stunned myocardium as the underlying cause of the LV dysfunction. In the case of scarred myocardium, there will be no change in the percent LV defect size from rest to redistribution. On the other hand, if hibernating but viable myocardium, the percent LV defect size will get smaller from rest to redistribution images. For stunned myocardium, the pattern of "reverse redistribution" will be present, especially when the images are acquired during the acute phase of myocardial injury following either a spontaneous, pharmacologic, or mechanical intervention.

Histomorphologic evidence for structural alterations in the extracellular matrix of remodeled areas of the LV from a patient with stable chronic ischemic heart disease and severe LV dysfunction who underwent orthotopic cardiac transplantation. On gross pathology (*top left*), there is evidence for myocardial scarring in the anterior extending to the anteroseptal region and hypertrophy of the remaining myocardial regions secondary to LV remodeling. Thallium tomogram acquired prior to cardiac transplantation (*top right*) shows severe defects in the corresponding scarred anterior and anteroseptal regions and normal uptake in the remodeled lateral region of the myocardium. Histomorphologic analysis of infarct and noninfarct myocardial segments (*bottom*), using picrosirius red stain, confirms transmural collagen replacement in the infarct region (*bottom left*) as was detected by both gross pathology and thallium SPECT. However, in the noninfarct, remodeled myocardium, layers of collagen replacement within the extracellular matrix of morphologically normal appearing myocytes are seen that could not be detected by thallium SPECT or gross pathology. (*Adapted from* Dilsizian [34].)

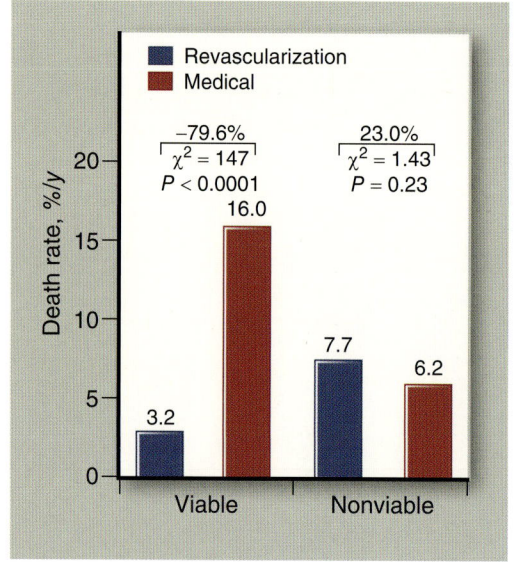

Figure 9-27. Prognostic implications of myocardial viability testing in patients with coronary artery disease and left ventricular dysfunction. Data from meta-analysis of 3088 patients (mean left ventricular ejection fraction, 32%, followed for 25 ± 10 months) demonstrates that in patients with preserved myocardial viability, the annual mortality rate was significantly lower in those who were treated with revascularization (3.2%) compared with those treated with medical therapy alone (16%). This represents a 79.6% decrease in annual mortality for patients with viability treated with revascularization ($P < 0.0001$). Moreover, there was a direct relationship between severity of left ventricular dysfunction and magnitude of benefit from revascularization among patients with myocardial viability ($P < 0.001$). In contrast, among patients without evidence of viable myocardium, there was no incremental benefit of revascularization over medical therapy. These data support the role of myocardial viability testing for the management of patients with chronic left ventricular dysfunction and in guiding therapeutic decisions for revascularization. (*Adapted from* Allman *et al.* [35].)

218 Atlas of Nuclear Cardiology

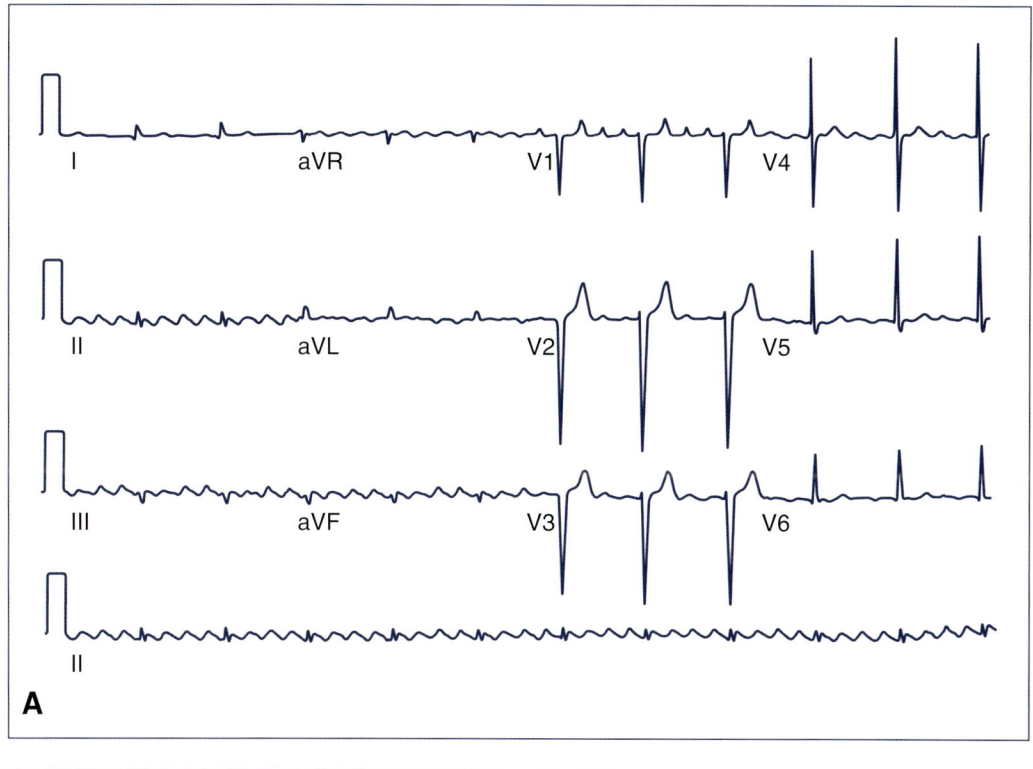

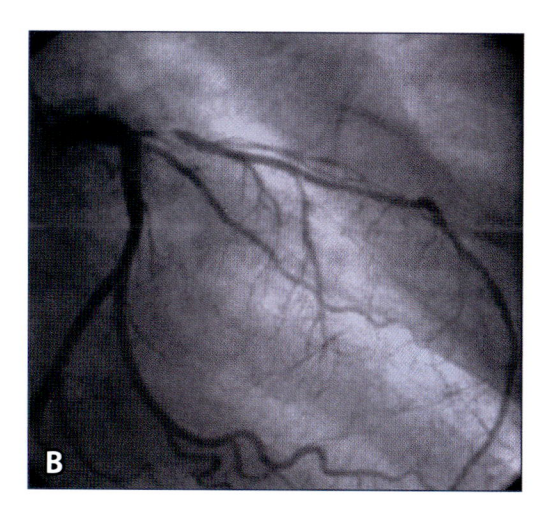

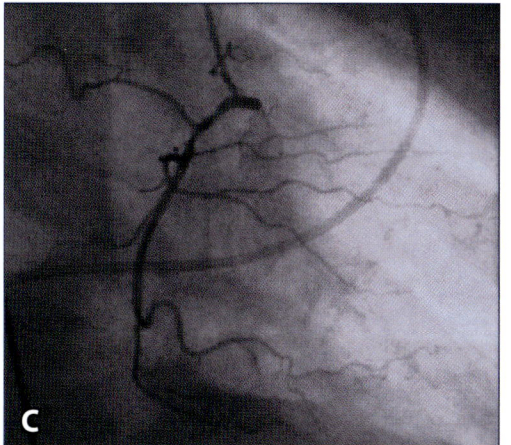

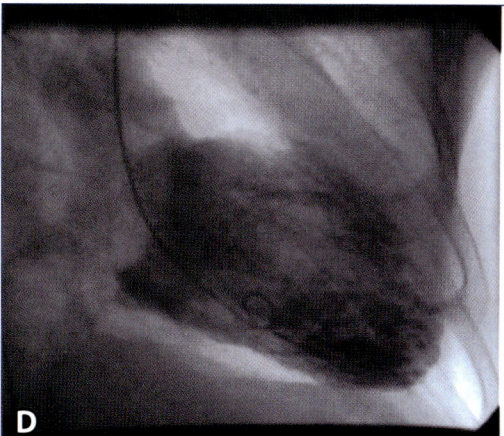

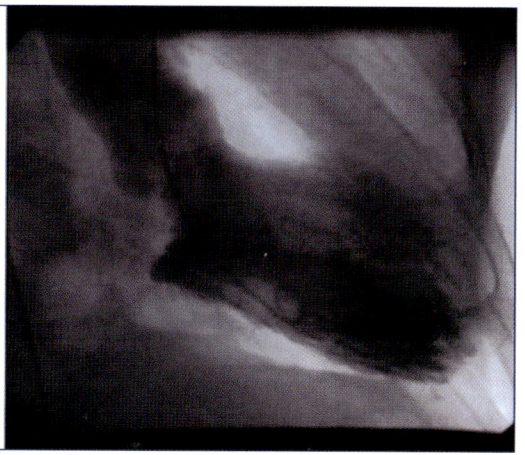

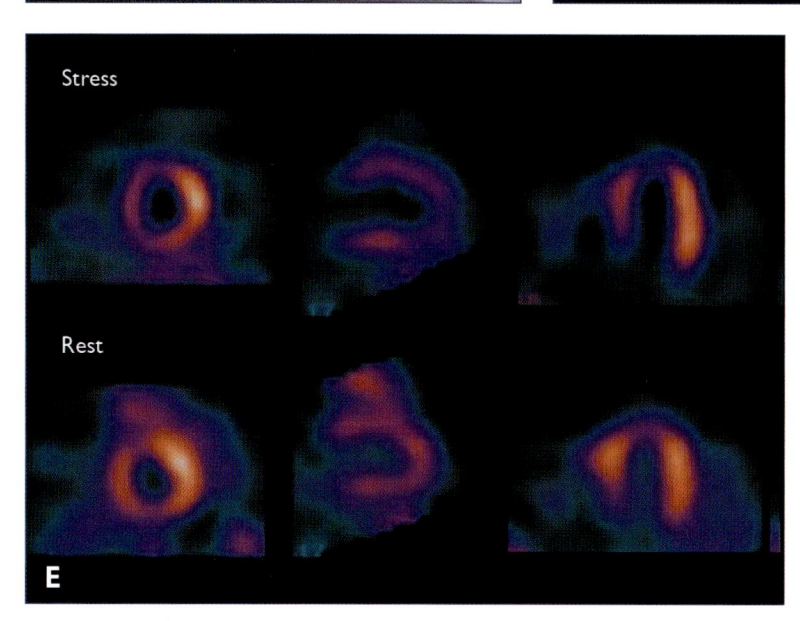

Figure 9-28. Example of a patient with ischemic cardiomyopathy. A patient with prior history of hypertension and diabetes mellitus presented with 1-week history of shortness of breath and leg swelling. His physical examination was consistent with congestive heart failure. The electrocardiogram showed atrial flutter (**A**) while the coronary angiogram show two-vessel disease: subtotal occlusion of the proximal left anterior descending (LAD) coronary artery (**B**) and significant narrowing of the proximal right coronary artery (RCA) (**C**). The left ventriculogram shows severe diffuse hypokinesis and moderate-to-severe left ventricular dysfunction (**D**, *left panel* = diastole and *right panel* = systole). Adenosine pharmacologic dual-isotope gated SPECT images show extensive ^{99m}Tc sestamibi perfusion defects in the anterior, septal, apical, and inferior regions that become reversible on the rest thallium images, providing evidence for ischemic and viable myocardium in the LAD and RCA vascular territories (**E**). The extensive reversible defects are associated with abnormally increased lung uptake and transient ischemic cavity dilatation. These scintigraphic findings in the setting of heart failure symptoms secondary to ischemic left ventricular dysfunction portend good outcome after revascularization.

Nuclear Investigation in Heart Failure and Myocardial Viability

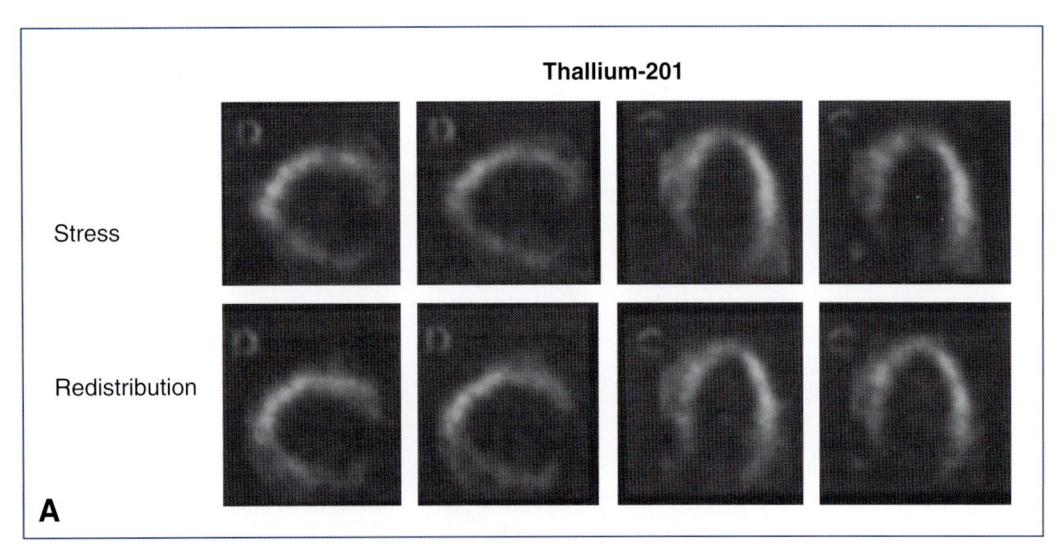

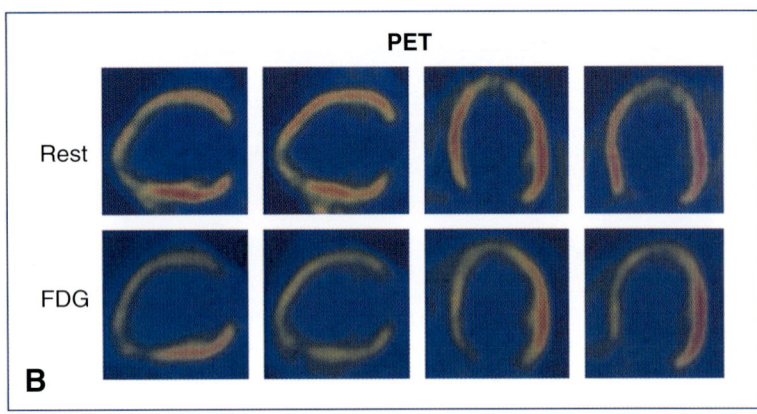

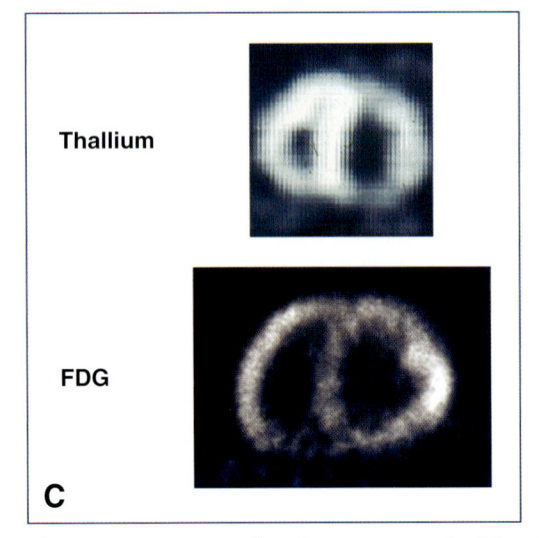

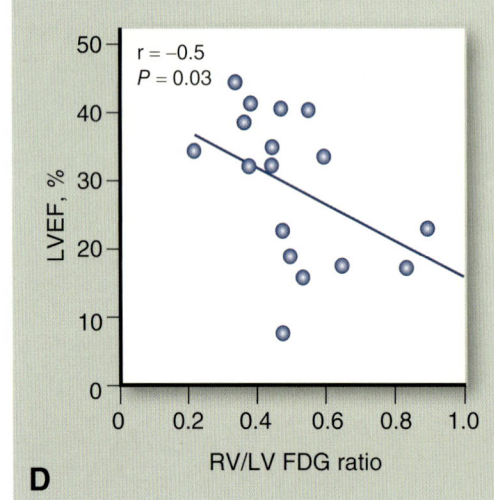

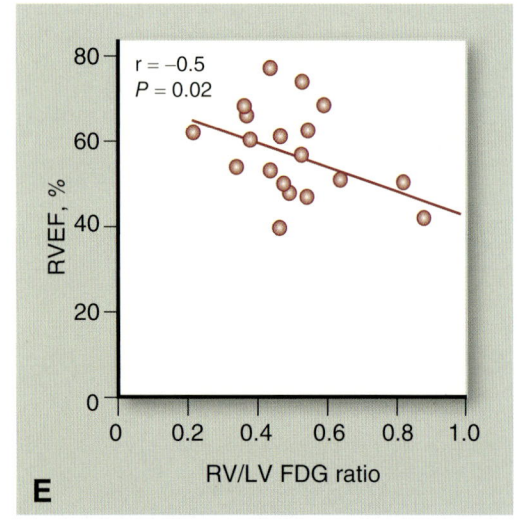

Figure 9-29. Example of a patient with dilated, nonischemic, cardiomyopathy. A patient with no risk factors for coronary artery disease presented with symptoms of progressive severe dyspnea and orthopnea. His physical examination was consistent with congestive heart failure. Stress-redistribution thallium SPECT images (**A**) show severely dilated left ventricular (LV) cavity without regional reversible or fixed perfusion defects. Rest ^{13}N ammonia and fluorodeoxyglucose (FDG) PET images (**B**) show severely dilated LV cavity with homogeneous distribution of myocardial blood flow at rest and glucose utilization (metabolism) after glucose loading. Right heart catheterization showed right ventricular (RV) pressure of 60/20, right atrial pressure of 13 mm Hg, pulmonary artery pressure of 56/30, pulmonary capillary wedge pressure of 28 mm Hg, and pulmonary vascular resistance of 3.2 wood units. Chronic persistent LV dysfunction, whether secondary to ischemic or nonischemic cardiomyopathy, may lead to increased pulmonary artery pressure. Chronically elevated pulmonary vascular resistance imposes RV overload, which is compensated by RV hypertrophy and ultimately resulting in RV dysfunction. Examples of patients with prominent RV myocardial uptake, reflecting RV hypertrophy, are shown in **C** with thallium SPECT (*top*) and FDG PET (*bottom*). The patient with FDG PET has left ventricular ejection fraction (LVEF) of 22% and right ventricular ejection fraction (RVEF) of 20%. The relation between RV/LV FDG ratio (as an index of RV hypertrophy) and LVEF is shown in **D**. There is an inverse relationship between RV/LV FDG ratio and severity of LV dysfunction. Similarly, the relation between RV/LV FDG ratio and RVEF is shown in **E**. There is an inverse relationship between RV/LV FDG ratio and severity of RV dysfunction [36,37].

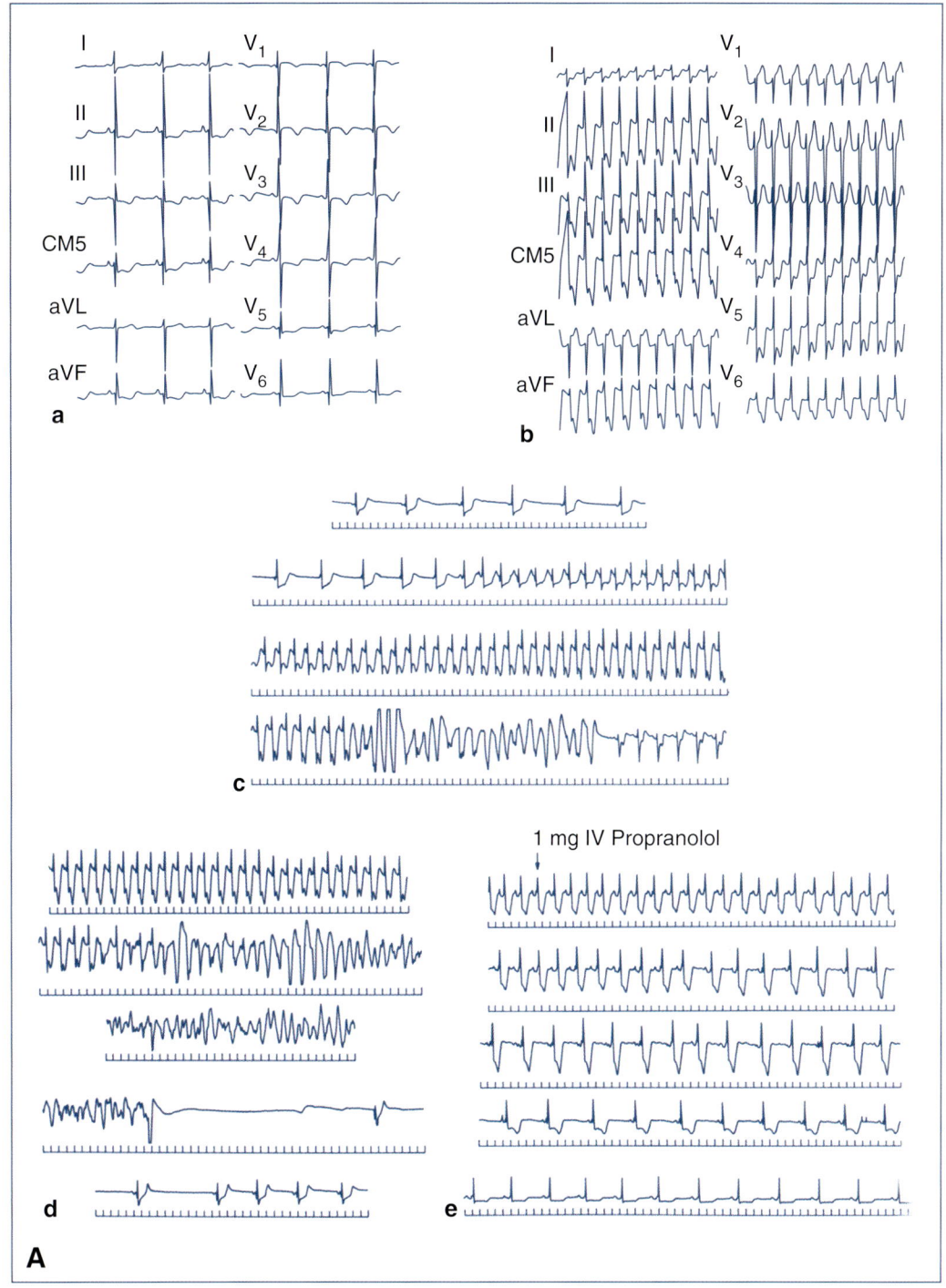

Figure 9-30. Example of a patient with hypertrophic cardiomyopathy. Angina and myocardial ischemia are prominent features of hypertrophic cardiomyopathy in adult patients, and evidence suggests that ischemia can be present even in young asymptomatic patients [38]. Electrocardiogram (ECG) recordings from an 11-year-old boy with history of recurrent cardiac arrests are shown in **A**. At baseline (*a*) the ECG shows minor ST-T wave abnormalities commonly seen in hypertrophic cardiomyopathy patients. During exercise on a treadmill (*b*), 12-mm ST segment depression developed in the inferolateral leads. Serial telemetry ECG recordings from the same patient at rest (*c*) reveal the development of sinus tachycardia first associated with a significant ST segment depression followed by a non-sustained polymorphic ventricular tachycardia. ECG recordings during a presyncopal episode (*d*), which shows sustained polymorphic ventricular tachycardia that was terminated by an electric shock from an implantable cardiac defibrillator. ECG recording in *e* shows another episode of marked ST segment depression that was associated with hypotension (brachial arterial pressure 60/40 mm Hg) and lightheadedness that was treated successfully with intravenous infusion of 1 mg of propranolol [38].

Myocardial ischemia, as assessed by reversible exercise-induced regional thallium abnormalities, is a prominent feature of hypertrophic carrdiomyopathy and has been associated with potentially lethal arrhythmias. That thallium abnormalities observed in hypertrophic cardiomyopathy represent myocardial ischemia is supported by the concordance of these abnormalities and abnormal lactate metabolism during rapid atrial pacing [39]; improvement of thallium abnormalities after medical therapy, such as verapamil; surgical relief of left ventricular outflow obstruction [40]; and excellent concordance with ^{99m}Tc sestamibi, whose uptake is independent of the active Na-K ATPase transport system. Thallium tomograms at baseline and after verapamil therapy in a patient with prior cardiac arrest is shown in **B**. Short-axis tomograms from apex to base are displayed for stress (*top row*) and thallium reinjection (*bottom row*). In the *left panel*, before verapamil therapy, there are extensive exercise-induced thallium abnormalities in the anterior, septal, and inferior regions that normalize on reinjection images 3 to 4 hours later, consistent with reversible myocardial ischemia. In the *right panel*, after verapamil therapy, exercise-induced thallium abnormalities are improved [38].

Continued on the next page

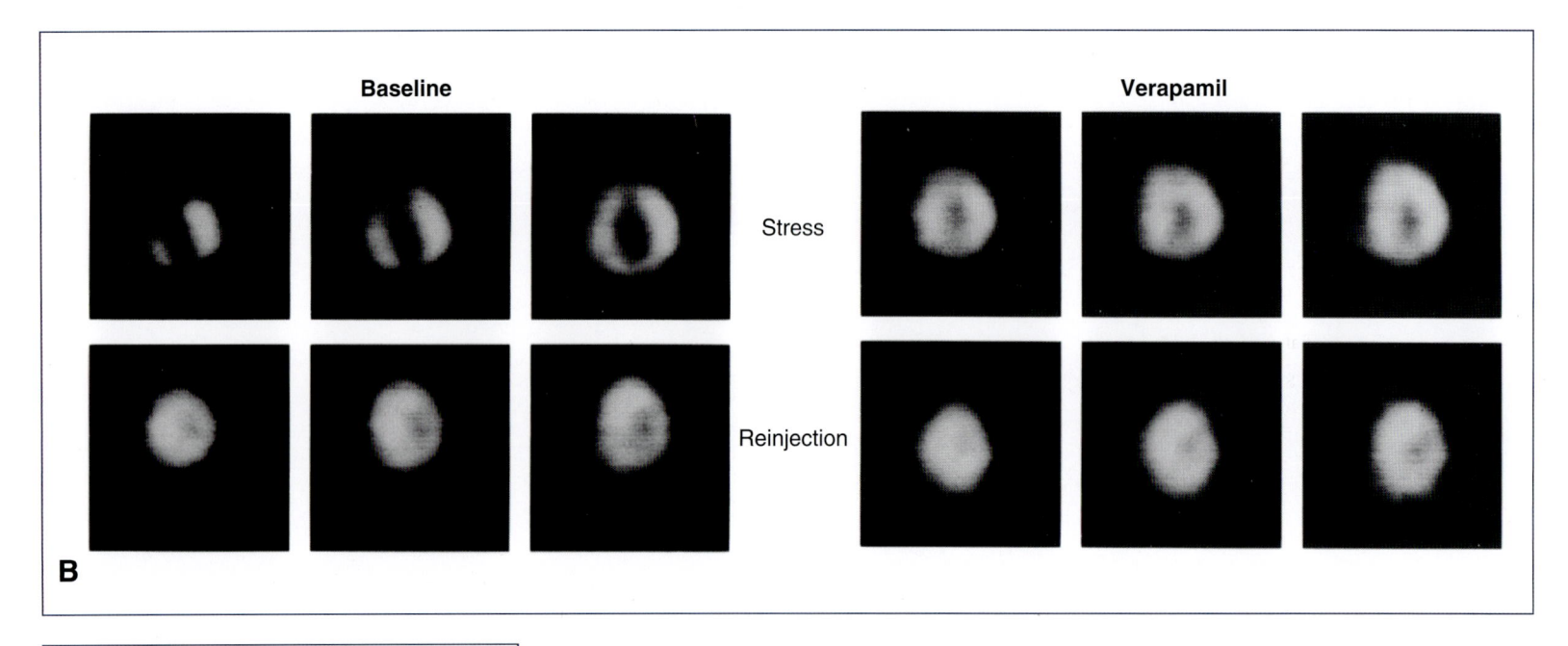

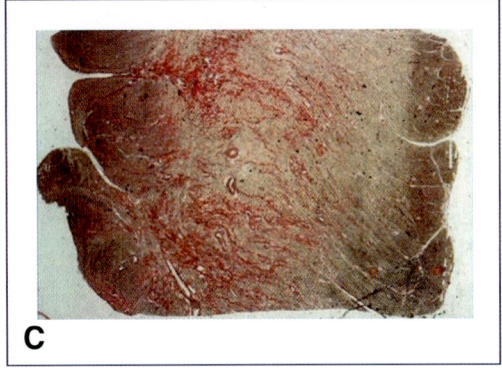

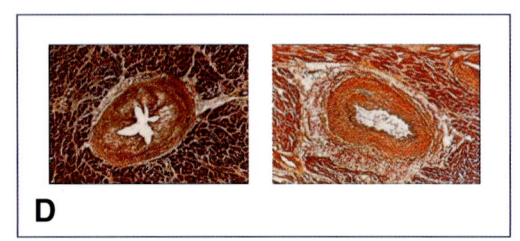

Figure 9-30. *(Continued)* Possible mechanisms for the development of myocardial ischemia in such patients may relate to inadequate myocardial blood flow and increased myocardial oxygen demand during exercise. Myocardial ischemia in the absence of epicardial coronary artery stenosis may be due to intramural small-vessel abnormalities, abnormal myocellular architecture, inadequate capillary density in regions of massive hypertrophy, and systolic compression of tunneled, bridged segments of large intramyocardial coronary arteries. Postmortem ventricular septal tissue from a patient with hypertrophic cardiomyopathy who died from sudden cardiac arrest shows morphologically abnormal and substantially increased size of the left ventricular collagen matrix (**C**), and abnormally narrowed and thickened intramural coronary arteries that have been shown to be more prevalent in areas of scarred myocardium (**D**) [41]. Impaired left ventricular relaxation and elevated end-diastolic filling pressures during diastole may result in compressive effects on the coronary microcirculation and restrict coronary artery blood flow. In addition, coronary vasodilator response may be limited by abnormalities of the intramural small coronary arteries that are characteristic of hypertrophic cardiomyopathy. Myocardial ischemia could be further aggravated by the increases in oxygen demand associated with myocardial hypertrophy and, in some patients, due to elevated systolic pressures as a result of outflow tract obstruction. Such recurrent myocardial ischemia may cause myocardial injury and scarring, which potentially can reduce the threshold for ventricular arrhythmias. Recently, important advances have been made in our understanding of the genetic and molecular abnormalities in hypertrophic cardiomyopathy. With further advances, a more refined explanation of the pathophysiologic mechanisms responsible for myocardial ischemia in this disease may be possible. (**C** and **D**, *from* Shirani *et al.* [41]; with permission.)

References

1. Jessup M, Abraham WT, Casey DE, *et al.*: 2009 Focused Update: ACC/AHA guidelines for the evaluation and management of chronic heart failure in the adult. A report of the American College of Cardiology/American Heart Association Task Force on Practice Guidelines. *Circulation* 2009, 119:1977–2016.

2. Narula J, Zaret BL: Epilogue: development of novel imaging techniques for ultimately superior management of congestive heart failure. *J Nucl Cardiol* 2002, 9(5 Suppl):81S–86S.

3. Swedberg K, Eneroth P, Kjekshus J, *et al.*: Effects of enalapril and neuroendocrine activation on prognosis in severe congestive heart failure (follow-up of the CONSENSUS trial). *Am J Cardiol* 1990, 66:40D–44D.

4. Shirani J, Narula J, Eckelman WC, *et al.*: Early imaging in heart failure: exploring novel molecular targets. *J Nucl Cardiol* 2007, 14:100–110.

5. Hirsch AT, Talsness CE, Schunkert H, *et al.*: Tissue-specific activation of cardiac angiotensin converting enzyme in experimental heart failure. *Circ Res* 1991, 69:475–482.

6. Lindpaintner K, Lu W, Niedermajer N, *et al.*: Selective activation of cardiac angiotensinogen gene expression in post-infarction ventricular remodeling in the rat. *J Mol Cell Cardiol* 1993, 25:133–143.

7. Meggs LG, Coupet J, Huang H, *et al.*: Regulation of angiotensin II receptors on ventricular myocytes after myocardial infarction in rats. *Circ Res* 1993, 72:1149–1162.

8. Harada K, Sugaya T, Murakami K, *et al.*: Angiotensin II type 1A receptor knockout mice display less left ventricular remodeling and improved survival after myocardial infarction. *Circulation* 1999, 100:2093–2099.

9. Dilsizian V, Eckelman WC, Loredo ML, *et al.*: Evidence for tissue angiotensin-converting-enzyme in explanted hearts of ischemic cardiomyopathy using targeted radiotracer technique. *J Nucl Med* 2007, 48:182–187.

10. Verjans JW, Lovhaug D, Narula N, et al.: Noninvasive imaging of myocardial angiotensin receptors in heart failure. *J Am Coll Cardiol Imag* 2008, 1:345–362.

11. Borne SVD, Isobe S, Verjans JW, et al.: Molecular imaging of interstitial alterations in remodeling myocardium after myocardial infarction. *J Am Coll Cardiol* 2008, 52:2017–2028.

12. Borne SVD, Isobe S, Fujimoto S, et al.: Effect of angiotensin-aldosterone axis suppression on cardiac remodeling assessed by molecular imaging by targeting collagen deposition using integrin-seeking radiolabeled probes. *J Am Coll Cardiol Imag* 2009, 2:187–198.

13. Verjans JW, Wolters SL, Lax M, et al.: Imaging αvβ3/β5 integrin upregulation in patients after myocardial infarction. *Circulation* 2007, 116:11–740.

14. Taegtmeyer H, Sharma S, Golfman L, et al.: Linking gene expression to function: metabolic flexibility in normal and diseased heart. *Ann N Y Acad Sci* 2004, 1015:1–12.

15. Depre C, Taegtmeyer H: Metabolic aspects of programmed cell survival and cell death in the heart. *Cardiovasc Res* 2000, 45:538–548.

16. Kim HD, Kim DJ, Lee IJ, et al.: Human fetal heart development after mid-term: morphometry and ultrastructural study. *J Mol Cell Cardiol* 1992, 24:949–965.

17. Zhao M, Zhang H, Robinson TF, et al.: Profound structural alterations of the extracellular collagen matrix in postischemic dysfunction ("stunned") but viable myocardium. *J Am Coll Cardiol* 1987, 10:1322–1334.

18. Taegtmeyer H: Modulation of responses to myocardial ischemia: metabolic features of myocardial stunning, hibernation, and ischemic preconditioning. In *Myocardial Viability: A Clinical and Scientific Treatise*. Edited by Dilsizian V. Armonk, New York: Futura; 2000:25–36.

19. Risk stratification and survival after myocardial infarction. *N Engl J Med* 1983, 309:331–336.

20. Mock MB, Ringqvist I, Fisher LD, et al.: Survival of medically treated patients in the coronary artery surgery study (CASS) registry. *Circulation* 1982, 66:562–568.

21. Alderman EL, Fisher LD, Litwin P, et al.: Results of coronary artery surgery in patients with poor left ventricular function (CASS). *Circulation* 1983, 68:785–795.

22. Bonow RO, Dilsizian V: Thallium-201 for assessment of myocardial viability. *Sem Nucl Med* 1991, 21:230–241.

23. Elefteriades JA, Tolis G Jr, Levi E, et al.: Coronary artery bypass grafting in severe left ventricular dysfunction: excellent survival with improved ejection fraction and functional state. *J Am Coll Cardiol* 1993, 22:1411–1417.

24. Rahimtoola SH: A perspective on the three large multicenter randomized clinical trials of coronary bypass surgery for chronic stable angina. *Circulation* 1985, 72(suppl V):V123–V135.

25. Braunwald E, Kloner RA: The stunned myocardium: prolonged, postischemic ventricular dysfunction. *Circulation* 1982, 66:1146–1149.

26. Heyndrickx GR, Millard RW, McRitchie RJ, et al.: Regional myocardial functional and electrophysiological alterations after brief coronary artery occlusion in conscious dogs. *J Clin Invest* 1975, 56:978–985.

27. Matsuzaki M, Gallagher KP, Kemper S, et al.: Sustained regional dysfunction produced by prolonged coronary stenosis: gradual recovery after reperfusion. *Circulation* 1983, 68:170–182.

28. Arnado LC, Gerber BL, Gupta SN, et al.: Accurate and objective infarct sizing by contrast-enhanced magnetic resonance imaging in a canine myocardial infarction model. *J Am Coll Cardiol* 2004, 44:2383–2389.

29. Klein C, Nekolla SG, Bengel FM, et al.: Assessment of myocardial viability with contrast-enhanced magnetic resonance imaging: comparison with positron emission tomography. *Circulation* 2002, 105:162–167.

30. Kim RJ, Wu E, Rafael A, et al.: The use of contrast-enhanced magnetic resonance imaging to identify reversible myocardial dysfunction. *N Engl J Med* 2000, 343:1445–1453.

31. Perrone-Filardi P, Pace L, Prastaro M, et al.: Assessment of myocardial viability in patients with chronic coronary artery disease. Rest-4-hour-24-hour 201Tl tomography versus dobutamine echocardiography. *Circulation* 1996, 94:2712–2719.

32. Kitsiou AN, Srinivasan G, Quyyumi AA, et al.: Stress-induced reversible and mild-to-moderate irreversible thallium defects: Are they equally accurate for predicting recovery of regional left ventricular function after revascularization? *Circulation* 1998, 98:501–508.

33. Dilsizian V, Rocco TP, Freedman NM, et al.: Enhanced detection of ischemic but viable myocardium by the reinjection of thallium after stress-redistribution imaging. *N Engl J Med* 1990, 323:141–146.

34. Dilsizian V: Cardiac magnetic resonance versus SPECT: are all non-infarct myocardial regions created equal? *J Nucl Card* 2007, 14:9–14.

35. Allman KC, Shaw LJ, Hachamovitch R, Udelson JE: Myocardial viability testing and impact of revascularization on prognosis in patients with coronary artery disease and left ventricular dysfunction: a meta-analysis. *J Am Coll Cardiol* 2002, 39:1151–1158.

36. Khin M, Panza JA, Ernst IR, et al.: Right ventricular fluorodeoxyglucose uptake in patients with chronic ischemic heart disease: relation to severity of left ventricular dysfunction. *J Nucl Med* 2001, 42:171.

37. Khin M, Carson J, Miller-Davis C, et al.: Does right ventricular fluorodeoxyglucose uptake reflect the severity of left and right ventricular dysfunction? *J Nucl Cardiol* 2001, 8:S127.

38. Dilsizian V, Bonow RO, Epstein SE, Fananapazir L: Myocardial ischemia detected by thallium scintigraphy is frequently related to cardiac arrest and syncope in young patients with hypertrophic cardiomyopathy. *J Am Coll Cardiol* 1993, 22:796–804.

39. Cannon RO, Dilsizian V, O'Gara PT, et al.: Myocardial metabolic, hemodynamic and electrocardiographic significance of reversible thallium-201 abnormalities in hypertrophic cardiomyopathy. *Circulation* 1991, 83:1660–1667.

40. Cannon RO, Dilsizian V, O'Gara PT, et al.: Impact of surgical relief of outflow obstruction on thallium perfusion abnormalities in hypertrophic cardiomyopathy. *Circulation* 1992, 85:1039–1045.

41. Shirani J, Pick R, Roberts WC, Maron BJ: Morphology and significance of the left ventricular collagen network in young patients with hypertrophic cardiomyopathy and sudden cardiac death. *J Am Coll Cardiol* 2000, 35:36–44.

Diagnosis and Risk Stratification in Acute Coronary Syndromes

10

James E. Udelson

Since the 1970s, radionuclide myocardial perfusion imaging (MPI) has played an important role in diagnosis as well as in risk stratification for patients suffering from acute ischemic coronary syndromes (ACS). Early studies using planar ^{201}Tl imaging documented the superior ability of this technique to assess both the presence and location of myocardial infarction (MI) and to predict the site of coronary disease involvement in unstable syndromes more accurately than electrocardiogram (ECG) findings alone [1]. More recently, the use of ^{99m}Tc-based agents such as sestamibi in the early hours of an infarct has provided important information on areas at risk in the setting of the coronary occlusion, while a follow-up study done several days later provided information on final infarct size and myocardial salvage when both sets of images were compared [2].

Stress MPI in the early aftermath of both unstable angina syndromes as well as acute MI carries powerful prognostic information for risk-stratifying stable post-ACS patients. Imaging for ischemia has been incorporated into numerous randomized clinical trials to better define the roles of different ACS management strategies [3,4]. Over the past few years, MPI has also been used to rule ACS in or out among patients with chest pain syndromes who do not have diagnostic ischemic ECG changes upon presentation to the emergency department. Several published studies now consistently demonstrate very high negative predictive value for ruling out acute ischemia, as well as powerful risk stratification information for those with positive tests in the emergency department setting [5–8]. Thus, single photon emission computed tomography (SPECT) MPI techniques are widely used in the setting of ACS, both for initial detection of abnormal blood flow underlying the clinical syndrome, and for decision making regarding conservative versus invasive interventional management.

Recent advances in hardware and software technology have allowed the combined assessment of stress and rest MPI with measures of regional and global left ventricular function using gated SPECT imaging [9]. Based on the wide availability of gated SPECT MPI of both perfusion and left ventricular function, obtaining the incremental value of adding functional information to the perfusion information in ACS is now routine.

In this chapter, the role of radionuclide imaging techniques in the broad setting of ACS will be reviewed, with emphasis on decision points where the imaging data has been shown to enhance the clinician's information base in order to optimally manage patients in this setting. Also reviewed will be imaging techniques under development but not yet widely available that may have potential clinical utility in some of the clinical settings of ACS.

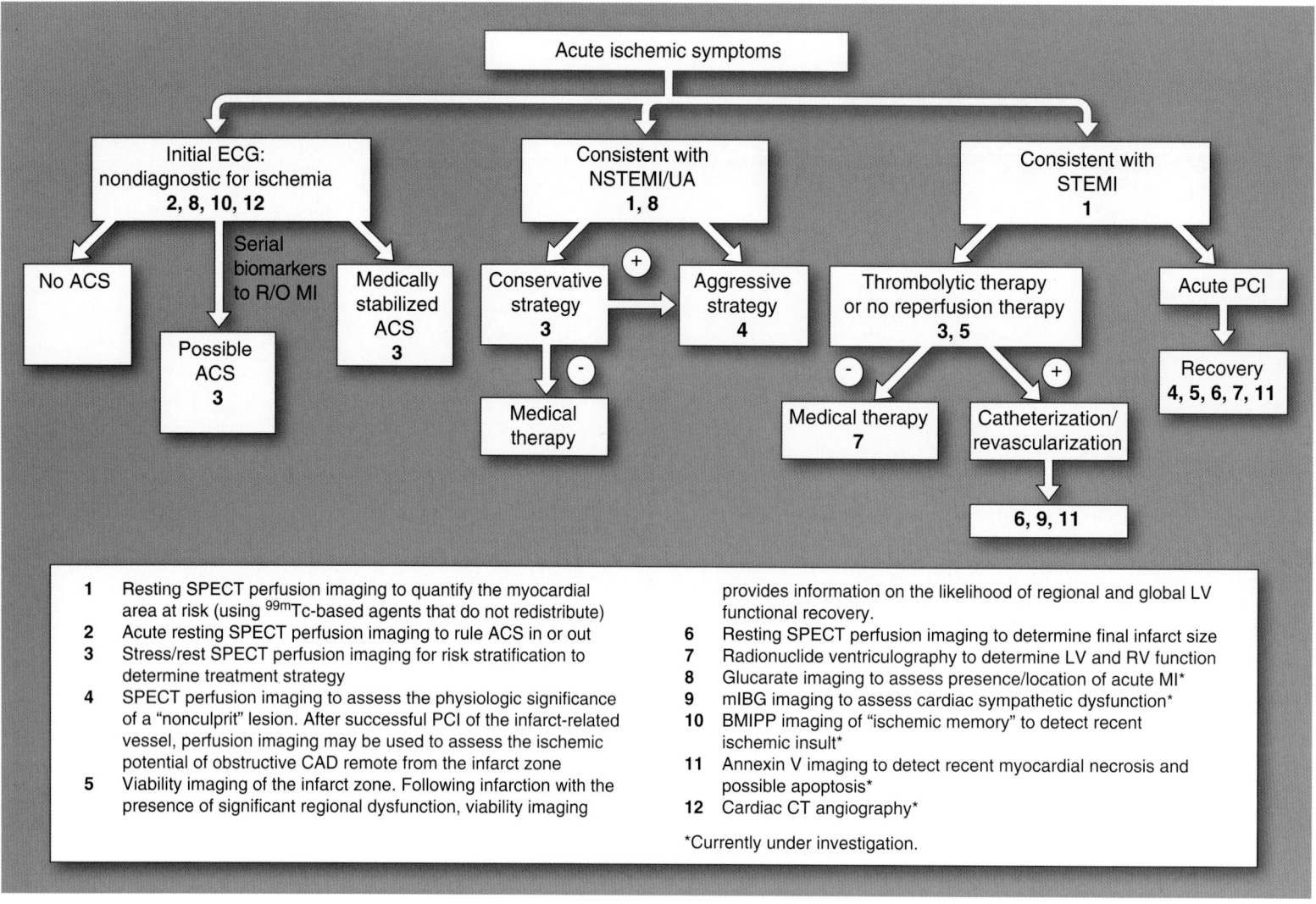

Figure 10-1. Diagnostic and therapeutic decision points in three categories of acute ischemic coronary syndromes (ACS). This schematic demonstrates the role of radionuclide techniques in patients seen in the emergency department with suspected ACS who have nondiagnostic electrocardiogram (ECG) changes, patients with non–ST segment elevation myocardial infarction/unstable angina (NSTEMI/UA), and patients with ST segment elevation myocardial infarction (STEMI). Radionuclide imaging techniques that have been applied in either a research or clinical setting are listed, keyed to the appropriate clinical time points where they would be most useful. BMIPP—15-(p-[iodine-123] iodophenyl)-3-(R,S) methylpentadecanoic acid; CAD—coronary artery disease; LV—left ventricle; mIBG—metaiodobenzylguanidine; PCI—percutaneous coronary intervention; RV—right ventricle; SPECT—single photon emission computed tomography.

Flowchart content:

Acute ischemic symptoms →
- Initial ECG: nondiagnostic for ischemia (2, 8, 10, 12)
  - No ACS
  - Serial biomarkers to R/O MI → Possible ACS (3)
  - Medically stabilized ACS (3)
- Consistent with NSTEMI/UA (1, 8)
  - Conservative strategy (3) → (+) Aggressive strategy (4)
  - (−) Medical therapy
- Consistent with STEMI (1)
  - Thrombolytic therapy or no reperfusion therapy (3, 5)
    - (−) Medical therapy (7)
    - (+) Catheterization/revascularization → 6, 9, 11
  - Acute PCI → Recovery (4, 5, 6, 7, 11)

1. Resting SPECT perfusion imaging to quantify the myocardial area at risk (using ^{99m}Tc-based agents that do not redistribute)
2. Acute resting SPECT perfusion imaging to rule ACS in or out
3. Stress/rest SPECT perfusion imaging for risk stratification to determine treatment strategy
4. SPECT perfusion imaging to assess the physiologic significance of a "nonculprit" lesion. After successful PCI of the infarct-related vessel, perfusion imaging may be used to assess the ischemic potential of obstructive CAD remote from the infarct zone
5. Viability imaging of the infarct zone. Following infarction with the presence of significant regional dysfunction, viability imaging provides information on the likelihood of regional and global LV functional recovery.
6. Resting SPECT perfusion imaging to determine final infarct size
7. Radionuclide ventriculography to determine LV and RV function
8. Glucarate imaging to assess presence/location of acute MI*
9. mIBG imaging to assess cardiac sympathetic dysfunction*
10. BMIPP imaging of "ischemic memory" to detect recent ischemic insult*
11. Annexin V imaging to detect recent myocardial necrosis and possible apoptosis*
12. Cardiac CT angiography*

*Currently under investigation.

Assessment of Patients with Suspected Acute Coronary Syndromes

Figure 10-2. Initial classification of patients presenting to the emergency department (ED) with symptoms suspicious for acute coronary syndrome (ACS). Patients with initial electrocardiograms (ECGs) demonstrating obvious ST segment elevation or ST segment depression (approximately 25% of all patients presenting with symptoms of possible ischemia) should be admitted promptly and managed according to contemporary practice guidelines [10,11]. In surveys of ED patients with chest pain syndromes, approximately 10% have symptoms that are very unlikely to be due to ischemia after initial history and examination. The remaining population of patients whose initial ECGs are not diagnostic for ACS (60%–70% of all patients presenting to EDs with possible ischemic symptoms) are candidates for acute resting myocardial perfusion imaging (MPI) to better stratify those patients whose symptoms are likely to be ischemic from those whose symptoms are most likely not due to ischemia. The former group (abnormal scan) may be considered candidates for more aggressive therapy, while the latter group (normal resting perfusion scan) may be considered candidates for early discharge from the ED.

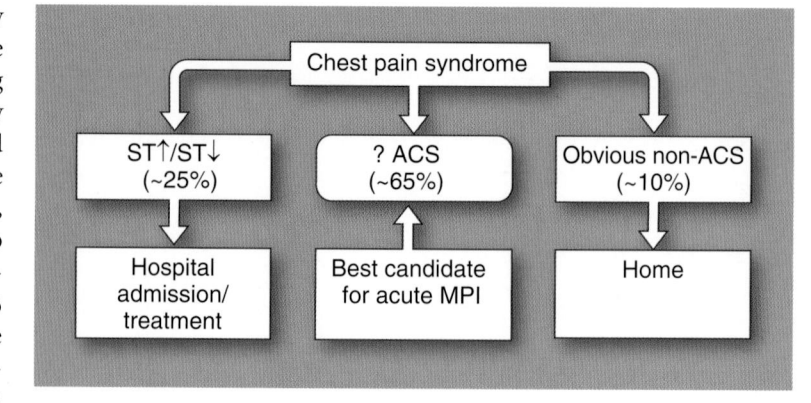

Chest pain syndrome →
- ST↑/ST↓ (~25%) → Hospital admission/treatment
- ? ACS (~65%) → Best candidate for acute MPI
- Obvious non-ACS (~10%) → Home

226 Atlas of Nuclear Cardiology

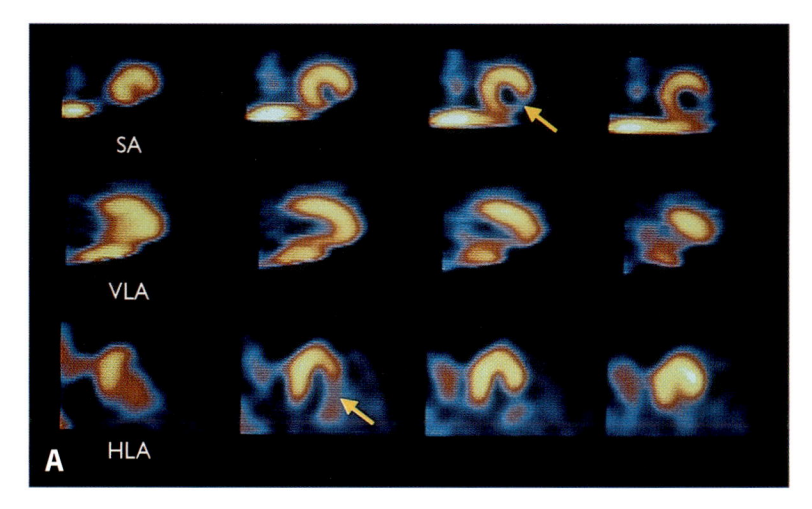

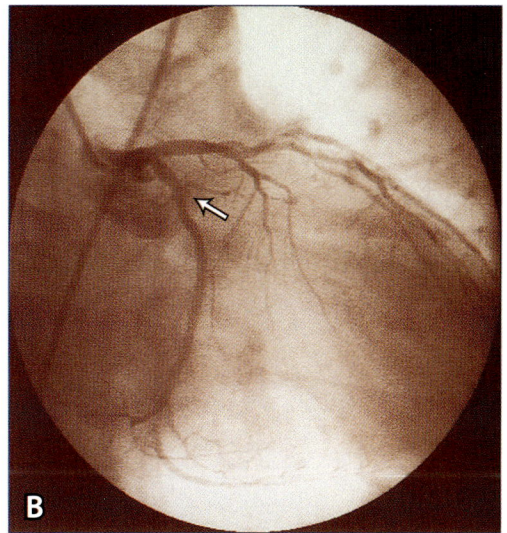

Figure 10-3. Significant myocardial perfusion abnormalities in patients with chest pain but nondiagnostic electrocardiographic alterations. **A,** Short-axis (SA), vertical long-axis (VLA), and horizontal long-axis (HLA) resting single photon emission computed tomography (SPECT) myocardial perfusion images (MPIs) of a 39-year-old-man who presented to the emergency department (ED) with chest pain atypical for angina and a normal initial electrocardiogram (ECG). He was injected with ^{99m}Tc-sestamibi at rest in the ED and underwent SPECT imaging soon thereafter. The images show a dense inferolateral resting perfusion defect (*arrows*), which in the setting of ongoing symptoms was most suggestive of resting ischemia and acute coronary syndrome (ACS). He was immediately triaged to the catheterization laboratory.

B, Right anterior oblique view of the left coronary artery injection showing an occluded left circumflex artery (*arrow*) in the patient in **A**. Ischemia or infarct resulting from left circumflex occlusions are not always well seen on the standard 12-lead ECG. The patient subsequently underwent successful percutaneous coronary intervention of the left circumflex artery, with an excellent anatomic result. Had MPI not been performed, he may have been admitted for observation, and serial enzyme analysis may have been positive for a myocardial infarction. The use of MPI likely allowed significantly earlier intervention in this case.

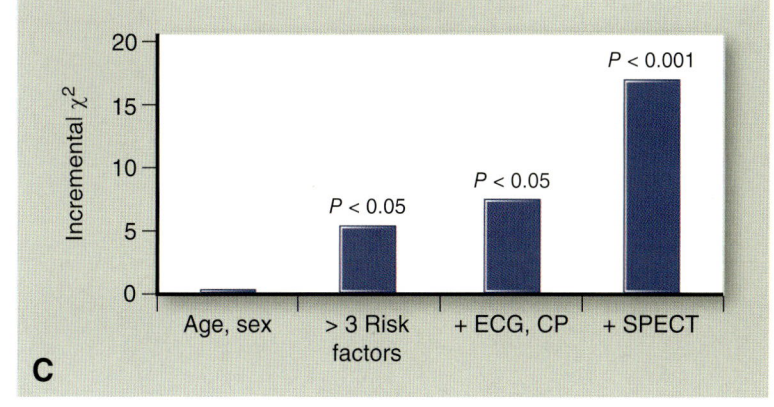

C, Analysis of the incremental value of resting MPI data to predict cardiac events in patients presenting to the ED with suspected ischemia. The incremental χ^2 value measures the strength of the association between individual factors added to a clinician's knowledge base in incremental fashion and unfavorable cardiac events. Addition of resting SPECT MPI data (+ SPECT) in the ED setting adds highly statistically significant value on detection of ACS and events even given knowledge of age, sex, multiple (> three) risk factors for coronary artery disease, and ECG changes and the presence or absence of chest pain (CP). (**C,** *adapted from* Heller *et al.* [8].)

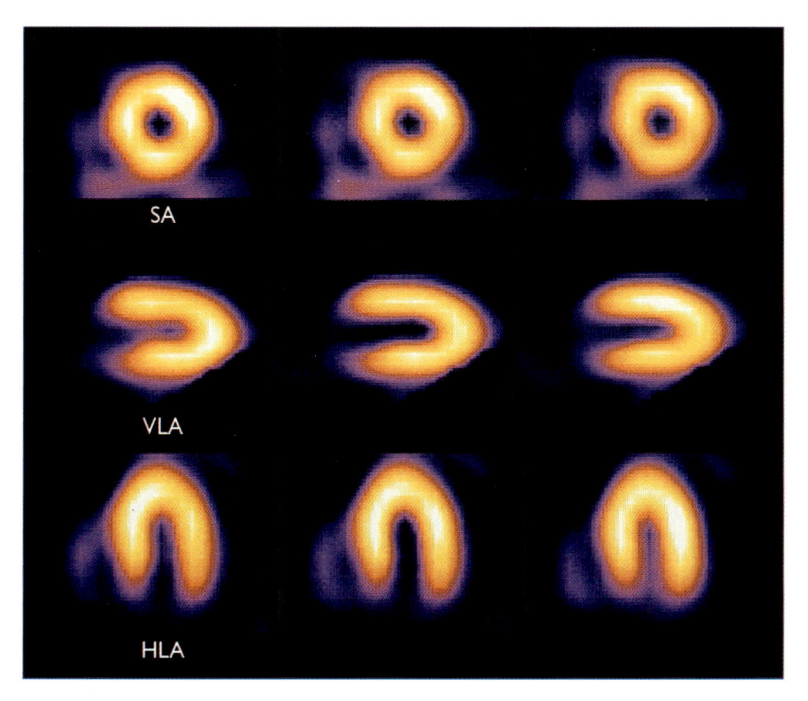

Figure 10-4. Absence of myocardial perfusion abnormality in a patient presenting with chest pain but nondiagnostic electrocardiogram changes. Short-axis (SA), vertical long-axis (VLA), and horizontal long-axis (HLA) single photon emission computed tomography (SPECT) images of a 52-year-old-man who presented to the emergency department (ED) with chest pain atypical for angina and an initial electrocardiogram with nonspecific ST segment abnormalities not diagnostic for acute ischemia. He was injected with ^{99m}Tc-sestamibi at rest in the ED and underwent SPECT imaging soon thereafter. The images show a completely normal resting perfusion pattern, and the gated SPECT imaging of resting left ventricular function (not shown) was also normal. This finding is associated with a very low probability of myocardial infarction and acute ischemic syndrome (*see* Fig. 10-5), suggesting that such a patient may be discharged directly from the ED.

Major Clinical Studies Involving Myocardial Perfusion in Acute Chest Pain

Author	Number	Sensitivity	Specificity	PPV	NPV	Endpoint
Wackers et al. [1]	203	100	63	55	100	MI
Bilodeau et al. [12]	45	96	76	86	94	CAD (by angiography)
Varetto et al. [5]	64	100	67	43	100	MI
		100	92	90	100	CAD
Hilton et al. [6]	102	100	78	38	99	MI
		94	83	44	99	All events
Tatum et al. [7]	438	100	78	7	100	MI
		82	83	32	98	MI, revasc
Kontos et al. [13]	532	93	71	15	99	MI
		81	76	40	95	MI, revasc
Heller et al. [8]	357	90	60	12	99	MI
Duca et al. [14]	75	100	73	33	100	MI
		73	93	89	81	CAD
Kosnik et al. [15]	69	71	92	50	97	MI, revasc, or cardiac death

Figure 10-5. Summary of major clinical studies [1,5–8,12–15] involving myocardial perfusion imaging for endpoint events in patients with chest pain syndromes but nondiagnostic electrocardiograms. All published studies demonstrate a very high negative predictive value (NPV), suggesting that when such a patient has a normal resting perfusion study (as in Fig. 10-4), the risk of myocardial infarction (MI) or ischemic event is relatively small. CAD—coronary artery disease; PPV—positive predictive value; revasc—revascularization by coronary artery bypass grafting or percutaneous transluminal coronary angioplasty.

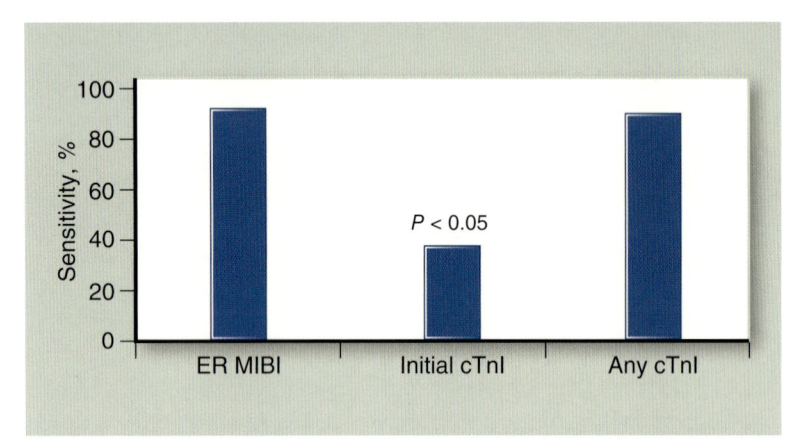

Figure 10-6. Comparative role of myocardial perfusion imaging (MPI) and serial analysis of cardiospecific enzymes in patients with chest pain in the emergency room (ER) setting. ^{99m}Tc-sestamibi MPI (ER MIBI) was performed and serial analysis of cardiac troponin I (cTnI) was undertaken in patients presenting with suspected acute coronary syndrome (ACS) but no obvious ischemic electrocardiogram changes (low to moderate risk for ACS). The sestamibi perfusion studies, performed very early during the initial evaluation, had 92% sensitivity to detect myocardial infarction, while the initial troponin I value, drawn at a similarly early time in the evaluation, had a sensitivity of only 39%. The sensitivity of any troponin I value on serial testing over 24 hours ultimately achieved similar sensitivity as the perfusion study. This study illustrates that in the presence of ACS, MPI likely will be positive earlier than serial analysis of enzymes, allowing the opportunity for earlier intervention. (*Adapted from* Kontos et al. [13].)

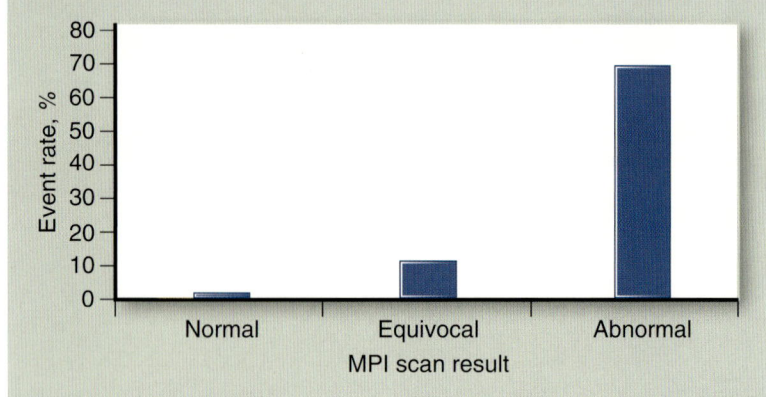

Figure 10-7. Cardiac event rate as a function of results of resting ^{99m}Tc-sestamibi single photon emission computed tomography myocardial perfusion imaging (MPI) in patients presenting to the emergency department with suspected ischemia. Patients with a normal scan demonstrate a very low event rate, and patients with an abnormal scan had a significantly higher event rate [6], consistent with numerous studies from the literature in this population. Patients with "equivocal" results on resting MPI, ie, results that were neither completely normal nor definitely abnormal, likely reflect some patients whose scans were influenced by attenuation artifacts, or those who had small areas of ischemia or infarct, driving an intermediate event rate. Based on such data, equivocal scans should be considered mildly positive for purposes of clinical decision making because the event rate is not as low as with patients who have a "normal" scan. (*Adapted from* Hilton et al. [6].)

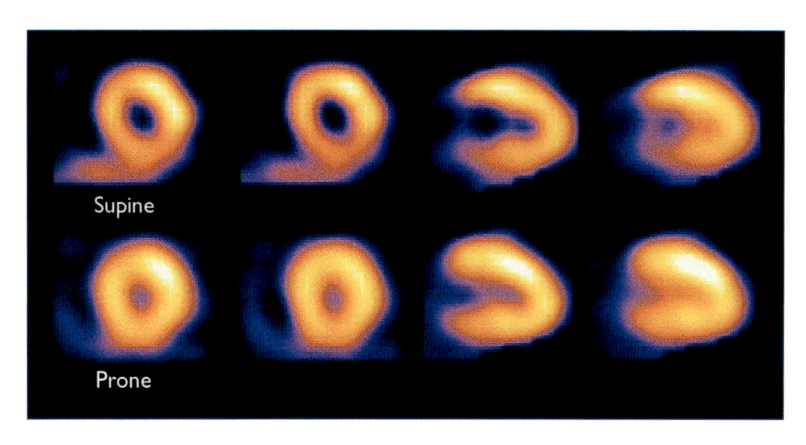

Figure 10-8. Characterization of equivocal myocardial perfusion study results. Various strategies can be employed for clarification of equivocal studies. For instance, in a patient who presented to the emergency department with symptoms suspicious for ischemia but a nondiagnostic electrocardiogram, initial supine resting ^{99m}Tc-sestamibi imaging demonstrated a possible inferobasal defect consistent with either acute ischemia in that territory or diaphragmatic attenuation artifact (*top row*). Subsequently, imaging was performed in the prone position (*bottom row*). In this set of images, inferobasal myocardial perfusion appears normal, suggesting that the initial study represented diaphragmatic attenuation artifact and not ischemia. Other alternatives to clarify equivocal images include using attenuation correction algorithms in laboratories with the appropriate equipment and experience.

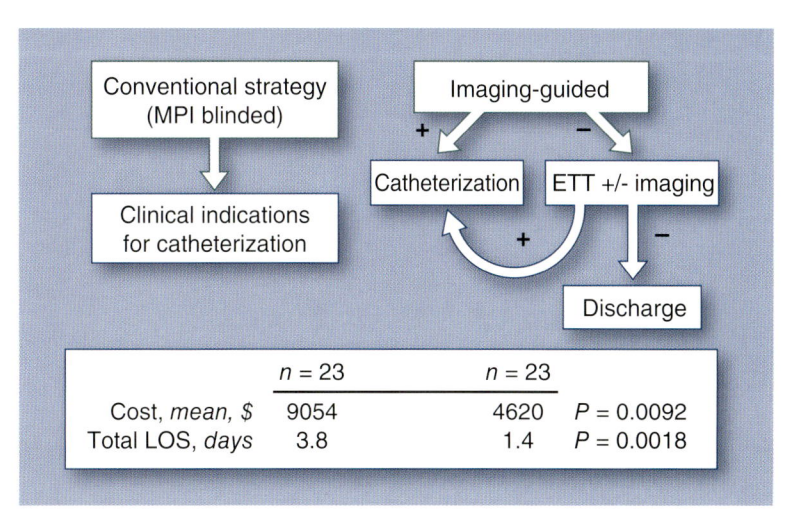

Figure 10-9. Myocardial perfusion imaging (MPI) and the management of patients with nondiagnostic electrocardiogram changes. Although MPI has been shown in observational studies to have very high negative predictive value for ruling out acute coronary syndrome (ACS) (*see* Fig. 10-5), in none of those studies was the imaging information allowed to affect the management, *ie*, the triage decision on whether to admit the patient to the hospital for observation or to discharge directly home from the emergency department. In order to optimally assess the value of imaging (or any test) in this setting, a randomized trial is needed to compare the decisions made using imaging with those made with a strategy not incorporating imaging. In one such study, a small group of patients presenting to an emergency deparment with a suspected ischemic syndrome were randomized to an imaging-guided strategy or a conventional strategy (control) not incorporating imaging. In the imaging-guided strategy, perfusion studies were reviewed and management was based on the results; in the control arm, imaging results were kept blinded. The study endpoints included length of hospital stay (LOS) and overall costs of care, with the hypothesis that both would be lower if imaging were used to guide decisions. Among patients randomized to the test arm, LOS as well as costs were reduced by approximately 50% because fewer patients underwent catheterization. The results suggest that MPI could favorably affect management and lower costs in the setting of suspected ACS. ETT—exercise tolerance testing. (*Adapted from* Stowers et al. [16].)

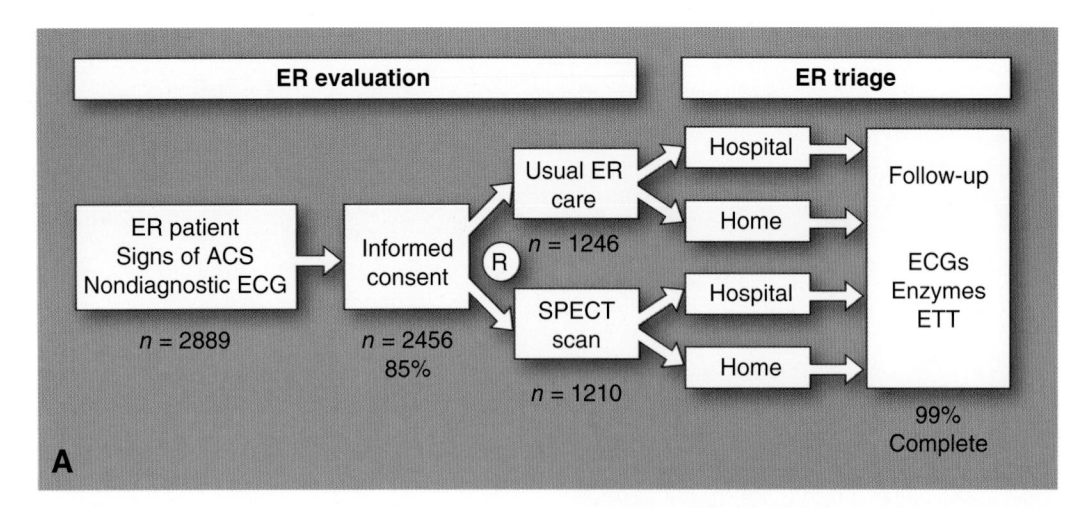

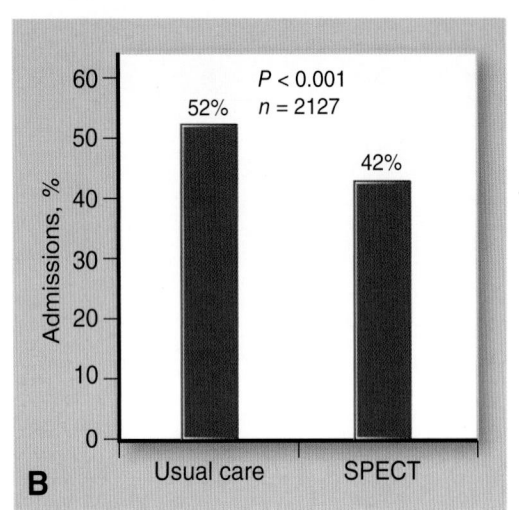

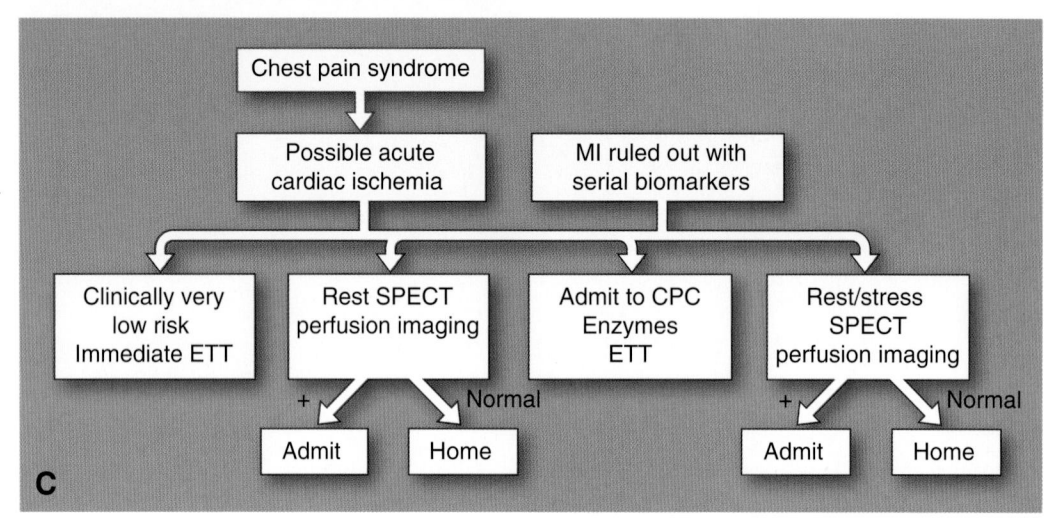

Figure 10-10. Assessment of the role of myocardial perfusion imaging (MPI) to improve clinical decision making in patients with chest pain with nondiagnostic electrocardiogram (ECG) changes. **A,** In a large prospective, randomized study, the ERASE (Emergency Room Assessment of Sestamibi for the Evaluation of Chest Pain) trial [17], investigators at seven sites enrolled 2475 patients with chest pain or other symptoms suggestive of acute cardiac ischemia and a normal or nondiagnostic initial ECG in the emergency department (ED). Patients were randomly assigned to receive either the usual ED evaluation strategy or the usual strategy supplemented by results from acute resting ^{99m}Tc-sestamibi single photon emission computed tomography (SPECT) imaging. The physician incorporated the imaging information into the decision-making either to admit the patient to the hospital for observation or to discharge directly home from the ED. The "correctness" of that decision was based on all follow-up information (available in 99% of patients at 1 month after presentation), so that the effect of incorporating the imaging information on clinical decision making could be assessed rigorously [17].

B, For those patients ultimately determined not to have acute cardiac ischemia as the presenting syndrome, hospitalization was reduced from 52% with usual care to 42% with ^{99m}Tc-sestamibi imaging (odds ratio 0.68), ie, imaging was associated with a 32% reduction in the odds of being admitted unnecessarily to the hospital for admission or observation. On 30-day follow-up, there were no differences in outcomes between the usual care group or imaging group. This study demonstrated that the incorporation of ^{99m}Tc-sestamibi imaging into ED triage decision making provided a clear benefit in reducing unnecessary hospital admissions without inappropriately reducing admission for patients with acute ischemia [17]. Data from these randomized trials provide sufficient evidence to result in level "1-A" evidence for guidelines (see Fig. 10-13).

C, Rest SPECT MPI has been studied rigorously for application in the ED setting, specifically for patients with suspected acute coronary syndrome (ACS) but a nondiagnostic initial ECG. There are several acceptable evaluation strategies for such patients: the "chest pain center" (CPC) protocol (serial evaluation of cardiac-specific enzymes over 12 to 24 hours followed by exercise tolerance testing [ETT] if negative), very early stress testing for clinically very low-risk patients, and a full stress and rest imaging protocol. MPI in this setting potentially can allow earlier triage than serial enzyme evaluation, but it must be performed with meticulous attention to high-quality acquisition, be interpreted by experienced readers, and be associated with prompt reporting of results, as well as good follow-up after discharge. The data suggest that if MPI studies are normal, the risk of ACS or negative events is very low, and early discharge from the ED to home may be considered. If imaging tests suggest acute infarction or ischemia, then rapid admission and entry into an appropriate evidence-based treatment pathway for ACS is in order. MI—myocardial infarction.

Figure 10-11. Potential use of fatty acid imaging for identifying patients later after symptom resolution: imaging of "ischemic memory". Following an ischemic insult, fatty acid metabolism may be suppressed for a prolonged time, far beyond the time when flow returns to normal and signs and symptoms of regional ischemia have resolved. Thus, there is potential for imaging the ongoing abnormality in fatty acid metabolism as a signal of ischemic memory. In the aftermath of the acute ischemic symptoms, a radioiodinated fatty acid analogue, 15-(p-[iodine-123] iodophenyl)-3-(R,S) methylpentadecanoic acid (BMIPP), has been used to assess fatty acid utilization in the myocardium. In one study of 111 patients presenting with symptoms of acute coronary syndrome but no myocardial infarction, BMIPP single photon emission computed tomography (SPECT) imaging performed 1 to 5 days after presentation was more sensitive than rest myocardial perfusion imaging (MPI) (performed within 24 hours of presentation) in identifying the presence and site of the culprit coronary stenosis or spasm (74% vs 38%, respectively; $P < 0.05$) at similar high specificity [18]. In this example from a more recent clinical trial, BMIPP SPECT images were obtained in a patient with suspected acute coronary syndrome whose initial electrocardiogram was nondiagnostic and whose initial troponin measurement was within normal limits. BMIPP was injected approximately 8 hours after symptoms had subsided. A single set of SPECT images was obtained beginning approximately 10 minutes after injection of the tracer. The *top row* demonstrates short-axis (SA) SPECT images reflecting fatty acid metabolism, and show a lateral wall defect (*arrows*). In the *bottom row*, the horizontal long-axis (HLA) images also show that defect (*arrows*). The imaging data suggest prolonged suppression of fatty acid metabolism in the lateral wall, consistent with recent ischemia in the left circumflex distribution. Subsequently, the patient had a stress SPECT MPI study demonstrating inducible ischemia in the lateral wall. Thus, this technique may provide earlier risk stratification information based on the magnitude of abnormal fatty acid metabolism compared with follow-up stress SPECT studies, to the extent that it may reflect the recent extent of ischemia during the symptomatic episode, using rest imaging alone without the need for a stress test. This concept is currently under study in multicenter trials.

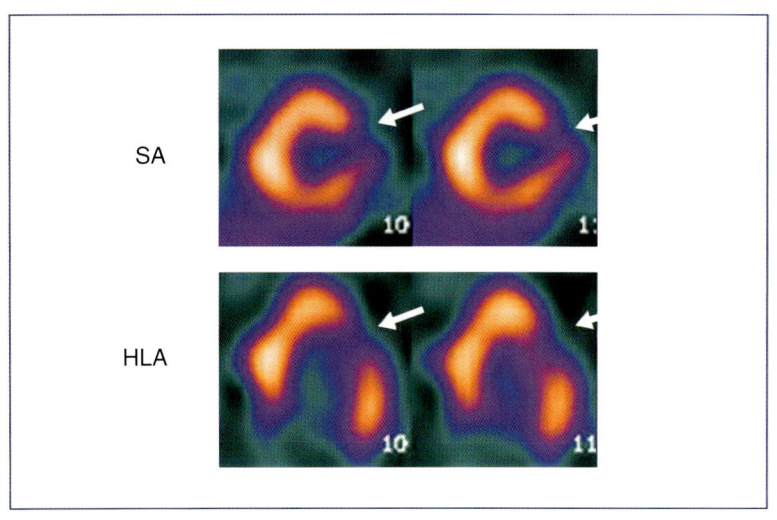

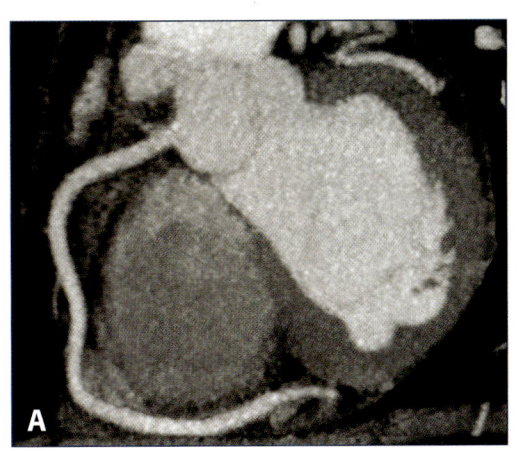

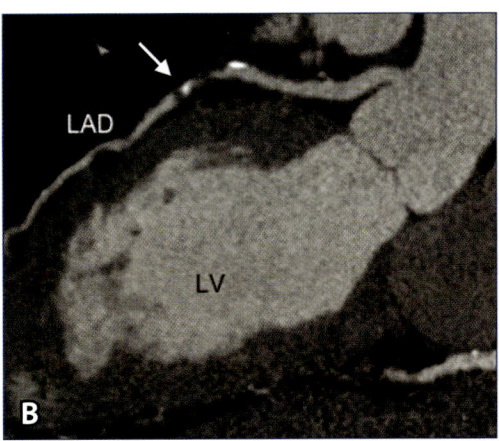

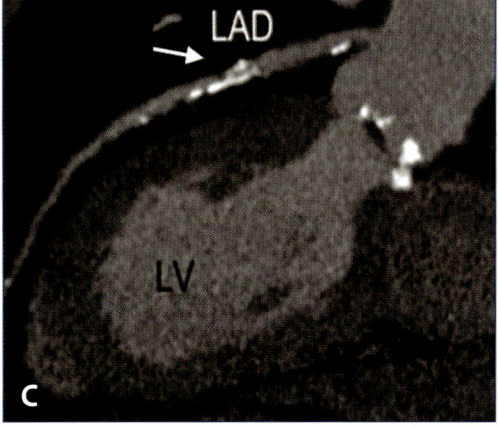

Figure 10-12. Use of cardiac computed tomographic angiography (CCTA) in patients with suspected acute coronary syndromes (ACS) in the emergency department (ED). Given the strong performance characteristics of CCTA for detecting or ruling out coronary stenoses ≥ 50% in comparison to invasive angiography in many recent publications, it is conceptually attractive to apply this technology to ED patients with suspected ACS. Shown are three examples of CCTA images in such patients. **A**, A patient with normal coronary arteries (the right coronary artery is shown). It is unlikely that the representing symptoms represent an ACS with unstable plaque, given the high negative predictive value for stenosis known for CCTA. **B**, A severe, complex stenosis of the left anterior descending (LAD) artery (*arrow*). In this patient, even in the absence of electrocardiogram changes or an initially positive troponin, the likelihood of ACS is high, and admission is warranted. **C**, A calcified plaque of apparently moderate severity in terms of luminal narrowing (*arrow*). In this patient, it is not clear from the anatomic information provided by the CCTA image whether or not the patient's symptoms represent an ACS, and it is likely that having identified the presence of coronary artery disease but still with an intermediate probability of an ACS, that admission for further testing is necessary.

Continued on the next page

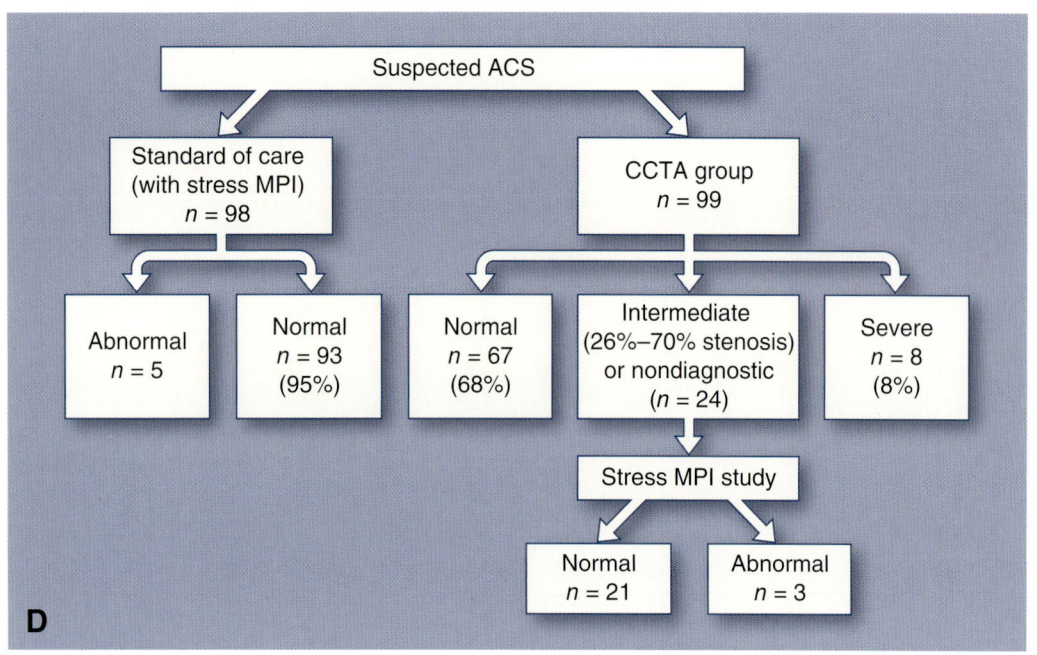

```
                        Suspected ACS
                              │
              ┌───────────────┴───────────────┐
              ▼                               ▼
      Standard of care                   CCTA group
      (with stress MPI)                    n = 99
          n = 98
              │                               │
        ┌─────┴─────┐           ┌─────────────┼─────────────┐
        ▼           ▼           ▼             ▼             ▼
    Abnormal    Normal      Normal      Intermediate     Severe
     n = 5      n = 93      n = 67    (26%–70% stenosis)  n = 8
               (95%)        (68%)      or nondiagnostic    (8%)
                                           (n = 24)
                                              │
                                              ▼
                                      Stress MPI study
                                              │
                                       ┌──────┴──────┐
                                       ▼             ▼
                                    Normal       Abnormal
                                    n = 21         n = 3
```
D

Figure 10-12. *(Continued)* **D**, Data from a small randomized trial in which patients with suspected ACS were randomized to have evaluation performed by stress myocardial perfusion imaging (MPI) or to a strategy of CCTA imaging. Among the patients randomized to the stress MPI evaluation strategy, the vast majority (95%) were normal (typical for this low-to-intermediate likelihood population), and work-up was complete. Among patients randomized to the CCTA strategy, a clear management direction was provided in the 68% of patients with normal coronaries as well as the 8% with evidence of severe disease. However, in 24% of the patients there were either intermediate stenoses of unclear clinical relevance to the presenting symptoms, or nondiagnostic images. All of these patients required further testing with stress MPI to clarify management, and the majority were normal. Moreover, a substantial number of patients who were screened for participation could not be randomized to CCTA for technical reasons including pulmonary disease, atrial fibrillation, or contrast allergy. Thus, while CCTA may have a role in this clinical situation, the anatomic information may often not be sufficient to initially establish low probability for ACS. Larger multicenter trials will explore the place of CCTA in this setting. LV—left ventricle. (**A–C**, *courtesy of* Udo Hoffmann, MD; **D**, *adapted from* Goldstein *et al.* [19].)

ACC/AHA/ASNC Guideline Recommendations for Radionuclide Imaging in Patients with Suspected ACS Presenting to the Emergency Department

Patient Subgroup	Imaging Modality	Recommendation/Evidence Level
Assessment of risk in suspected ACS with nondiagnostic initial ECG	Rest MPI	I, A
Diagnosis of CAD in suspected ACS with nondiagnostic ECG and negative biomarkers or normal rest MPI	Stress/rest MPI	I, B

Figure 10-13. American College of Cardiology (ACC)/American Heart Association (AHA)/American Society of Nuclear Cardiology (ASNC) guideline recommendations for radionuclide imaging in patients with suspected acute coronary syndrome (ACS) presenting to the emergency department. Based on the growing literature regarding imaging in patients with suspected ACS, recent guidelines have recommended the use of myocardial perfusion imaging (MPI) with a class I recommendation for specific situations. First, in patients who present with symptoms consistent with ACS but with a nondiagnostic initial electrocardiogram (ECG), rest MPI will supply substantial risk stratification information to inform clinical decision regarding triage decision, *ie*, does the patient need to be admitted or are they safe to discharge home. Secondly, among patients who have been observed and have negative serial biomarkers, stress/rest MPI can be strongly recommended for detection of coronary artery disease (CAD) as well as risk stratification.

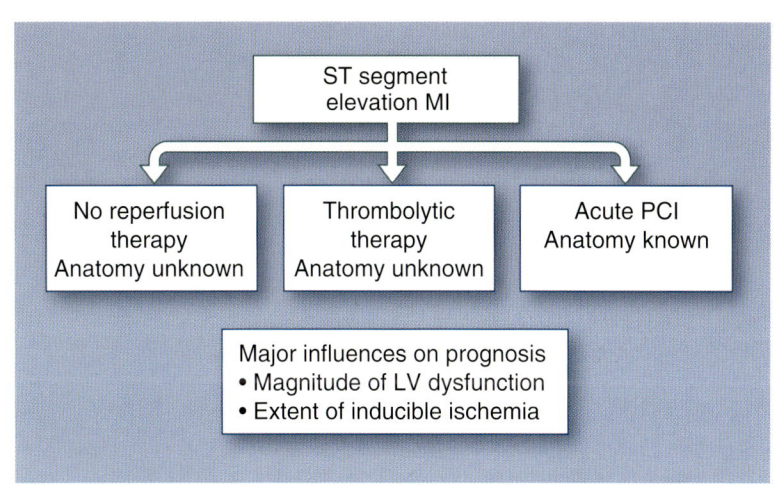

Assessment of Patients with ST Segment Elevation Myocardial Infarction

Figure 10-14. Therapeutic pathways for patients with ST segment elevation myocardial infarction. In the contemporary therapeutic era, patients with acute ST segment elevation myocardial infarction (MI) may be classified by the initial treatment strategy to assess the potential application of imaging modalities to subsequent management strategy. Based on numerous factors, some patients may receive no initial reperfusion therapy and may not have initial catheterization data; therefore, their anatomy will be unknown. Others may be treated with thrombolytic therapy and not sent to the catheterization laboratory, while a third group may be managed with primary percutaneous coronary intervention (PCI) of the infarct-related vessel, and thus full coronary anatomic information will be at hand. For all groups, however, post-MI prognosis is predicted by the magnitude of residual left ventricular (LV) dysfunction and the presence and magnitude of inducible ischemia. An imaging study in the post-MI setting can assess these variables, which in turn may allow classification and risk stratification of patients regarding potential long-term post-MI outcomes, information that readily translates into clinical management strategies. Thus, imaging techniques can provide data that can be used specifically to direct patient management.

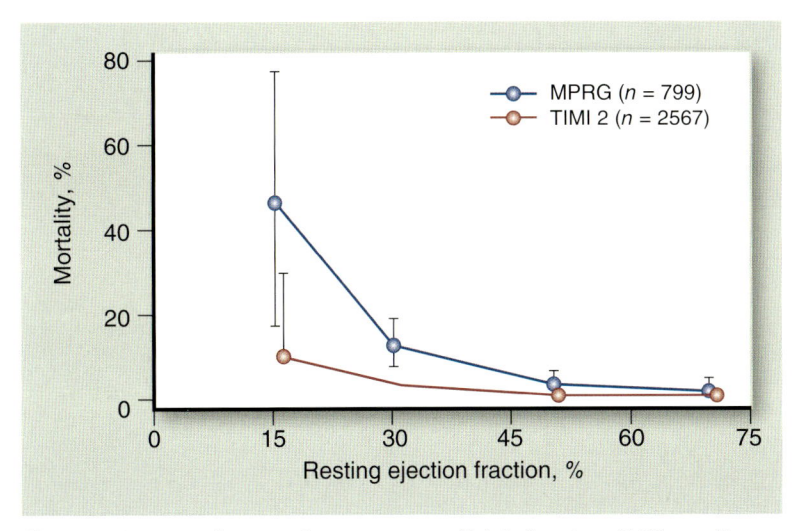

Figure 10-15. Relation of post–myocardial infarction (MI) cardiovascular mortality to resting ejection fraction in the pre- and post-thrombolytic era. Data from the MPRG (Multicenter Post Infarction Research Group) and the TIMI 2 (Thrombolysis in Myocardial Infarction Phase 2) trials demonstrate that as the magnitude of left ventricular dysfunction increases, the late mortality post-MI increases. At any given ejection fraction, the mortality is lower in patients receiving thrombolytic reperfusion therapy, but a relation between ejection fraction and survival remains evident in the thrombolytic era. (*Adapted from* Zaret *et al.* [20].)

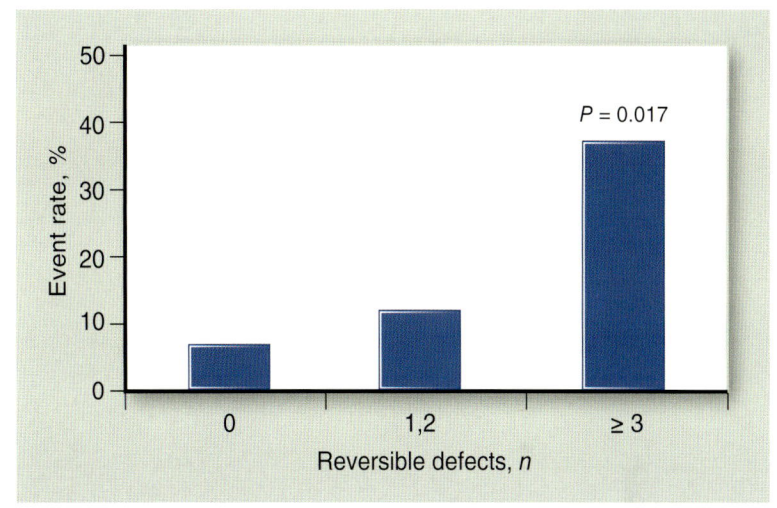

Figure 10-16. Relation between the post–myocardial infarction (MI) extent of inducible ischemia and the cardiac event rate. Patients with more extensive ischemia (documented as the number of reversible perfusion defects on ^{99m}Tc-sestamibi imaging) are at progressively higher risk of unfavorable outcome during late post-MI follow-up. These data, confirming the value of knowledge of the extent of ischemia in patients after MI, suggest that patients with a significant degree of inducible ischemia after MI are at risk of death or reinfarction, and thus are candidates for a more aggressive interventional post-MI treatment strategy. (*Adapted from* Travin *et al.* [21].)

Diagnosis and Risk Stratification in Acute Coronary Syndromes

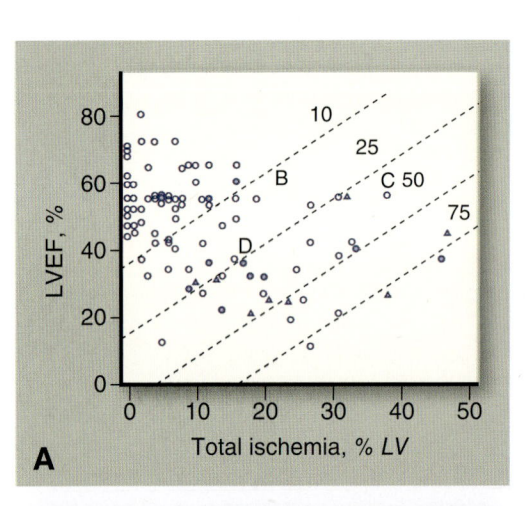

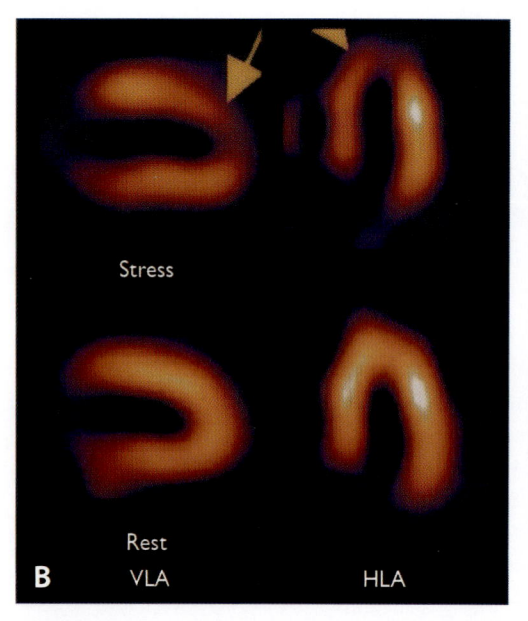

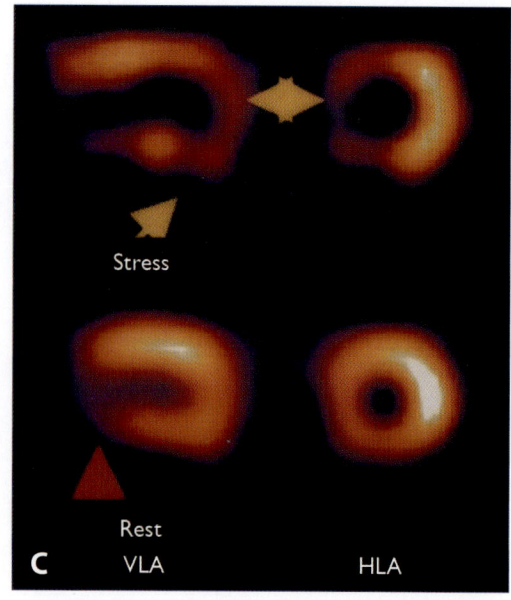

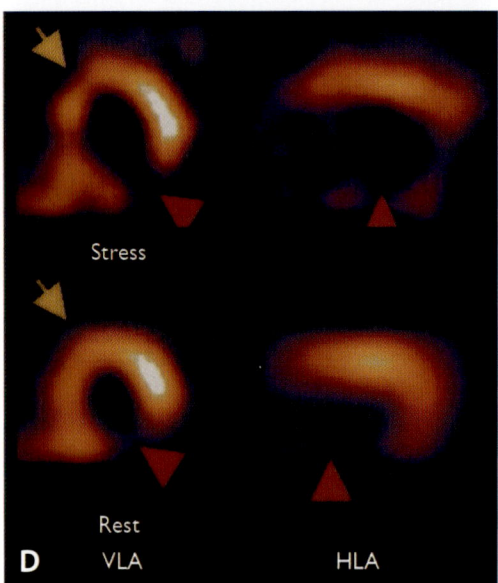

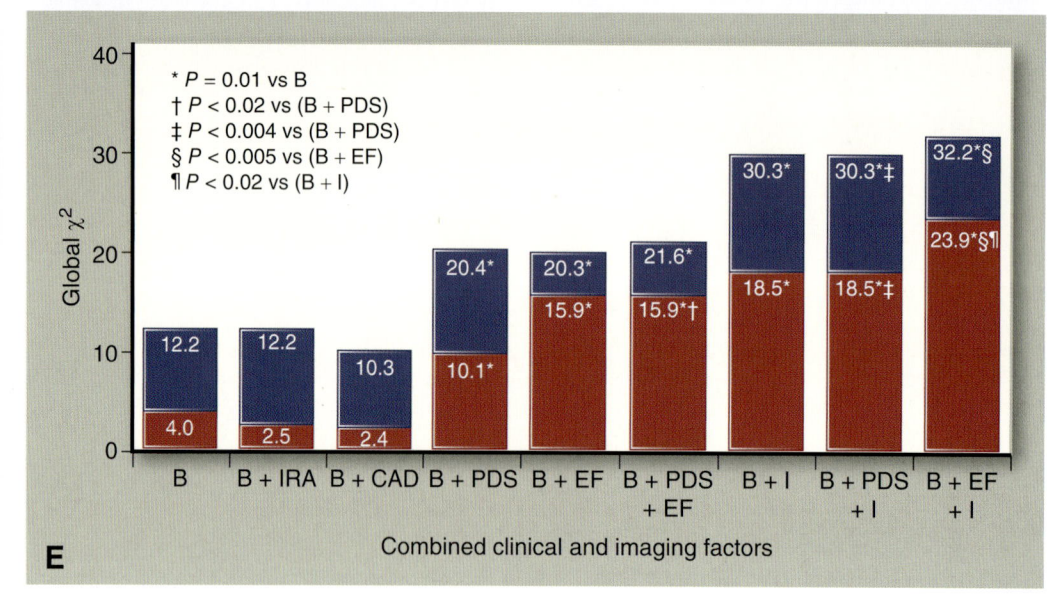

Figure 10-17. The independent but complementary nature of the information provided by imaging evaluation of the extent of inducible ischemia and the magnitude of left ventricular (LV) dysfunction. **A,** Graph of post–myocardial infarction (MI) natural history risk of death and nonfatal reinfarction based on Cox regression models displaying 1-year risk for cardiac event according to left ventricular ejection fraction (LVEF, y-axis) and total LV ischemia (x-axis) [22]. *Diagonal lines* denote representative isobars of percent risk of event. Patient risk for death and nonfatal reinfarction increases as total LV ischemia increases and LVEF decreases. For any given LVEF, risk varies widely depending on the extent of ischemia. Patients are plotted according to death (*triangles*), nonfatal reinfarction (*solid circles*), or neither of these events (*open circles*). These data suggest that comprehensive knowledge of LV function and the extent of inducible ischemia, information supplied in one test by gated single photon emission computed tomography (SPECT) myocardial perfusion imaging, in the post-MI setting creates a powerful and comprehensive basis for risk stratification and delineation of subsequent management strategies.

B–D, Examples of patients with different scintigraphic patterns and degrees of LV functional impairment post-MI, with mapping of the perfusion and function information to obtain a risk estimate in **A**, denoted by the letters *B*, *C*, and *D*. **B,** Stress (*top row*) and rest (*bottom row*) vertical long axis (VLA) and horizontal long axis (HLA) SPECT images demonstrate significant reversible defects consistent with extensive inducible ischemia (*yellow arrows*), quantitatively representing 25% total LV ischemia in a patient who presented with an anterior ST segment elevation MI and who received thrombolytic therapy early after symptom onset. The gated SPECT functional data revealed preserved LVEF at 58%. When this patient's ischemia and function data are plotted back in **A** (point B on the graph), estimated risk of reinfarction or death at 1 year is approximately 25%, a high risk, driving a decision towards catheterization and potential revascularization. **C,** Extensive anterior, apical, septal, and inferior ischemia (*yellow arrows*), with a small inferobasal fixed defect (*red arrowhead*) in the VLA and short-axis (SA) views, the latter consistent with infarction. Quantitated extent of ischemia was 42% of the LV and LVEF was 48%. The estimated 1 year risk of death or reinfarction is approximately 50% (point C on graph in **A**). **D,** A large fixed inferior and inferolateral defect consistent with infarction (*red arrowheads*), as well as septal and anterior ischemia. The LV EF was 33% by gated SPECT, with 16% total LV ischemia, resulting in a risk estimate of 25% to 50% (point D on graph in **A**).

Continued on the next page

Figure 10-17. *(Continued)* **E,** Incremental prognostic power of perfusion variables and ejection fraction information over baseline clinical variables (B) for predicting all events (*entire bar*) or death and reinfarction (*orange portion of bar*). The χ^2 analysis represents the quantified risk of outcome event after MI, based on individual or combined clinical and imaging factors. LVEF and perfusion defect size (PDS), as well as extent of inducible ischemia (I), independently and incrementally predict risk beyond the baseline clinical model. Also, extent of ischemia improved the predictive power of the combined baseline clinical model and PDS (B+PDS) or baseline model and LVEF (B+EF) for all events and for death and reinfarction. LVEF added significant power to the combined baseline model and PDS (B+PDS), as well as to the baseline model and extent of ischemia (B+I) for predicting death and reinfarction. These data confirm that knowledge of the magnitude of LV dysfunction as well as the scintigraphic extent of inducible ischemia carry powerful as well as independent prognostic value in the post-MI setting. CAD—coronary artery disease; IRA—infarct related artery. (*Adapted from* Mahmarian *et al.* [22].)

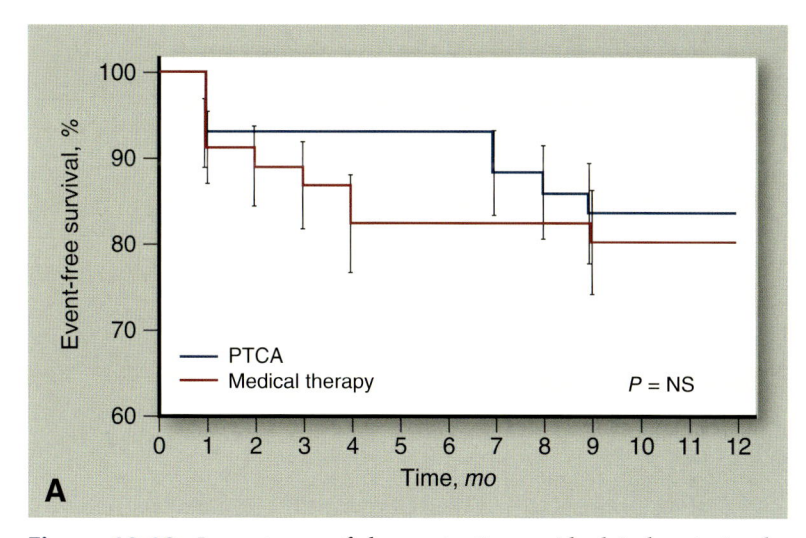

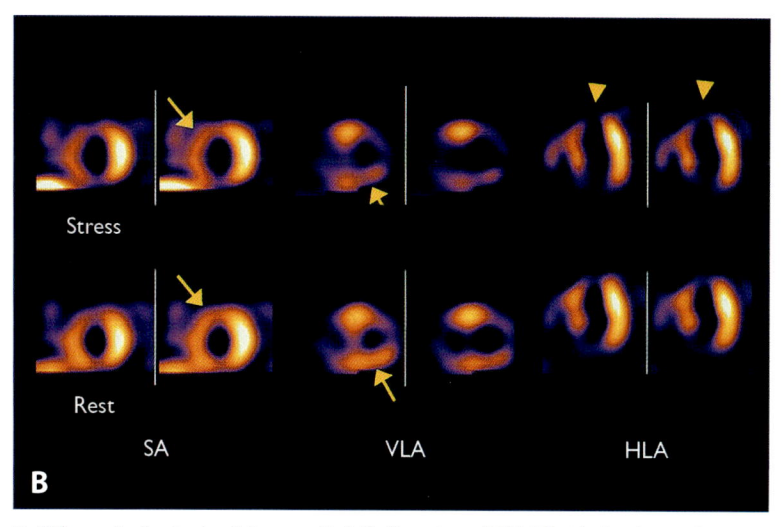

Figure 10-18. Importance of demonstrating residual ischemia in the infarct zone after thrombolytic therapy as a guide to the potential benefit of revascularization. **A,** Some cardiologists advocated angioplasty of any residual stenosis present after the administration of thrombolytic therapy. In a study designed to rigorously assess that notion [23], patients who had received thrombolytic therapy for acute myocardial infarction (MI) and also had a residual stenosis of the infarct-related artery but no inducible ischemia in the infarct territory by myocardial perfusion imaging were randomized to either a strategy of percutaneous transluminal coronary angioplasty (PTCA) of the residual stenosis or a strategy of no PTCA. Shown is a plot of actuarial freedom from cardiac death, MI, coronary bypass surgery, or PTCA after randomization to PTCA or medical therapy. There is no difference in outcome between the groups. Hence, identification of inducible ischemia (or lack thereof) within the infarct zone by myocardial perfusion imaging after acute MI and reperfusion therapy can guide management decisions regarding revascularization strategy. In the absence of any residual infarct-zone ischemia, there appears to be little benefit from a strategy of revascularization. This concept was readdressed in the more contemporary era by the OAT (Open Artery Trial), in which patients with an occluded infarct artery in the weeks following MI were randomized to a strategy of contemporary medical therapy versus percutaneous coronary intervention (PCI) to open the occluded infarct-related artery, in the absence of extensive ischemia. There was no difference in long-term natural history outcomes between the group randomized to optimal contemporary medical therapy versus those randomized to PCI of the occluded infarct artery plus optimal medical therapy [24].

B, To address the concept that all patients in the aftermath of acute MI treated with thrombolytic therapy should be catheterized, the TIMI 2 (Thrombolysis in Myocardial Infarction [TIMI] 2) [25] study randomized such patients to a strategy of catheterization in the days after presentation, with PTCA or coronary artery bypass grafting based on anatomic considerations, or to an "ischemia-guided" strategy, in which patients underwent noninvasive imaging to detect ischemia within or remote from the infarct zone, with subsequent catheterization based on the presence and extent of ischemia. At 6 months' follow-up, there was no difference between the groups in any outcome measure, and fewer patients in the ischemia-guided group underwent catheterization and revascularization, suggesting lower costs. These data suggest that routine catheterization after initial thrombolytic reperfusion strategy in all patients will not necessarily lead to better outcomes. In this figure, stress and resting SPECT images from a 74-year-old patient who presented with an anterior ST segment elevation MI are depicted. The patient initially had been treated with thrombolytic therapy with subsequent stabilization clinically, with no heart failure, recurrent ischemic symptoms, or arrhythmias. The SPECT study demonstrates an apical fixed defect consistent with infarction (*arrowheads*), but also evidence of extensive inducible ischemia involving the septum and inferior walls (*arrows*), as well as a partially reversible defect of the anterior wall (consistent with ischemia within the infarct zone. Ejection fraction was 38% by gated SPECT imaging. Thus, in this case the post-MI risk stratification SPECT study suggested very high outcome risk based on the extent of inducible ischemia and the left ventricular dysfunction. Despite the stable clinical state, this patient was referred for catheterization and revascularization (as anatomically feasible) with the expectation of improved long-term outcome. HLA—horizontal long axis; SA—short axis; VLA—vertical long axis. (**A,** *adapted from* Ellis *et al.* [23].)

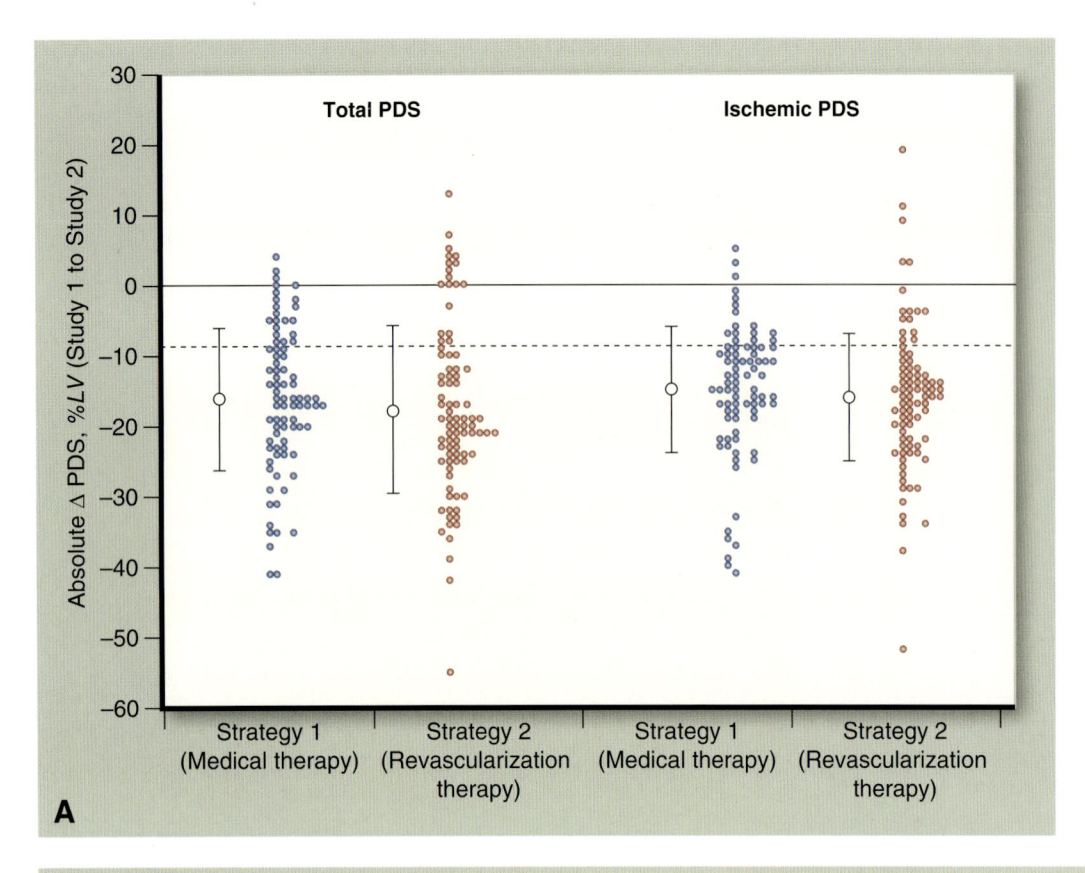

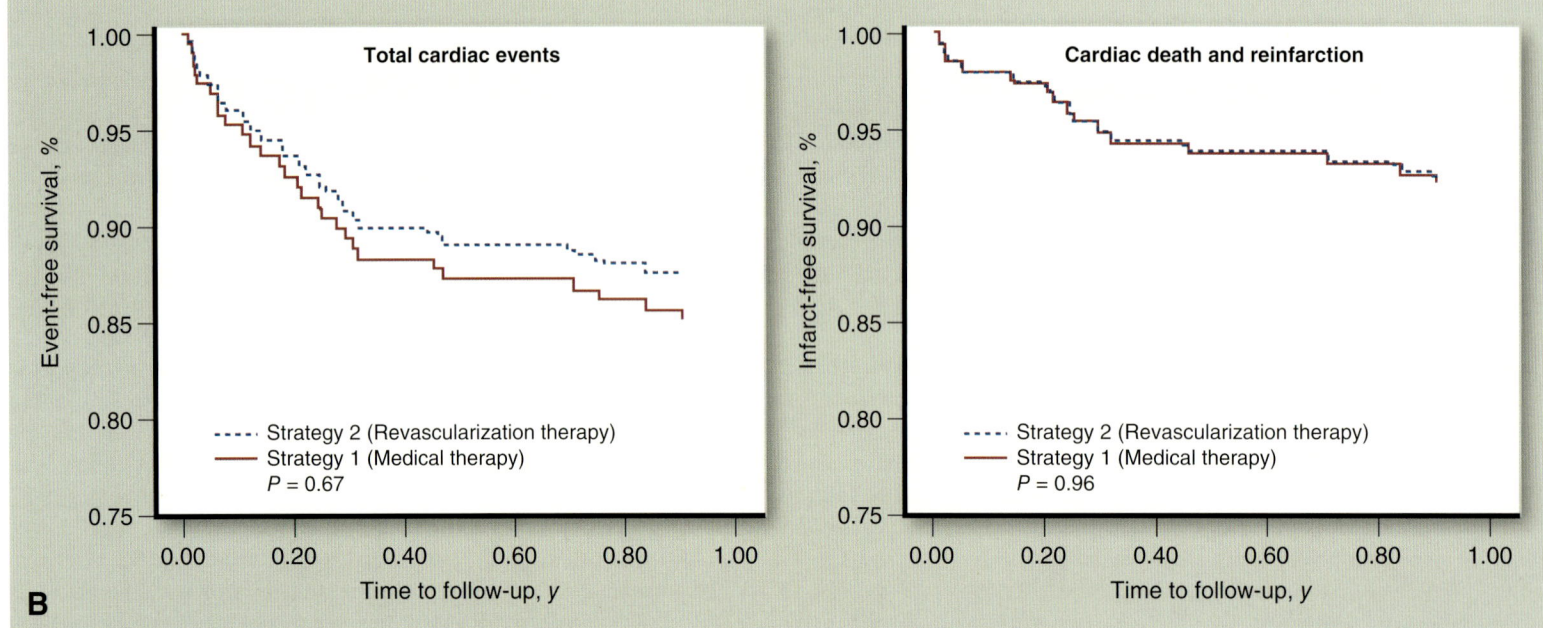

Figure 10-19. Suppression of ischemia by medical or interventional therapies after myocardial infarction (MI) and subsequent outcome events. While many studies have demonstrated an important correlation between the presence and extent of ischemia and subsequent outcome after acute MI, the specificity of such determinations is often low. Among patients with "high-risk" scintigraphic or clinical signs, only a minority will suffer an important cardiac event during follow-up, while the majority of patients categorized in this way will remain event free. Thus, to the extent that common practice dictates that most if not all of these "high-risk" patients should undergo catheterization and intervention, many patients are being intervened upon who would otherwise not have an event in order to prevent such events in the minority. This may be particularly relevant in the contemporary era of aggressive secondary prevention, resulting in a greater degree of plaque stabilization than may have been present in past studies prior to the aggressive use of statins and other therapies in the post-MI setting.

A, In a multicenter randomized trial study designed to address this question (the INSPIRE [Adenosine Sestamibi SPECT Post-Infarction Evaluation] trial), Mahmarian et al. [26] reported on 205 stable survivors of acute MI (ST elevation or non-ST elevation MI) who underwent adenosine SPECT myocardial perfusion imaging (MPI) within 10 days after MI. These patients had large total (> 20% of the left ventricle [LV]) and ischemic (>10% of the LV) perfusion defect size on single photon emission computed tomography (SPECT) quantitative analysis, and LV ejection fraction (EF) > 35%, *ie*, they were "high-risk" patients based on the MPI results and who would usually be referred for revascularization. These patients were randomized to either aggressive and intensive medical therapy, or to revascularization by either percutaneous coronary intervention or bypass surgery. Changes in total and in ischemic perfusion defect size (PDS) during repeat adenosine SPECT imaging 6 weeks following randomization to medical or invasive therapy are shown. Similar reduction in PDS was achieved in both groups, suggesting that in post-MI patients with evidence of extensive ischemia, aggressive contemporary therapy can result in similar suppression of ischemia as does revascularization.

Continued on the next page

Figure 10-19. *(Continued)* **B**, Outcome events among the patients randomized to either aggressive medical therapy or to revascularization in the INSPIRE trial. Over 1 year of follow-up after randomization to one of the two management strategies, there was no apparent difference in outcome events between the two groups, either total cardiac events or a composite of cardiac death and reinfarction. Based on the small population studied and the small number of events, these data should be considered to generate an important hypothesis for future, larger studies. That is, aggressive contemporary medical therapy may result in similar outcomes as revascularization in patients with evidence of scintigraphic ischemia post-MI. This provocative notion is worthy of further testing. *(Adapted from Mahmarian et al. [26].)*

Validation of ^{99m}Tc-sestamibi Tomographic Infarct Size

Method for Measuring Infarct Size	R Value	P Value
Discharge ejection fraction	−0.8	< 0.0001
6-week ejection fraction	−0.81	< 0.0001
1-year ejection fraction	−0.78	< 0.0001
Discharge regional wall motion	−0.75	< 0.0001
6-week regional wall motion	−0.81	< 0.0001
1-year end-systolic volume	0.80	< 0.0001
Peak creatinine kinase levels	0.78	0.002
^{201}Tl perfusion defect	0.73	0.002
Human disease	0.91	0.002

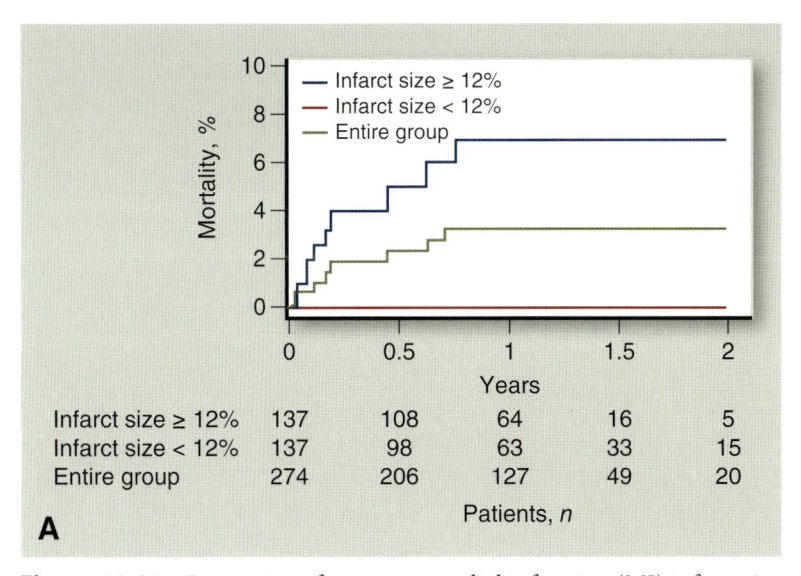

Figure 10-20. Estimation of post–myocardial infarction (MI) infarct size and clinical outcomes. A substantial body of literature exists supporting the concept that estimation of infarct size by quantitative single photon emission computed tomography (SPECT) ^{99m}Tc myocardial perfusion imaging (MPI) has powerful prognostic value in the aftermath of acute MI. Miller *et al.* [27] studied 274 patients with acute MI who underwent imaging prior to reperfusion therapy (to measure the area of myocardium at risk) and at discharge (to measure final infarct size and myocardial salvage). **A**, Mortality curves are shown for the entire group and those with final infarct size 12% or greater of the left ventricle and less than 12% of the left ventricle by quantitative analysis. The magnitude of infarct size was associated significantly with subsequent mortality. Based on studies such as this, detection of final infarct size by SPECT MPI may be used as an intermediate surrogate marker in trials of new reperfusion strategies in acute MI. Therapies that are shown to result in smaller final infarct size by this technique in phase 2 studies have a higher probability of success in subsequent phase 3 outcome studies. **B**, Validation of ^{99m}Tc-sestamibi tomographic infarct size. Final infarct size using SPECT MPI has been correlated with several other measures reflective of outcome after MI. (**A**, *adapted from* Miller *et al.* [27]; **B**, *adapted from* Christian [28].)

Figure 10-21. Vertical long-axis single photon emission computed tomography images in a patient following acute anterior myocardial infarction treated with primary percutaneous coronary intervention. The stress and rest images demonstrate a very large, severe, fixed defect in the anterior wall and apex *(arrows)* with evidence of inducible ischemia of the inferior wall *(arrowhead)*. The severity of the anterior wall and apical defect would suggest that very little myocardial viability exists in those territories, and the large infarct size would suggest high-risk for mortality, based on data depicted in Figure 10-20.

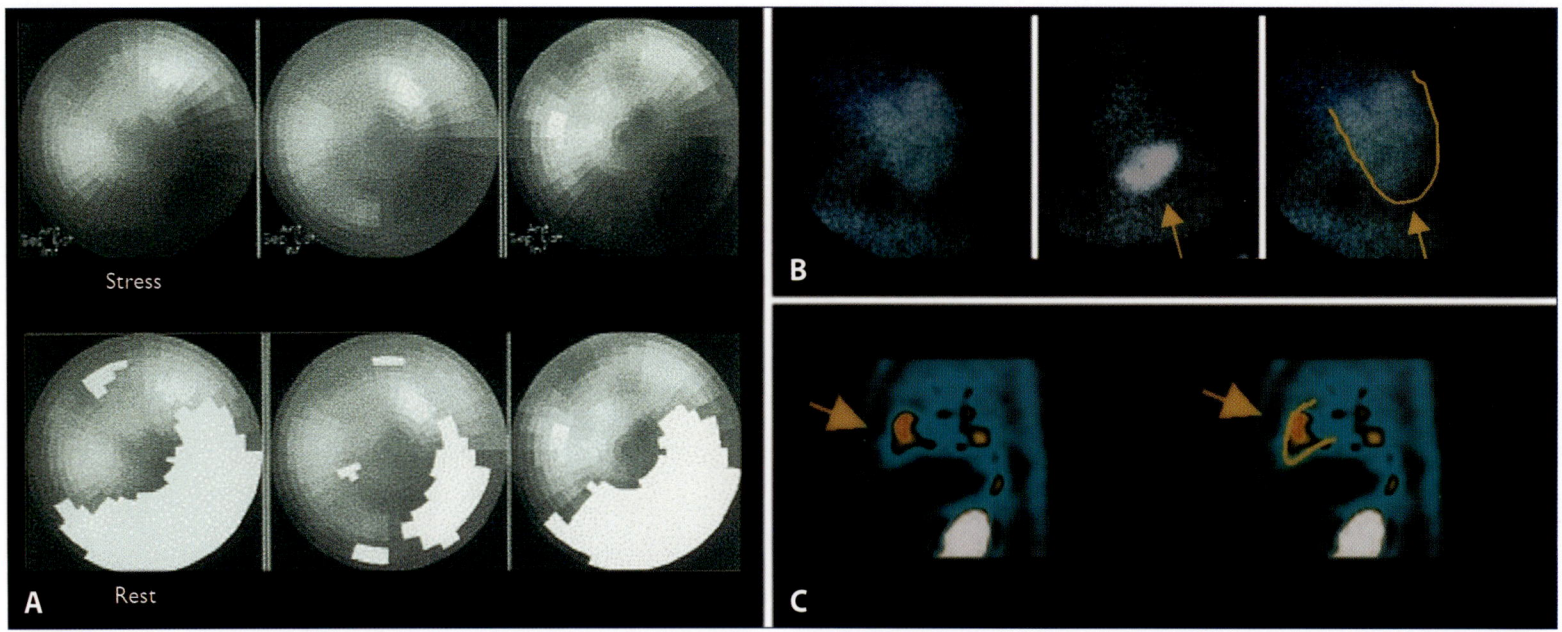

Figure 10-22. Several scintigraphic approaches to assess patients with infarction are under investigation. **A**, ^{123}I metaiodobenzylguanidine (mIBG) imaging. An intriguing area of scintigraphic risk stratification in the post–myocardial infarction (MI) setting involves the use of ^{123}I mIBG imaging of cardiac sympathetic innervation. In the post-MI setting, several studies have shown that the territory of abnormal ^{123}I mIBG uptake, corresponding to sympathetic denervation, may often exceed the final infarct size, and that such patients may be at higher risk for subsequent ventricular arrhythmias. Matsunari *et al.* [29], using single photon emission computed tomography (SPECT) ^{99m}Tc-sestamibi imaging of infarct risk area and final infarct size as well as ^{123}I mIBG imaging in patients with acute MI, demonstrated that the territory of sympathetic denervation (^{123}I mIBG defect, *right column*) corresponded more closely to the initial MI risk area (*left column*) than the final infarct size (*middle column*). Should such findings in the contemporary therapeutic era prove prognostic for late post-MI outcomes, as suggested by earlier studies, ^{123}I mIBG imaging may prove useful in selecting post-MI patients who may optimally benefit from implantable defibrillators. *Top row*, Polar maps of imaging data depict inferior and lateral defects (darker areas). *Bottom row*, White areas represent defect sizes. The mIBG defect is similar in magnitude to the initial myocardium at risk than to the final infarct size.

B and **C**, In addition to the role of myocardial perfusion imaging, methods for early scintigraphic identification of myocardial necrosis are under investigation. ^{99m}Tc-glucarate may be taken up by early necrotic myocardium relatively soon after the onset of ischemia, and far earlier than older techniques using antimyosin antibodies or pyrophosphate [27]. In experimental models, ^{99m}Tc-glucarate may be taken up by infarcting myocardium as early as 30 to 60 minutes after onset of necrosis. In contrast, ^{99m}Tc-pyrophosphate may require up to 48 hours after onset of infarction to turn positive, while antimyosin antibodies, highly specific for myocardial necrosis, may take 12 to 48 hours, both for uptake and blood pool clearance. In **B**, uptake of ^{99m}Tc-glucarate is shown in a rabbit model of coronary occlusion, with the *yellow arrow* in the *middle* and *right panels* indicating the apex. Uptake is substantial by 30 minutes after injection of the tracer, as shown in the *middle panel*. In **C**, a sagittal image from reconstructed SPECT of ^{99m}Tc-glucarate uptake taken 2 hours after tracer injection shows focal uptake in the anteroapex (*yellow arrows, yellow outline* = cardiac outline). The patient was injected 11 hours after onset of chest pain and electrocardiogram showed ST elevation anterior MI.

An exciting potential approach to evaluating patients following the onset of myocardial necrosis utilizes ^{99m}Tc-labeled annexin V for in vivo visualization of apoptosis [30,31]. Should the role of apoptosis in acute MI be confirmed in larger studies, it will allow development of novel therapeutic approaches to attenuate impending myocellular death. (**B**, *courtesy of* Ban-An Khaw, PhD; **C**, *courtesy of* Lynne Johnson, MD).

Patient Subgroup/Indication	Imaging Modality	Recommendation/Evidence Level
Assessment of LV function (all patients)	Rest RNA or gated SPECT	I, B
Detection of inducible ischemia and myocardium at risk in patients after thrombolytic therapy who do not undergo catheterization	Stress MPI with gated SPECT	I, B
Assessment of infarct size and myocardial viability post-MI	Rest RNA and/or stress MPI with gated SPECT	I, B
Assessment of RV function in suspected RV MI	Rest RNA or FP RNA	IIa, B

Figure 10-23. American College of Cardiology (ACC)/American Heart Association (AHA)/American Society of Nuclear Cardiology (ASNC) guideline recommendations for radionuclide imaging in diagnosis, risk assessment, prognosis, and assessment of therapy after acute ST segment elevation myocardial infarction (MI). Based on the totality of data that have been published over the years, guidelines have summarized recommendations for the use of radionuclide imaging in patients with acute ST segment elevation MI. Radionuclide assessment of left ventricular (LV) function (by resting radionuclide angiography [RNA] or gated single photon emission computed tomography [SPECT]) is recommended at a class I level, and is particularly useful when quantitative assessment is indicated. Risk stratification by stress/rest myocardial perfusion imaging (MPI) gated SPECT in stable patients in the aftermath of acute ST segment elevation MI who receive thrombolytic reperfusion therapy and who are not routinely undergoing angiography provides information on two of the most important parameters defining risk: the extent and severity of inducible ischemia and the status of LV function. Imaging after rest injection with single photon agents now has substantial literature supporting its use for quantitation of infarct size as well as defining regional viability in the setting of regional dysfunction. Finally, in the appropriate setting, assessment of right ventricular (RV) function, by first-pass (FP) or equilibrium RNA, is given a class IIa recommendation, *ie*, indicated in most circumstances.

Assessment of Patients with Non–ST Segment Elevation Myocardial Infarction/Unstable Angina

Figure 10-24. Use of perfusion imaging for identification of non–ST elevation in patients with acute coronary syndrome (ACS) likely to benefit from intervention. In patients presenting with symptoms consistent with ACS in whom the diagnosis is clear on initial presentation (*ie*, there are clear ischemic initial electrocardiogram [ECG] changes such as ST segment depression or T-wave inversion), initial management consists of aspirin (ASA), intravenous heparin, β-blockers, and nitrates [11]. The current evidence-based paradigm suggests that such patients may derive overall benefit from an "invasive" management strategy, with administration of intravenous platelet inhibitors and referral to catheterization with subsequent revascularization, particularly for the subset of patients with elevated troponin levels or other higher-risk clinical markers, such as the TIMI (Thrombolysis in Myocardial Infarction) Risk Score [32].

The role of radionuclide imaging is predominantly within the "conservative" strategy, wherein patients are risk stratified, followed by more selective referral to catheterization and revascularization based on the extent of inducible ischemia. In the TACTICS (Treat Angina with Aggrastat and Determine Cost of Therapy with an Invasive or Conservative Strategy)–TIMI 18 trial [33], patients with symptoms of ACS and ECG changes supportive of the diagnosis received the platelet inhibitor tirofiban and were randomized to an "early invasive" management strategy (referral to catheterization and revascularization based on anatomic findings at angiography) or an "early conservative" strategy (stress testing with referral to catheterization based on the extent of ischemia or on the basis of spontaneous ischemia). In this contemporary trial, outcomes favored the invasive strategy. Because the absolute benefit of the invasive management strategy was relatively small, subgroup analysis was performed to examine whether any clinical findings could identify a subgroup in which the benefits were larger (or smaller). Subgrouping by troponin status suggested that most of the benefit of the invasive strategy was seen in the subgroup of patients identified by elevated troponins or a higher TIMI risk score, and that TACTICS-type patients without elevation of troponin derived little benefit from the invasive strategy. These latter patients may be best managed by a more conservative approach, with risk stratification using imaging techniques followed by more selective referral to catheterization. GP— glycoprotein; IV—intravenous; MPI—myocardial perfusion imaging. -, absence of significant inducible ischemia; +, presence of significant inducible ischemia.

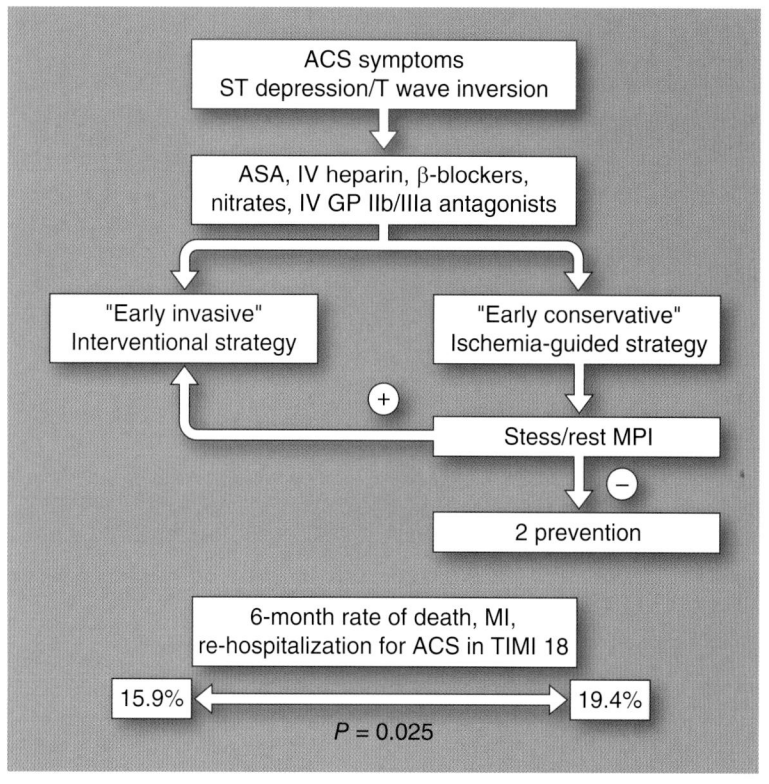

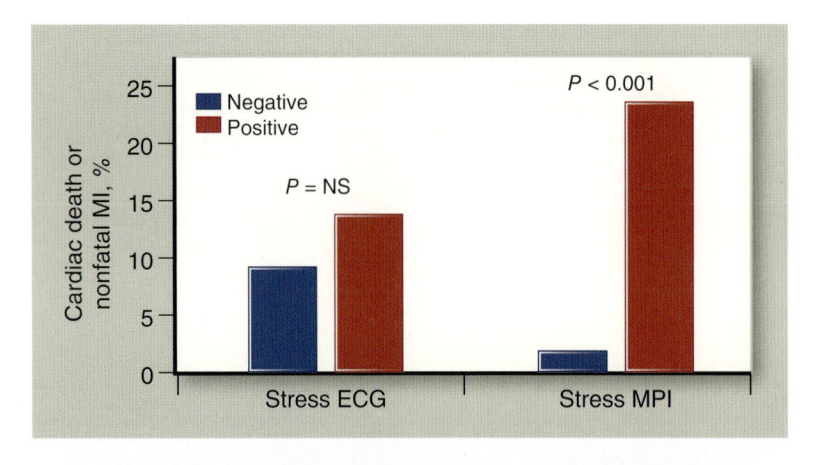

Figure 10-25. Use of myocardial perfusion imaging (MPI) as the decision point in a "conservative" management strategy in non–ST segment elevation acute coronary syndrome. The predictive value of stress MPI and stress electrocardiogram (ECG) is shown in patients studied after initial stabilization of unstable angina with medical therapy. This figure summarizes the results of three studies in which the incidence of cardiac death or nonfatal myocardial infarction (MI) were assessed as endpoints during follow-up after stabilization of unstable angina. The presence of reversible perfusion defects reflective of ischemia ("positive" stress MPI) was strongly predictive of cardiac events in this setting. The absence of inducible ischemia on MPI ("negative" stress MPI) identifies a low-risk group, suggesting that such patients can be managed conservatively. Data are less consistent on the use of exercise ECG in this setting. NS—not significant. (*Adapted from* Brown [34].)

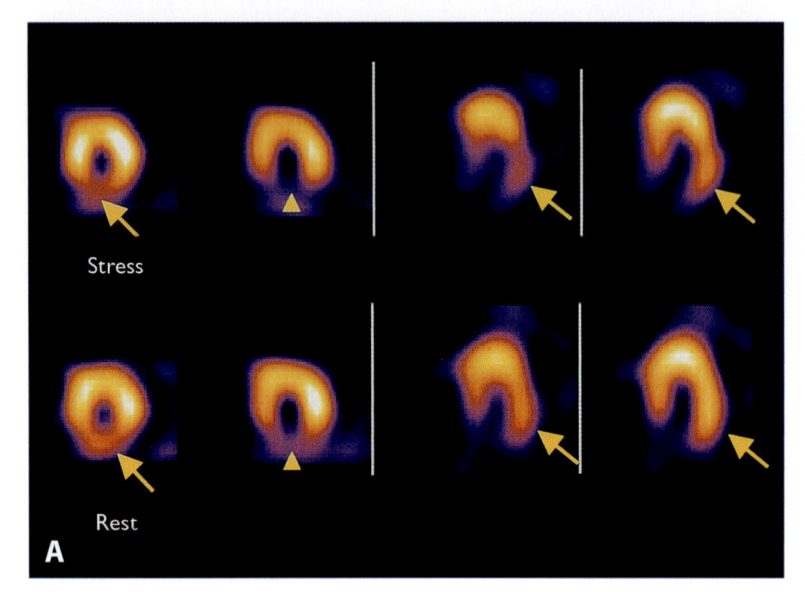

Figure 10-26. Examples of myocardial perfusion imaging (MPI) in non–ST elevation acute coronary syndrome. **A**, Positive MPI study in a patient with medically stabilized unstable angina. After presentation, the patient's symptoms were controlled with initial medical therapy, and stress MPI was performed. There is evidence of an inferobasal infarct (*arrowhead*), but the extent of inducible ischemia involving the inferoapical and lateral walls (*arrows*) suggests the patient is at high risk for future events, and the patient was subsequently referred to catheterization. **B**, Normal stress and rest single photon emission computed tomography MPI in a 63-year-old woman who presented with a clinical syndrome consistent with unstable angina but nonspecific electrocardiographic changes. Symptoms abated after treatment with aspirin, heparin, β-blockers, and nitrates. The normal MPI study suggests a very low risk for subsequent ischemic events, and catheterization/revascularization is unlikely to improve that risk. In clinical trials of unstable angina, up to 30% of some populations of patients are found to have normal or near-normal coronary arteries after routine catheterization. In a nonclinical high-risk patient, MPI will allow more optimal selection for catheterization based on the risk stratification information inherent in the image results. HLA—horizontal long axis; SA—short axis; VLA—vertical long axis.

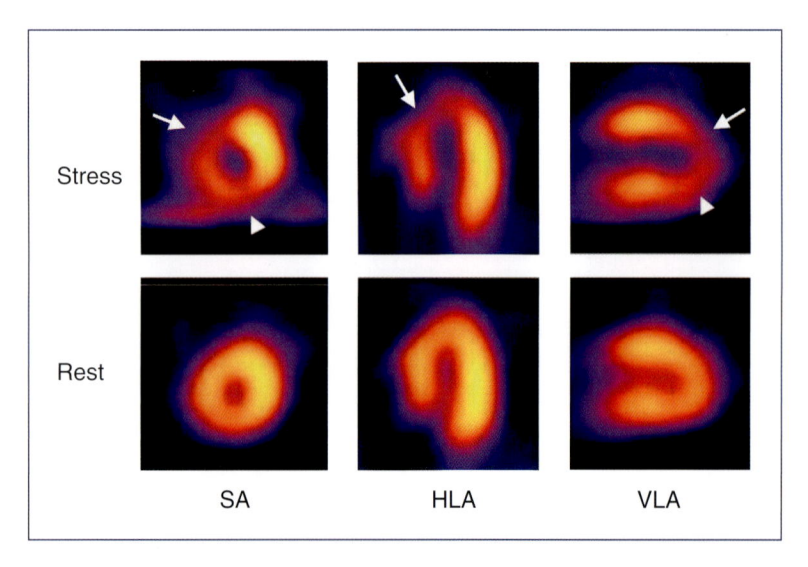

Figure 10-27. Stress single photon emission computed tomography myocardial perfusion imaging (MPI) can provide risk stratification information to help guide management in complex cases using principles derived from the published literature. In this example, an elderly woman was admitted with a non–ST elevation myocardial infarction with positive troponins. On the basis of most trials and guidelines, an interventional strategy would be warranted. However, there were several complicating factors, including extensive peripheral vascular disease and renal insufficiency, making the risk of catheterization higher than usual. It is not likely that such a complicated patient would have been enrolled in randomized acute coronary syndrome trials. In order to better define the risk–benefit ratio for moving ahead with an interventional strategy, stress MPI was performed. Extensive reversible defects on the left anterior descending and right coronary territories (*arrow* and *arrowhead*, respectively), as well as transient ischemic dilatation are seen, findings all consistent with very extensive and severe coronary artery disease. Thus, the potential benefit of an interventional strategy is high, putting the higher risk into context for clinical decision making. HLA—horizontal long axis; SA—short axis; VLA—vertical long axis.

240 Atlas of Nuclear Cardiology

ACC/AHA/ASNC Guideline Recommendations for Radionuclide Imaging in Risk Assessment/Prognosis in Patients With Non–ST Segment Elevation MI and Unstable Angina

Patient Subgroup/Indication	Imaging Modality	Recommendation/Evidence Level
Identification of inducible ischemia in patients at low or intermediate clinical risk	Stress MPI with gated SPECT	I, B
Identification of inducible ischemia in patients whose angina has been stabilized medically	Stress MPI with gated SPECT	I, A
Identification of hemodynamic significance of a coronary stenosis after angiography	Stress MPI with gated SPECT	I, B
Assessment of LV function	Rest RNA or gated SPECT	I, B
Identification of the severity/extent of ischemia/CAD in patients with ongoing suspected ischemia symptoms when ECG changes are nondiagnostic	Rest MPI	IIa, B

Figure 10-28. American College of Cardiology (ACC)/American Heart Association (AHA)/American Society of Nuclear Cardiology (ASNC) guideline recommendations for radionuclide imaging in risk assessment/prognosis in patients with non–ST segment elevation myocardial infarction (MI) and unstable angina. Current guidelines recommend radionuclide assessment of perfusion and/or function in various situations for patients with non–ST segment elevation MI or unstable angina [35]. Most commonly imaging is used and supported by randomized trials of strategies in patients with "medically stabilized" acute coronary syndrome in whom the clinical signs or laboratory tests (such as troponin levels) do not suggest clear benefit from an "invasive" strategy (direct to catheterization with revascularization as appropriate). Stress/rest gated single photon emission computed tomography (SPECT) myocardial perfusion imaging (MPI) can provide information on the extent and severity of inducible ischemia (which directly relates to subsequent natural history risk), as well as the status of left ventricular (LV) function. This information can guide decisions on the potential benefit of revascularization, or whether a "conservative" strategy (no catheterization with aggressive risk factor control) is appropriate. Among patients who are catheterized and have lesions identified of unclear significance, stress/rest imaging is recommended to assess the impact of the stenosis on coronary flow reserve. CAD—coronary artery disease; ECG—electrocardiogram; RNA—radionuclide angiography.

References

1. Wackers FJ, Lie KI, Liem KL, et al.: Potential value of thallium-201 scintigraphy as a means of selecting patients for the coronary care unit. *Br Heart J* 1979, 41:111–117.

2. Gibbons RJ, Verani MS, Behrenbeck T, et al.: Feasibility of tomographic 99mTc-hexakis-2-methoxy-2-methylpropyl-isonitrile imaging for the assessment of myocardial area at risk and the effect of treatment in acute myocardial infarction. *Circulation* 1989, 80:1277–1286.

3. Boden WE, O'Rourke RA, Crawford MH, et al.: Outcomes in patients with acute non–Q-wave myocardial infarction randomly assigned to an invasive as compared with a conservative management strategy [published correction appears in *N Engl J Med* 1998, 339:1091]. *N Engl J Med* 1998, 338:1785–1792.

4. Effects of tissue plasminogen activator and a comparison of early invasive and conservative strategies in unstable angina and non–Q-wave myocardial infarction: results of the TIMI IIIB trial: Thrombolysis in Myocardial Ischemia. *Circulation* 1994, 89:1545–1556.

5. Varetto T, Cantalupi D, Altieri A, et al.: Emergency room technetium-99m sestamibi imaging to rule out acute myocardial ischemic events in patients with nondiagnostic electrocardiography. *J Am Coll Cardiol* 1993, 22:1804–1808.

6. Hilton TC, Thompson RC, Williams H, et al.: Technetium-99m sestamibi myocardial perfusion imaging in the emergency room evaluation of chest pain. *J Am Coll Cardiol* 1994, 23:1016–1022.

7. Tatum JL, Jesse Rl, Kontos MC, et al.: Comprehensive strategy for the evaluation and triage of the chest pain patient. *Ann Emerg Med* 1997, 29:116–125.

8. Heller GV, Stowers SA, Hendel RC, et al.: Clinical value of acute rest technetium-99m tetrofosmin tomographic myocardial perfusion imaging in patients with acute chest pain and nondiagnostic electrocardiograms. *J Am Coll Cardiol* 1998, 31:1011–1017.

9. Jafary F, Udelson JE: Assessment of myocardial perfusion and left ventricular function in acute coronary syndromes: implications for gated SPECT imaging. In *Clinical Gated Cardiac SPECT*. Edited by Germano G, Berman DS. Armonk, NY: Futura; 1999.

10. Antman EM, Anbe DT, Armstrong PW, et al.: ACC/AHA guidelines for the management of patients with ST-elevation myocardial infarction: a report of the American College of Cardiology/American Heart Association Task Force on Practice Guidelines (Committee to Revise the 1999 Guidelines for the Management of Patients With Acute Myocardial Infarction). 2004. Available at www.acc.org/clinical/guidelines/stemi/index.pdf.

11. Braunwald E, Antman EM, Beasley JW, et al.: ACC/AHA guidelines for the management of patients with unstable angina and non-ST-segment elevation myocardial infarction: a report of the American College of Cardiology/American Heart Association Task Force on Practice Guidelines (Committee on the Management of Patients with Unstable Angina). *J Am Coll Cardiol* 2000, 36:970–972.

12. Bilodeau L, Theroux P, Gregoire J, et al.: Technetium-99m sestamibi tomography in patients with spontaneous chest pain: correlations with clinical, electrocardiographic and angiographic findings. *J Am Coll Cardiol* 1991, 18:1684–1691.

13. Kontos MC, Jesse RL, Anderson P, et al.: Comparison of myocardial perfusion imaging and cardiac troponin I in patients admitted to the emergency department with chest pain. *Circulation* 1999, 99:2073–2078.

14. Duca MD, Giri S, Wu AHB, et al.: Comparison of acute rest myocardial perfusion imaging and serum markers of myocardial injury in patients with chest pain syndromes. *J Nucl Cardiol* 1999, 6:570–576.

15. Kosnik JW, Zalenski RJ, Shamsa F, et al.: Resting sestamibi imaging for the prognosis of low-risk chest pain. *Acad Emerg Med* 1999, 6:998–1004.

16. Stowers SA, Eisenstein EL, Wackers FJ, et al.: An economic analysis of an aggressive diagnostic strategy with single photon emission computed tomography myocardial perfusion imaging and early exercise stress testing in emergency department patients who present with chest pain but nondiagnostic electrocardiograms: results from a randomized trial. *Ann Emerg Med* 2000, 35:17–25.

17. Udelson JE, Beshansky JR, Ballin DS, et al.: Myocardial perfusion imaging for evaluation and triage of patients with suspected acute cardiac ischemia: a randomized controlled trial. *JAMA* 2002, 288:2693–2700.

18. Kawai Y, Tsukamoto E, Nozaki Y, et al.: Significance of reduced uptake of iodinated fatty acid analogue for the evaluation of patients with acute chest pain. *J Am Coll Cardiol* 2001, 38:1888–1894.

19. Goldstein JA, Gallagher MJ, O'Neill WW, et al.: A randomized controlled trial of multi-slice coronary computed tomography for evaluation of acute chest pain. *J Am Coll Cardiol* 2007, 49:863–871.

20. Zaret BL, Wackers FJ, Terrin ML, et al.: Value of radionuclide rest and exercise left ventricular ejection fraction in assessing survival of patients after thrombolytic therapy for acute myocardial infarction: results of Thrombolysis in Myocardial Infarction (TIMI) phase II study. *J Am Coll Cardiol* 1995, 26:73–79.

21. Travin MI, Dessouki A, Cameron T, Heller GV: Use of exercise technetium-99m sestamibi SPECT imaging to detect residual ischemia and for risk stratification after acute myocardial infarction. *Am J Cardiol* 1995, 75:665–669.

22. Mahmarian JJ, Mahmarian AC, Marks GF, *et al.*: Role of adenosine thallium-201 tomography for defining long-term risk in patients after acute myocardial infarction. *J Am Coll Cardiol* 1995, 25:1333–1340.

23. Ellis SG, Mooney MR, George BS, *et al.*: Randomized trial of late elective angioplasty versus conservative management for patients with residual stenoses after thrombolytic treatment of myocardial infarction (TOPS trial). *Circulation* 1992, 86:1400–1406.

24. Hochman JS, Lamas GA, Buller CE, *et al.*: Coronary intervention for persistent occlusion after myocardial infarction. *N Engl J Med* 2006, 355:2395–2407.

25. The TIMI Study Group: Comparison of invasive and conservative strategies after treatment with intravenous tissue plasminogen activator in acute myocardial infarction. Results of the thrombolysis in myocardial infarction (TIMI) phase II trial. *N Engl J Med* 1989, 320:618–627.

26. Mahmarian JJ, Dakik HA, Filipchuk NG, *et al.*, for the INSPIRE Investigators: An initial strategy of intensive medical therapy is comparable to that of coronary revascularization for suppression of scintigraphic ischemia in high-risk but stable survivors of acute myocardial infarction. *J Am Coll Cardiol* 2006, 48:2458–2462.

27. Miller TD, Christian TF, Hopfenspirger MR, *et al.*: Infarct size after acute myocardial infarction measured by quantitative tomographic 99mTc sestamibi imaging predicts subsequent mortality. *Circulation* 1995, 92:334–341.

28. Christian TF: The use of perfusion imaging in acute myocardial infarction: applications for clinical trials and clinical care. *J Nucl Cardiol* 1995, 2:423–436.

29. Matsunari I, Schricke U, Bengel FM, *et al.*: Extent of cardiac sympathetic neuronal damage is determined by the area of ischemia in patients with acute coronary syndromes. *Circulation* 2000, 101:2579–2585.

30. Narula J, Petrov A, Pak KY, *et al.*: Very early noninvasive detection of acute experimental nonreperfused myocardial infarction with 99mTc-labeled glucarate. *Circulation* 1997, 95:1577–1584.

31. Hofstra L, Liem IH, Dumont EA, *et al.*: Visualisation of cell death in vivo in patients with acute myocardial infarction. *Lancet* 2000, 356:209–212.

32. Antman EM, Cohen M, Bernink PJ, *et al.*: The TIMI risk score for unstable angina/non-ST elevation MI: a method for prognostication and therapeutic decision making. *JAMA* 2000, 284:835–842.

33. Cannon CP, Weintraub WS, Demopoulos LA, *et al.*: Comparison of early invasive and conservative strategies in patients with unstable coronary syndromes treated with the glycoprotein IIb/IIIa inhibitor trofiban. *N Engl J Med* 2001, 344:1879–1887.

34. Brown KA: Management of unstable angina: the role of noninvasive risk stratification. *J Nucl Cardiol* 1997, 4:S164–S168.

35. Klocke FJ, Baird MG, Bateman TM, *et al.*: ACC/AHA/ASNC guidelines for the clinical use of cardiac radionuclide imaging—executive summary: a report of the American College of Cardiology/American Heart Association Task Force on Practice Guidelines (ACC/AHA/ASNC Committee to Revise the 1995 Guidelines for the Clinical Use of Radionuclide Imaging). Available at http://www.acc.org/qualityandscience/clinical/guidelines/radio/exec_summary.pdf

Myocardial Innervation

Markus Schwaiger, Antti Saraste, and Frank M. Bengel

The heart is innervated by sympathetic and parasympathetic nerve fibers, which modify cardiac performance to respond quickly and effectively to changing demands on cardiovascular performance. The sympathetic nervous system is considered stimulatory, yielding positive inotropic and chronotropic effects, whereas the parasympathetic nervous system exerts primarily negative chronotropic responses [1]. The autonomic innervation is divided into presynaptic and postsynaptic arms, which interact by release of neurotransmitters. The predominant sympathetic neurotransmitter is norepinephrine, which is synthesized, stored, and metabolized within the sympathetic nerve terminal. Upon neurostimulation, the neurotransmitter is released by exocytosis. Within the synaptic cleft, a small portion of the released neurotransmitter interacts with α- and β-adrenergic receptors, predominantly β-1 receptors in the heart. The majority of the released neurotransmitter undergoes reuptake in the nerve terminals (uptake 1); this norepinephrine transporter (NET, a sodium/chloride-dependent transport protein) has a high affinity to amines (catecholamines and catecholamine analogues). Uptake 2 refers to nonneuronal uptake of catecholamines in cardiac tissue. Inside the nerve terminal, norepinephrine is either metabolized by monoamine oxidase or sequestered in vesicles by the vesicular monoamine transporter, a proton-dependent transport protein localized in the vesicle membrane. The amine transport system (uptake 1) regulates the extraneuronal concentration of adrenergic neurotransmitters and plays an important physiologic and pathophysiologic role in modifying signal transduction and extraneuronal catecholamine concentration. This regulatory role includes the reuptake of locally released norepinephrine as well as the uptake and metabolism of circulating catecholamines, which enter the extracellular space. This high affinity uptake system is of significance in protecting the heart from the deleterious effects of elevated levels of circulating catecholamines [2,3].

The density of sympathetic nerve terminals is highest in the right and left ventricles. Sympathetic nerve fibers travel along the vascular structures, penetrating the myocardial wall from the epicardial surface toward the endocardium. A heterogeneous distribution of nerve terminals has been reported in animals and humans, with a gradient from the base to the apex of the left ventricle [4,5]. In contrast, parasympathetic nerve fibers are found most predominantly in the atria. The nerve fibers travel along endocardial layers within the right and left ventricles. There is a high density of muscarinic receptors (predominantly M_2) that interact with the parasympathetic neurotransmitter acetylcholine released by the parasympathetic nerve terminals.

The scintigraphic evaluation of cardiac innervation using radiopharmaceutical agents developed for positron emission tomography or single-photon emission CT allows a unique pathophysiologic evaluation of disease processes that affect the autonomic nervous system. This article gives an overview of the tracers and nuclear imaging methodology used to study autonomic innervation of the heart together with their clinical applications. In addition to being a valuable research tool, recent clinical studies indicate potential for prognostic assessment of heart failure patients.

Autonomic Nervous System

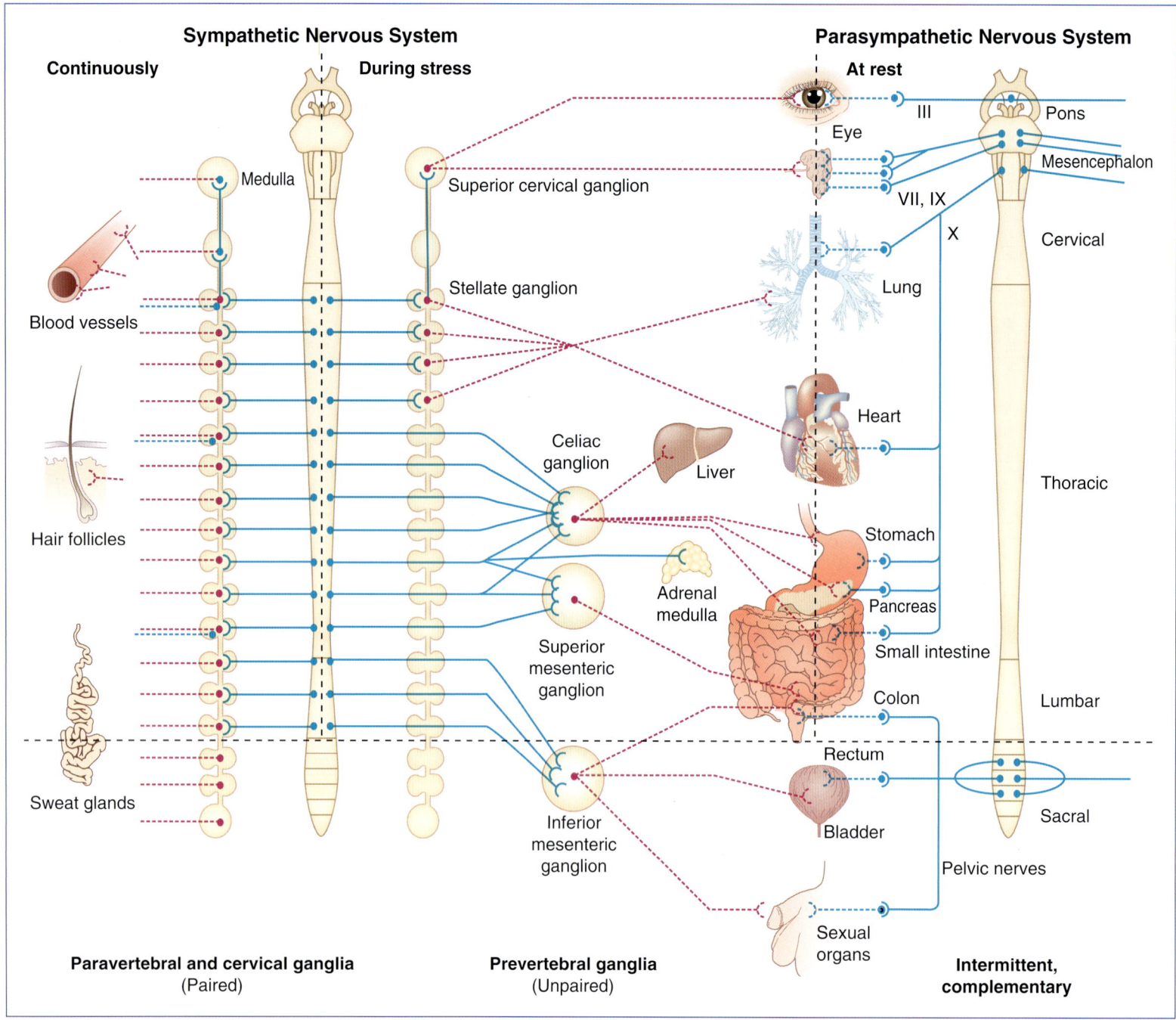

Figure 11-1. Structure of the autonomic nervous system (ANS). The ANS is historically divided in two major efferent components, the sympathetic (cervicothoracic, SNS) and parasympathetic (craniosacral, PNS) nervous systems. In either case, end-organ innervation is provided by nerve fibers originating from autonomic ganglia located outside the central nervous system (CNS), driven by preganglionic cholinergic input from the CNS (*solid blue lines*). Main differences consist of the types of principal transmitter used by postganglionic fibers (PNS: acetylcholine [dotted blue]; SNS: norepinephrine [dotted red]), the location of the ganglia (PNS: near or within the end organs; SNS: near the spinal cord, either paravertebral [22 pairs] or prevertebral [unpaired]), the degree of divergence and convergence of preganglionic input to postganglionic neurons (PNS: very little; SNS: considerable), and their respective functional roles. Most internal organs receive input from both PNS and SNS (*center*). Important exceptions include skin and blood vessels (pilomotor and sudomotor) functions, which are exclusively controlled by noradrenergic and cholinergic postganglionic fibers of SNS origin only (*left*), and the adrenal gland, which functions as the equivalent of a sympathetic ganglion, causing systemic catecholamine release (80% epinephrine, 20% norepinephrine) in response to preganglionic cholinergic stimulation. In the case of most internal organs, SNS and PNS exert opposite effects. PNS effects normally prevail at rest, whereas SNS effects predominate during stress or exercise ("flight or fight" response). In genitourinary organs, SNS and PNS functions are complementary; for example, PNS mediates erection, SNS mediates ejaculation. (*Adapted from* Bannister and Mathias [6].)

244 Atlas of Nuclear Cardiology

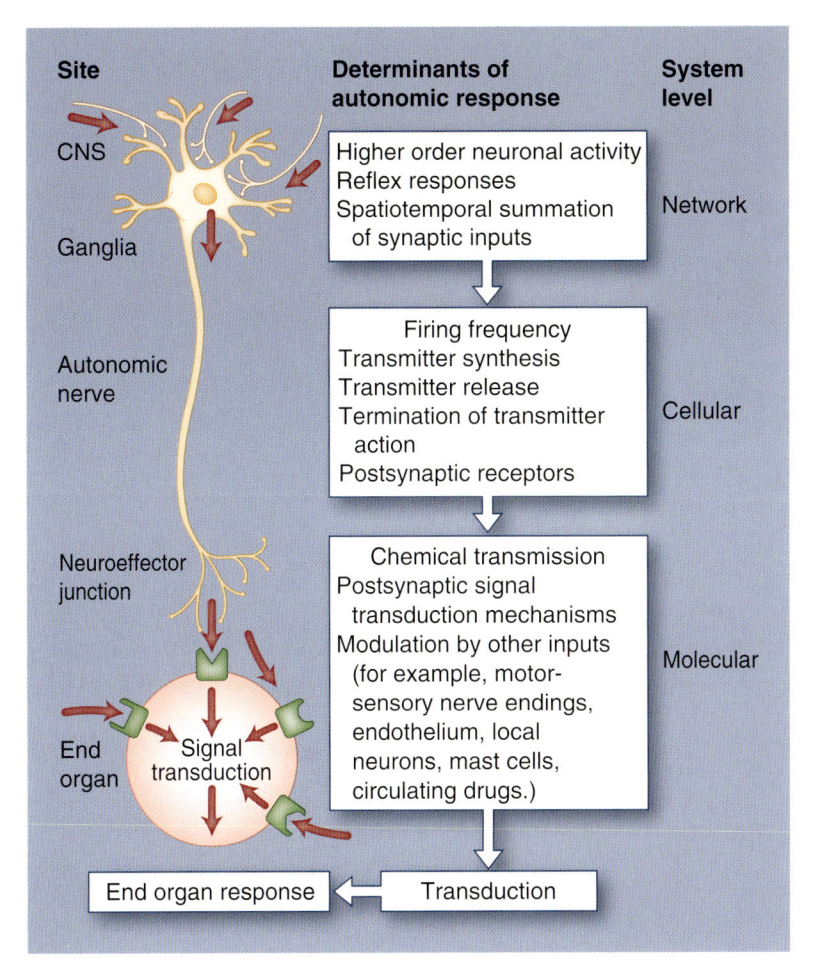

Figure 11-2. Determinants of end-organ control by the autonomic nervous system (ANS). Control mechanisms operate concurrently at different system levels. At a neural network level, processing and integration of patterns of neuronal activity (including reflex responses) determine the firing frequency of autonomic efferent nerve fibers. Cellular mechanisms operative at the level of nerve terminals determine the types, amounts, and fates of chemical transmitters released at autonomic synapses and neuroeffector junctions. At a molecular level, membrane receptor and postsynaptic signal transduction mechanisms determine the types and magnitude of cellular effector responses. At each of these system levels, various interactions occur between distinct functional divisions of the ANS (sympathetic, parasympathetic, afferent, enteric, and local neuronal systems) involving classic (cholinergic and adrenergic) transmitters as well as a variety of nonclassic neurotransmitter systems. CNS—central nervous system. (*Adapted from* Milner and Burnstock [7].)

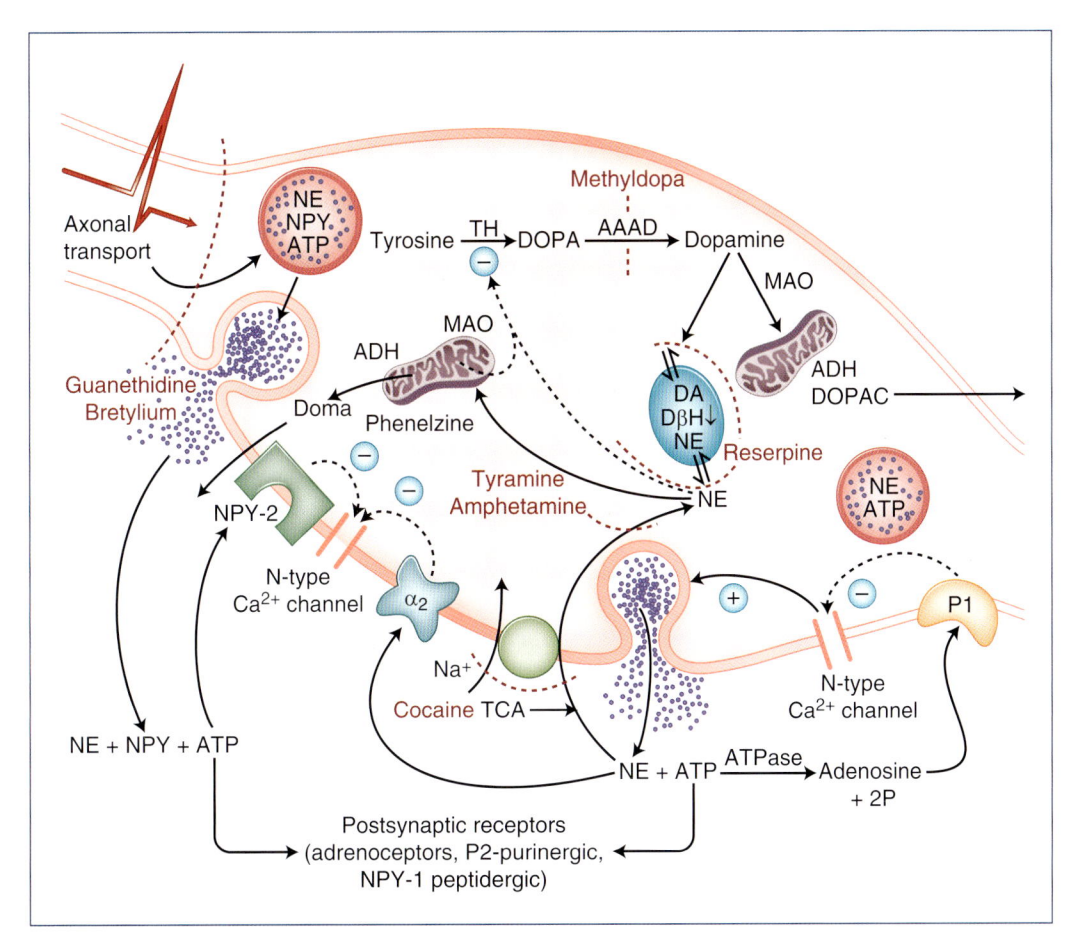

Figure 11-3. Neurotransmitter synthesis and release at adrenergic nerve terminals. Mechanisms controlling transmitter synthesis and release at adrenergic nerve terminals. Transmitters are stored in two types of synaptic vesicles: small vesicles containing only the principal transmitter norepinephrine (NE) and cotransmitter adenosine triphosphate (ATP) (each synthesized within the nerve terminal itself), and larger dense-core vesicles containing the polypeptide cotransmitter neuropeptide Y (NPY) and chromogranin (both of which are exclusively synthesized in the cell soma) as well as NE and ATP. The rate-limiting step for NE synthesis in the nerve terminal is tyrosine hydroxylase (TH) enzyme activity, which is negatively controlled by the cytoplasmic concentration of NE. The TH enzymatic product dopa is decarboxylated to dopamine by (unspecific) aromatic L-amino acid decarboxylase (AAAD) in a step subject to therapeutic interference by provision of the "false" substrate methyldopa (resulting in the eventual formation of the "false transmitter" methyl-NE). Dopamine is to equal proportions either deaminated and excreted as 3,4-dihydroxyphenylacetic acid (DOPAC) or taken up into dopamine-β-hydroxylase (DβH)-containing storage vesicles via a reserpine-sensitive active uptake process and hydroxylated to NE.

Continued on the next page

Myocardial Innervation 245

Figure 11-3. *(Continued)* The cytoplasmic concentration of NE is determined by a dynamic equilibrium established between diffusion (leakage) out of storage vesicles, reserpine-sensitive (active) reuptake into storage vesicles, cytoplasmic displacement and extrusion by indirect sympathomimetics such as tyramine and amphetamine, reuptake from the extracellular space via a Na$^+$-dependent cotransport mechanism sensitive to inhibition by cocaine or tricyclic antidepressants (TCAs), and elimination after metabolizing to 3,4-dihydroxymandelic acid (DOMA) by mitochondrial monoamine oxidase (MAO) and aldehyde dehydrogenase (ADH), a pathway sensitive to inhibition by MAO inhibitors such as phenelzine. In adrenal medullary neurons, 80% of cytoplasmic NE is methylized by N-methyl transferase into epinephrine before being packaged into storage vesicles. Nerve stimulation–evoked physiologic transmitter release occurs via fusion of synaptic storage vesicles with the cell membrane after the invasion of the nerve terminal by propagated action potentials (sensitive to blockade by guanethidine or bretylium) and the resulting increase in cytoplasmic Ca^{2+} through activation of voltage-sensitive (predominantly N-type) Ca^{2+} channels. Upon release, ATP, NE, and NPY produce neuroeffector responses through actions on postsynaptic membrane receptors. In addition, all three transmitters inhibit further release through action on presynaptic (P1, 2-adrenergic, NPY-2) receptors [8,9]. Transmitter actions are terminated by hydrolysis (ATP), reuptake into nerve terminals (NE), uptake into nonneuronal tissue and metabolism by catechol-O-methyl transferase (COMT) (NE), and diffusion away from the terminal and into the bloodstream (NE, NPY). *(Adapted from* Nicholls *et al.* [10].)

Radiotracers

Several radiolabeled compounds have been synthesized to probe the sympathetic and parasympathetic nervous system at the pre- and postsynaptic levels [11]. These tracers can be divided into radiolabeled catecholamines and catecholamine analogues. The most commonly employed single-photon emission CT (SPECT) tracer is metaiodobenzylguanidine (mIBG), which represents an analogue of the antihypertensive drug guanethidine [12]. Radiolabeled catecholamine analogues for positron emission tomography (PET) include metaraminol, metahydroxyephedrine, and phenylephrine [13–15]. These "false adrenergic neurotransmitters" share the same reuptake mechanism and endogenous storage with the true neurotransmitters, but are not metabolized and display a decreased affinity for postsynaptic receptor proteins.

Although there is little tissue uptake of mIBG involving the nonneuronal transport process as well as passive diffusion, retention of mIBG in the myocardium has been found to be specific for sympathetic nerve terminals [16]. Imaging studies involve a two-step protocol, with early image acquisition after tracer injection followed by delayed imaging (4 or more hours after injection). By comparing initial uptake and delayed retention, regional distribution of nerve terminals as well as washout kinetics can be determined. There is indirect evidence that the rate of mIBG washout from the myocardium represents a parameter of neuronal function [17–19]. Planar and SPECT images are usually acquired, and an activity ratio can be determined by using regions of interest placed over the myocardium and the mediastinum [20]. Most commonly, radiolabeling of mIBG is performed using isotopic exchange reactions. More recently, a non–carrier-added synthesis of ^{123}I-mIBG has been described. This labeling procedure yields a higher specific activity of ^{123}I-mIBG, which may affect the tissue kinetics. However, studies have shown that even in the carrier-added synthesis method, specific activity is high enough to avoid mass effects on the neuronal uptake mechanism [21,22].

The most successful PET radiopharmaceutical agent for the imaging of presynaptic function is C-11 hydroxyephedrine (^{11}C-HED) [23,24]. ^{11}C-HED is produced by N-methylation of metaraminol using C-11 methyliodide. In contrast to mIBG, this tracer uptake primarily reflects the transport by NET (a sodium/chloride-dependent transport protein). Vesicular storage seems to occur, but binding inside the vesicle is weaker compared with norepinephrine due to its higher lipid solubility. Based on experimental observations, myocardial retention reflects a continuing release and reuptake of ^{11}C-HED in the nerve terminal. Tracer retention is commonly quantified by calculating the retention index or retention fraction (which reflects myocardial activity at 40 minutes) normalized to the integral of the arterial input function [18]. More recently, a tracer kinetic model for ^{11}C-HED kinetics has been developed that allows calculation of the distribution volume within the myocardium. As an alternative tracer to ^{11}C-HED, C-11 epinephrine has been proposed as a naturally occurring transmitter. Myocardial retention of this tracer represents uptake, metabolism, and storage of catecholamines [25].

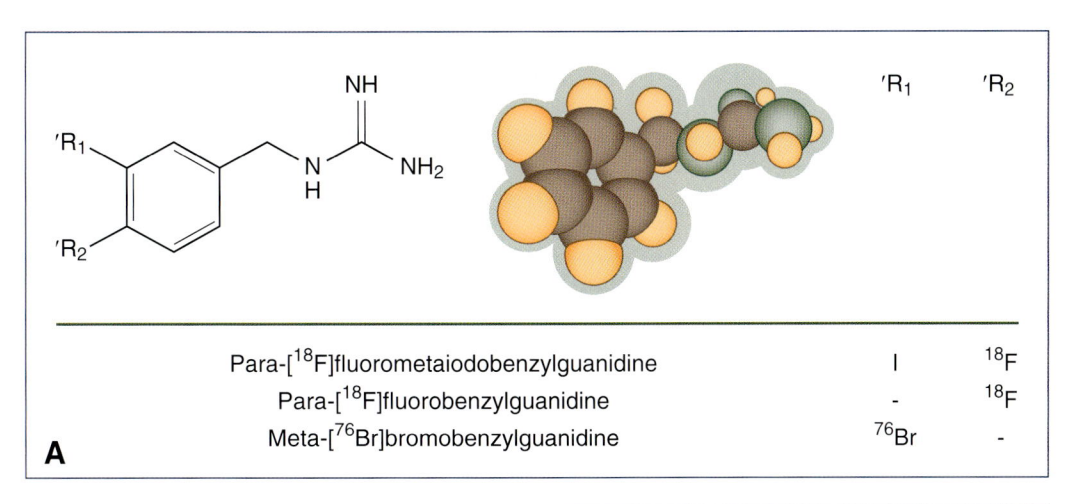

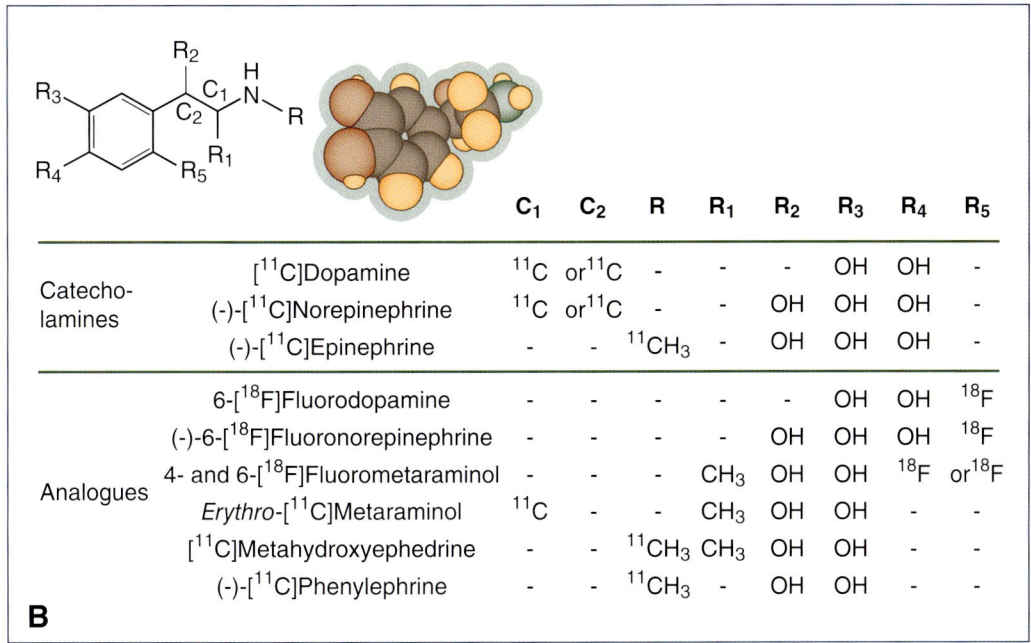

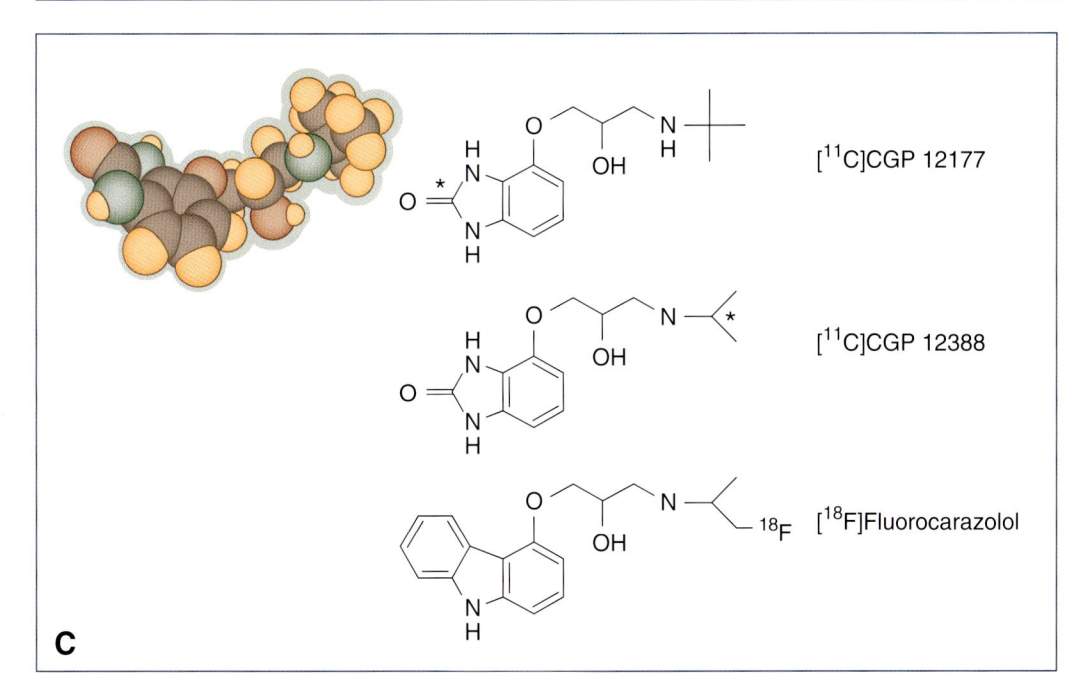

Figure 11-4. Positron emission tomography radiotracers for mapping of cardiac sympathetic neurons. The radiotracers used for the evaluation of the sympathetic nervous system can be classified into three categories: radiolabeled analogues of benzylguanidine (**A**), radiolabeled catecholamines or catecholamine analogues (**B**), and β-adrenoceptor ligands (**C**). The common lead structure and a computed model of the prototypic compounds are provided. The ^{11}C-carbon position in *panel A* is indicated by 'R$_1$ and 'R$_2$ and in *panel B* by C$_1$ and C$_2$. The radiolabeled compounds are listed under the lead structures and computed models.

Myocardial Innervation 247

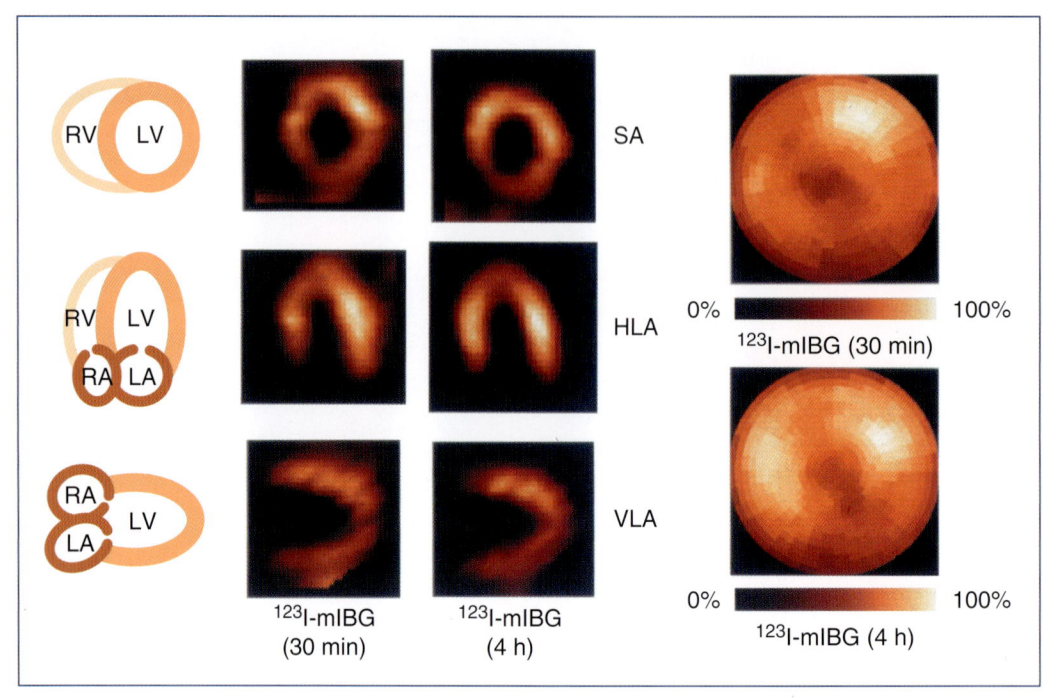

Normal Myocardial Innervation

Figure 11-5. I-123 Metaiodobenzylguanidine (^{123}I-mIBG) distribution in normal myocardium. Tomographic single-photon emission CT images were obtained at 180° in a healthy volunteer 30 minutes after intravenous injection of 10 mCi ^{123}I-mIBG. Data acquisition was repeated 4 hours later. Regional myocardial tracer retention is displayed in short-axis (SA), horizontal long-axis (HLA), and vertical long-axis (VLA) views. There is homogeneous uptake of the tracer throughout the myocardium of the left ventricle (LV). The right ventricle (RV), right atrium (RA), and left atrium (LA) are not seen due to their thin walls. Polar maps represent the three-dimensional distribution of the tracer within the LV. The activity at the apex is displayed at the center of the map whereas the basal parts of the LV represent the outer rings. The activity is normalized to maximal activity within the LV. The regional tracer retention was determined by circumferential radial search for activity maxima. The individual circumferential profiles of several myocardial slices are then combined into one representative polar map. Note the relatively low activity of ^{123}I-mIBG in the inferior and inferoseptal areas, showing the known heterogeneity of neuronal distribution [4,5]. The same distribution pattern can be found in the 4-hour images, which are also normalized to their own maxima. The relative washout of activity between 30 minutes and 4 hours averages around 20% to 30% in healthy people [18]. The late images are considered specific for the relative distribution of sympathetic nerve terminals, while the washout has been used as a marker of neuronal integrity or sympathetic tone.

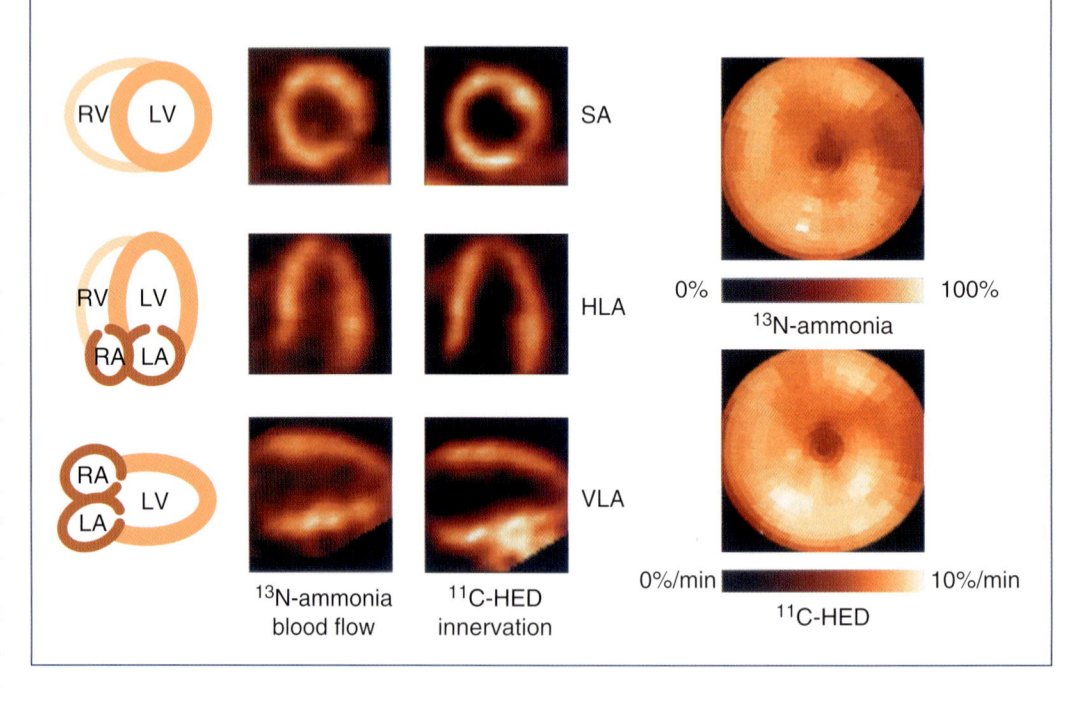

Figure 11-6. C-11 hydroxyephedrine (^{11}C-HED) distribution in normal myocardium. Positron emission tomography (PET) images in short-axis (SA), horizontal long-axis (HLA), and vertical long-axis (VLA) views were obtained following an injection of 20 mCi ^{13}N-ammonia as blood flow marker and about 40 minutes after the intravenous injection of 20 mCi ^{11}C-HED. The myocardial blood flow is homogeneous throughout the left ventricle (LV), paralleled by homogeneous uptake of ^{11}C-HED in all segments of the LV. Polar maps using circumferential profile analysis display homogeneous distribution of ^{13}N-ammonia and ^{11}C-HED. The polar maps of flow are normalized to their own maxima, whereas the ^{11}C-HED data are expressed by retention index. This index represents the activity at 40 minutes normalized to arterial input function, derived from a region of interest placed over left ventricular activity. Dynamic PET images allow for generation of myocardial and blood time-activity curves. LA—left atrium; RA—right atrium; RV—right ventricle.

248 Atlas of Nuclear Cardiology

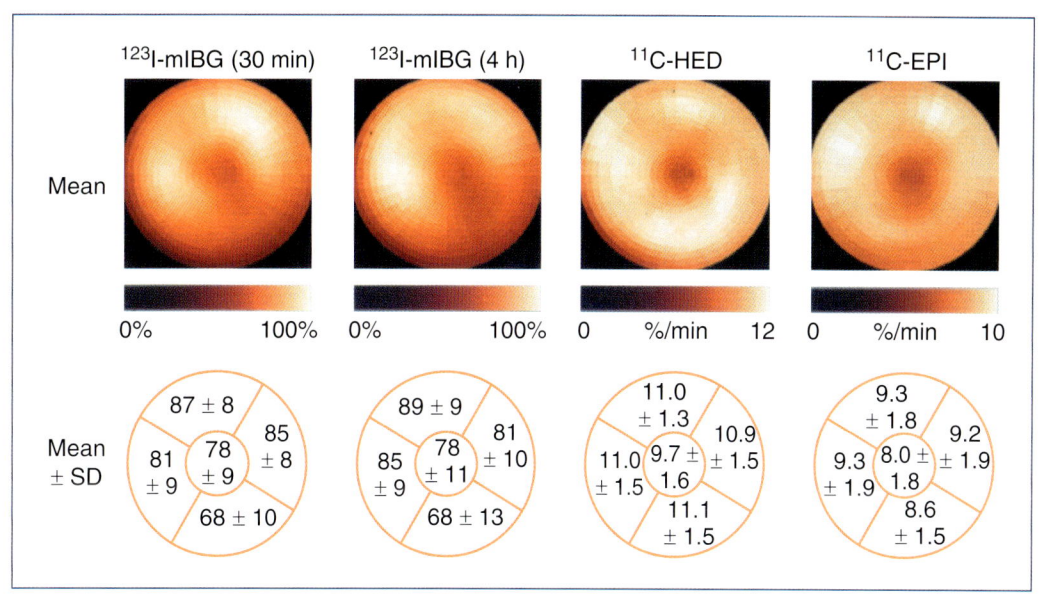

Figure 11-7. Comparison of normal tracer distribution of I-123 metaiodobenzylguanidine (^{123}I-mIBG), C-11 hydroxyephedrine (^{11}C-HED), and C-11 epinephrine (^{11}C-EPI) in normal myocardium. For each tracer distribution, 10 patients were imaged following intravenous injection of 10 mCi ^{123}I-mIBG, 20 mCi ^{11}C-HED, and 20 mCi ^{11}C-EPI. The relative tracer distribution normalized to the individual maximum in each patient is displayed in the *lower panel*. Note the slight heterogeneity of tracer retention at 30 minutes and 4 hours after ^{123}I-mIBG injection. The relative activity in the inferior segments of the left ventricle including the apex show significantly lower values as compared with the anteroseptal and anterolateral segments. This may represent an attenuation artifact, but inhomogeneous density of sympathetic nerve terminals in normal myocardium cannot be ruled out. The C-11 tracer retention is expressed as retention index, which represents tracer activity 40 minutes after tracer injection, normalized to the arterial input function obtained after placing a region of interest over the cavity of the left ventricle [24]. The retention index is expressed as percent per minute (%/min). ^{11}C-EPI retention was obtained 30 minutes after tracer injection and expressed as myocardial retention index.

These measurements of myocardial positron emission tomography (PET) tracer uptake display greater homogeneity compared with mIBG data. The lower retention index in the apex of the left ventricle most likely represents partial volume effect during nongated PET data acquisition. PET data are acquired with attenuation correction; however, there may be biologic differences in affinity for uptake 1 between mIBG and HED.

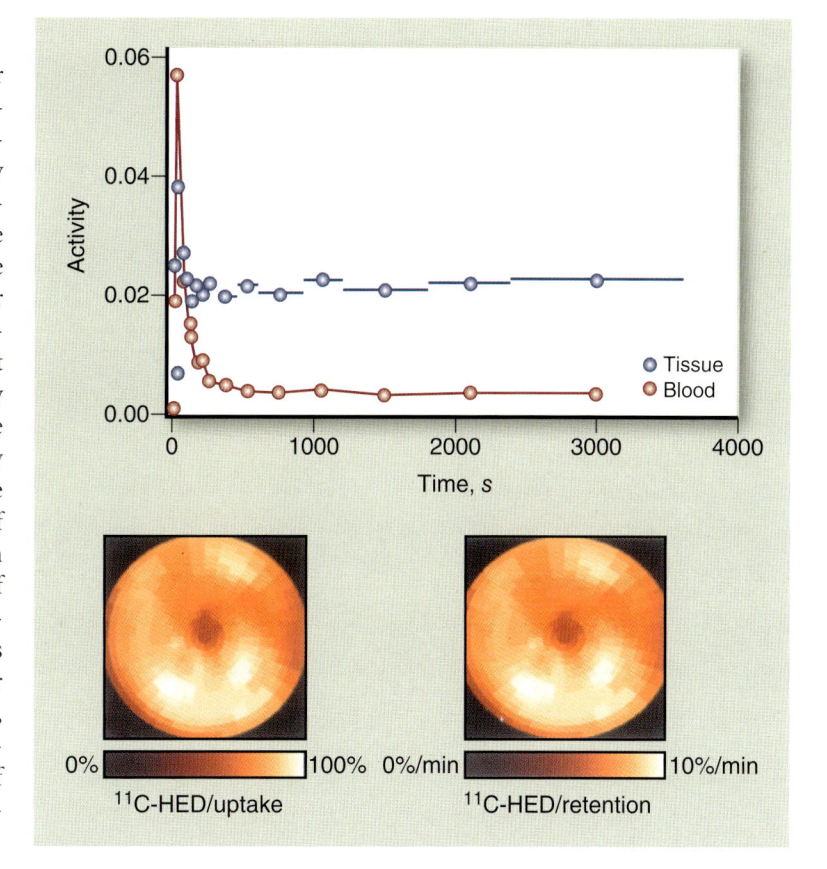

Figure 11-8. Time-activity curve obtained after intravenous injection of 20 mCi of the tracer C-11 hydroxyephedrine (^{11}C-HED) in a healthy volunteer. Dynamic positron emission tomography imaging with short framing rate allows the determination of tracer time-activity curves of tissue and blood pool. The time-activity curves were determined using regions of interest placed over the chamber of the left ventricle for the determination of blood activity and placed over the left ventricular myocardium for the tissue activity distribution. The tracer rapidly clears from the blood, resulting in little residual blood activity minutes after tracer injection. In contrast, the activity obtained from the myocardial region of interest shows stable retention in the myocardium over the time of observation. The initial peak of myocardial tracer activity measured reflects contamination by blood pool activity. Dividing this activity measured 30 to 40 minutes after tracer injection by the integral of the input function, which reflects the available tracer to the myocardium during this time, yields the calculation of the myocardial retention index. This index averages over 12% in the normal heart.

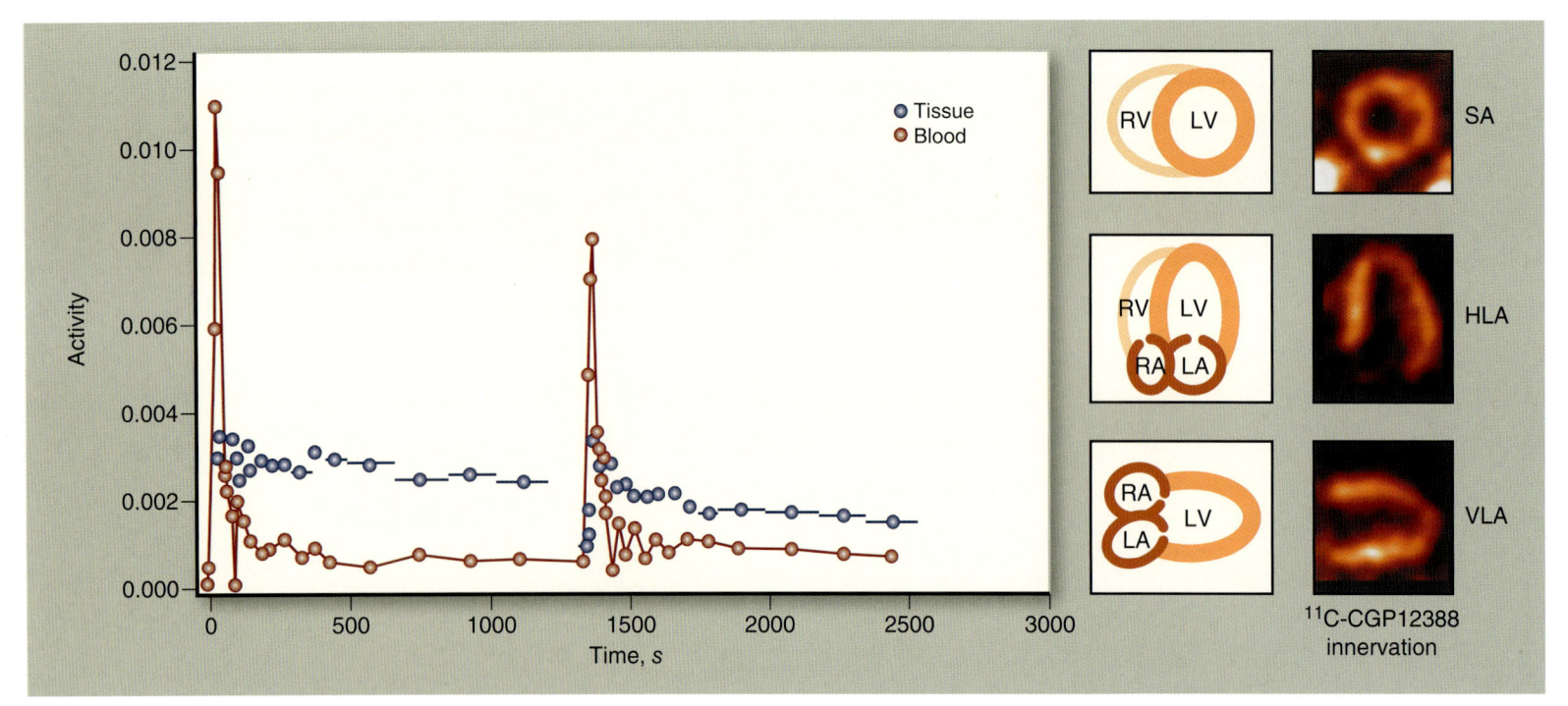

Figure 11-9. β-Receptor distribution in normal myocardium. Positron emission tomography images following the intravenous injection of β-receptor antagonist ¹¹C-CGP12388 are shown in short-axis (SA), horizontal long-axis (HLA), and vertical long-axis (VLA) images. Images were obtained 40 minutes after tracer injection and show high contrast between myocardial and nonmyocardial tissue. Pretreatment of patients with cold β-blocker β-receptor antagonists showed reduced tracer retention, suggesting high specific binding to the receptors. However, the shown retention images at 40 minutes primarily represent the delivery of tracer to the myocardium, which is determined by blood flow. To calculate the density of β-receptors in the myocardium, a tracer kinetic model has been proposed by Delforge et al. [26]. A comparison of ¹¹C-CGP measurements with β-receptor density measured in vitro resulted in a linear correlation with high correlation coefficients. Using a tracer kinetic model consisting of two tracer injections with different specific activities, the receptor density can be calculated by curve-fitting procedures of tissue and blood pool–time-activity curves [26]. LA—left atrium; LV—left ventricle; RA—right atrium; RV—right ventricle.

Heart Failure

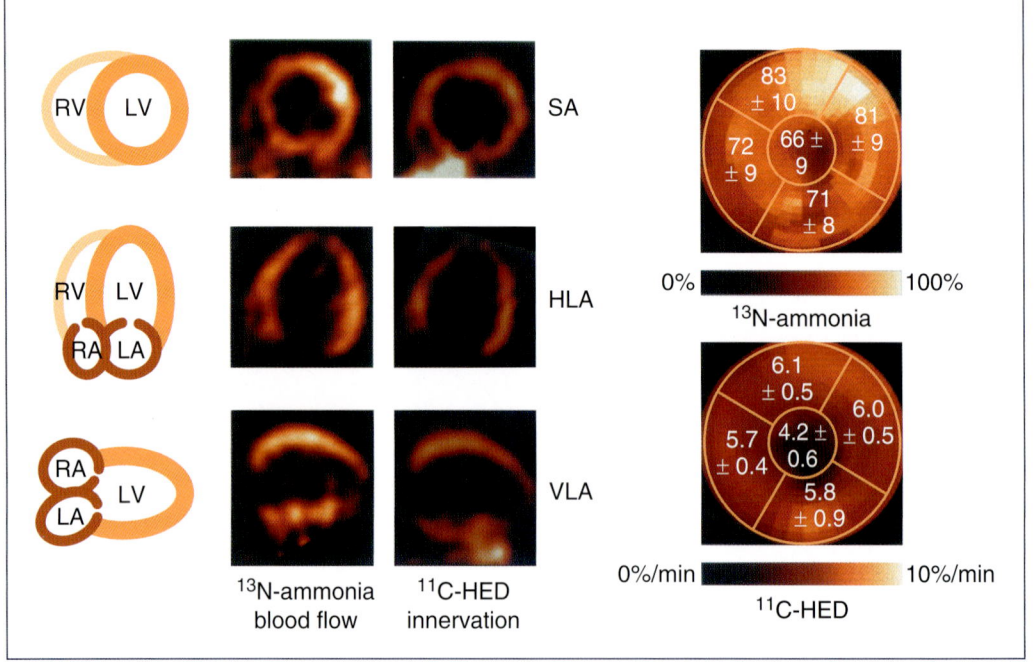

Figure 11-10. An increased activity of the sympathetic nervous system is a hallmark of heart failure. Plasma levels of noradrenaline are elevated, myocardial norepinephrine reuptake is reduced, and myocardial β-receptors are downregulated, reflecting generalized adrenergic activation [2,3]. Enhanced sympathetic activity increases myocardial contractility and heart rate and—via increased preload—activates the Frank-Starling mechanism. These responses are capable of maintaining ventricular performance and cardiac output for a limited period of time. However, adrenergic activation eventually contributes to deterioration of cardiac function and progression of heart failure.

In comparison to healthy subjects, retention of C-11 hydroxyephedrine (¹¹C-HED) and I-123 metaiodobenzylguanidine (¹²³I-mIBG) are abnormally reduced in heart failure patients [20,27,28]. In this example, a patient with dilated cardiomyopathy and reduced left ventricular function was imaged with positron emission tomography following the injection of ¹³N-ammonia and 40 minutes after the injection of ¹¹C-HED. The tomographic slices are displayed in short-axis (SA), horizontal long-axis (HLA), and vertical long-axis (VLA) views. There is relatively homogeneous distribution of ¹³N-ammonia, indicating integrity of myocardial perfusion. However, there is markedly reduced retention of ¹¹C-HED, indicating partial denervation of the left ventricle (LV). The quantitative retention index of ¹¹C-HED is reduced to 6% (normal values > 12%). The area of denervation is most evident in the distal anterior wall and apical area of the LV, consistent with the injury of the autonomic nervous system being a heterogeneous process in patients with congestive heart failure [27]. Furthermore, a mismatch between pre- and postsynaptic sympathetic function with more pronounced reduction of ¹¹C-HED retention compared with β-adrenergic receptor density as assessed by β-receptor antagonist ¹¹C-CGP12177 is common in patients with ischemic heart failure [28]. LA—left atrium; RA—right atrium; RV—right ventricle.

250 Atlas of Nuclear Cardiology

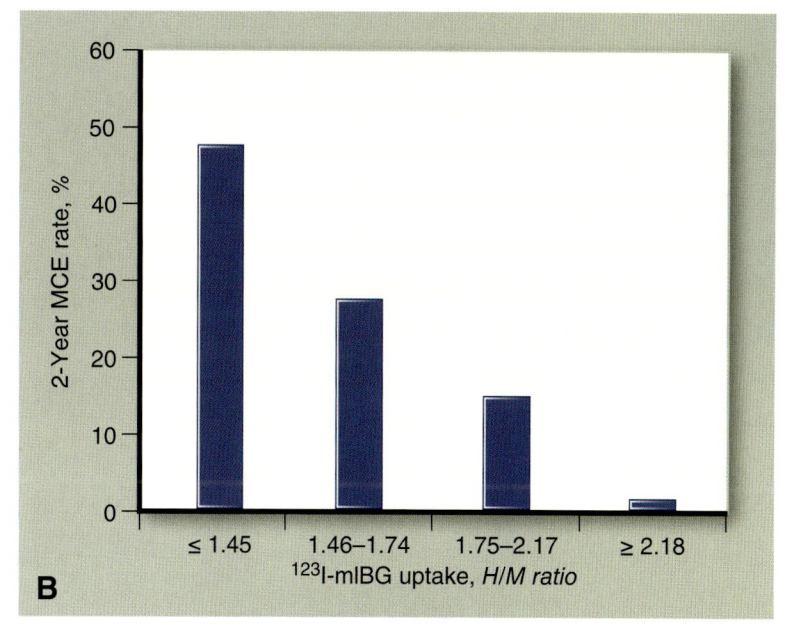

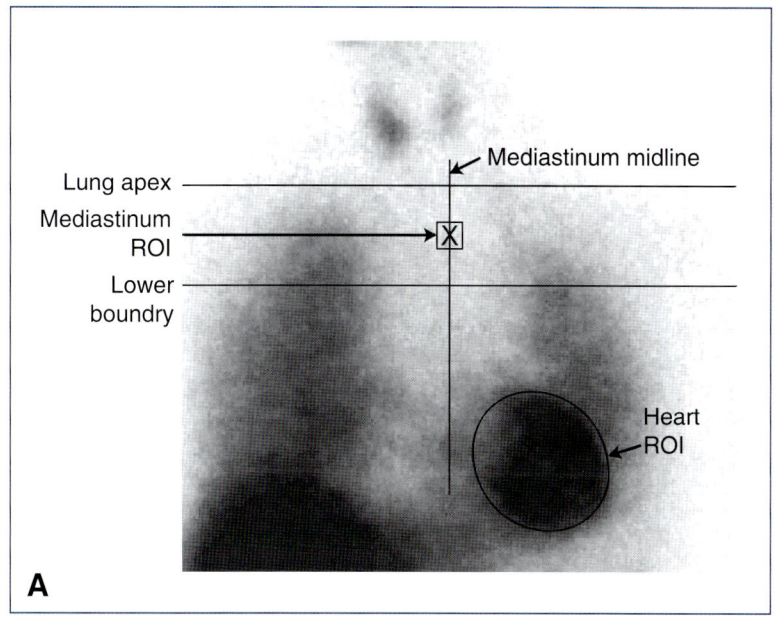

Figure 11-11. Several studies have provided evidence that I-123 metaiodobenzylguanidine (^{123}I-mIBG) imaging offers prognostic information in heart failure patients. A meta-analysis of single-center studies indicated that decreased heart-to-mediastinum (H/M) ratio in late ^{123}I-mIBG images as well as increased washout of ^{123}I-mIBG were associated with a high risk of cardiac events [29]. Some of the studies indicate predictive value for cardiac death that is superior to conventional parameters, such as left ventricular ejection fraction. Application of these findings to clinical patient management have been constrained due to relatively small sample sizes, limited standardization of the imaging techniques among studies, and the lack of optimal cutoff value for pathologic H/M ratio. A recent retrospective, multicenter study addressed these issues by applying standardized methodology to reanalyze late H/M ratios in ^{123}I-mIBG images of 290 heart failure patients obtained in six European centers [30,31]. **A,** Determination of H/M ratio in a late, planar myocardial ^{123}I-mIBG image from this study [30]. Regions of interest (ROI) were placed over the myocardium and the mediastinum and the H/M ratio calculated by dividing the mean counts per pixel in the heart by that in the mediastinum. The positioning of the mediastinum ROI was standardized in relation to the lung apex, the lower boundary of the upper mediastinum, and the midline between the lungs. The H/M ratios interpreted by three blinded observers were highly consistent (inter-reader correlation, 0.99), with changes in the ROIs requested during the reanalysis resulting in change in H/M ratio greater than 0.1 in only less than 1% of studies. However, H/M ratios were influenced by some technical factors, such as type of collimation as well as duration and timing of acquisition, pointing to the need of imaging technology standardization to improve universal clinical applicability of ^{123}I-mIBG imaging [31].

B, The multicenter study demonstrated a strong relationship between H/M ratios and the occurrence of major cardiac events including 13 cardiac deaths, 44 cardiac transplantations, and eight life-threatening arrhythmias during the 2-year follow-up period after the ^{123}I-mIBG imaging [30]. Optimal H/M ratio for predicting cardiac events was 1.75, providing sensitivity of 84%, specificity of 60%, and area under the receiver operating characteristic (ROC) curve of 0.77. The 2-year event-free survival was 62% for H/M ratio less than 1.75 and 95% for H/M ratio greater than 1.75. The image illustrates the rate of major cardiac events (MCE) in relation to quartiles of H/M ratios of ^{123}I-mIBG uptake. The relationship between H/M ratios and events remained significant irrespective of the left ventricular systolic function. Although outcome events in the study were dominated by cardiac transplantations, there was also a significant relationship between cardiac death and the H/M ratio. While 10 deaths occurred in patients with H/M ratio less than 1.75, only three deaths occurred in patients with H/M ratio greater than 1.75 and none of them in patients with H/M ratio greater than 2.18. A large prospective multicenter international trial (ADMIRE-HF) that included almost 1000 New York Heart Association class 2/3 heart failure subjects with left ventricular ejection fraction ≤ 35% recently confirmed the prognostic significance of the H/M ratio on ^{123}I-mIBG imaging. Using a binary categorization of < 1.60 and ≥ 1.60, the hazard ratio for occurrence of a composite of heart failure progression, arrhythmic events, and cardiac death was 0.40, with 2-year even rates of 37% for subjects with H/M < 1.60 compared with 15% for subjects with H/M ≥ 1.60. Two-year cardiac death rate was 11.2% for subjects with H/M < 1.60 compared with 1.8% for those with H/M ≥ 1.60 [32].

Drugs counteracting activation of the neurohormonal pathways, *ie*, drugs inhibiting the renin-angiotensin system or cardiac sympathetic activity, slow down the progression of heart failure and improve patient survival. Treatment with angiotensin-converting enzyme inhibitors [33], angiotensin-receptor blockers [34], β-receptor antagonists [35–37], spironolactone [38], and cardiac resynchronization therapy [39–41] is associated with an improvement in cardiac ^{123}I-mIBG retention. The extent of this improvement correlated with reversal of structural remodeling of the left ventricle after treatment with the β-blocker carvedilol or spironolactone [36,38]. The baseline levels of ^{123}I-mIBG retention have also been shown to predict the therapeutic response to β-blockers [36,37] or cardiac resynchronization [39]. These studies suggest that in addition to risk stratification, ^{123}I-mIBG imaging may be useful for guiding and monitoring of therapeutic response to treatment in heart failure. (**A** and **B,** *adapted from* Agostini *et al.* [30].)

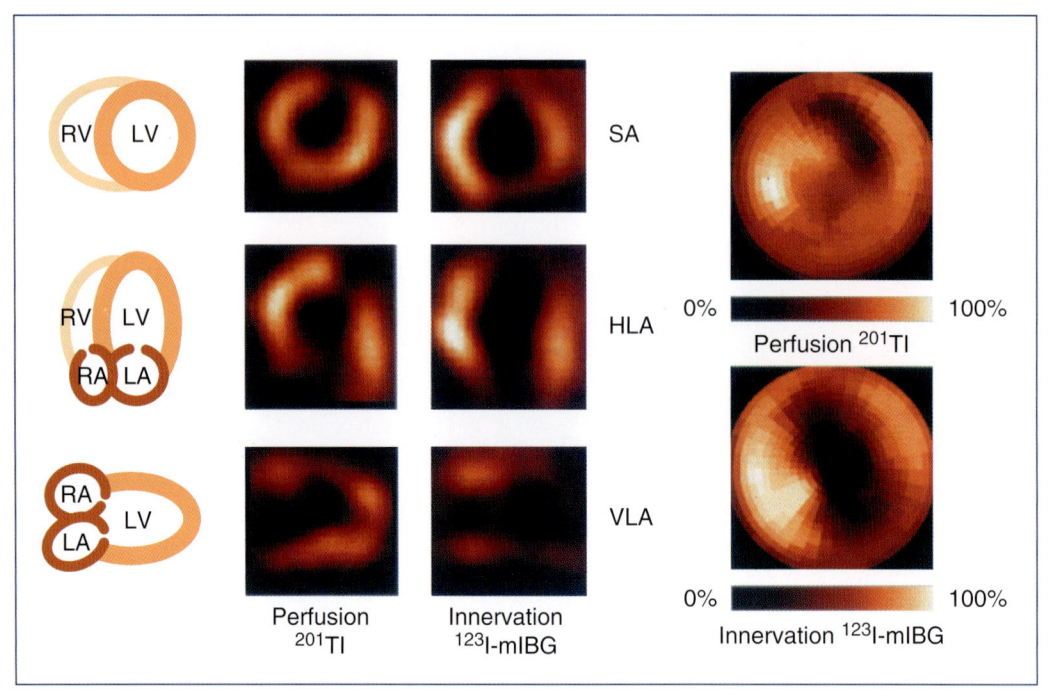

Ischemic Heart Disease

Figure 11-12. Sympathetic nerve terminals are susceptible to ischemic damage as illustrated in these single-photon emission CT images that were obtained in a patient within 14 days of an anterior myocardial infarction [42–44]. The tomographic slices are displayed in short-axis (SA), horizontal long-axis (HLA), and vertical long-axis views (VLA). Regional retention of 10 mCi I-123 metaiodobenzylguanidine (^{123}I-mIBG) after 4 hours was compared with the myocardial perfusion as assessed from images acquired 20 minutes after injection of 2 mCi of thallium-201 (^{201}Tl). There is a perfusion abnormality in the ^{201}Tl images involving the anterolateral wall of the left ventricle (LV). The images obtained after ^{123}I-mIBG injection reveal a markedly larger area of reduced ^{123}I-mIBG retention involving the anterolateral wall as well as the distal inferior wall. Polar maps display the disparity of perfusion and neuronal abnormality, reflecting the infarct size and area of denervation. This mismatch between perfusion and ^{123}I-mIBG retention is present in almost 80% of patients after acute myocardial infarction and indicates that sympathetic neurons are more sensitive to ischemia than the myocytes [43]. Although reduced C-11 hydroxyephedrine (^{11}C-HED) retention was found in an experimental model of chronically ischemic hibernating myocardium, the dependency of the ^{11}C-HED retention on resting myocardial blood flow or flow reserve was small in patients with chronic coronary artery disease [44]. LA—left atrium; RA—right atrium; RV—right ventricle.

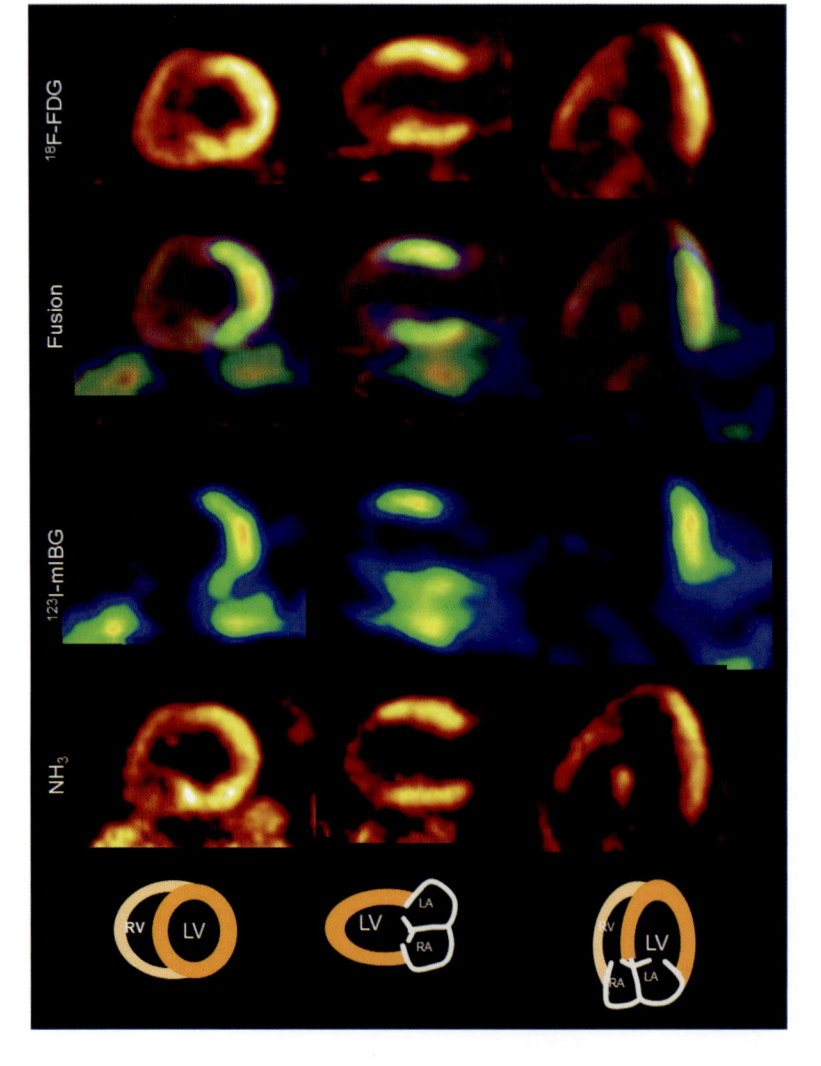

Figure 11-13. It has been proposed that denervated but viable myocardium can form a substrate for ventricular arrhythmias after myocardial infarction. The mismatch pattern of innervation and viability has been shown to correlate with abnormal electrophysiological findings [45–48]. However, its relationship to clinical arrhythmic events remains unclear at present [45]. The figure demonstrates detailed assessment of viability, perfusion, and sympathetic innervation by evaluation of fluorodeoxyglucose (^{18}F-FDG) uptake with positron emission tomography (PET), ^{13}N-ammonia (NH$_3$) PET, and I-123 metaiodobenzylguanidine (^{123}I-mIBG) single-photon emission CT in a patient with a previous anterior myocardial infarction and sustained ventricular tachycardia considered for ablation.

Ventricular Arrhythmias

Figure 11-14. Experimental and clinical studies have linked pre- and postsynaptic sympathetic nervous function and the presence of ventricular arrhythmias [49–51]. Innervation imaging has demonstrated abnormalities in patients with primary arrhythmic cardiac disorders in the absence of structural heart disease, such as right ventricular outflow tract tachycardia, Brugada syndrome, and idiopathic ventricular fibrillation [52–55]. **A**, I-123 metaiodobenzylguanidine (^{123}I-mIBG) single-photon emission CT images were obtained in a 54-year-old man with idiopathic right ventricular outflow tract tachycardia. The tomographic slices are displayed in short-axis (SA), horizontal long-axis (HLA), and vertical long-axis (VLA) views. ^{123}I-mIBG images acquired 4 hours following injection show a marked ^{123}I-mIBG retention defect in the midventricular and basal inferior walls (*arrows*), suggesting regional sympathetic denervation. Unfortunately, the right ventricle cannot be imaged by radionuclide techniques due to thin myocardial walls. **B**, Schematic display illustrating a proposed pathophysiologic mechanism of tachycardia in patients with idiopathic right ventricular outflow tract tachycardia. Impairment of catecholamine clearance contributes to reduced clearance of neurotransmitter from the synaptic cleft and thus to myocardial catecholamine overexposure. The resulting pre- and postsynaptic imbalance is thought to contribute to electronic instability and arrhythmogenesis. Assuming that stimulatory G proteins (G) are upregulated in connection with downregulated β-adrenoceptors, an acute increase in synaptic norepinephrine concentration would increase cyclic adenosine 3′,5′-monophosphate (cAMP) via activation of adenylyl cyclase (AC). The increase in cAMP will produce a rise in intracellular Ca^{2+} levels by activation of protein kinase A (PKA), and will eventually trigger ventricular tachycardia. ATP—adenosine triphosphate; NE—norepinephrine; RE—release; UP—uptake.

Figure 11-15. Internal cardioverter defibrillators (ICDs) capable of recording electrocardiogram at the time of arrhythmias provide an opportunity to study the association between I-123 metaiodobenzylguanidine (^{123}I-mIBG) imaging findings and ventricular arrhythmias [55–57]. Nagahara *et al.* [57] prospectively followed 53 patients treated with ICD for 15 months after ^{123}I-mIBG imaging [57]. Most patients (*n* = 39) had an underlying structural heart disease, including nine patients with idiopathic dilated cardiomyopathy and eight patients with ischemic heart disease. Patients who had appropriate ICD discharges due to life-threatening ventricular arrhythmias (*n* = 21) or died of cardiac causes had significantly lower heart-to-mediastinum (H/M) ratios than the other patients. The H/M ratio of 1.95 was the optimal cutoff value that identified arrhythmias (area under the receiver operating characteristic [ROC] curve, 0.68) independently of many other variables, including LV ejection fraction (EF) and plasma brain natriuretic peptide (BNP) level. The event rates among quartiles of H/M ratio are shown in the figure. When H/M ratio was combined with either EF or BNP, their sensitivities were 67% and 45% with specificities of 70% and 94%, respectively. These are better than those provided by left ventricular EF only, but the value of ^{123}I-mIBG imaging in improving the selection of patients for treatment with ICD remains to be established in future trials involving larger numbers of patients representative of the common underlying etiologies of heart failure, particularly ischemic heart disease. (*Adapted from* Nagahara *et al.* [57].)

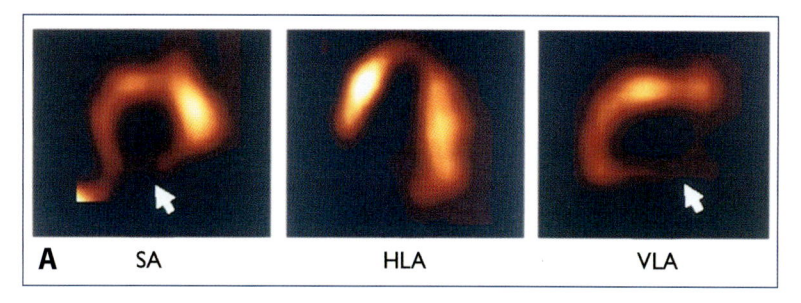

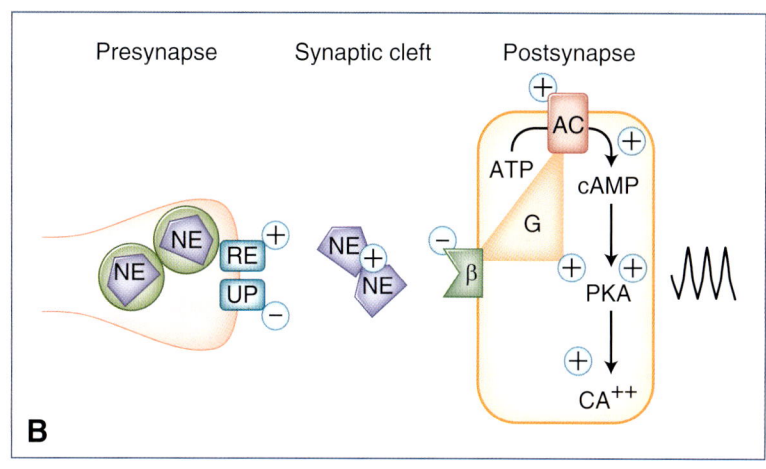

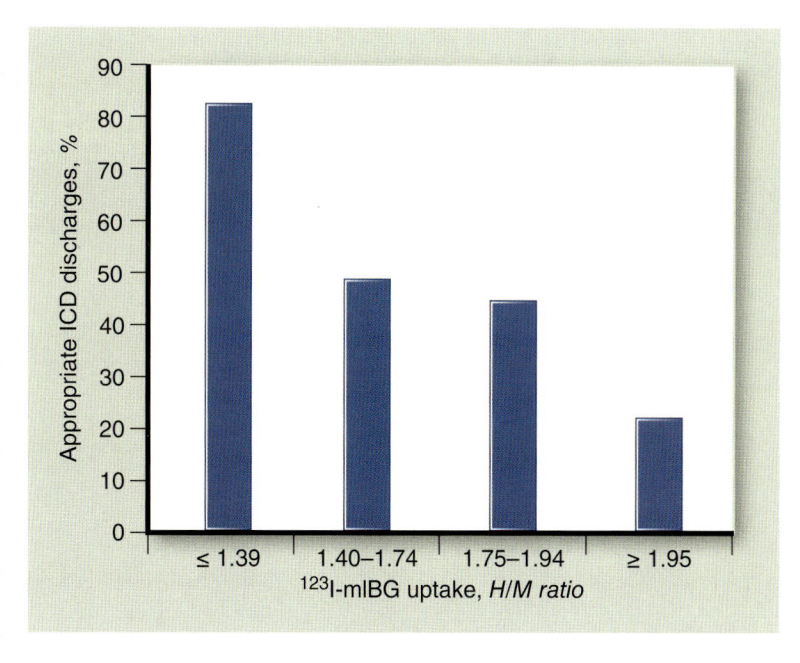

Diabetes

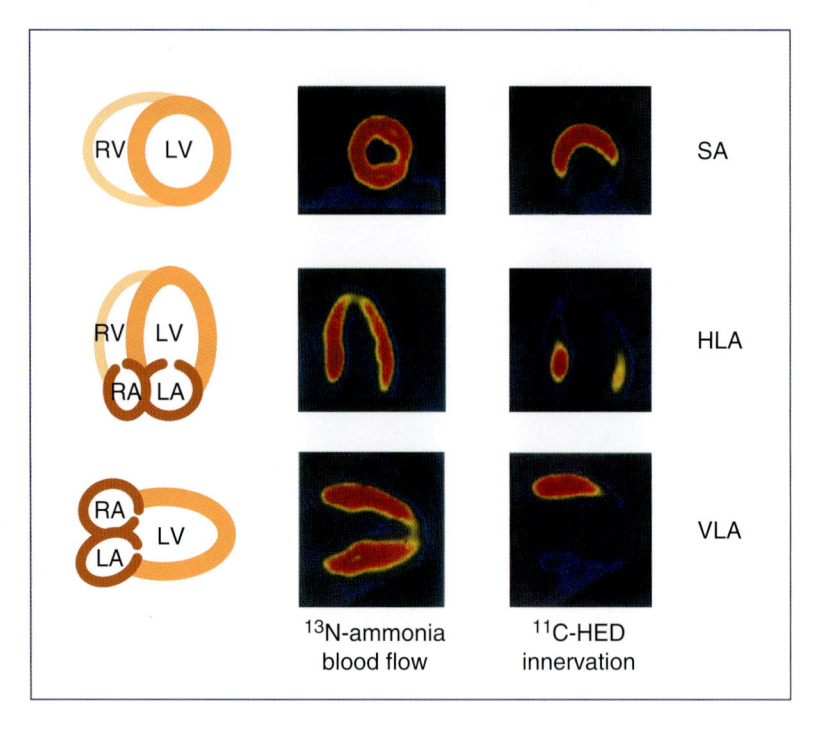

Figure 11-16. Myocardial neuropathy in diabetes. Positron emission tomography images were obtained in a patient with advanced diabetic neuropathy as defined by functional testing. Following the injection of C-11 hydroxyephedrine (^{11}C-HED), short-axis (SA), horizontal long-axis (HLA), and vertical long-axis (VLA) views were obtained. The regional retention of ^{11}C-HED is compared with the regional perfusion as assessed by ^{13}N-ammonia. There is heterogeneous denervation in patients with diabetic neuropathy. The ^{11}C-HED retention is reduced most prominently in the distal aspects of the anterior wall, apex, and inferior wall of the left ventricle (LV). As the process of neuropathy proceeds, denervation starts at the apex and extends to the basal aspects of the left ventricle. The proximal, anterior, and anterolateral wall segments are most protected from the disease process. This heterogeneity of denervation has been linked to the increased incidence of sudden cardiac death in patients with diabetic neuropathy of the heart [58]. A correlation has been established between the degree of cardiac denervation and clinical parameters of autonomic dysfunction [59,60]. The scintigraphic determination of presynaptic tracer uptake appears to be more sensitive than clinical parameters in detecting early involvement of the heart in diabetic neuropathy. However, no prospective data are available defining the prognostic value of neuronal imaging for detection of patients with increased incidence of cardiovascular complications [58,59,61–63]. LA—left atrium; RA—right atrium; RV—right ventricle.

Cardiac Transplantation

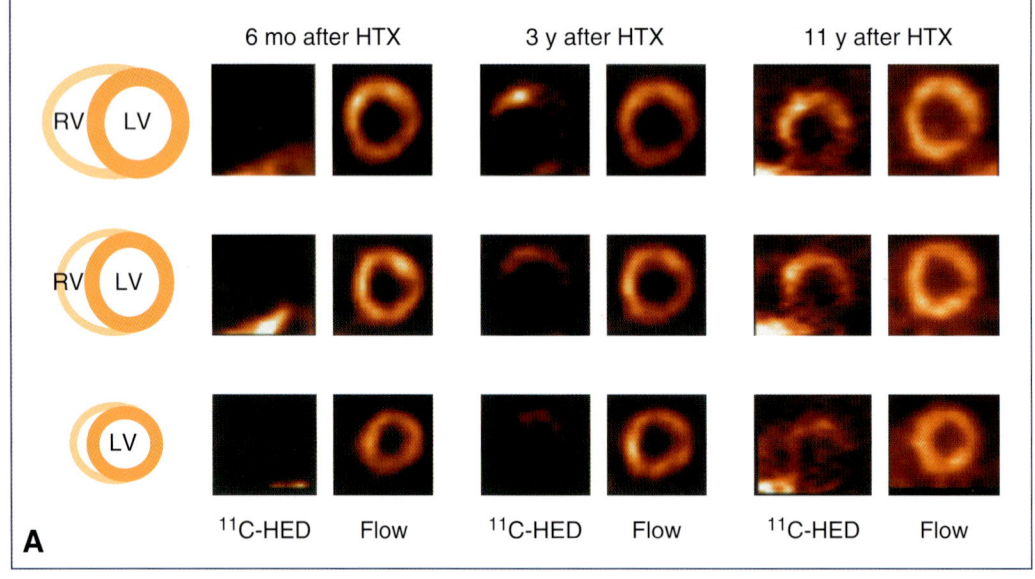

Figure 11-17. Reinnervation of cardiac allograft. Cardiac transplantation (HTX) represents the best model of cardiac denervation because the neuronal fibers are cut during the transplantation surgery. However, as time after cardiac transplantation passes, there is evidence for regional reinnervation [24]. Uptake of radiolabeled catecholamines in the anterior wall, septum, and base of the left ventricle (LV) indicates the reappearance of functioning sympathetic nerve terminals. The pharmacologic integrity of these nerve terminals has been demonstrated by studies of neurotransmitter released following the intracoronary injection of tyramine [64]. A study linking regional tracer uptake with exercise capacity indicates that the reinnervation process is beneficial for the exercise performance of patients following heart transplantation [65]. **A,** Neuronal imaging with C-11 hydroxyephedrine (^{11}C-HED) obtained 6 months after transplantation shows little retention of the tracer in the myocardium 40 minutes after tracer injection in comparison to the myocardial perfusion assessed with ^{13}N-ammonia. In a patient studied 3 years after heart transplantation, myocardial perfusion is homogeneous throughout the LV, but the ^{11}C-HED images obtained 40 minutes after injection reveal reappearance of regional ^{11}C-HED retention in the anteroseptal area of the LV. The area of reinnervation appears larger in a patient studied 11 years after transplantation, but regional denervation remains detectable in the inferior aspects of the LV that display normal perfusion. These examples of positron emission tomography (PET) images at different time points after transplantation depict the reinnervation process occurring in about 40% to 50% of the patients. The reinnervation process does not result in complete reinnervation but shows regional reappearance of sympathetic nerve terminals. Functional studies have shown that patients with reinnervation show greater heart rate variability, better exercise tolerance, and improved LV function with exercise [65].

Continued on the next page

Figure 11-17. *(Continued)* **B**, PET–^{11}C-HED polar maps of cardiac transplantation patients at various time points after surgery. Early after transplantation, the retention index is reduced throughout the entire left ventricular myocardium. Using a threshold of 7%/min retention index, no reinnervated area can be detected. At 3 years after transplantation, the anteroseptal areas show reinnervated territories (about 18% of the LV). The PET images obtained 11 years after transplantation show a reinnervated area of 48% of the LV, illustrating the progress of the reinnervation process in the anterior septal wall towards the apex. However, the inferior inferolateral wall remains denervated as seen in most of the patients undergoing neuronal imaging late after cardiac transplantation [65–67]. RV—right ventricle.

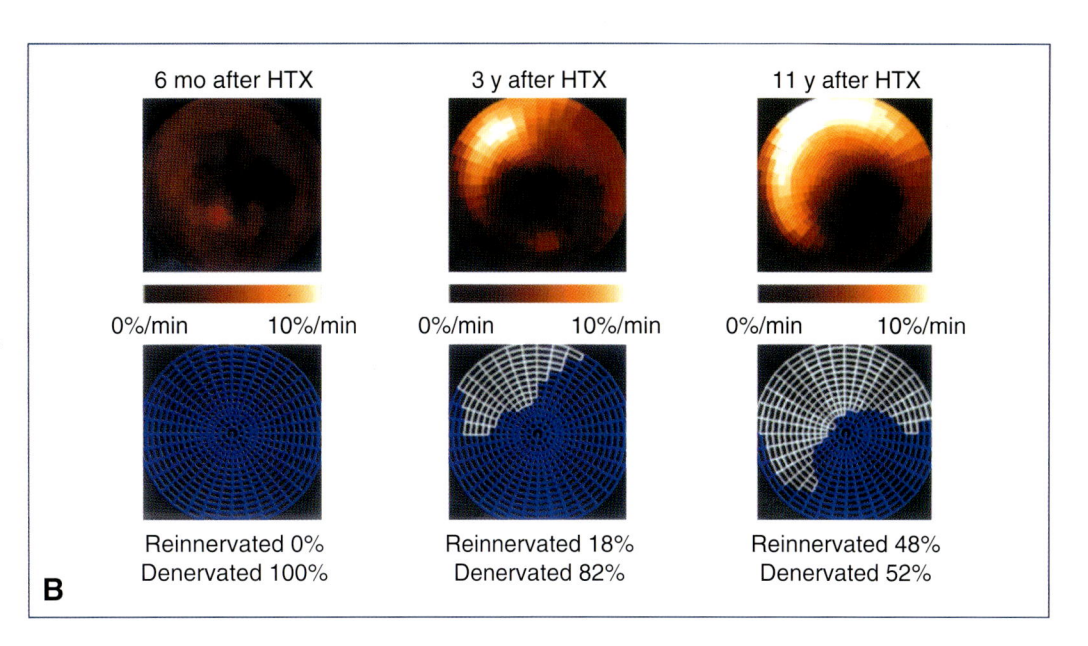

References

1. Levy M: Sympathetic-parasympathetic interaction in the heart. In *Neurocardiology*. New York: Futura Publishing Co.; 1988:85–98.

2. Bristow MR, Minobe W, Rasmussen R, et al.: Beta-adrenergic neuroeffector abnormalities in the failing human heart are produced by local rather than systemic mechanisms. *J Clin Invest* 1992, 89:803–815.

3. Bristow MR, Anderson FL, Port JD, et al.: Differences in beta-adrenergic neuroeffector mechanisms in ischemic versus idiopathic dilated cardiomyopathy. *Circulation* 1991, 84:1024–1039.

4. Somsen GA, Verberne HJ, Fleury E, Righetti A: Normal values and within-subject variability of cardiac I-123 MIBG scintigraphy in healthy individuals: implications for clinical studies. *J Nucl Cardiol* 2004, 11:126–133.

5. Momose M, Tyndale-Hines L, Bengel FM, Schwaiger M: How heterogeneous is the cardiac autonomic innervation? *Basic Res Cardiol* 2001, 96:539–546.

6. Bannister R, Mathias CJ: Introduction and classification of autonomic disorders. In *Autonomic Failure*. Edited by Bannister R, Mathias CJ. New York: Oxford University Press; 1992:1–12.

7. Milner P, Burnstock G: Neurotransmitters in the autonomic nervous system. In *Handbook of Autonomic Nervous System Dysfunction*. Edited by Korczyn AD. New York: Marcel Dekker; 1995:5–32.

8. Lipscombe D, Kongsamut S, Tsien RW, et al.: Adrenergic inhibition of sympathetic neurotransmitter release mediated by modulation of N-type calcium-channel gating. *Nature* 1989, 340:639–642.

9. Toth PT, Bindokas VP, Bleakman D, et al.: Mechanism of presynaptic inhibition by neuropeptide Y at sympathetic nerve terminals. *Nature* 1993, 364:635–639.

10. Nicholls JG, Martin AR, Wallace BG, et al.: *From Neuron to Brain: A Cellular and Molecular Approach to the Function of the Nervous System*. Sunderland, MA: Sinauer Associates; 1992.

11. Langer O, Halldin C: PET and SPECT tracers for mapping the cardiac nervous system. *Eur J Nucl Med* 2002, 29:416–434.

12. Kline RC, Swanson DP, Wieland DM, et al.: Myocardial imaging in man with I-123 meta-iodobenzylguanidine. *J Nucl Med* 1981, 22:129–132.

13. Wieland DM, Rosenspire KC, Hutchins GD, et al.: Neuronal mapping of the heart with 6-[18F]fluorometaraminol. *J Med Chem* 1990, 33:956–964.

14. Rosenspire KC, Haka MS, Van Dort ME, et al.: Synthesis and preliminary evaluation of carbon-11-meta-hydroxyephedrine: a false transmitter agent for heart neuronal imaging. *J Nucl Med* 1990, 31:1328–1334.

15. Raffel DM, Corbett JR, del Rosario RB, et al.: Clinical evaluation of carbon-11-phenylephrine: MAO-sensitive marker of cardiac sympathetic neurons. *J Nucl Med* 1996, 37:1923–1931.

16. Degrado TR, Zalutsky MR, Vaidyanathan G: Uptake mechanisms of meta-[123I]iodobenzylguanidine in isolated rat heart. *Nucl Med Biol* 1995, 22:1–12.

17. Nakajima K, Taki J, Tonami N, Hisada K: Decreased 123I-MIBG uptake and increased clearance in various cardiac diseases. *Nucl Med Commun* 1994, 15:317–323.

18. Bengel FM, Barthel P, Matsunari I, et al.: Kinetics of 123I-MIBG after acute myocardial infarction and reperfusion therapy. *J Nucl Med* 1999, 40:904–910.

19. Yamada T, Shimonagata T, Fukunami M, et al.: Comparison of the prognostic value of cardiac iodine-123 metaiodobenzylguanidine imaging and heart rate variability in patients with chronic heart failure: a prospective study. *J Am Coll Cardiol* 2003, 41:231–238.

20. Patel A, Iskandrian A: MIBG imaging. *J Nucl Cardiol* 2002, 9:75–94.

21. Farahati J, Bier D, Scheubeck M, et al.: Effect of specific activity on cardiac uptake of iodine-123-MIBG. *J Nucl Med* 1997, 38:447–451.

22. DeGrado TR, Zalutsky MR, Coleman RE, Vaidyanathan G: Effects of specific activity on meta-[(131)I]iodobenzylguanidine kinetics in isolated rat heart. *Nucl Med Biol* 1998, 25:59–64.

23. Schwaiger M, Kalff V, Rosenspire K, et al.: Noninvasive evaluation of sympathetic nervous system in human heart by positron emission tomography. *Circulation* 1990, 82:457–464.

24. Schwaiger M, Hutchins GD, Kalff V, et al.: Evidence for regional catecholamine uptake and storage sites in the transplanted human heart by positron emission tomography. *J Clin Invest* 1991, 87:1681–1690.

25. Munch G, Nguyen N, Nekolla S, et al.: Evaluation of sympathetic nerve terminals with [(11)C] epinephrine and [(11)D]hydroxyephedrine and positron emission tomography. *Circulation* 2000, 101:516–523.

26. Delforge J, Syrota A, Lancon JP, et al.: Cardiac beta-adrenergic receptor density measured in vivo using PET, CGP 12177, and a new graphical method [published erratum appears in J Nucl Med 1994, 35(5):921]. *J Nucl Med* 1991, 32:739–748.

27. Hartmann F, Ziegler S, Nekolla S, et al.: Regional patterns of myocardial sympathetic denervation in dilated cardiomyopathy: an analysis using carbon-11 hydroxyephedrine and positron emission tomography. *Heart* 1999, 81:262–270.

28. Caldwell JH, Link JM, Levy WC, et al.: Evidence for pre- to postsynaptic mismatch of the cardiac sympathetic nervous system in ischemic congestive heart failure. *J Nucl Med* 2008, 49:234–241.

29. Verberne HJ, Brewster LM, Somsen GA, van Eck-Smit BL: Prognostic value of myocardial 123I-metaiodobenzylguanidine (MIBG) parameters in patients with heart failure: a systematic review. *Eur Heart J* 2008, 29:1147–1159.

30. Agostini D, Verberne HJ, Burchert W, et al.: I-123-mIBG myocardial imaging for assessment of risk for a major cardiac event in heart failure patients: insights from a retrospective European multicenter study. *Eur J Nucl Med Mol Imaging* 2008, 35:535–546.

31. Verberne HJ, Habraken JB, van Eck-Smit BL, et al.: Variations in 123I-metaiodobenzylguanidine (MIBG) late heart mediastinal ratios in chronic heart failure: a need for standardisation and validation. *Eur J Nucl Med Mol Imaging* 2008, 35:547–553.

32. Jacobson AF, Senior R, Weiland F, et al.: Prognostic significance of 123I-mIBG myocardial scintigraphy in heart failure patients: results from the Prospective Multicenter International ADMIRE-HF Trial. Late-Breaking Clinical Trial. *American College of Cardiology 58th Annual Scientific Sessions*. Orlando, FL; March 31, 2009.

33. Somsen GA, van Vlies B, de Milliano PA, et al.: Increased myocardial [123I]-metaiodobenzylguanidine uptake after enalapril treatment in patients with chronic heart failure. *Heart* 1996, 76:218–222.

34. Kasama S, Toyama T, Kumakura H, et al.: Effects of candesartan on cardiac sympathetic nerve activity in patients with congestive heart failure and preserved left ventricular ejection fraction. *J Am Coll Cardiol* 2005, 45:661–667.

35. Suwa M, Otake Y, Moriguchi A, et al.: Iodine-123 metaiodobenzylguanidine myocardial scintigraphy for prediction of response to beta-blocker therapy in patients with dilated cardiomyopathy. *Am Heart J* 1997, 133:353–358.

36. Kasama S, Toyama T, Hatori T, et al.: Evaluation of cardiac sympathetic nerve activity and left ventricular remodelling in patients with dilated cardiomyopathy on the treatment containing carvedilol. *Eur Heart J* 2007, 28:989–995.

37. Cohen-Solal A, Rouzet F, Berdeaux A, et al.: Effects of carvedilol on myocardial sympathetic innervation in patients with chronic heart failure. *J Nucl Med* 2005, 46:1796–1803.

38. Kasama S, Toyama T, Kumakura H, et al.: Effect of spironolactone on cardiac sympathetic nerve activity and left ventricular remodeling in patients with dilated cardiomyopathy. *J Am Coll Cardiol* 2003, 41:574–581.

39. Erol-Yilmaz A, Verberne HJ, Schrama TA, et al.: Cardiac resynchronization induces favorable neurohumoral changes. *Pacing Clin Electrophysiol* 2005, 28:304–310.

40. Nishioka SA, Martinelli Filho M, Brandão SC, et al.: Cardiac sympathetic activity pre and post resynchronization therapy evaluated by 123I-MIBG myocardial scintigraphy. *J Nucl Cardiol* 2007, 14:852–859.

41. Gould PA, Kong G, Kalff V, et al.: Improvement in cardiac adrenergic function post biventricular pacing for heart failure. *Europace* 2007, 9:751–756.

42. Allman KC, Wieland DM, Muzik O, et al.: Carbon-11 hydroxyephedrine with positron emission tomography for serial assessment of cardiac adrenergic neuronal function after acute myocardial infarction in humans. *J Am Coll Cardiol* 1993, 22:368–375.

43. Matsunari I, Schricke U, Bengel FM, et al.: Extent of cardiac sympathetic neuronal damage is determined by the area of ischemia in patients with acute coronary syndromes. *Circulation* 2000, 101:2579–2585.

44. Frickel E, Frickel H, Eckert S, et al.: Myocardial sympathetic innervation in patients with chronic coronary artery disease: Is reduction in coronary flow reserve correlated with sympathetic denervation? *Eur J Nucl Med Mol Imaging* 2007, 34:206–211.

45. Yukinaka M, Nomura M, Ito S, Nakaya Y: Mismatch between myocardial accumulation of 123I-MIBG and 99mTc-MIBI and late ventricular potentials in patients after myocardial infarction: association with the development of ventricular arrhythmias. *Am Heart J* 1998, 136:859–867.

46. Simões MV, Barthel P, Matsunari I, et al.: Presence of sympathetically denervated but viable myocardium and its electrophysiologic correlates after early revascularised, acute myocardial infarction. *Eur Heart J* 2004, 25:551–557.

47. Calkins H, Allman K, Bolling S, et al.: Correlation between scintigraphic evidence of regional sympathetic neuronal dysfunction and ventricular refractoriness in the human heart. *Circulation* 1993, 88:172–179.

48. Sasano T, Abraham MR, Chang KC, et al.: Abnormal sympathetic innervation of viable myocardium and the substrate of ventricular tachycardia after myocardial infarction. *J Am Coll Cardiol* 2008, 51:2266–2275.

49. Schwartz PJ: The autonomic nervous system and sudden death. *Eur Heart J* 1998, 19:F72–F80.

50. Meredith IT, Broughton A, Jennings GL, Esler MD: Evidence of a selective increase in cardiac sympathetic activity in patients with sustained ventricular arrhythmias. *N Engl J Med* 1991, 325:618–624.

51. Rubart M, Zipes DP: Mechanisms of sudden cardiac death. *J Clin Invest* 2005, 115:2305–2315.

52. Wichter T, Schafers M, Rhodes CG, et al.: Abnormalities of cardiac sympathetic innervation in arrhythmogenic right ventricular cardiomyopathy: quantitative assessment of presynaptic norepinephrine reuptake and postsynaptic beta-adrenergic receptor density with positron emission tomography. *Circulation* 2000, 101:1552–1558.

53. Schafers M, Lerch H, Wichter T, et al.: Cardiac sympathetic innervation in patients with idiopathic right ventricular outflow tract tachycardia. *J Am Coll Cardiol* 1998, 32:181–161.

54. Kies P, Wichte T, Schafers M, et al.: Abnormal myocardial presynaptic norepinephrine recycling in patients with Brugada syndrome. *Circulation* 2004, 110:3017–3022.

55. Paul M, Schäfers M, Kies P, et al.: Impact of sympathetic innervation on recurrent life-threatening arrhythmias in the follow-up of patients with idiopathic ventricular fibrillation. *Eur J Nucl Med Mol Imaging* 2006, 33:866–870.

56. Arora R, Ferick K, Nakata T, et al.: I-123 MIBG imaging and heart rate variability analysis to predict the need for an implantable cardioverter defibrillator. *J Nucl Cardiol* 2003, 10:121–131.

57. Nagahara D, Nakata T, Hashimoto A, et al.: Predicting the need for an implantable cardioverter defibrillator using cardiac metaiodobenzylguanidine activity together with plasma natriuretic peptide concentration or left ventricular function. *J Nucl Med* 2008, 49:225–233.

58. Langen KJ, Ziegler D, Weise F, et al.: Evaluation of QT interval length, QT dispersion and myocardial m-iodobenzylguanidine uptake in insulin-dependent diabetic patients with and without autonomic neuropathy. *Clin Sci* 1997, 93:325–333.

59. Stevens MJ, Raffel DM, Allman KC, et al.: Cardiac sympathetic dysinnervation in diabetes: implications for enhanced cardiovascular risk. *Circulation* 1998, 98:961–968.

60. Pop-Busui R, Kirkwood I, Schmid H, et al.: Sympathetic dysfunction in type 1 diabetes: association with impaired myocardial blood flow reserve and diastolic dysfunction. *J Am Coll Cardiol* 2004, 44:2368–2374.

61. Allman KC, Stevens MJ, Wieland DM, et al.: Noninvasive assessment of cardiac diabetic neuropathy by carbon-11 hydroxyephedrine and positron emission tomography. *J Am Coll Cardiol* 1993, 22:1425–1432.

62. Ziegler D, Weise F, Langen KJ, et al.: Effect of glycaemic control on myocardial sympathetic innervation assessed by [123I]metaiodobenzylguanidine scintigraphy: a 4-year prospective study in IDDM patients. *Diabetologia* 1998, 41:443–451.

63. Wei K, Dorian P, Newman D, Langer A: Association between QT dispersion and autonomic dysfunction in patients with diabetes mellitus. *J Am Coll Cardiol* 1995, 26:859–863.

64. Odaka K, von Scheidt W, Ziegler SI, et al.: Reappearance of cardiac presynaptic sympathetic nerve terminals in the transplanted heart: correlation between PET using (11)C-hydroxyephedrine and invasively measured norepinephrine release. *J Nucl Med* 2001, 42:1011–1016.

65. Bengel FM, Ueberfuhr P, Schiepel N, et al.: Effect of sympathetic reinnervation on cardiac performance after heart transplantation. *N Engl J Med* 2001, 345:731–738.

66. De Marco T, Dae M, Yuen-Green MS, et al.: Iodine-123 metaiodobenzylguanidine scintigraphic assessment of the transplanted human heart: evidence for late reinnervation. *J Am Coll Cardiol* 1995, 25:927–931.

67. Estorch M, Camprecios M, Flotats A, et al.: Sympathetic reinnervation of cardiac allografts evaluated by 123I-MIBG imaging. *J Nucl Med* 1999, 40:911–916.

Molecular Imaging of Atherosclerosis: A Biological Roadmap

12

Farouc A. Jaffer and Jagat Narula

Significant advances have been made toward the management of coronary disease, but it is not yet possible to clinically identify patients likely to develop an acute coronary event. Although the presence of risk factors and circulating biomarkers enable the identification of vulnerable patients, it is necessary to prospectively recognize the rupture-prone atherosclerotic plaque to prevent occurrences of acute events. For such a strategy to be successful, emphasis needs to be placed on the structural and molecular characteristics underlying plaques of interest. The majority of acute coronary syndromes arise from disrupted plaques that may not necessarily be significantly obstructive. Histopathologic data reveal that "vulnerable plaques" are generally voluminous with significant expansive remodeling, contain bulky necrotic cores with neovascularization and intraplaque hemorrhage, and are covered by attenuated and inflamed fibrous caps. They are usually not heavily calcified. It has been proposed that the outwardly remodeled vascular segments and low attenuation plaques can be detected by multislice CT with reasonable diagnostic accuracy. On the other hand, plaque volumes, lipid accumulation, and intraplaque hemorrhage have been identified by MRI at least in large and immobile noncoronary vasculature. The assessment of the thickness of the cap has required invasive instrumentation such as optical coherence tomography. The fibrous cap and subintimal inflammation, apoptosis, and angiogenesis are amenable to molecular imaging [1–4].

The role of inflammation in driving and defining plaque vulnerability is well-established [5]. Recent trials have demonstrated that the circulating biomarkers of inflammation help predict likelihood of acute vascular events even when cholesterol levels are not very high. While biomarkers allow an assessment of the inflammatory state in general, it will be attractive to recognize inflamed plaques locally in clinically relevant vascular beds (coronary and carotid arteries), to both refine risk prediction and to guide novel therapeutic strategies targeted for local intervention and primary prevention of acute vascular events.

Pathologic Substrates for Imaging Vulnerable Plaques

Plaque rupture is responsible for up to 75% of acute coronary events [3,4]. The rupture of the fibrous cap exposes a thrombogenic core to the luminal blood and leads to acute thrombosis. Disrupted plaques have distinct pathologic characteristics; they are generally large both cross-sectionally and longitudinally. These voluminous plaques may not necessarily impose significant luminal obstruction because the arterial wall at the lesion site is outwardly (positive or expansively) remodeled. These plaques contain large necrotic cores. The disrupted fibrous caps are thin and infiltrated by foamy macrophages.

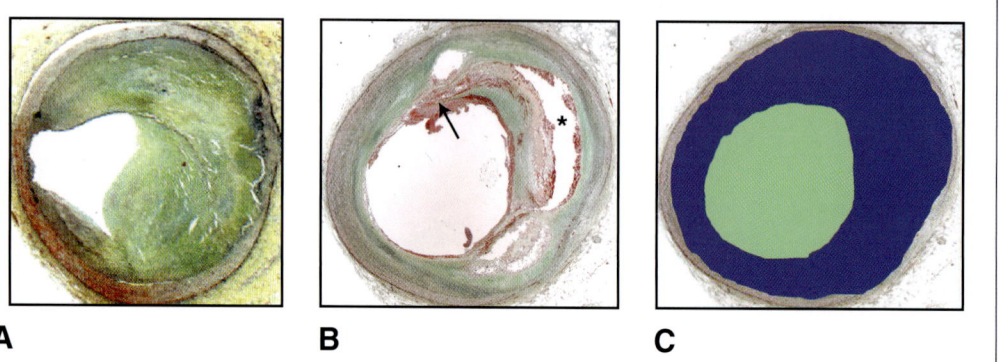

Figure 12-1. Pathologic characteristics of a stable plaque and a ruptured plaque. The stable plaque is rich in collagen and smooth muscle with minimal lipid accumulation (**A**). On the other hand, ruptured plaque is formed predominantly by a large necrotic core (*asterisk*) and covered by a thin fibrous cap (**B**). The site of plaque rupture (*arrow*) exposes the necrotic core to luminal blood and allows thrombotic occlusion of the vessel. The pathologic examination of culprit plaques from the victims of acute coronary syndrome reveals that these plaques are usually significantly voluminous. In the schematic representation of the ruptured plaque (**C**), the plaque area has been colored *blue* and the luminal area as *green*. Up to 80% of the disrupted plaques demonstrate greater than 50% cross-sectional vascular area involvement (*blue area* divided by *blue + green area*) and about 50% of the ruptured plaques occupy more than 75% of the cross-sectional area of the vessel. This is in contrast to angiographic reports in patients presenting with acute coronary events that have traditionally demonstrated nonocclusive culprit plaques [6,7]. The discrepancy between the angiographic and pathologic data has been explained by the positive remodeling of the vessel, which allows outwardly plaque expansion without luminal encroachment. Positive remodeling is not seen in stable plaques that have smaller or no lipid cores; their predominantly fibrotic content may in fact result in negative remodeling (or vascular shrinkage) [3,4]. (*Adapted from* Shapiro et al. [4].)

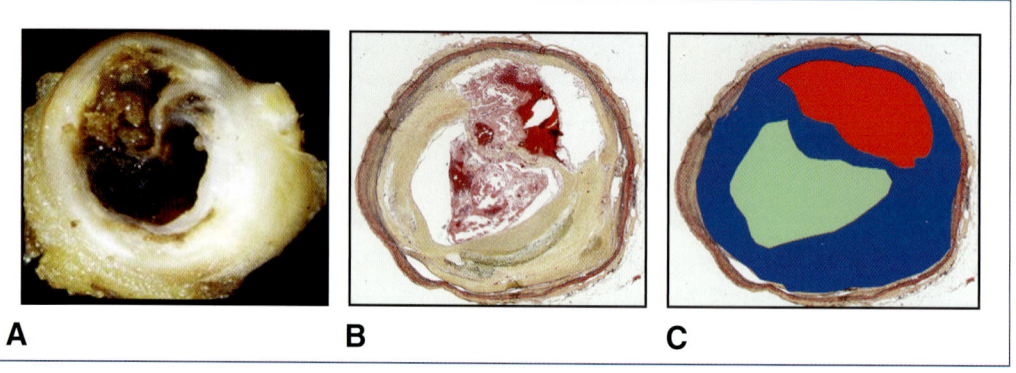

Figure 12-2. **A–C**, Disrupted plaques usually demonstrate large necrotic cores (NC). This figure shows gross morphology of a culprit coronary lesion (**A**), histopathologic characteristics (**B**), and schematic presentation of the NC in *red* (**C**). In the culprit plaques, the NC usually occupy greater than 25% of the plaque area (*red area* divided by *blue area*) and show more than 120° circumferential involvement of the vessel in at least 75% of instances. The NC extend 2 to 22 mm in longitudinal dimension (median, 9 mm). The larger the plaque area and the larger the NC size, the higher the likelihood of plaque instability [3,4]. (*Adapted from* Shapiro et al. [4].)

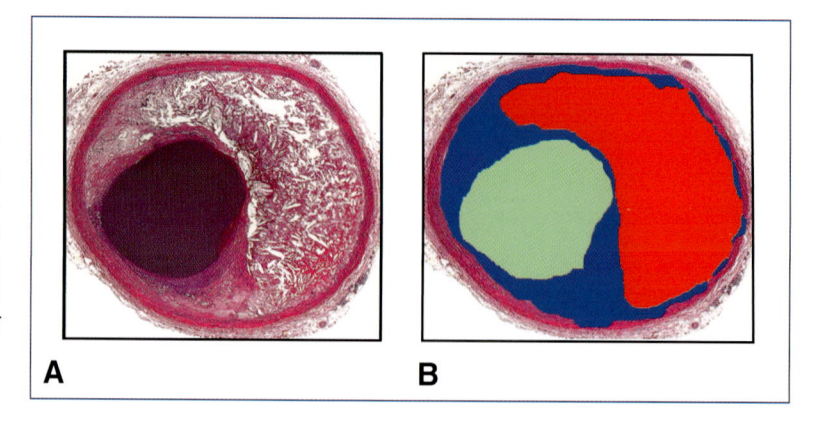

Figure 12-3. Histologic features of a vulnerable plaque or thin-cap fibroatheroma (**A**). It is reasonable to presume that before the acute event, plaques vulnerable to rupture harbor the same histopathologic signatures, except that the thin fibrous cap is still intact. Schematic presentation (**B**) with *blue plaque* and *green lumen* again demonstrates plaque occupying more than 75% of cross-sectional vascular area. The lumen is not obstructed and the large plaque volume is accommodated by positive remodeling of the vessel. Necrotic core shaded in *red* occupies almost entire plaque area. (*Adapted from* Shapiro et al. [4].)

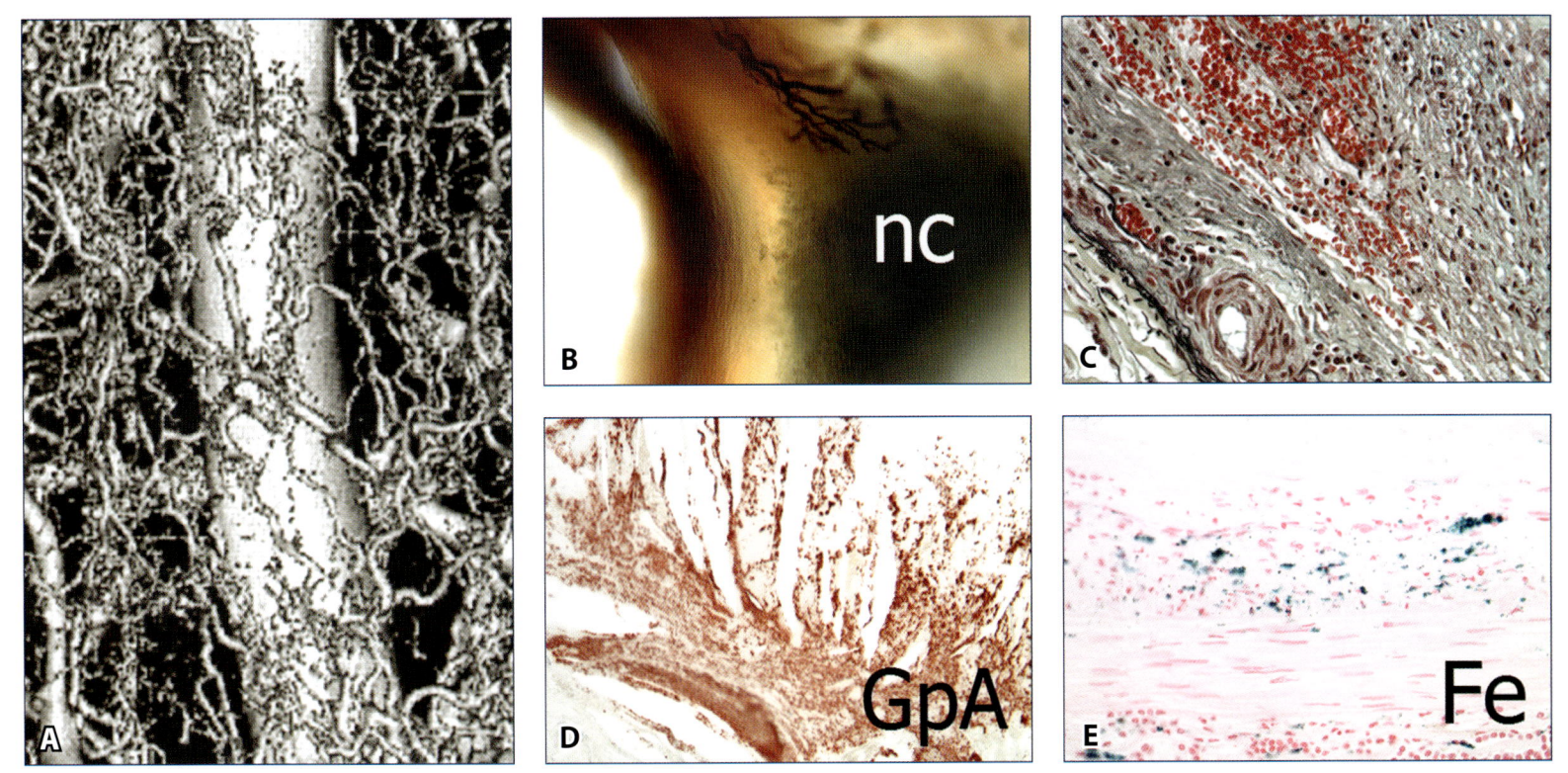

Figure 12-4. A–E, Evolution of necrotic core (NC) in the plaque. The ongoing death of lipid laden macrophages contributes to the formation of the NC in atherosclerotic plaques. Worsening hypoxia in the enlarging plaque perpetuates macrophage death, enlarges the NC, and promotes neovascularization (**B**) [14]. These nascent vessels are inherently leaky and allow extravasation of red blood cells (RBC) into the plaque (**C**). It is well appreciated that the cholesterol content of erythrocyte membranes exceeds that of most other cells in the body and likely contributes to the cholesterol pool of the growing NC. Intraplaque hemorrhage (**C**) due to the rupture of these immature vessels further leads to the accumulation of a large number of RBC and hence cholesterol. The plaque hemorrhages are common in the coronary arteries in patients dying from plaque rupture. The extent of iron deposits (**E**) in the plaque (Fe) and that of glycophorin A (**D**) (GpA, a protein exclusively associated with RBC membrane) staining is directly proportional to the size of the NC [15,16].

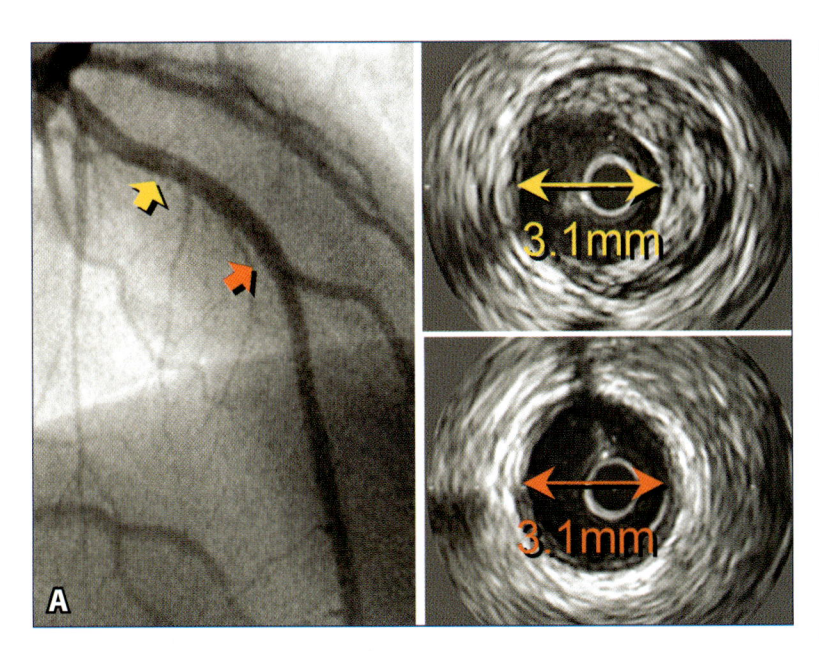

Plaque neovascularization is accompanied by proliferation of vasa vasorum (**A**) [16,17]. Disrupted plaques have a fourfold higher vasa vasorum density compared with stable plaques with severe luminal narrowing. Microvessels that perforate from the adventitial layer to the medial layer are well formed with the smooth muscle cell (SMC) envelope, unlike those that extend to the neointima, which appear immature and leaky. Abundant T-helper cells found at the medial wall perforation site likely inhibit SMC proliferation through interferon. The density of vasa vasorum, measured by micro-CT, increases markedly during hypercholesterolemia and resolves with statin treatment. The increase in vasa vasorum is associated with vascular endothelial growth factor expression in the neointima and neoangiogenesis. Interestingly, erythrocyte membrane-derived cholesterol is elevated in patients presenting with acute coronary syndromes and is sensitive to statin therapy. (**A,** *adapted from* Kwon et al. [14]; **B,** *adapted from* Kolodgie et al. [17].)

Figure 12-5. Imaging of morphologic characteristics of atherosclerotic plaques. Intravascular ultrasound (IVUS) and CT angiography (CTA) offer excellent assessment of the magnitude of the plaque and necrotic core size and the extent of positive remodeling; thin fibrous caps can be quantitatively characterized by optical coherence tomography (OCT). **A,** The IVUS examination of the left anterior descending coronary artery in the given example reveals an apparently normal lumen in the presence of a large atherosclerotic plaque burden [8]. The region with a large eccentric plaque (*yellow arrow*) shows same lumen size as in the normal segment of the artery (*orange arrow*) distal to the plaque area. A strong association of positive vascular remodeling with culprit lesions in acute coronary syndromes has been widely reported. IVUS in patients presenting with acute coronary syndromes demonstrated positive vascular remodeling and plaques containing relatively signal-free necrotic cores. IVUS imaging of coronary arteries has often demonstrated actual plaque rupture sites. Plaque rupture of the infarct-related vessel occurred in two thirds of patients presenting with acute myocardial infarction [9]. It was therefore proposed that intact plaques with similar findings should be deemed vulnerable, and this presumption has been validated in follow-up after IVUS examination; the lesions that lead to an acute coronary event over time were characteristically large, containing prominent and shallow echolucent zones [10]. (**A,** *adapted from* Glagov et al. [8].)

Continued on the next page

Molecular Imaging of Atherosclerosis: A Biological Roadmap 259

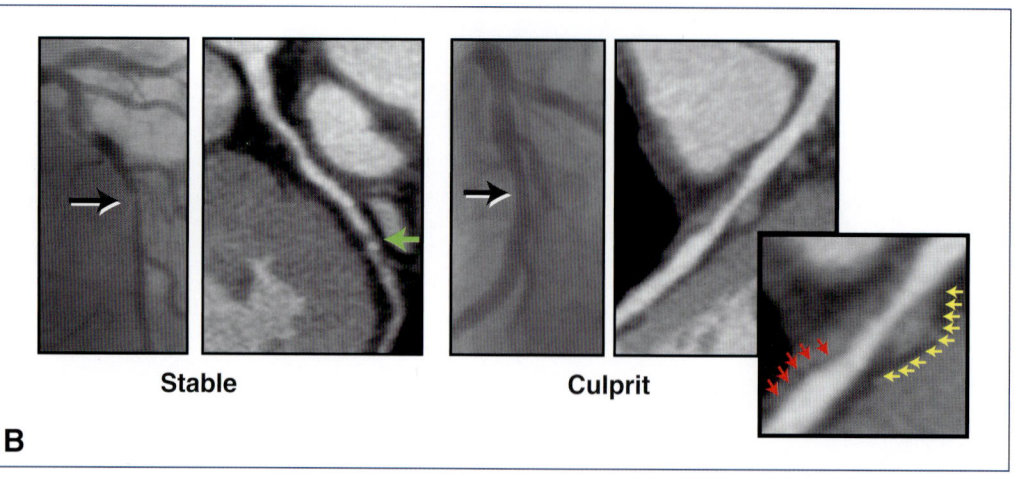

Figure 12-5. *(Continued)* **B,** Multislice CTA of culprit and stable coronary lesions with invasive coronary angiogram. The culprit lesion is outwardly remodeled (*yellow arrows* in inset) compared with the proximal normal vessel, and contains low attenuation (likely soft) plaque (*red arrows*) [11]. The stable lesion is not remodeled and shows intermediate attenuation (likely fibrous) plaque (*green arrow*). The culprit lesions have also been demonstrated to be more frequently associated with spotty calcific deposits but not large calcific plates. If plaques with similar CTA characteristics are identified incidentally, up to one fourth of them may develop acute coronary syndrome during a 2-year follow-up period [12]. Plaques with stable characteristics are associated with a less than 0.5% likelihood of an acute cardiac event. The fibrous caps are significantly attenuated in the vulnerable plaques and are disrupted at the weakest site in an acute coronary event. Based on a large set of disrupted plaques postmortem, it was proposed that fibrous cap thickness of less than 65 microns predicts vulnerability to plaque rupture. The fibrous cap thickness can be accurately measured by OCT [13]. (**B,** *adapted from* Motoyama et al. [11].)

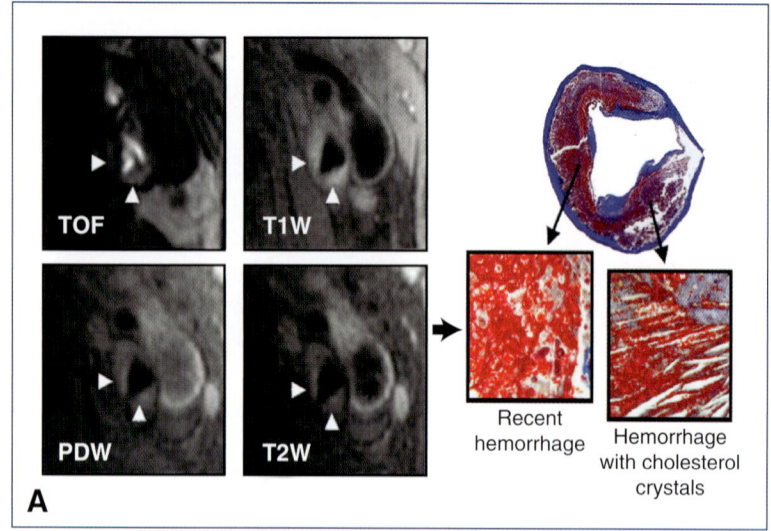

Figure 12-6. Noninvasive imaging for vasa vasorum and plaque hemorrhage. **A,** Magnetic resonance T1-weighted imaging of carotid arteries has demonstrated high diagnostic accuracy for histologically verified plaque hemorrhage in resected carotid endarterectomy specimens [18]. It has been demonstrated that the plaques with intraplaque hemorrhage almost invariably demonstrate an increase in plaque volume on follow-up even if treated with high doses of statins. In addition, patients with no plaque hemorrhage frequently decrease their plaque volume after statin treatment. On the other hand, the T2* values are lower in carotid lesions with intraplaque hemorrhage [19]. **B,** Ultrasound microbubble studies have identified increased vasa vasorum and vessel wall vascularity in patients with carotid atherosclerosis [20]. A longitudinal image of a carotid artery has become well visualized after contrast administration and distinguishes the intimal-medial thickness of the anterior and posterior walls. Note the striking pattern of vasa vasorum neovascularization leading to the core of the atherosclerotic plaque (*arrow*). This patient had diabetes and was not receiving statin therapy. Subsequent to the recording of these images, the patient underwent a carotid endarterectomy for symptomatic cerebral vascular disease; the endarterectomy specimen revealed a plethora of microvasculature within the matrix of the plaque, and residual deposits of hemosiderin resulting from prior hemorrhage (*inset*).

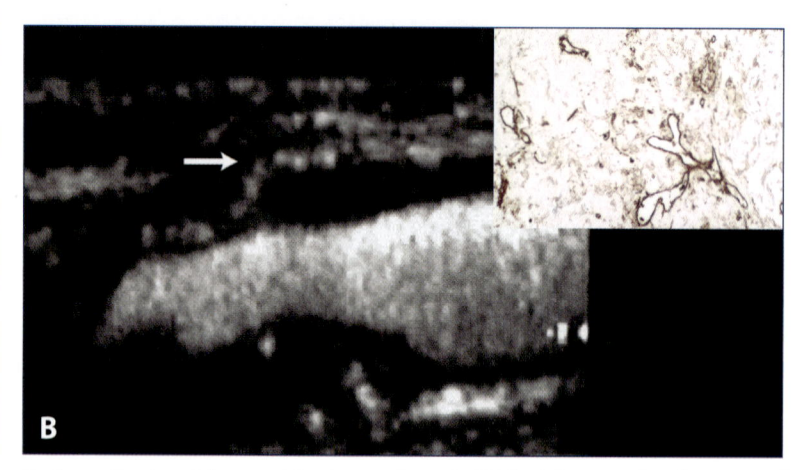

260 Atlas of Nuclear Cardiology

Inflammation, Plaque Vulnerability, and Molecular Imaging

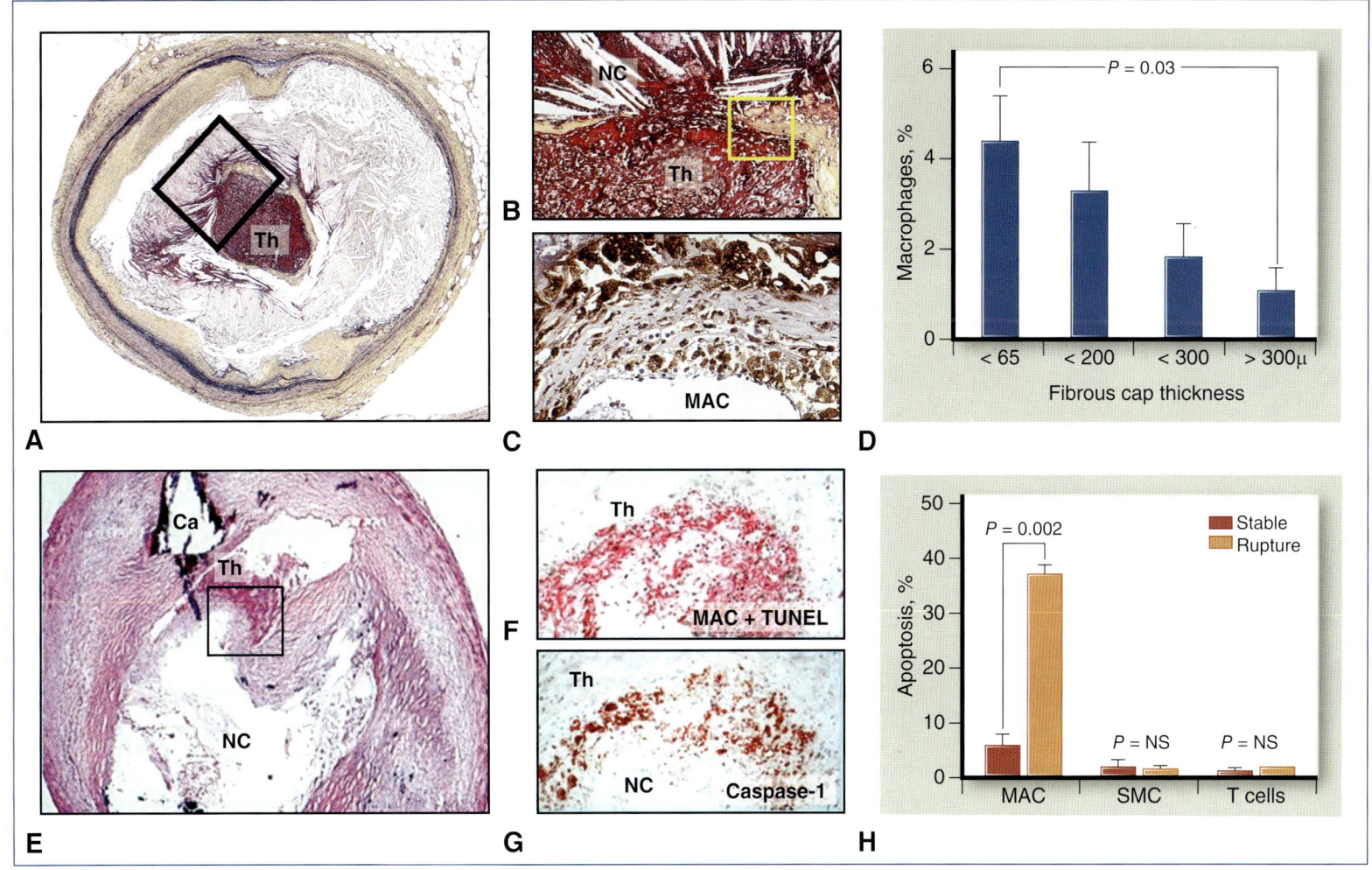

Figure 12-7. Fibrous cap inflammation in ruptured plaques. The thin fibrous caps of the ruptured or vulnerable plaques are markedly inflamed with monocyte-macrophage infiltration. In a histologic section of coronary vessel obtained from a sudden death victim, a huge concentric plaque and cholesterol crystal-rich necrotic core (NC) are seen. The thin fibrous cap is disrupted and thrombus (Th) occludes the lumen. The area enclosed by the *black square* in **A** is magnified in **B**; the *yellow boxed area* is further magnified and stained for macrophages (MAC) (**C**) [4]. The disrupted site is significantly inflamed. Analysis of fibrous caps demonstrates that macrophages are the most dominant cellular population in ruptured and vulnerable plaques, whereas smooth muscle cells (SMC) are dominant in stable atherosclerotic lesions. Higher numbers of macrophages are associated with thinner fibrous caps (**D**).

A large proportion of these macrophages in the vulnerable and disrupted plaques undergo cell death by the process of apoptosis. The histopathologic characterization of another ruptured coronary plaque (**E**) shows huge occlusive plaque, large necrotic core, spotty calcification (Ca) and attenuated fibrous cap. The severely narrowed lumen is partially obstructed by the thrombus. Further evaluation of the *boxed area* in **E** shows apoptotic macrophages in the fibrous cap (**F**; dual staining for macrophages and DNA fragmentation) with abundant caspase-1 expression (**G**); approximately 40% of macrophages undergo apoptosis in disrupted plaques (**H**). (*Adapted from* Shapiro *et al.* [4].)

Molecular Imaging of Atherosclerosis: A Biological Roadmap

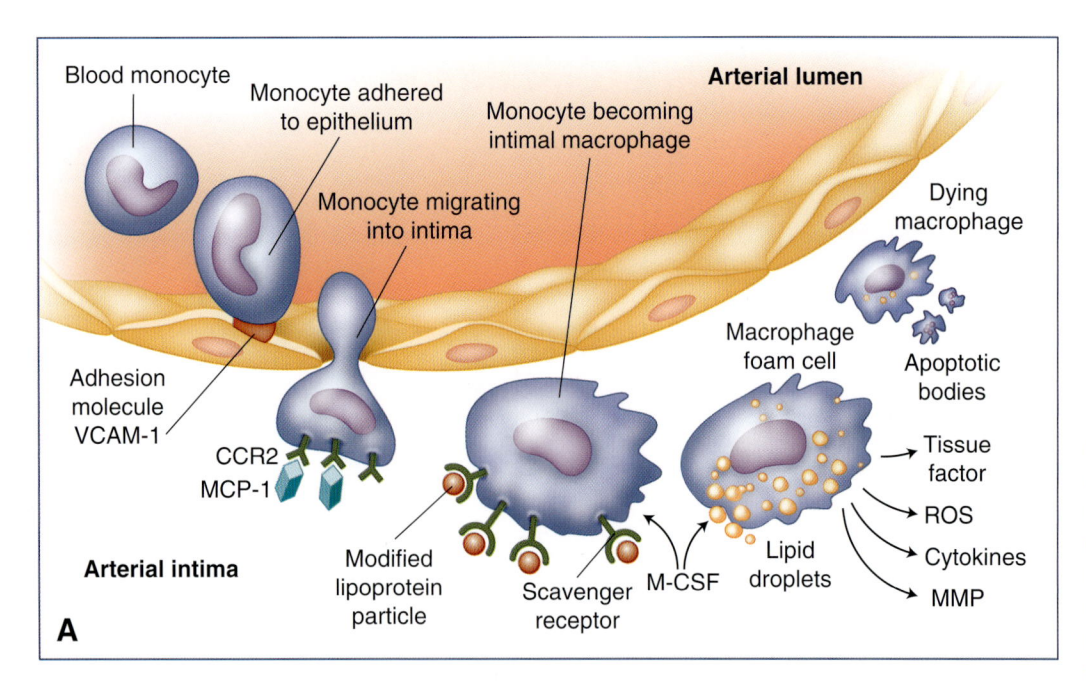

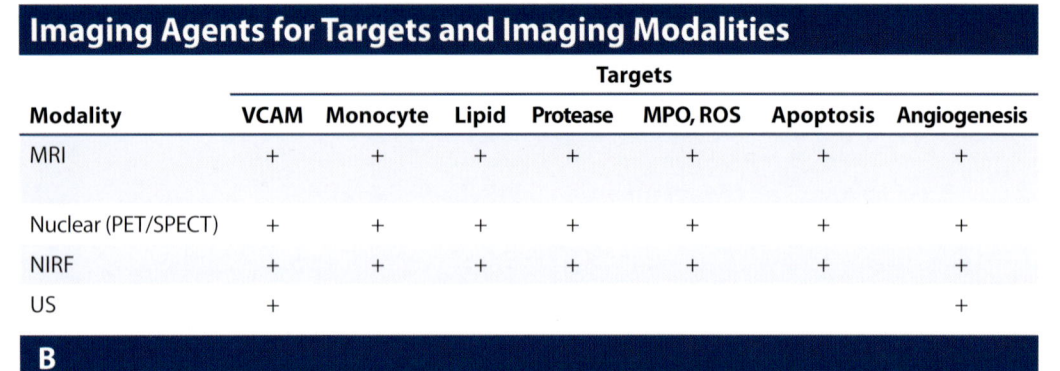

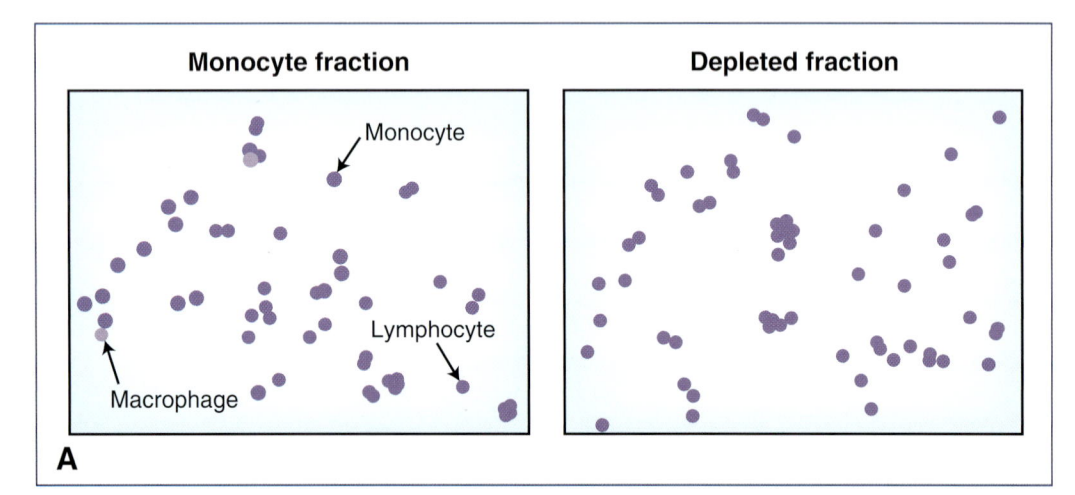

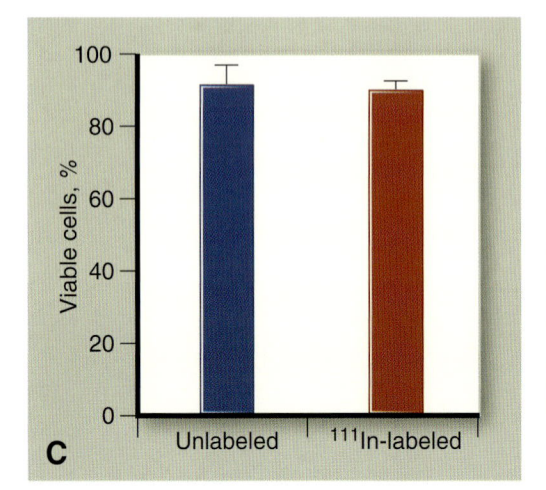

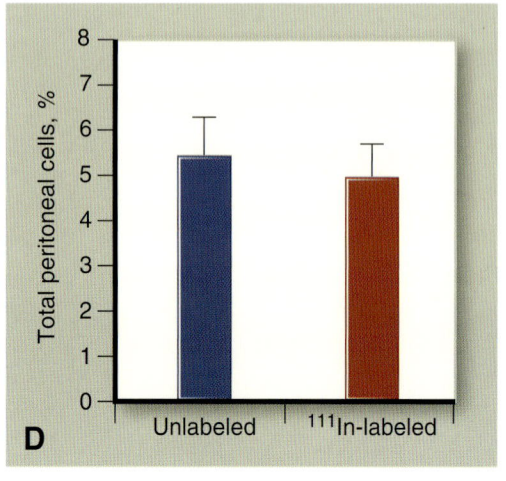

Figure 12-8. Strategies for targeting of inflammation in atherosclerosis. In vivo identification of inflammation has been best exploited by molecular imaging of monocyte-macrophages [1–4]. These techniques have targeted upregulation of surface molecules or secreted products that are uniquely expressed by the imflammatory cells associated with unstable plaques. **A**, This road map identifies important targets for molecular imaging. **B**, Imaging agents are available for an array of targets and imaging modalities, and several agents have been tested in clinical studies. CCR2—chemokine (CC motif) receptor 2; MCP—monocyte chemoattractant protein; M-CSF—monocyte colony-stimulating factor; MMP—matrix metalloproteinase; MPO—myeloperoxidase; NIRF—near infrared fluorescence; ROS—reactive oxygen species; US—ultrasound; VCAM—vascular cell adhesion molecule. (*Adapted from* Libby [21].)

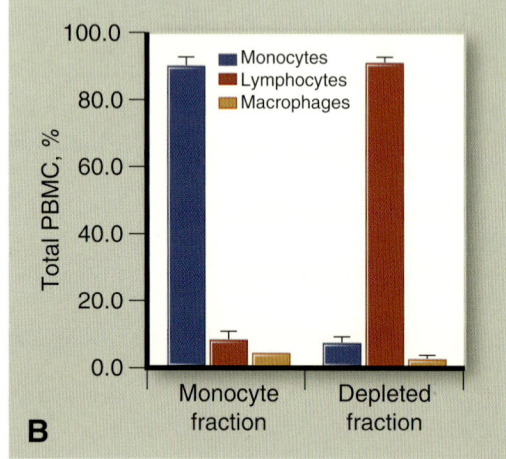

Figure 12-9. Imaging of monocyte trafficking in atheroma. Purified peripheral blood mononuclear cells (PBMC) (precursors of tissue macrophages) were labeled with ^{111}In oxine, a clinical radiotracer, and injected into atherosclerotic apoE$^{-/-}$ mice. **A**, Cytospin and Wright-Giemsa staining of purified mononuclear cells revealed a well-separated monocyte fraction (*left*) and corresponding depleted fraction (*right*). **B**, Cytospin slides revealed that more than 90% of the population was purely monocytes. Lymphocytes were the next prevalent cell type. **C**, ^{111}In-oxine did not significantly affect trypan-blue stain–determined monocyte viability. **D**, ^{111}In-oxine also did not significantly alter monocyte recruitment in vivo in a peritonitis model.

Continued on the next page

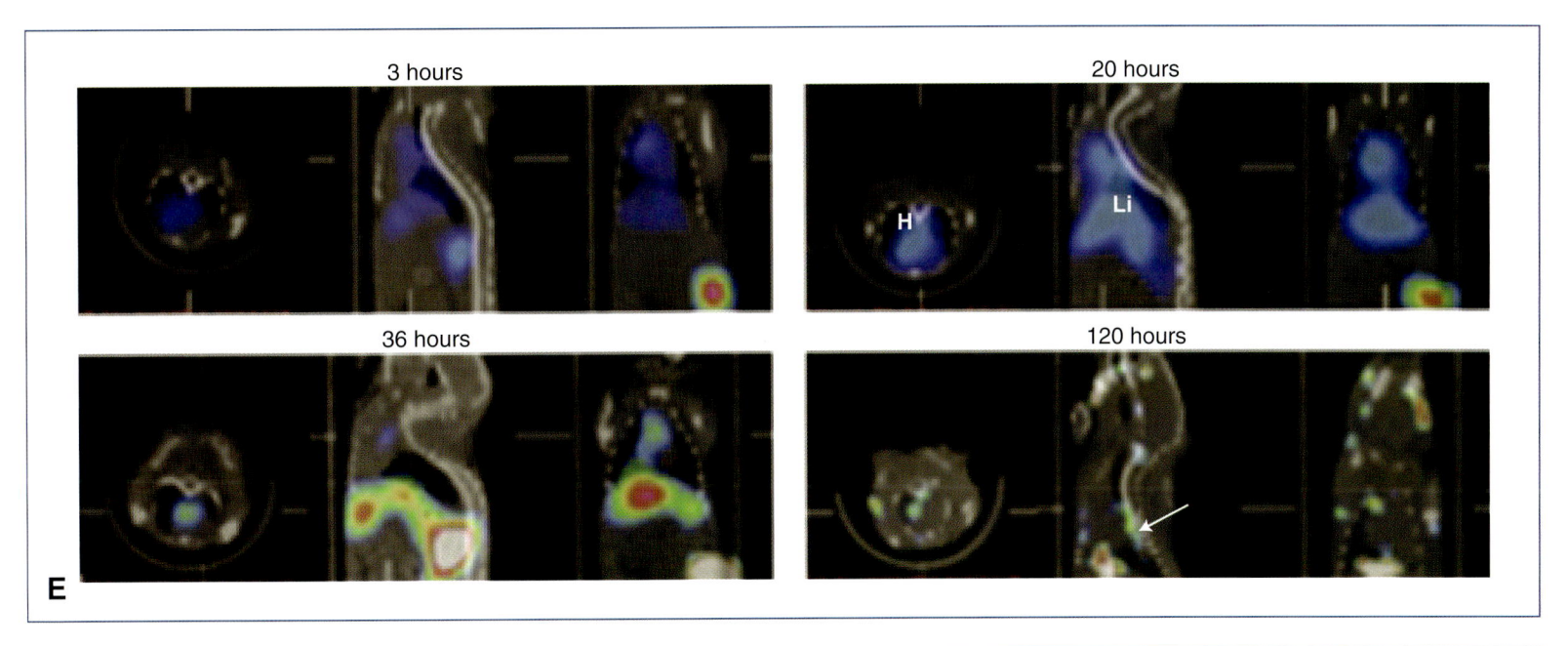

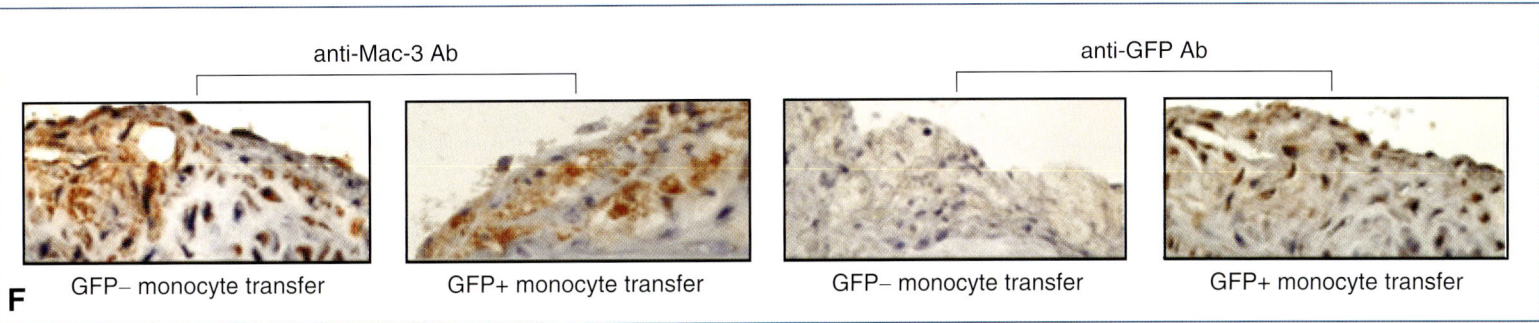

Figure 12-9. *(Continued)* **E**, In vivo SPECT/CT imaging of ^{111}In-oxine labeled monocytes in atherosclerosis (heart [H]; liver [Li]). SPECT signal emerged in the heart and lungs at 24 hours, followed by the liver and spleen at 36 hours, with accumulation in atherosclerotic lesions by 120 hours (*arrow*). **F**, In atherosclerotic plaques resected 5 days after injection of green fluorescence protein- (GFP) or GFP+ monocytes, numerous macrophages (Mac) were detectable on immunohistochemical staining (*left*). In contrast anti-GFP stains (*right*) demonstrated strong signal only in GFP+ monocytes. (*Adapted from* Kircher et al. [22].)

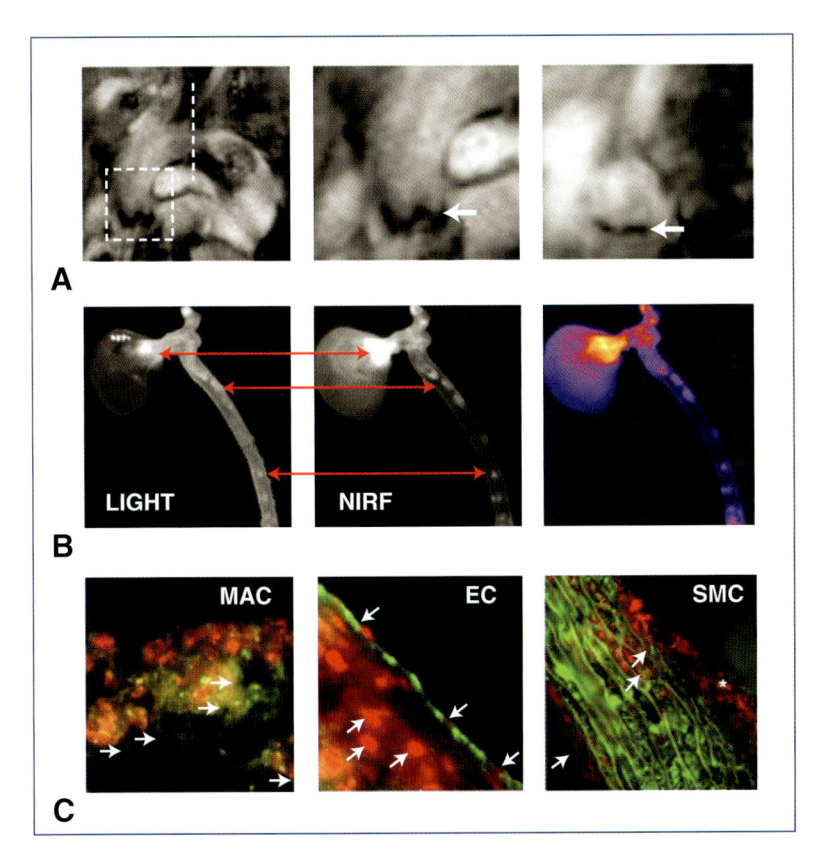

Figure 12-10. Exploiting the phagocytic properties of macrophages (MAC) for tracer localization. MRI and fluorescence imaging of plaque cellular inflammation employing a magnetofluorescent nanoparticle (MFNP) is shown. **A**, In vivo T2*-weighted aortic MRI of atherosclerotic apoE$^{-/-}$ mice 24 hours after nanoparticle injection (15 mg Fe/kg). *Left*, Long-axis cross-section of the aortic root (*dashed box*) and transverse aortic arch (*dashed line*) reveals focal MRI signal loss in aortic plaques. Compared with saline injected mice, the plaque contrast-to-noise ratio increased by more than threefold ($P < 0.001$). **B**, Ex vivo light (*left*) and near infrared fluorescence (NIRF) reflectance images (*middle* and pseudocolor on *right*) of resected aortas from apoE$^{-/-}$ mice. Plaques in the aortic root, aortic arch, and descending thoracic aorta (*arrows*, light image) demonstrated strong, matched NIRF signal. **C**, Fluorescence microscopy of plaques demonstrated MFNP uptake (*red*) preferentially in MAC (*left*); however, MFNP signal also deposited in endothelial cells (EC) (*middle*) and smooth muscle cells (SMC) (*right*). (*Adapted from* Jaffer et al. [23].)

Molecular Imaging of Atherosclerosis: A Biological Roadmap

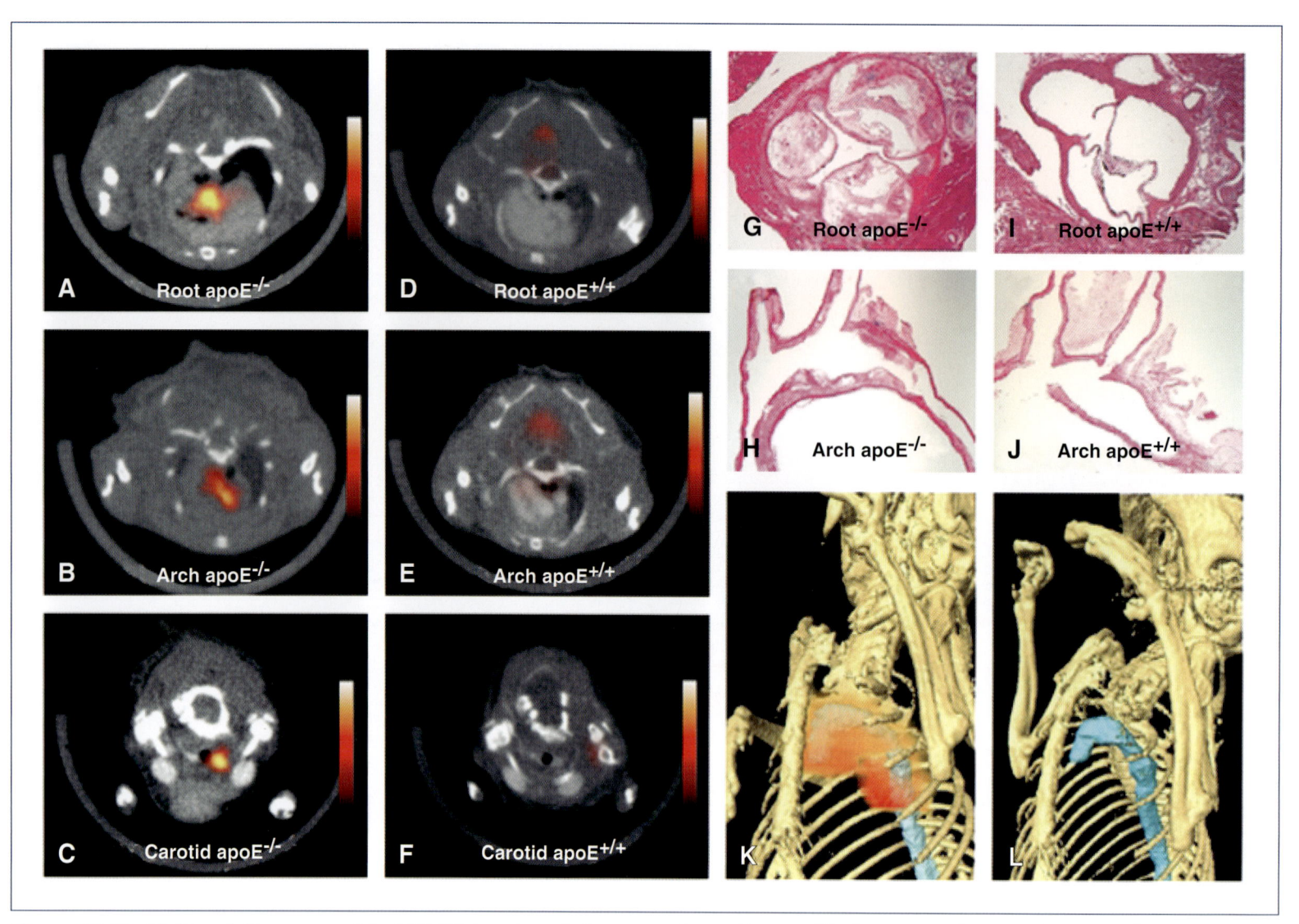

Figure 12-11. Multimodality nanoparticle PET-CT imaging of plaque macrophages. The macrophage-avid magnetic, radioactive, and fluorescent tri-modality nanoparticle (^{64}Cu-TNP, detectable on PET, MRI, and near infrared fluorescence [NIRF]) was injected into atherosclerotic apoE$^{-/-}$ mice and then imaged after 24 hours on an integrated PET-CT system. Contrast-mediated CT angiography was performed prior to PET imaging. Fused PET-CT images of atheroma of the aortic root (**A**), arch (**B**), and carotid artery (**C**) demonstrated strong plaque signal on PET images, in contrast to wild-type mice (**D,E,F**). Aortic root and arch plaque sections (× 100) confirmed plaque presence in apoE$^{-/-}$ (**G,H**) but not wild-type mice (**I,J**). Three-dimensional maximum intensity PET-CT reconstruction images revealed TNP-mediated PET signal (*red*) in the aorta (*blue*) of an apoE$^{-/-}$ mouse (**K**) but not of a wild-type mouse (**L**). (*Adapted from* Nahrendorf *et al.* [24].)

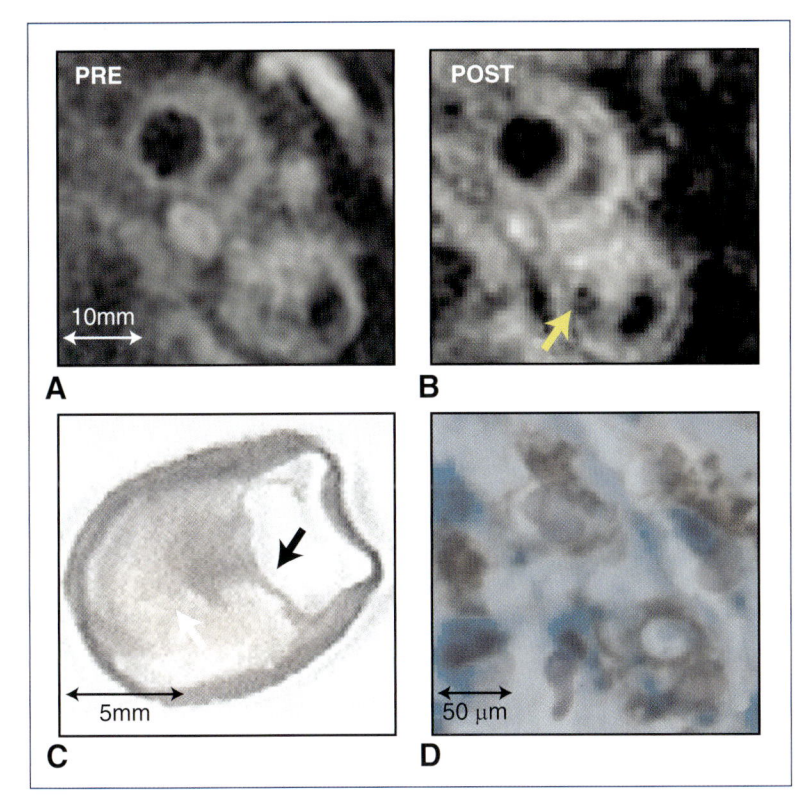

Figure 12-12. Clinical imaging of carotid arterial plaque inflammation using ultrasmall superparamagnetic iron oxide (USPIO) magnetic nanoparticles. Pre-USPIO (**A**) and post-USPIO (**B**) axial MR images localized 3 mm above the left carotid artery division. USPIO particles induced T2*-mediated signal loss within the plaque compared with the baseline (pre-injection) image. **C**, Plaque histology revealed a thin fibrous cap (*black arrowhead*) housing a large lipid core (*white arrowhead*). **D**, High-power double stain for USPIO and macrophages demonstrated colocalization of USPIO (*blue*) with plaque macrophages near the fibrous cap (*brown*; 40× magnification). (*From* Trivedi *et al.* [25]; with permission.)

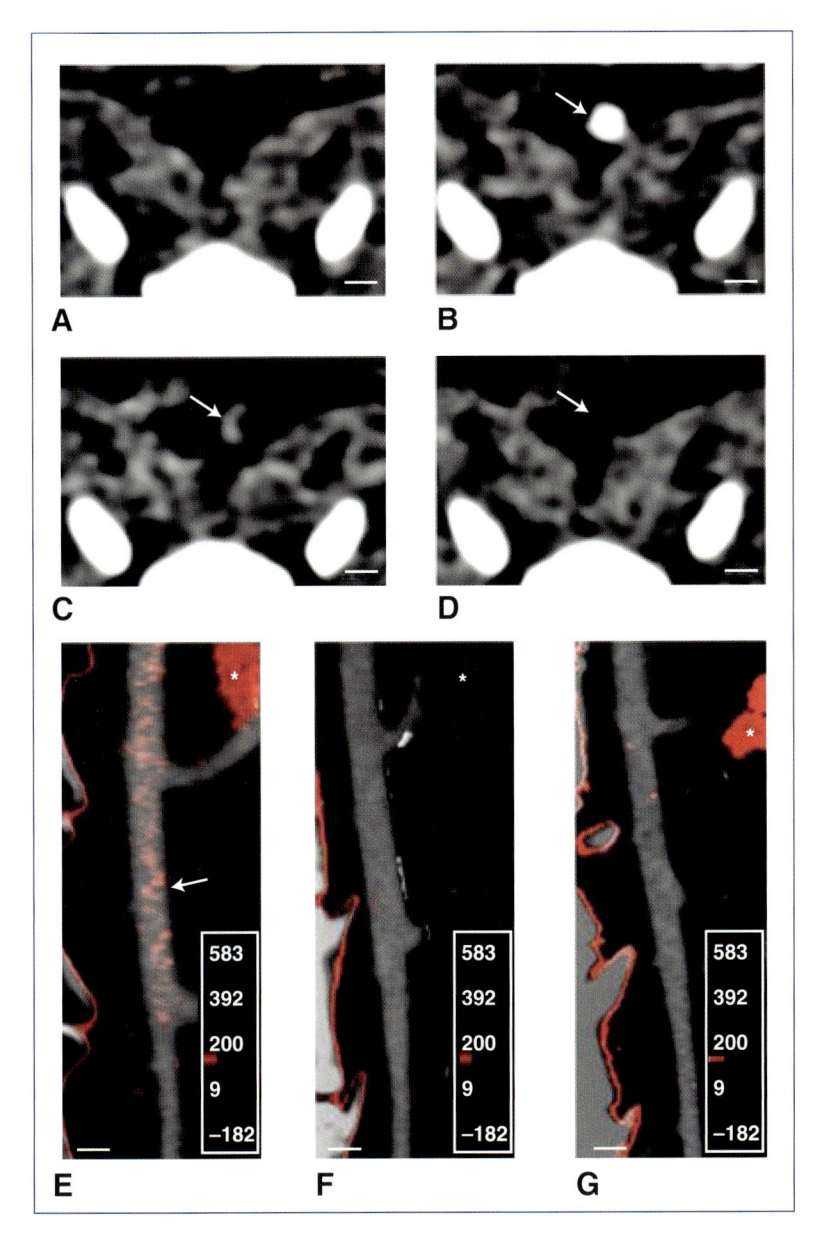

Figure 12-13. Molecular CT imaging using iodinated macrophage-targeted nanoparticles. The dispersed nanoparticle (NP, N1177) was intravenously injected into atherosclerotic and control rabbits (250 mg iodine/kg). The same atherosclerotic rabbits also received the control agent iopamidol, a conventional iodinated angiographic contrast agent, and underwent CT imaging 1 week prior to NP imaging. In the CT protocol, images were obtained during imaging agent infusion and then at 2 hours postinjection. Axial views (**A**–**C**) of the thoracic and abdominal aorta obtained by CT imaging before (**A**) and during (**B**) NP injection. During the infusion period, NP enabled a vascular angiogram, similar to a conventional contrast agent. **C**, At 2 hours post-NP injection, enhanced CT signal was detectable in atherosclerotic plaques. **D**, In contrast, plaque-specific enhancement did not occur in atherosclerotic rabbits injected with iopamidol on the 2-hour delayed CT image. **E**–**G**, Delayed aortic CT images (intensity pseudocolored *red*) superimposed on the initial CT angiogram image obtained during agent infusion. **E**, NP-injected rabbits showed strong plaque signal (*red*) scattered throughout the aorta. In contrast, minimal signal was present in both atherosclerotic rabbits injected with iopamidol (**F**), or control rabbits injected with NP (**G**). *White asterisk* indicates spleen. Scale bar, 5 mm. (*From* Hyafil *et al.* [26]; with permission.)

Molecular Imaging of Atherosclerosis: A Biological Roadmap 265

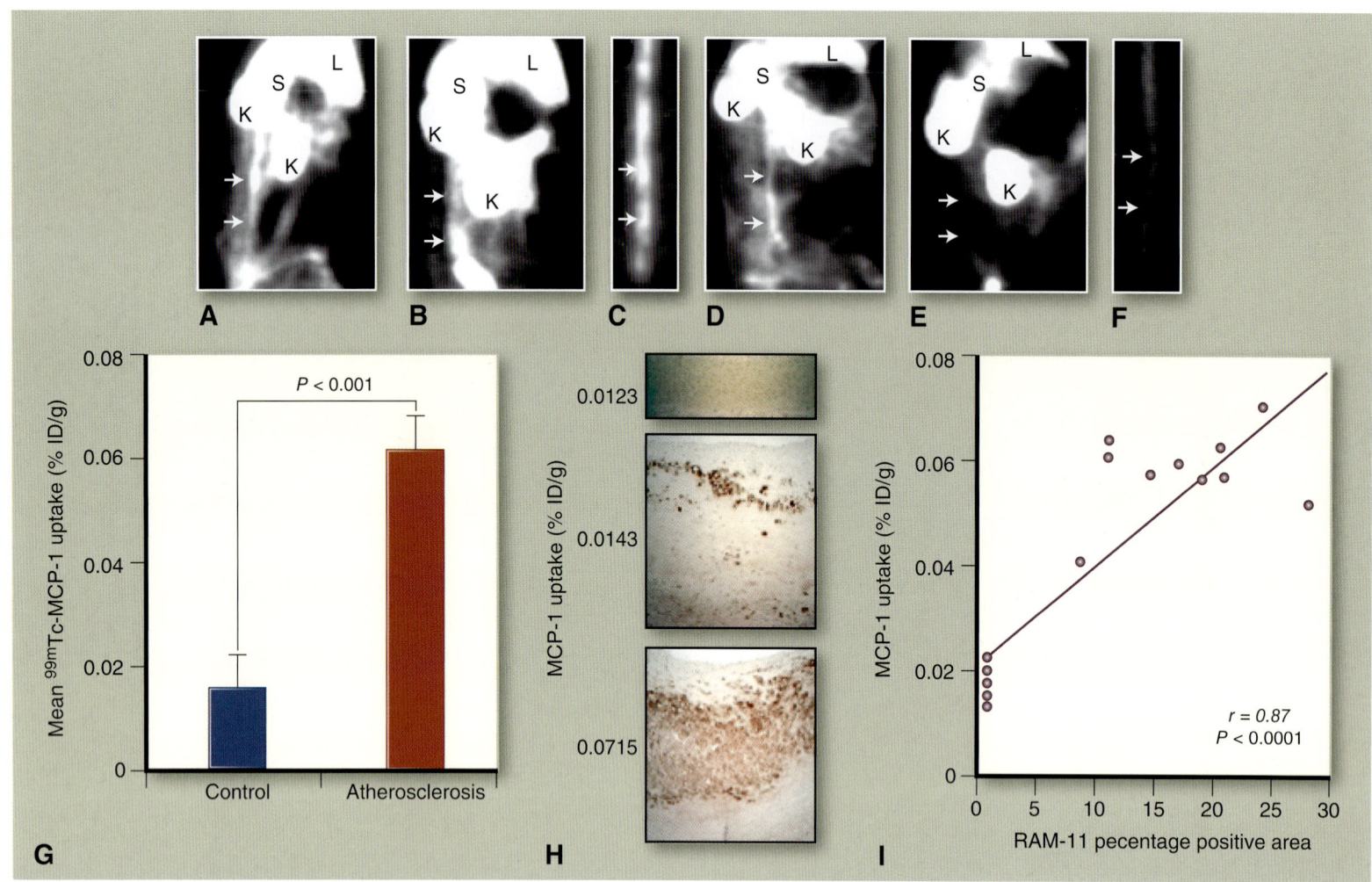

Figure 12-14. Exploiting unique receptor upregulation on infiltrating monocytes. Noninvasive imaging of monocyte chemoattractant protein (MCP)-1 receptor expression with radiolabeled ^{99m}Tc-MCP-1. MCP-1 plays a key role in the transmigration of mononuclear cells into nascent atheroma. Images obtained from both atherosclerotic (**A–C**) and control (nonatherosclerotic, **D–F**) rabbits. **A–C,** Planar images of an atherosclerotic rabbit. The image obtained immediately after intravenous MCP-1 injection outlines aortic blood-pool activity as a vascular angiogram (*arrows*) (**A**). Three hours after radiotracer administration, significant accumulation is detectable in the abdominal aorta (*arrows*) (**B**). Ex vivo images of resected aorta confirms in vivo evidence of MCP-1 uptake (*arrows*) (**C**). **D–F,** Planar images of a control rabbit show immediate postinjection blood pool signal (**D**) but lack of MCP-1 uptake in the abdominal aorta in vivo (**E**) and ex vivo (**F**) images (liver [L]; kidney [K]; spleen [S]). **G,** Bar graphs quantify ^{99m}Tc MCP-1 uptake within abdominal aortas of atherosclerotic and control animals. Radiolabeled MCP-1 uptake (% injected dose [ID]/g tissue) was significantly greater in atherosclerotic animals compared with control animals.

Correlation of MCP-1 uptake and macrophage content in abdominal aorta. **H,** RAM-11–positive macrophages in the neointima (×100) are visibly higher in an animal with high radiolabeled MCP-1 uptake (*bottom panel*). In addition, lower RAM-11–positive areas correlated with lower radiolabeled MCP-1 uptake (*middle panel*). Control aortic specimens show absent RAM-1–positive staining (*top panel*). **I,** Correlation between MCP-1 uptake and macrophage presence is strong. (*Adapted from* Hartung et al. [27].)

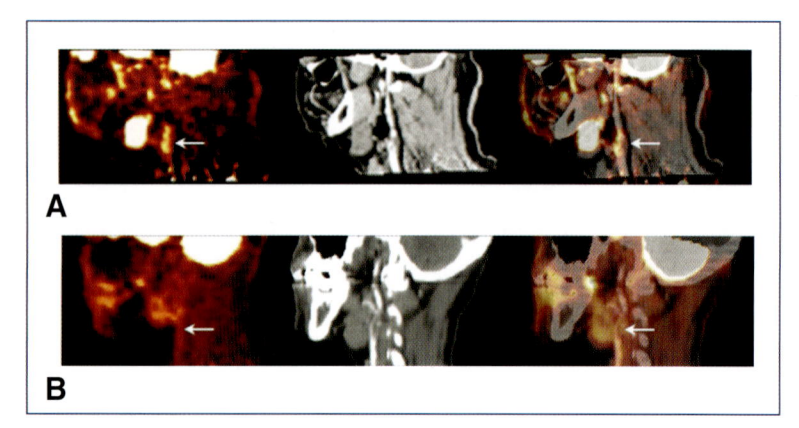

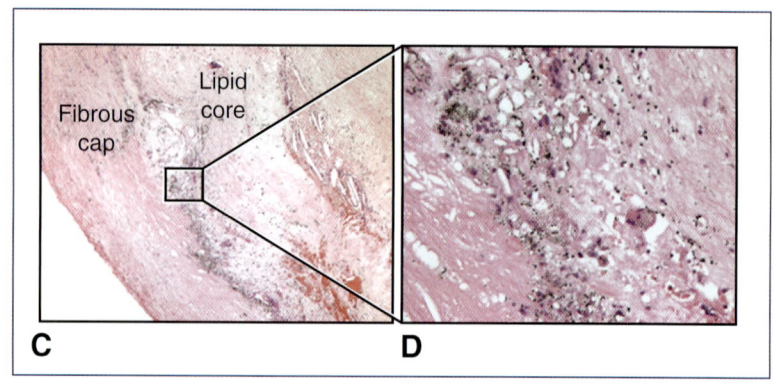

Figure 12-15. Exploiting macrophage metabolism for targeted imaging: ^{18}F-fluorodeoxyglucose (^{18}FDG)-based PET imaging. **A,** PET (*left*), contrast-enhanced CT (*middle*), and co-registered PET/CT (*right*) images of a symptomatic patient who received an intravenous bolus of ^{18}FDG (dose 370 MBq). The PET image demonstrates focal FDG signal within a right carotid plaque (*arrow*), as registered by the CT angiogram and seen on the fusion image. **B,** In contrast the carotid plaque of an asymptomatic patient injected with FDG shows weaker signal. **C** and **D,** A resected carotid plaque from a symptomatic patient was ex vivo incubated with tritiated deoxyglucose enabling microautoradiography. Autoradiography shows colocalization of silver grains (tritiated deoxyglucose) with plaque macrophages (**D,** anti-CD68 antibody, ×200) in areas of the fibrous cap and lipid core [28]. (*Courtesy of* J. Rudd and P. Weissberg, Addenbrooke's Hospital, Cambridge, UK.)

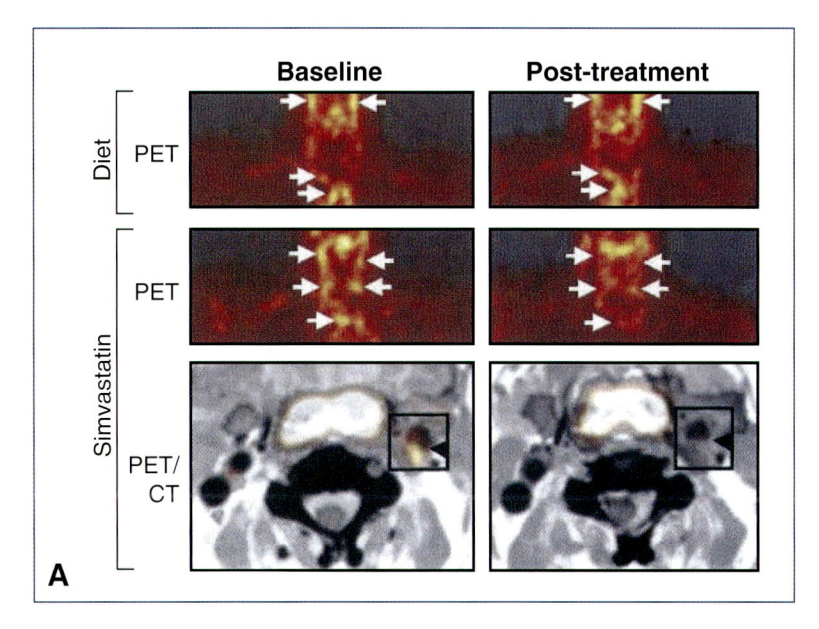

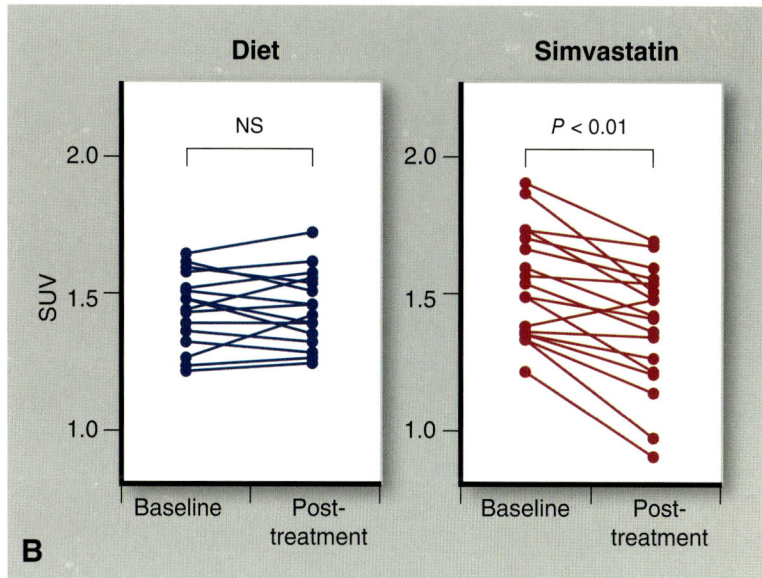

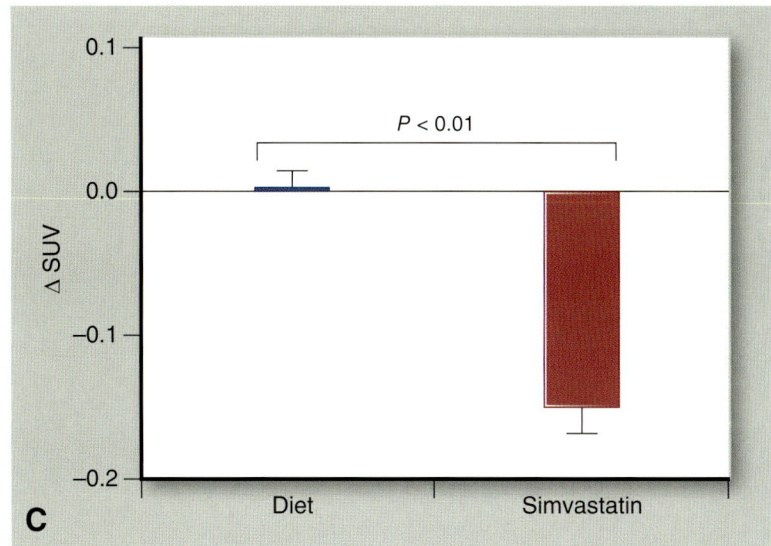

Figure 12-16. Serial fluorodeoxyglucose (FDG) imaging to evaluate the effect of statin therapy in subjects with carotid artery disease. Cancer patients with occult atherosclerosis detected on FDG staging scans were randomized to dietary change or dietary changes plus statin therapy (simvastatin) for 3 months. Patients underwent FDG-enhanced PET imaging of carotid artery plaque metabolism (dose 4.2 MBq), followed-by contrast-enhanced carotid CT angiography. **A**, In patients randomized to dietary changes alone, the carotid plaque FDG PET signal was similar at at baseline and after 3 months of treatment. In contrast, patients treated with dietary changes and simvastatin showed reduced FDG plaque signal in just 3 months. **B** and **C**, Quantification of the carotid plaque metabolic PET signal via maximum standardized uptake values (SUVs). Diet plus statin-treated patients showed reduced SUVs after 3 months of therapy, as opposed to the minimal SUV changes observed in the dietary group. Δ*SUV* indicates change in the SUV following treatment. *Bar* indicates 1 standard deviation. (*Adapted from* Tahara *et al.* [29].)

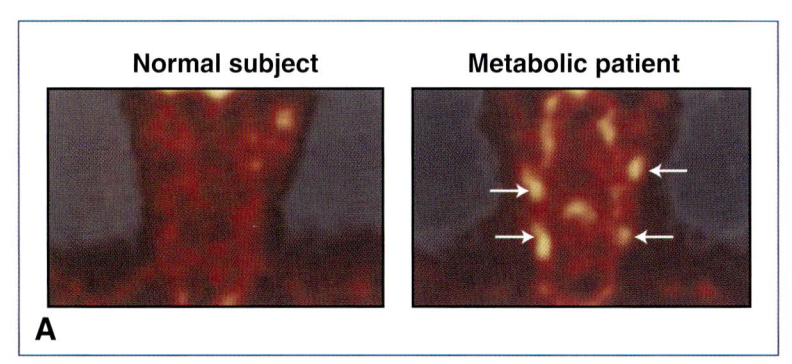

Figure 12-17. Fluorodeoxyglucose (FDG)-PET imaging of carotid plaques in the metabolic syndrome. **A**, Greater FDG uptake within the carotid arteries in a patient with the metabolic syndrome (*right*) compared with a control patient (*left*). **B**, Transaxial FDG-PET, contrast-enhanced CT, and the coregistration of PET and CT (PET/CT) images showing FDG uptake within the carotid artery of a metabolic syndrome patient. *Black arrow-arrowhead* denotes vessel wall or atherosclerotic plaque on CT. *Red arrow-arrowhead* indicates vascular FDG uptake. (*From* Tahara *et al.* [30]; with permission.)

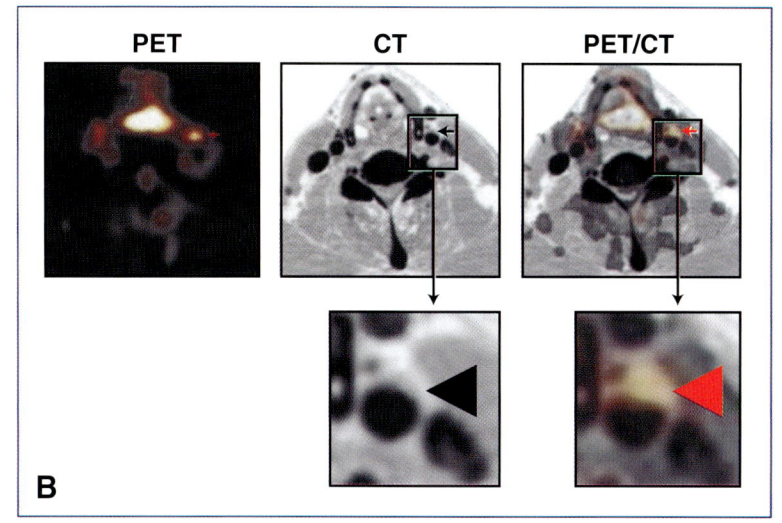

Molecular Imaging of Atherosclerosis: A Biological Roadmap

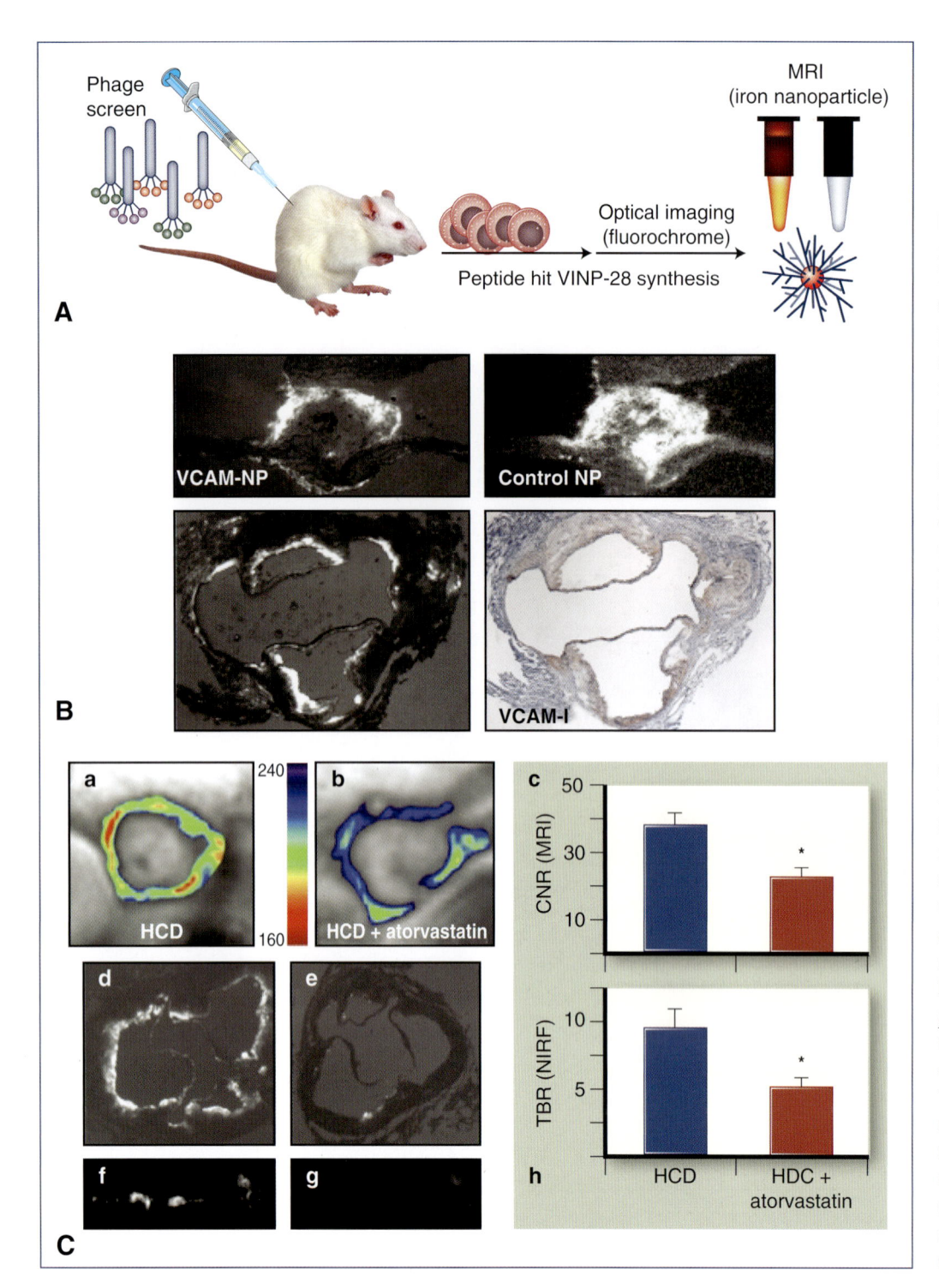

Figure 12-18. Imaging of upregulated adhesion molecule expression. Noninvasive MRI of vascular cell adhesion molecule-1 (VCAM-1) expression in atherosclerosis is modulated by statin pharmacotherapy. **A**, Discovery and synthesis of a VCAM-1 targeted nanoparticle agent. Iterative in vivo phage display of atheroma of apoE[-/-] mice produced a linear peptide with strong avidity for VCAM-1. An MRI and near infrared fluorescence (NIRF)-detectable ultrasmall superparamagnetic iron oxide (USPIO) nanoparticle (NP) was next conjugated to multiple copies of the VCAM-1 targeted peptide to form VCAM-NP (VINP-28). **B**, ApoE[-/-] mice were injected with both VCAM and a control NP, an underivatized and spectrally distinct USPIO nanoparticle. Multiwavelength microscopy revealed that VCAM-NP localized the superficial intimal layer (*top left*) in contrast to the broadly distributed control magnetic nanoparticles (MNP) (*top right*). On aortic plaque sections, VCAM-NP fluorescence (*bottom left*) colocalized with immunoreactive VCAM-1 (*bottom right*, original magnification, ×200). **C**, Noninvasive MRI assessment of VCAM-1 expression after short-term statin therapy. MRI of the aortic root of apoE[-/-] mouse on a high-cholesterol diet (HCD) reveals strong VCAM-NP uptake (*a*, reflected by lower MRI signal due to MNP deposition, *red pseudocolor*). In contrast, statin-treated animals (HCD + atorvastatin) showed less VCAM-NP uptake (*b, blue pseudocolor*, $P < 0.05$). Reduced VCAM-NP uptake and lower contrast-to-noise (CNR) ratio ($P < 0.05$) was evident in statin-treated animals (*c*). Fluorescence microscopy (*d*, HCD; *e*, HCD + statin) and macroscopic fluorescence reflectance images provided similar results (*f–h*). TBR—target-to-background ratio. (*Adapted from* Nahrendorf *et al.* [31].)

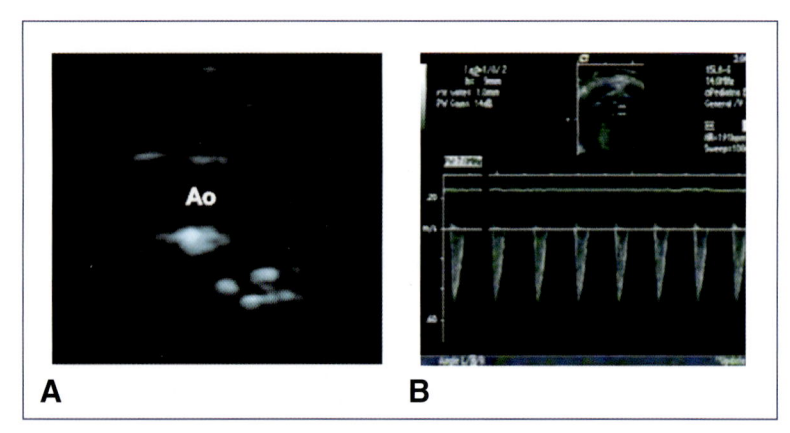

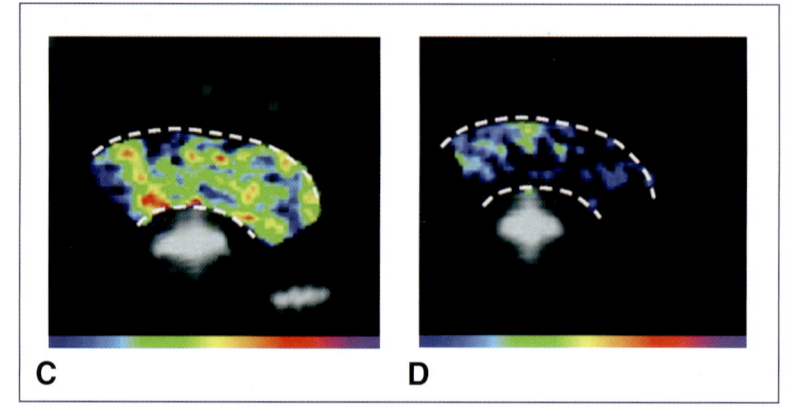

Figure 12-19. Ultrasound imaging of vascular cell adhesion molecule-1 (VCAM-1) expression in atheroma using targeted microbubbles. Representative images from an ApoE[-/-] mouse on a high-cholesterol diet. **A**, The aortic arch (Ao) on two-dimensional ultrasound imaging. **B**, Pulsed-wave Doppler imaging of the arch. **C** and **D**, Contrast-enhanced ultrasound aortic arch images 10 minutes after intravenous injection of VCAM-1 targeted microbubbles (**C**) demonstrates greater plaque signal than images from mice injected with control microbubbles (**D**). Each targeted image was adjusted for signal from freely circulating microbubbles. (*From* Kauffmann *et al.* [32]; with permission.)

268 Atlas of Nuclear Cardiology

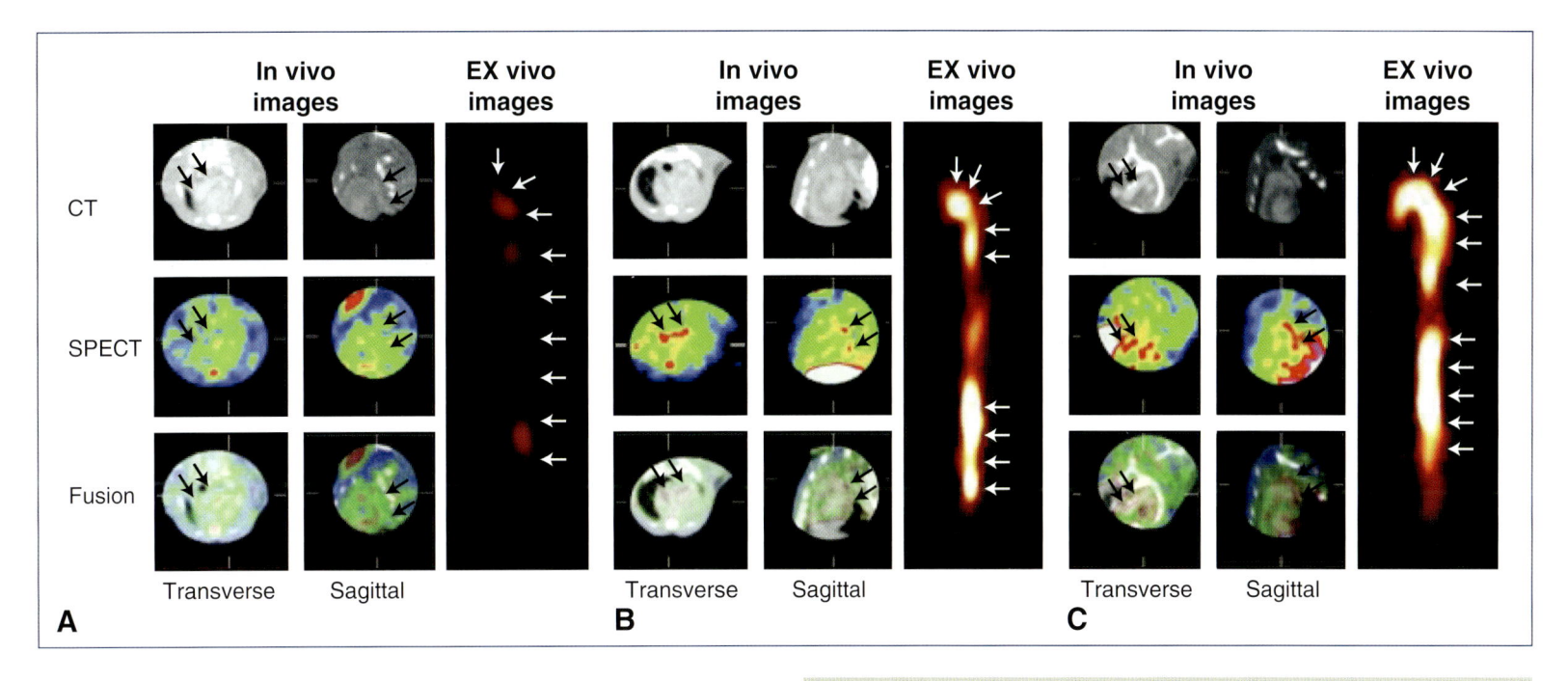

Figure 12-20. Exploiting imaging of macrophage death in atheroma. Noninvasive integrated micro-SPECT–micro-CT imaging of plaque apoptosis in apoE$^{-/-}$ mice. To bind phosphatidylserine residues on apoptotic cells, radiolabeled annexin A5 (^{99m}Tc-annexin A5, 175 MBq) was intravenously injected into aged apoE$^{-/-}$ mice (62 weeks old). Coregistered in vivo and ex vivo CT, SPECT, SPECT–CT fusion images, and ex vivo planar images of a control mouse (**A**); apoE$^{-/-}$ mouse without high-cholesterol diet (**B**); and apoE$^{-/-}$ mouse on a high-cholesterol diet (**C**). Mild annexin A5 signal was detected in control mice (**A**). Strong uptake was evident in plaques located in the aortic arch and abdominal aorta of chow-fed apoE$^{-/-}$ mice (**B**). Even greater annexin A5 signal was detected in cholesterol-fed (Ch) apoE$^{-/-}$ mice (**C**). CT-detected aortic arch calcification (**C**, transverse section, *arrows*) facilitated coregistration of the images. **D**, Significant aortic radioactivity differences were evident in the three experimental groups (% injected dose [ID]/g). (*Adapted from* Isobe *et al.* [33].)

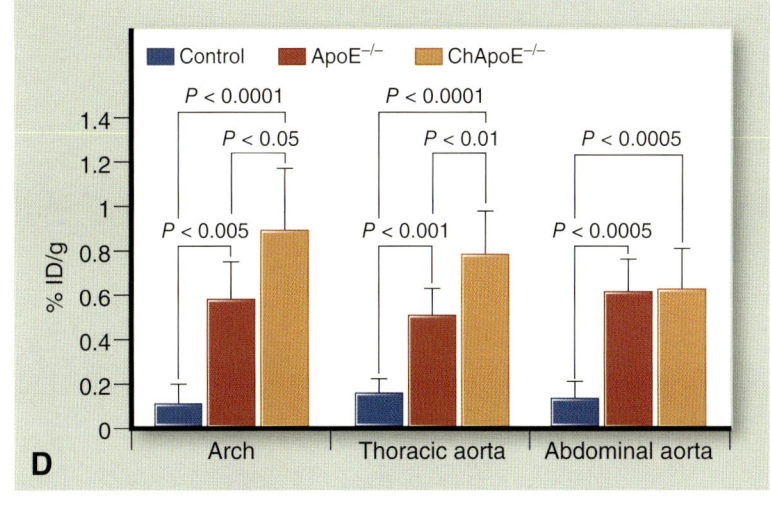

Figure 12-21. Noninvasive imaging of apoptosis by radiolabeled AA5 in a rabbit model of atherosclerosis. The atherosclerotic lesions were produced in rabbits by balloon deendothelialization of the abdominal aorta, following which they received a high-cholesterol, high-fat diet for 4 months. **A**, Left lateral oblique in vivo gamma image 2 hours after intravenous administration of ^{99m}Tc-AA5 (*L* and *K* mark liver and kidney activities, respectively). AA5 uptake is clearly visible in the abdominal aorta (*arrows, left*) subsequently confirmed in the ex vivo image of the explanted aorta (*middle*).

Continued on the next page

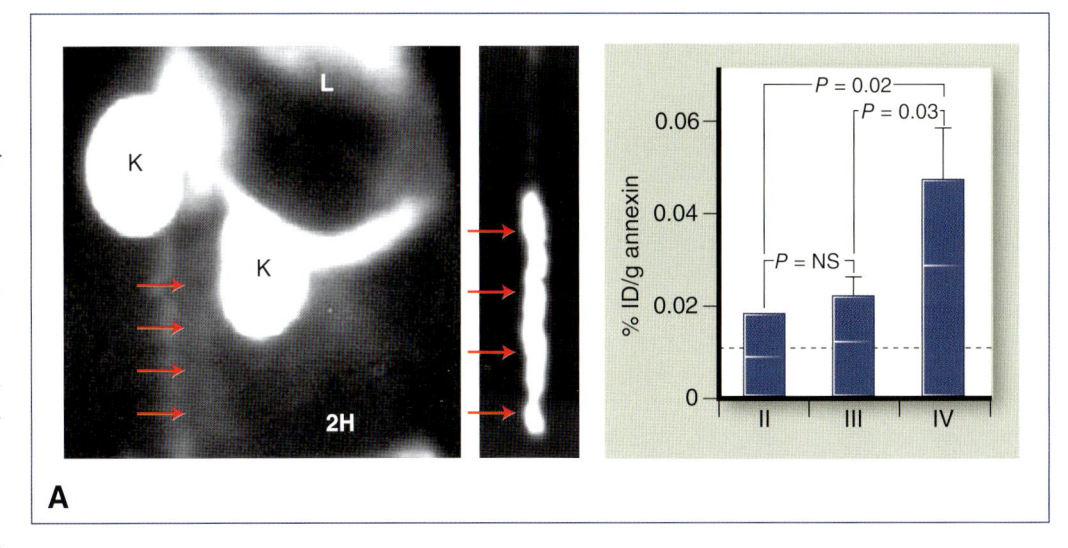

Molecular Imaging of Atherosclerosis: A Biological Roadmap 269

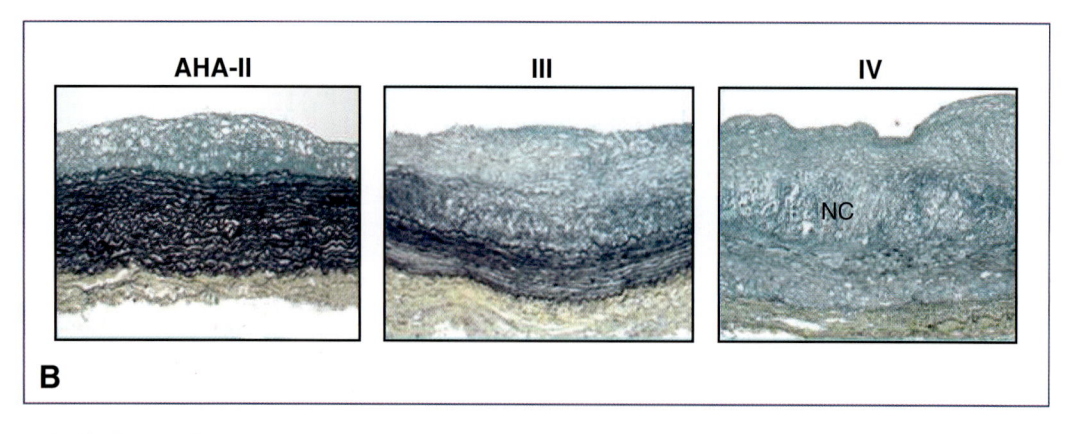

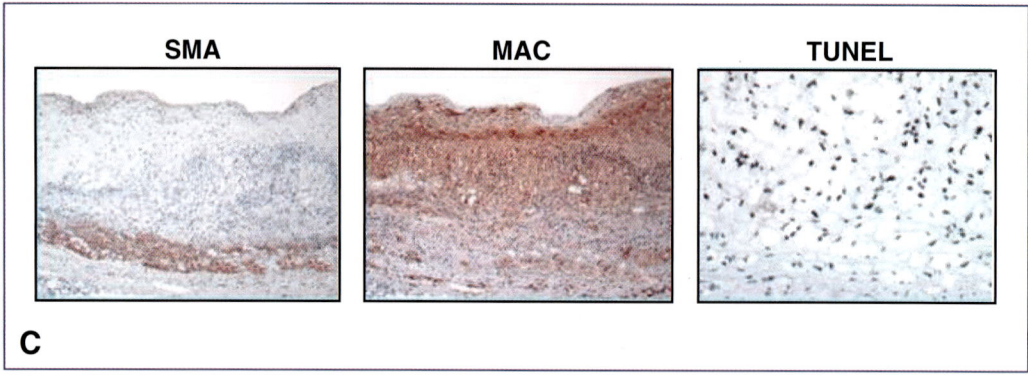

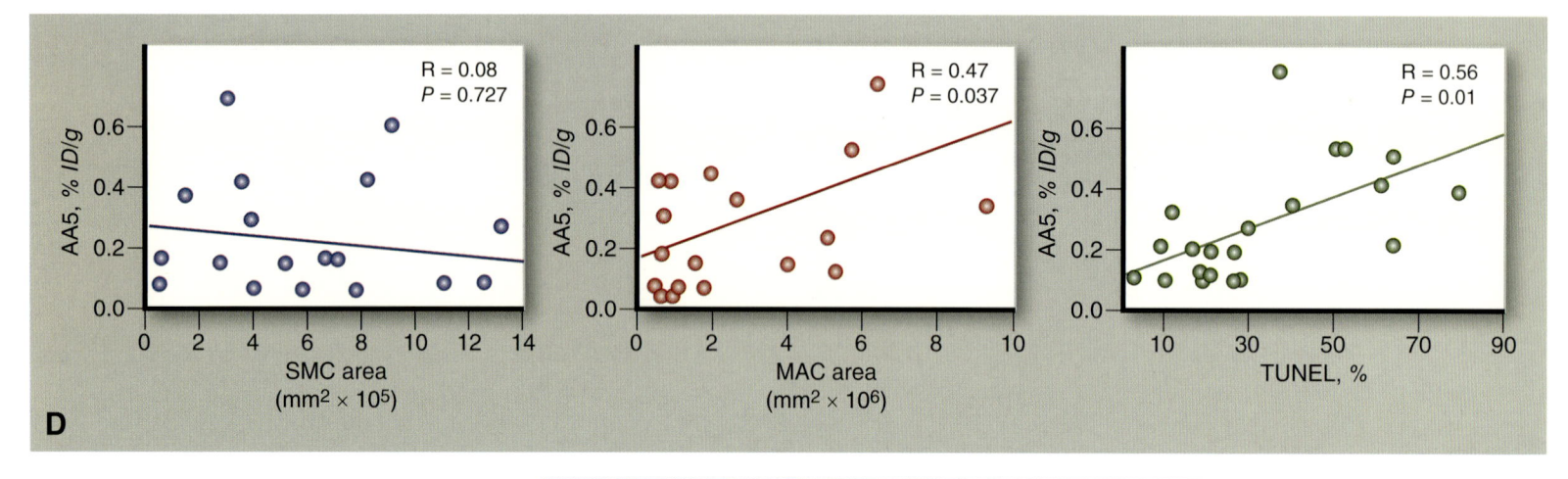

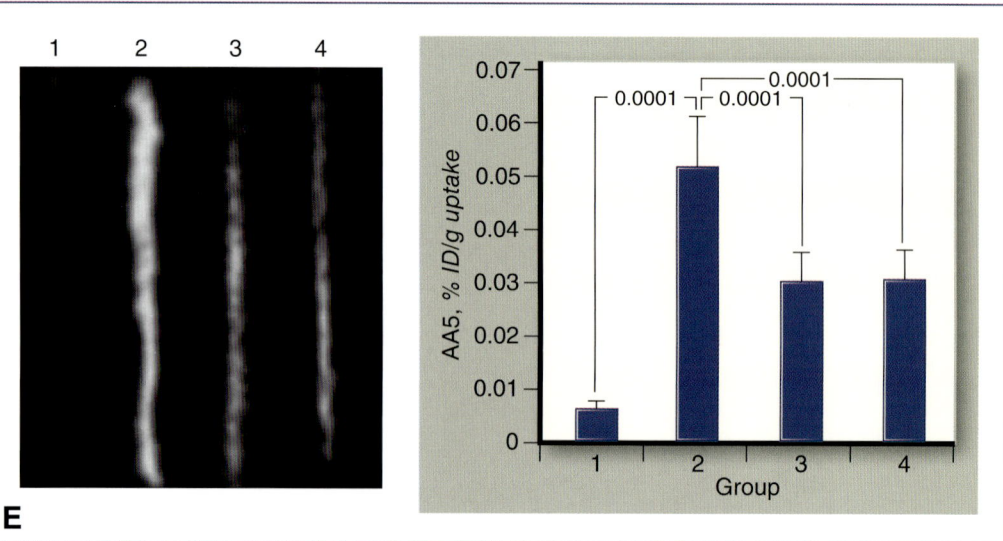

Figure 12-21. *(Continued)* No AA5 uptake was seen in the control unmanipulated animals and the aorta was indistinguishable from the background at 2 hours after AA5 administration (not shown). The atherosclerotic lesions were characterized using the American Heart Association (AHA) classification scheme (**B**) as AHA type II (× 100), III (× 100) and IV lesions (× 200). The AA5 uptake was significantly higher in type IV lesions; no differences in AA5 uptake were noted between types II and III lesions (**A**, *box plot*). **C**, Further characterization was performed for the presence of smooth muscle cells (SMA, brown staining with HHF-35 antibody), macrophages (MAC, brown staining with RAM-11 antibody), and apoptosis (blue-black nuclear TUNEL staining). Simple regression analyses (**D**) demonstrated no significant relationship between AA5 uptake and SMC burden but showed directly proportional relationships to the prevalence of macrophages and the extent of TUNEL-positive apoptosis cells.

Apoptosis is significantly reduced after dietary modification and statin therapy as assessed by radiolabeled AA5 uptake. **E**, Ex vivo images of explanted aortas (groups 1–4) show intense AA5 uptake in rabbits fed a high-cholesterol diet for 4 months (group 2); only negligible AA5 uptake is seen in the diet withdrawal (group 3) and statin therapy (group 4) groups. No annexin AA5 uptake is observed in control rabbits receiving normal chow diet for 4 months (group 1).

270 Atlas of Nuclear Cardiology

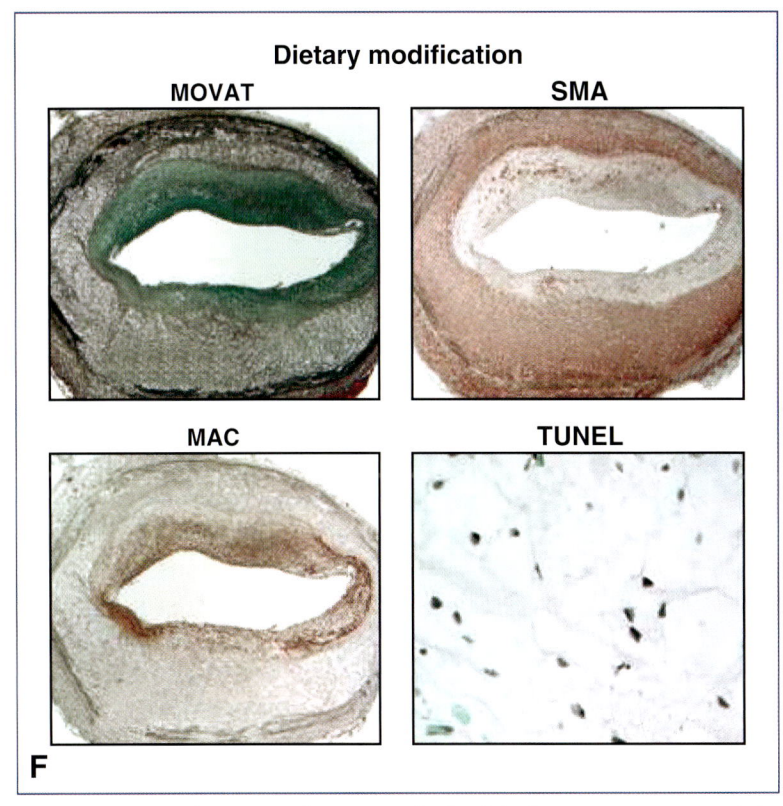

Figure 12-21. *(Continued)* Bar graph *(right)* shows quantitative AA5 uptake represented as mean ± SD and corresponds to the ex vivo images. Resolution of AA5 uptake also corresponds to decreased apoptosis (compare with the previous figure) observed after diet withdrawal (**F**) and statin therapy (**G**) (× 200). Micrographs of cross sections of abdominal aortas stained with Movat pentachrome, and those for SMC (× 30) and MAC (× 30) show decreased macrophage populations and increased SMC content, and represent histologic evidence of stabilization of plaques. (**A–D**, *adapted from* Kolodgie et al. [34]; **E–G**, *adapted from* Hartung et al. [35].)

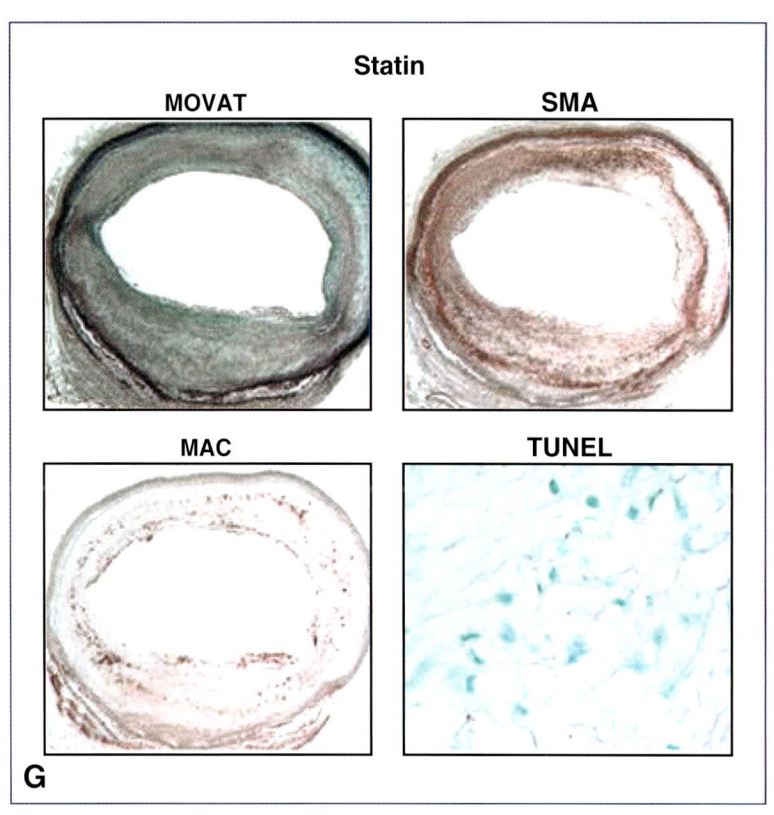

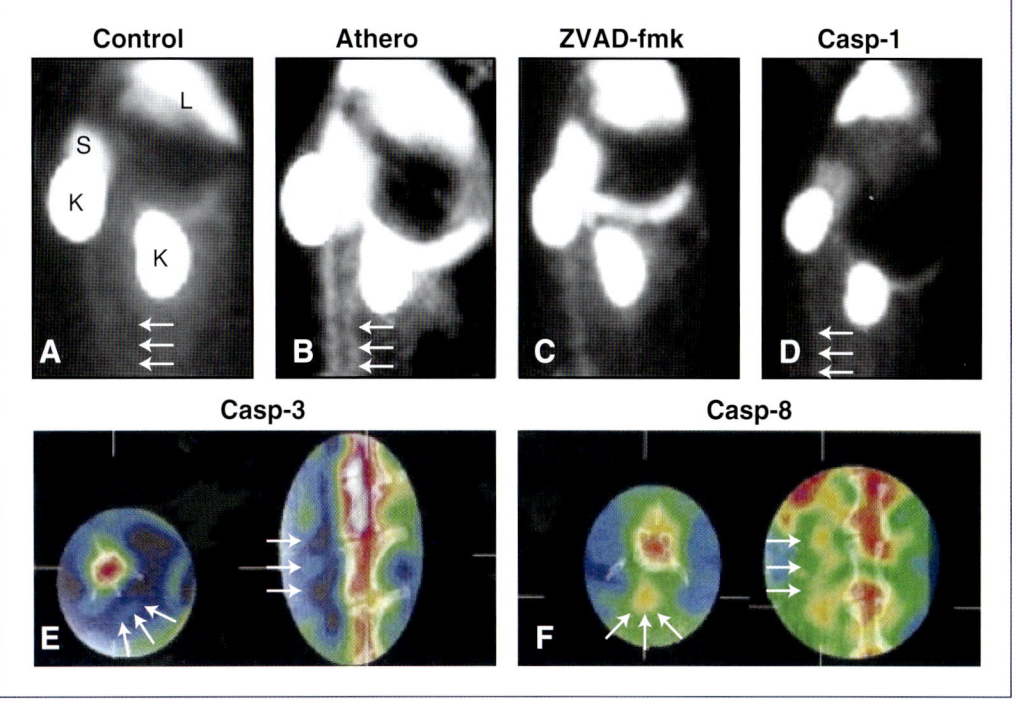

Figure 12-22. Noninvasive SPECT imaging of acute resolution of apoptosis by administration of caspase inhibitors. Radiolabeled annexin A5-enhanced SPECT images were obtained in both control (nonatherosclerotic) and atherosclerotic rabbits treated with or without caspase inhibitor therapy. **A–D,** Planar gamma images. **E** and **F,** Micro-SPECT images superimposed on anatomical micro-CT images. **A,** Absent annexin uptake in the region of the abdominal aorta (*arrows*) in a normal rabbit. Metabolism and excretion of annexin A5 results in signal from the liver (L), spleen (S), and kidney (K). **B,** In contrast to the control rabbit, significant annexin A5 accumulation is visible in the abdominal aorta (*arrows* in front of vertebral column activity) of a rabbit with experimental atherosclerotic lesions. Rabbits receiving a nonselective caspase inhibitor (ZVAD-fmk) (**C**) or selective caspase-1 inhibitor (**D**) demonstrate significant reductions of annexin plaque uptake. **E** and **F,** Transverse and sagittal fusion nuclear and CT images following treatment with a selective caspase-3 inhibitor and a caspase-8 inhibitor. While the caspase-3 inhibitor completely prevented annexin A5 uptake (*arrows*, identifying the aorta in front of vertebral uptake), caspase-8 inhibition did not affect annexin uptake or apoptosis. In caspase-8 inhibitor–treated animals, vivid uptake of radiotracer is seen in the abdominal aorta. Lack of effect of caspase-8 inhibitor, but efficacy of caspase-1, -9, and -3 inhibitors suggested the involvement of mitochondrial pathways of apoptosis. (*From* Sarai et al. [36]; with permission.)

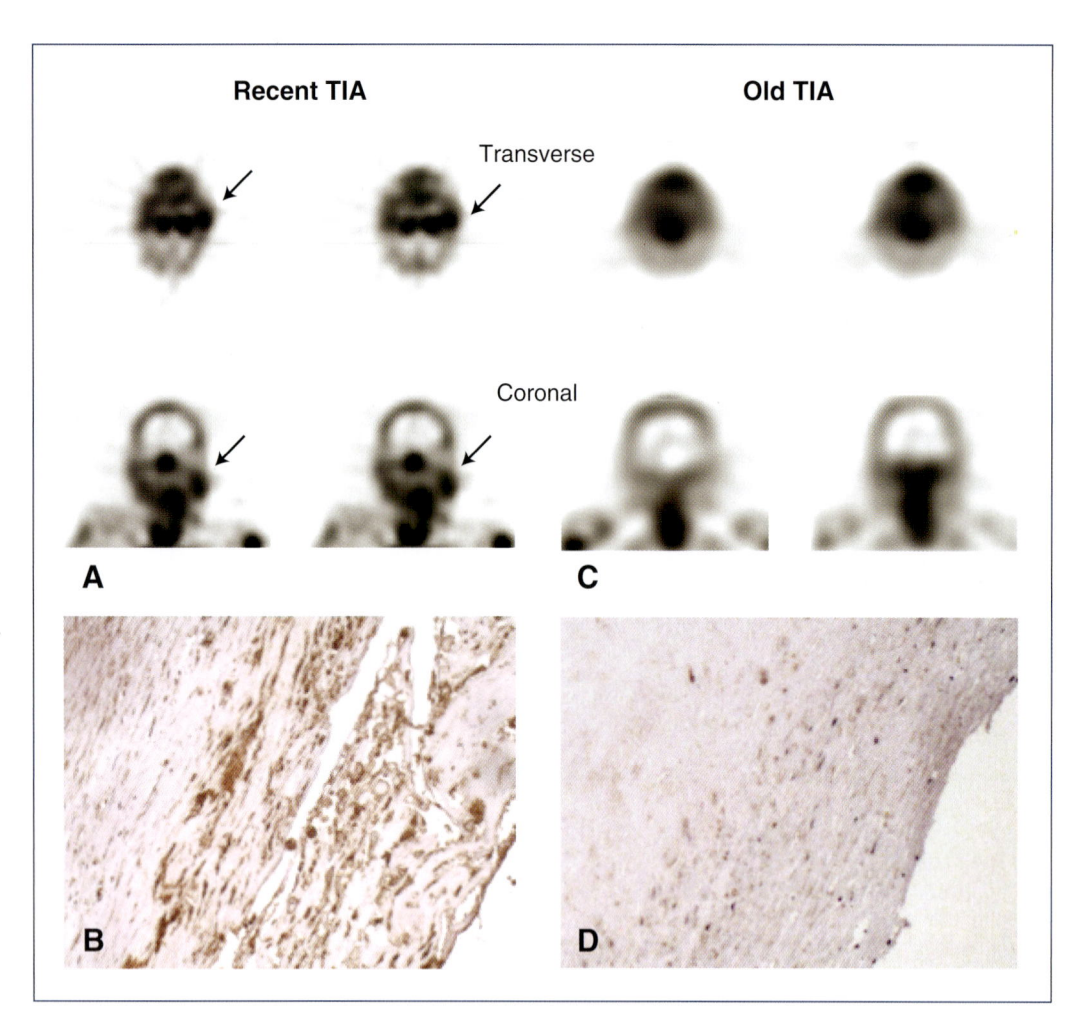

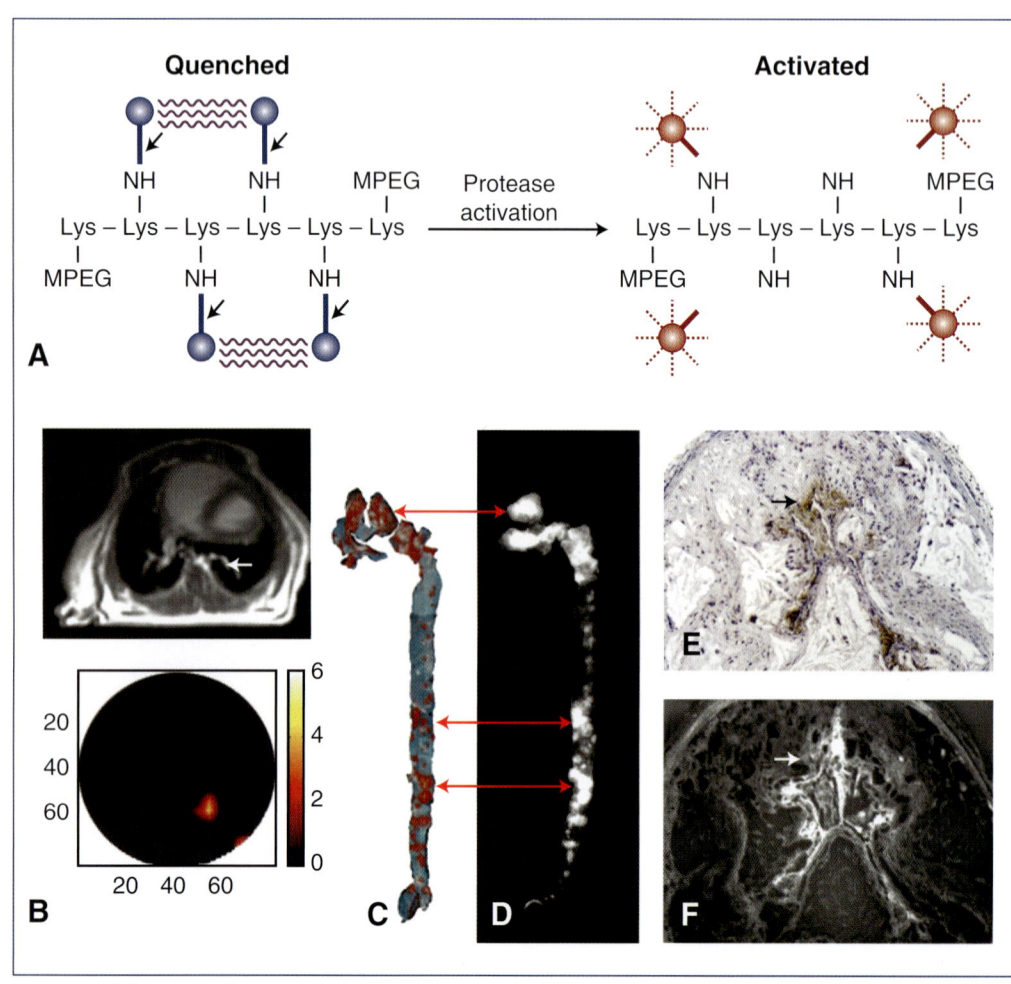

Figure 12-23. Clinical imaging of carotid plaque apoptosis. ^{99m}Tc-annexin A5 accumulated in a carotid lesion (**A**, SPECT images, *arrows*) of a patient with a recent transient ischemic attack (TIA). **B** and **D**, Annexin A5 in sections of the resected plaque stains (**B**, anti-annexin A5 polyclonal antibody, original magnification ×400) in a macrophage-rich area. In contrast, no annexin A5 uptake occurs (**C**) in the carotid artery of a patient with a remote TIA. **D**, Annexin A5 immunoreactivity is at a background level in the corresponding smooth muscle cell–rich lesion. (*Adapted from* Kietselaer et al. [37].)

Figure 12-24. Exploiting imaging of proteases released by inflammatory cells; near infrared fluorescence (NIRF) molecular imaging of augmented cysteine protease activity. **A**, Mechanism of activation for a lysine-cleavable protease-activatable agent. The injectable imaging agent is a long-circulating compound (~ 550 kD) that has been tested in clinical trials. Multiple NIR fluorochromes are then conjugated to the backbone. Due to the close proximity of the fluorochromes, self-quenching of the imaging agent occurs through fluorescence resonance energy transfer and favorably minimizes the background signal of the agent. Proteases at the target of interest then cleave the agent, liberating fluorescence and generating high target-to-background ratios. **B–F**, In vivo molecular imaging of augmented cysteine proteolytic activity in plaques of apoE$^{-/-}$ mice. **B**, Anatomical black-blood aortic MRI of an apoE$^{-/-}$ mouse (*arrow*). **C**, Following injection of the protease-activatable agent, noninvasive fluorescence-mediated tomography reveals a focal NIRF signal in the aorta consistent with plaque signal. Sudan IV fat staining of the aorta correlates well with NIR fluorescent plaques seen on ex vivo fluorescence reflectance imaging (**D**). **E**, Cathepsin B, a cysteine protease implicated in atherosclerosis and able to activate the imaging agent, colocalized with microscopic NIRF signal in atheromata (**F**). (*Adapted from* Chen et al. [38].)

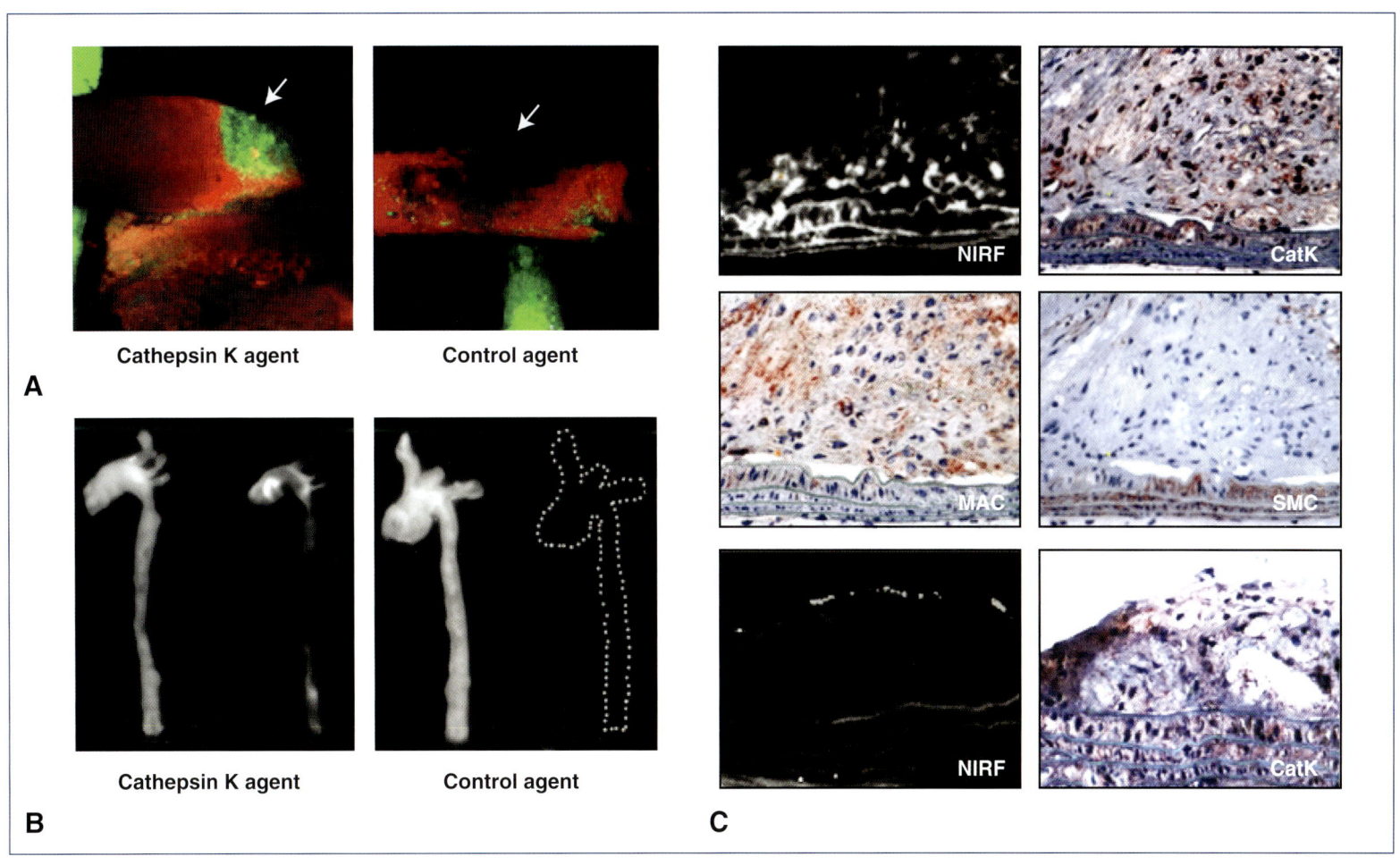

Figure 12-25. Intravital fluorescence microscopy (IVFM) of cathepsin K (CatK) protease activity. A CatK-activatable near infrared fluorescence (NIRF) agent (similar to the Prosense agent but modified with a CatK selective peptide), or control agent, was injected into apoE$^{-/-}$ mice. After 24 hours, plaques were surgically exposed and underwent multichannel, high-resolution IVFM (5× magnification, 13×13×10 micrometer resolution). **A**, Fusion image (*green* = CatK or control agent, *red* = intravascular agent) of a carotid artery demonstrated abundant CatK signal (*green*) in an atheroma involving the distal bifurcation. A separately injected intravascular agent provided an angiogram (*red*). In contrast, the control agent demonstrated a low 680-nm channel signal in carotid plaques, resulting in a filling defect on the fusion image (*arrow*). **B**, Corresponding light (*left side* of each panel) and NIRF reflectance images (*right side* of each panel) confirmed plentiful NIRF signal in the CatK agent group but not the control agent group. **C**, Fluorescence microscopy confirmed abundant NIRF signal in plaque sections in the CatK agent group (*top left*) but not in the control agent group (*lower left*). The NIRF signal indicating CatK activity arises from plaque macrophages (MAC) rather than smooth muscles cells (SMC). (Original magnification, ×400.) (*Adapted from* Jaffer *et al*. [39].)

Molecular Imaging of Atherosclerosis: A Biological Roadmap

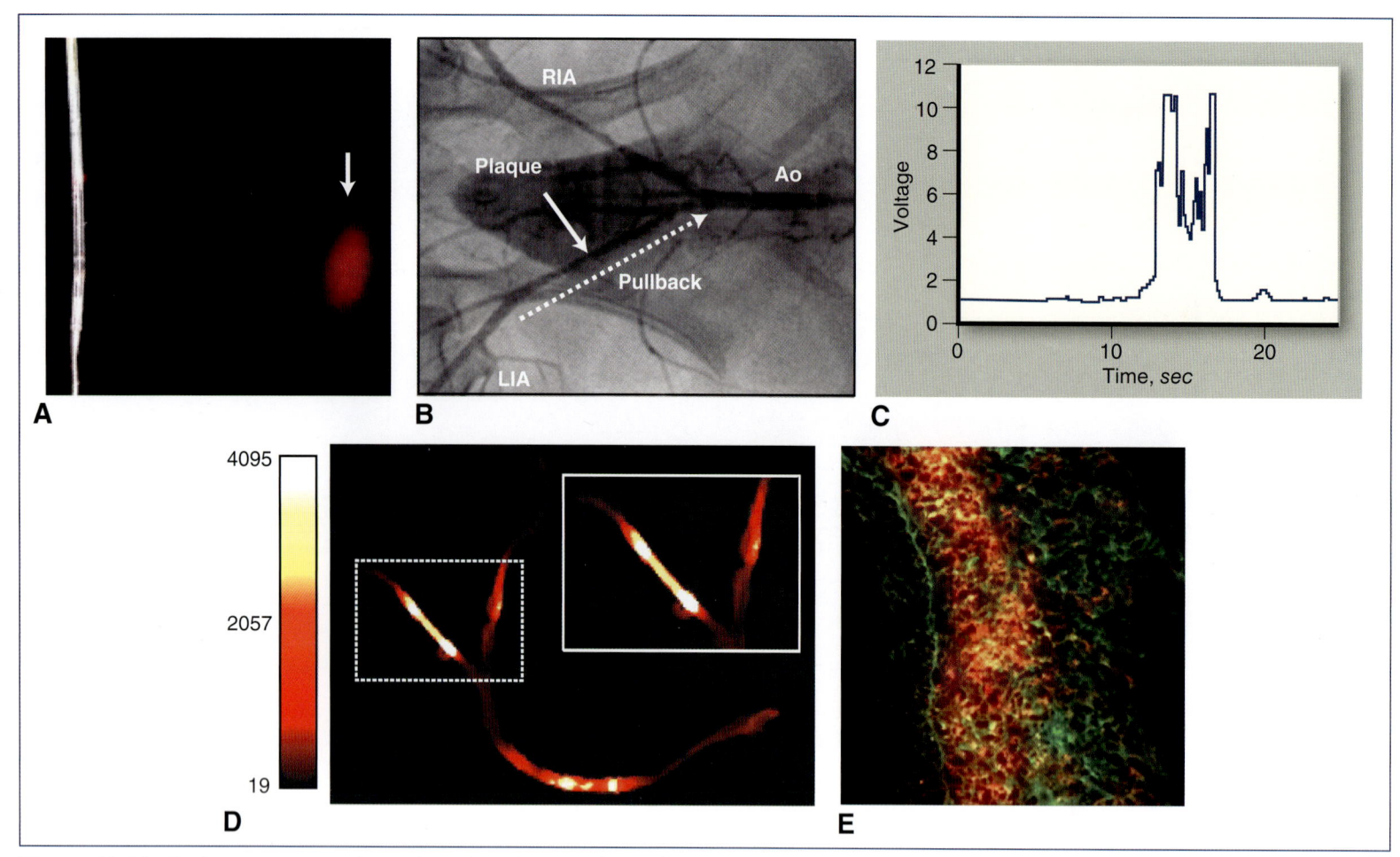

Figure 12-26. Real-time intravascular catheter-based near infrared fluorescence (NIRF) imaging of augmented protease activity. **A,** An intravascular catheter was re-engineered from a clinical optical coherence tomography (OCT) guidewire used in human coronary atherosclerosis imaging. NIR light (*red*) is emitted in a 90-degree arc and focused 2-mm away from the aperture. **B,** X-ray angiogram of atherosclerotic iliac arteries following balloon injury and hyperlipidemic diet in rabbits. After 24 hours following Prosense injection, the NIRF guidewire was advanced percutaneously into the left iliac artery (LIA). Pullback was performed manually over 20 seconds through blood, without flushing. Real-time NIRF voltage measurements (**C**) showed signal peaks in zones of plaques but not in control regions. **D,** Ex vivo NIRF images corroborated the in vivo imaging findings. **E,** Merged two-color fluorescence microscopy of a plaque section demonstrated NIRF (*orange*, cysteine protease activity) that was spatially distinct from 500-nm–based autofluorescence (*green*). Ao—aorta; RIA—right iliac artery. (*Adapted from* Jaffer *et al.* [40].)

274 Atlas of Nuclear Cardiology

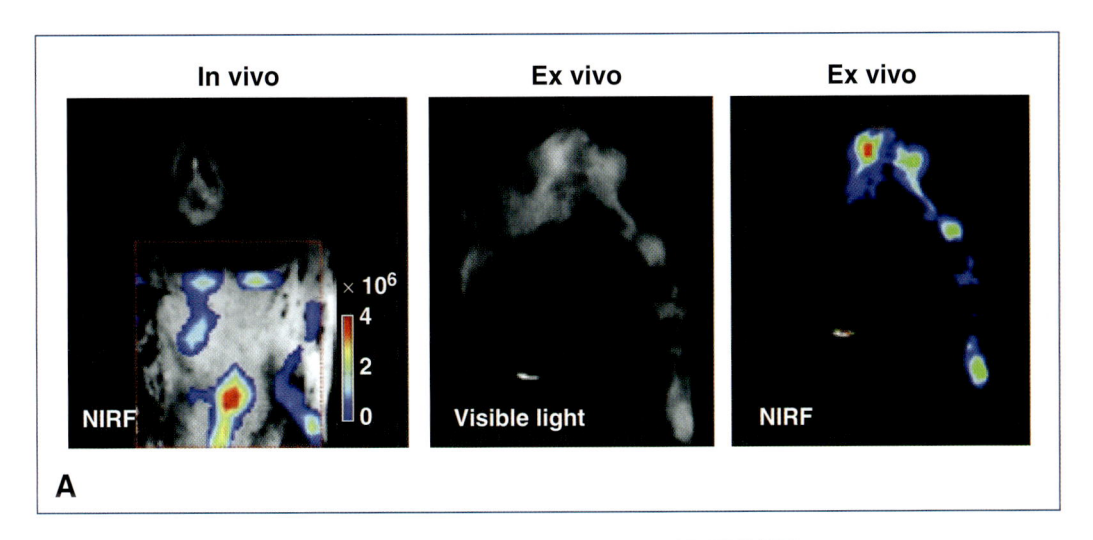

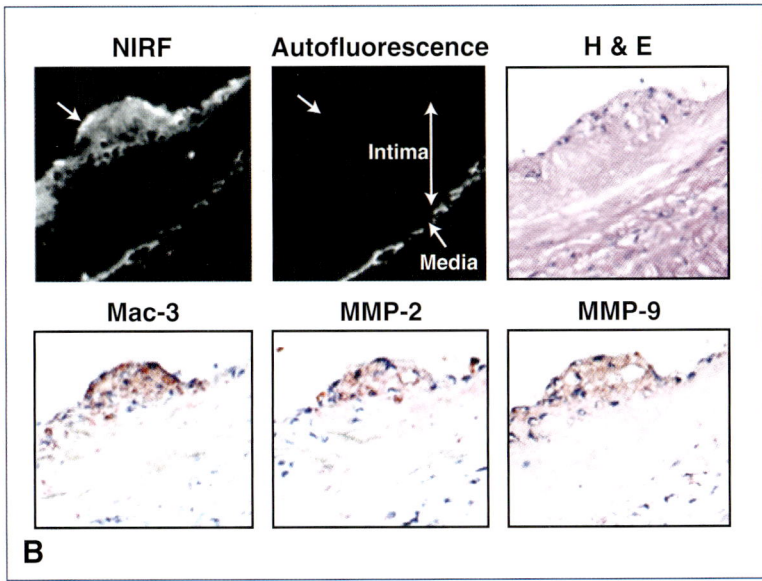

Figure 12-27. Noninvasive fluorescence molecular tomography (FMT) of matrix metalloproteinase (MMP) activity. ApoE$^{-/-}$ mice were injected a gelatinase (MMP-2 and MMP-9) activatable agent for near infrared fluorescence (NIRF) imaging, with similar activation mechanism as the cysteine protease-activatable agents. **A**, FMT of apoE$^{-/-}$ mice 24 hours after MMP-activatable NIRF imaging agent injection (excitation 675 nm, emission 694 nm). Strong NIRF signal (*left*) was visualized in the central chest housing the aortic root and ascending aorta, known prominent sites of atherosclerosis in apoE$^{-/-}$ mice. In vivo plaque signal findings were corroborated by ex vivo fluorescence reflectance imaging (*right*) and light image (*middle*). **B**, Plaque sections from mice injected with the gelatinase agent showed high NIRF signal in the superficial, cell-rich intimal zones. In a 480-nm control (autofluorescence) channel, minimal plaque signal was evident, confirming the specificity of the MMP-activatable NIRF agent. Macrophages (Mac-3), MMP-2, and MMP-9 colocalized with the NIRF signal. H & E—hematoxylin and eosin. (*Adapted from* Deguchi et al. [41].)

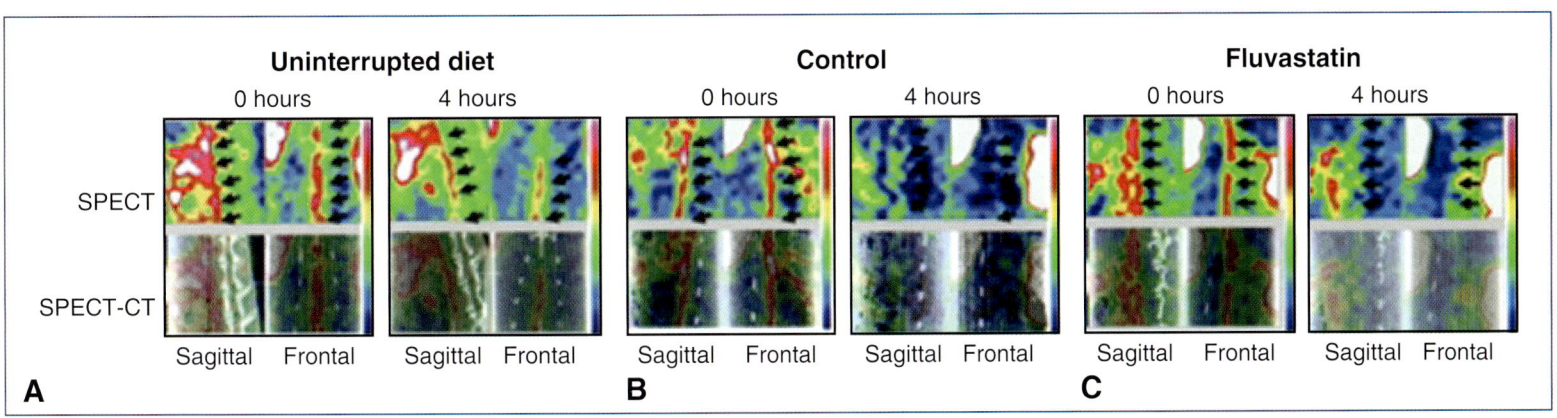

Figure 12-28. SPECT imaging of experimental atherosclerotic lesions using ^{99m}Tc–matrix metalloprotease inhibitor (MPI) in rabbits. **A–C**, Images in a two-by-two format display sagittal and frontal projections in columns, with each row displaying micro-SPECT and SPECT-CT fusion images. The *left* set of two columns displays images immediately postradiotracer administration (blood pool image). The *right set* displays 4-hour images (representing bound tracer uptake in target atheroma tissue). Images were obtained from an atherosclerotic rabbit on uninterrupted cholesterol-supplemented diet (**A**), a control rabbit (without atherosclerotic lesions) (**B**), and a fluvastatin-treated rabbit on a high-cholesteol diet (**C**). Blood pool (*left*) in all animals (**A–C**) is visible (*black arrows*) in front of vertebral column (as identified in the fusion images) in the early images. However, delayed images (*right*) obtained at 4 hours reveal intense MPI uptake only in an atherosclerotic animal on an uninterrupted high-cholesterol diet (**A**). Minimal MPI uptake is present in a control animal without lesions (**B**), and in a statin-treated animal (**C**). (*From* Fujimoto et al. [42]; with permission.)

Molecular Imaging of Atherosclerosis: A Biological Roadmap

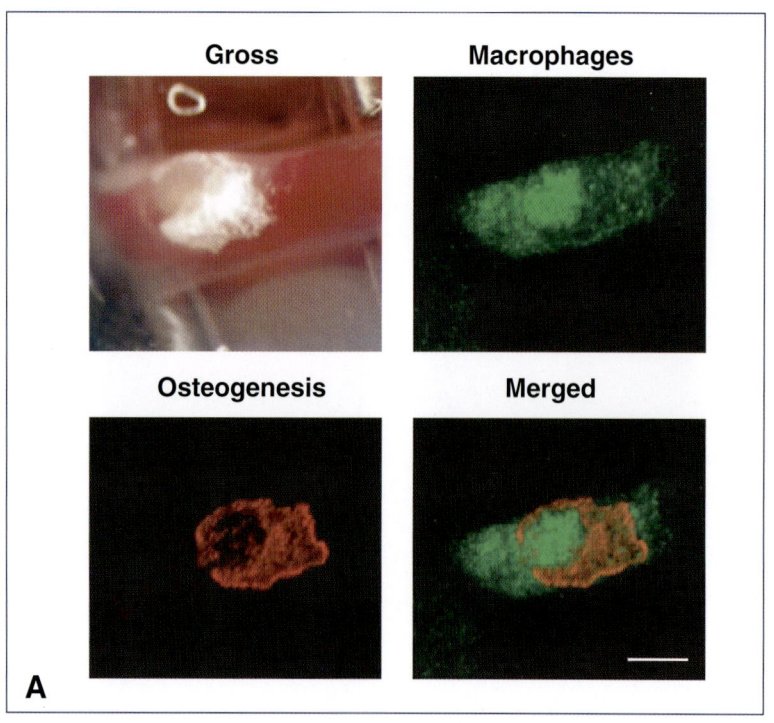

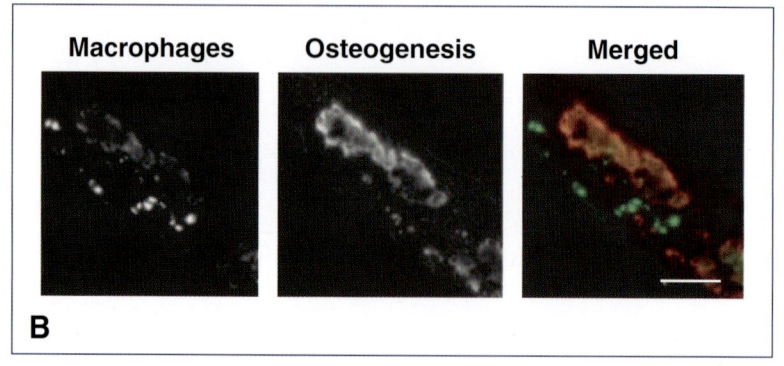

Figure 12-29. Molecular imaging of the spatial distribution of plaque osteogenic activity (microcalcification) and inflammation (macrophages) by multichannel intravital fluorescence microscopy (IVFM). **A**, Aged apoE$^{-/-}$ mice coinjected with a spectrally distinct macrophage-targeted and osteogenic-targeted near infrared fluorescence (NIRF) agent demonstrate plaque osteogenic signal that is spatially distinct from macrophages. Gross morphology of a calcified carotid artery plaque correlated in vivo with macrophages (*green*) and calcification (*red*) on a representative IVFM image (bar = 500 μm) and on cross-sectional fluorescence microscopy (**B**) (*left*, macrophage-targeted signal; *middle*, osteogenic NIRF signal; *right*, merged image) (bar = 200 μm). Calcification appears spatially distinct from macrophage accumulation within atheroma. (*From* Aikawa *et al.* [43]; with permission.)

Future Directions

Most of the molecular imaging studies have been conducted in the experimental models of atherosclerosis or clinically in large immobile vessels (such as carotid arteries, abdominal aorta, and iliofemoral vessels). Such studies have provided the proof of principle. Molecular imaging has hitherto suffered from the limitations of available hardware and the differentiation of target localization in coronary vessels from underlying blood pool tracer activity or myocardial tracer activity. Clinical studies of target localization in coronary vessels have just started to emerge in the literature and have infused tremendous enthusiasm in the imaging community [44].

References

1. Jaffer FA, Weissleder R: Molecular imaging in the clinical arena. *JAMA* 2005, 293:855–862.

2. Jaffer FA, Libby P, Weissleder R: Molecular imaging of cardiovascular disease. *Circulation* 2007, 116:1052–1061.

3. Narula J, Garg P, Achenbach S, *et al.*: Arithmetic of vulnerable plaques for noninvasive imaging. *Nat Cardiovasc Med* 2008, 5:S2–S10.

4. Shapiro E, Bush D, Motoyama S, *et al.*: Imaging atherosclerotic plaques vulnerable to rupture. In *Atlas of Cardiovascular Computed Tomography*. Edited by Budoff MJ, Achenbach S, Narula J. Philadelphia: Current Medicine Group; 2007:119–138.

5. Hansson GK: Inflammation, atherosclerosis, and coronary artery disease. *N Engl J Med* 2005, 352:1685–1695.

6. Ambrose JA, Winters SL, Stern A, *et al.*: Angiographic morphology and the pathogenesis of unstable angina pectoris. *J Am Coll Cardiol* 1985, 5:609–616.

7. Ambrose JA, Winters SL, Arora RR, *et al.*: Coronary angiographic morphology in myocardial infarction: a link between the pathogenesis of unstable angina and myocardial infarction. *J Am Coll Cardiol* 1985, 6:1233–1238.

8. Glagov S, Weisenberg E, Zarins CK, *et al.*: Compensatory enlargement of human atherosclerotic coronary arteries. *N Engl J Med* 1987, 316:1371–1375.

9. Hong MK, Mintz GS, Lee CW, et al.: Comparison of coronary plaque rupture between stable angina and acute myocardial infarction: a three-vessel intravascular ultrasound study in 235 patients. *Circulation* 2004, 110:928–933.

10. Yamagishi M, Terashima M, Awano K, *et al.*: Morphology of vulnerable coronary plaque: insights from follow-up of patients examined by intravascular ultrasound before an acute coronary syndrome. *J Am Coll Cardiol* 2000, 35:106–111.

11. Motoyama S, Kondo T, Anno H, *et al.*: Multi-slice compute tomographic characteristics of coronary lesions in acute coronary syndromes. *J Am Coll Cardiol* 2007, 50:319–326.

12. Motoyama S, Sarai M, Harigaya H, *et al.*: Computed tomography characteristics of atherosclerotic plaques subsequently resulting in acute coronary syndrome. *J Am Coll Cardiol* 2009, In press.

13. Jang IK, Tearney GJ, MacNeill B, *et al.*: In vivo characterization of coronary atherosclerotic plaque by use of optical coherence tomography. *Circulation* 2005, 111:1551–1555.

14. Kwon HM, Sangiorgi G, Ritman EL, *et al.*: Enhanced coronary vasa vasorum neovascularization in experimental hypercholesterolemia. *J Clin Invest* 1998, 101:1551–1556.

15. Kolodgie FD, Gold HK, Burke AP, *et al.*: Intraplaque hemorrhage and progression of coronary atheroma. *N Engl J Med* 2003, 349:2316–2325.

16. Virmani R, Kolodgie FD, Burke AP, *et al.*: Atherosclerotic plaque progression and vulnerability to rupture: angiogenesis as a source of intraplaque hemorrhage. *Arterioscler Thromb Vasc Biol* 2005, 25:2054–2061.

17. Kolodgie FD, Narula J, Yuan C, *et al.*: Elimination of neoangiogenesis for plaque stabilization: is there a role for local drug therapy? *J Am Coll Cardiol* 2007 49:2093–2101.

18. Takaya N, Yuan C, Chu B, *et al.*: Presence of intraplaque hemorrhage stimulates progression of carotid atherosclerotic plaques: a high-resolution magnetic resonance imaging study. *Circulation* 2005, 111:2768–2775.

19. Raman SV, Winner MW, Tran T, *et al.*: In vivo atherosclerotic plaque characterization using magnetic susceptibility distinguishes symptom-producing plaques. *J Am Coll Cardiol Imgaging* 2008, 1:49–57.

20. Feinstein SB: Contrast ultrasound imaging of the carotid artery vasa vasorum and atherosclerotic plaque neovascularization. *J Am Coll Cardiol* 2006, 48:236–243.

21. Libby P: Inflammation in atherosclerosis. *Nature* 2002, 420:868–874.

22. Kircher MF, Grimm J, Swirski FK, *et al.*: Noninvasive in vivo imaging of monocyte trafficking to atherosclerotic lesions. *Circulation* 2008, 117:388–395.

23. Jaffer FA, Nahrendorf M, Sosnovik D, *et al.*: Cellular imaging of inflammation in atherosclerosis using magnetofluorescent nanomaterials. *Mol Imaging* 2006, 5:85–92.

24. Nahrendorf M, Zhang H, Hembrador S, *et al.*: Nanoparticle PET-CT imaging of macrophages in inflammatory atherosclerosis. *Circulation* 2008, 117:379–387.

25. Trivedi RA, Graves MJ, Kirkpatrick PJ, *et al.*: Noninvasive imaging of carotid plaque inflammation. *Neurology* 2004, 63:187–188.

26. Hyafil F, Cornily JC, Feig JE, *et al.*: Noninvasive detection of macrophages using a nanoparticulate contrast agent for computed tomography. *Nat Med* 2007, 13:636–641.

27. Hartung D, Petrov A, Haider N, *et al.*: Radiolabeled Monocyte Chemotactic Protein 1 for the detection of inflammation in experimental atherosclerosis. *J Nucl Med* 2007, 48:1816–1821.

28. Rudd JH, Warburton EA, Fryer TD, *et al.*: Imaging atherosclerotic plaque inflammation with [18F]-fluorodeoxyglucose positron emission tomography. *Circulation* 2002, 105:2708–2711.

29. Tahara N, Kai H, Ishibashi M, *et al.*: Simvastatin attenuates plaque inflammation: evaluation by fluorodeoxyglucose positron emission tomography. *J Am Coll Cardiol* 2006, 48:1825–1831.

30. Tahara N, Kai H, Yamagishi S, *et al.*: Vascular inflammation evaluated by [18F]-fluorodeoxyglucose positron emission tomography is associated with the metabolic syndrome. *J Am Coll Cardiol* 2007, 49:1533–1539.

31. Nahrendorf M, Jaffer FA, Kelly KA, *et al.*: Noninvasive vascular cell adhesion molecule-1 imaging identifies inflammatory activation of cells in atherosclerosis. *Circulation* 2006, 114:1504–1511.

32. Kaufmann BA, Sanders JM, Davis C, *et al.*: Molecular imaging of inflammation in atherosclerosis with targeted ultrasound detection of vascular cell adhesion molecule-1. *Circulation* 2007, 116:276–284.

33. Isobe S, Tsimikas S, Zhou J, *et al.*: Noninvasive imaging of atherosclerotic lesions in apolipoprotein E-deficient and low-density-lipoprotein receptor-deficient mice with annexin A5. *J Nucl Med* 2006, 47:1497–1505.

34. Kolodgie FD, Petrov A, Virmani R, *et al.*: Targeting of apoptotic macrophages and experimental atheroma with radiolabeled annexin V: a technique with potential for noninvasive imaging of vulnerable plaque. *Circulation* 2003, 108:3134-3139.]

35. Hartung D, Sarai M, Petrov A, *et al.*: Resolution of apoptosis in atherosclerotic plaque by dietary modification and statin therapy. *J Nucl Med.* 2005, 46:2051-2056.

36. Sarai M, Hartung D, Petrov A, *et al.*: Broad and specific caspase inhibitor-induced acute repression of apoptosis in atherosclerotic lesions evaluated by radiolabeled annexin A5 imaging. *J Am Coll Cardiol* 2007, 50:2305–2312.

37. Kietselaer BL, Reutelingsperger CP, Heindendal GA, *et al.*: Noninvasive detection of plaque instability by radiolabeled annexin A5 in patients with carotid artery atherosclerosis. *N Engl J Med* 2004, 350:1472–1473.

38. Chen J, Tung CH, Mahmood U, *et al.*: In vivo imaging of proteolytic activity in atherosclerosis. *Circulation* 2002, 105:2766–2771.

39. Jaffer FA, Kim DE, Quinti L, *et al.*: Optical visualization of cathepsin K activity in atherosclerosis with a novel, protease-activatable fluorescence sensor. *Circulation* 2007, 115:2292–2298.

40. Jaffer FA, Vinegoni C, John MC, *et al.*: Real-time catheter molecular sensing of inflammation in proteolytically active atherosclerosis. *Circulation* 2008, 118:1802–1809.

41. Deguchi JO, Aikawa M, Tung CH, *et al.*: Inflammation in atherosclerosis: visualizing matrix metalloproteinase action in macrophages in vivo. *Circulation* 2006, 114:55–62.

42. Fujimoto S, Hartung D, Ohshima S, *et al.*: Molecular imaging of matrix metalloproteinase in atherosclerotic lesions: resolution with dietary modification and statin therapy. *J Am Coll Cardiol* 2008, 52:1847–1857.

43. Aikawa E, Nahrendorf M, Figueiredo JL, *et al.*: Osteogenesis associates with inflammation in early-stage atherosclerosis evaluated by molecular imaging in vivo. *Circulation* 2007, 116:2841–2850.

44. Rogers IS, Figueroa AL, Nasir KA, *et al.*: Assessment of coronary segment inflammation with combined 18F-FGD positron emission tomography and 64-slice multidetector computed tomography. *Circulation* 2007, 116:II-410.

Index

A

Acute coronary syndromes.
 See also specific disorders
 assessment of suspected, 226–232
 risk stratification and imaging in, 225–241
Adenosine, 63–69, 86, 91, 99, 156–157, 176
African American population
 cardiovascular disease in, 177–178
Age
 myocardial blood flow and, 90
Alpha particles, 2, 6
Angina, 193, 239–241
Angiography
 in cold pressor testing, 93–94
 computed tomography, 231–232
 coronary, 50, 157
 radionuclide, 122. *See also* specific techniques
Angiotensin receptor imaging, 206
Angiotensin-converting enzyme
 inhibitors, 205
Antioxidant therapy, 103
Aortic regurgitation, 123–125
Apoptosis imaging, 269–272
L-Arginine
 myocardial blood flow and, 92
Arrhythmias
 ventricular, 253
Artifacts, 28, 30, 32, 42
Atheroma, 262–263, 268–269
Atherosclerosis
 imaging of, 257–276
Atrial fibrillation, 155
Attenuation, 5, 42
 correction of, 20, 27–28
Autonomic nervous system, 244–246
AutoQuant quantitative perfusion
 assessment, 135–138

B

Backprojection, 15–16
Beta particles, 2, 6
Biventricular pacing, 127
Breast attenuation, 42
Bundle branch block, 124, 127, 152

C

Cameras. *See* Scintillation cameras
Carbon-11 acetate, 182, 189
Carbon-11 hydroxyephedrine, 248–250, 252, 254–255
Carbon-11 palmitate, 182, 187
Cardiac catheterization, 146, 157–158
Cardiac computed tomographic
 angiography, 231–232
Cardiac death, 149, 155, 157, 174–176

Cardiac events, 149, 151, 154, 176, 228, 236–237
Cardiac function assessment.
 See also Myocardial perfusion imaging; specific techniques
 blood pool imaging in, 110–130
 gated myocardial perfusion SPECT in, 131–138
 overview of, 109
Cardiac hypertrophy, 185–186
Cardiac metabolism imaging, 181–199
 overview of, 181
 PET in, 182, 187, 189–197
 radiotracers for, 182
 SPECT in, 182, 188, 194, 199
Cardiac transplantation, 254–255
Cardioverter defibrillators, 253
Caucasian population
 cardiovascular disease in, 177–178
Cellular viability requirements, 212
Center of rotation, 31
Chest pain assessment, 226–230
Circulation. *See also* Myocardial
 blood flow quantitation
 coronary, 80, 88–91
Cold pressor testing, 86–87, 91–96, 98–101, 103–104
Collimation and collimators, 12, 26
Collisions and collisional losses, 6
Compton scatter, 4
Compton window subtraction, 21
Computed tomographic angiography, 231–232, 259–260
Computed tomography, 264–267
Contrast resolution, 1, 11
Coronary angiography, 50, 157, 260
Coronary artery anatomy, 39, 79–104
Coronary artery bypass grafting, 138
Coronary artery disease
 atherosclerosis in, 257–276
 conventional *versus* nuclear imaging in, 141
 in high-risk populations, 170
 myocardial blood flow in, 39
 myocardial blood flow quantitation in, 97, 99–104
 myocardial perfusion imaging in, 37–55, 79–104, 225–241
 myocardial viability studies in, 193, 213–216, 218–219
 pharmacologic stress testing for, 61–75
 radiotracer uptake in, 40
 in renal failure, 198–199
 risk stratification in, 141–165, 226–241
 sensitivity of SPECT in, 44, 55
 stress testing in, 144–145, 225
Coronary calcium score, 162–165
Coronary endothelial dysfunction, 101
Coronary vasomotor function, 101

Cost effectiveness
 of stress testing, 74, 147–148
Crystal, 10
Curie, 3
Cyclotrons, 7

D

Decay curves, 3
Detector response, 12
Diabetes mellitus, 99, 153–154, 156, 174–177, 184, 254
Digital scintillation cameras.
 See Scintillation cameras
Dilated cardiomyopathy, 220
Dipyridamole, 63, 65, 67–70, 72–73, 86, 98–100, 177
Dobutamine, 63, 66–67, 69
Doxorubicin, 122

E

ECG gating. *See* Electrocardiographic gating
Echocardiography, 173–174
Ejection fraction
 left ventricular.
 See Left ventricular ejection fraction
 right ventricular, 124
Elderly population, 170, 177
Electrocardiographic gating
 assumptions in, 119
 in equilibrium gated blood pool imaging, 116
 myocardial perfusion imaging and, 50
 in SPECT myocardial perfusion imaging, 23, 131–138
Electronic collimation, 26
Electrons, 4, 6
Elution, 8
Energy peaking, 29
Equilibrium gated blood pool imaging, 110–111, 116–117, 121
Ethnicity
 cardiovascular disease and, 177–178
Exercise, 63, 67, 102, 113–114, 124, 144, 147

F

Fatty acids, 185, 194, 231
Fibrous cap, 261
Filling phase indices, 120
Filtered backprojection reconstruction, 15–16
First pass blood pool imaging
 advantages and disadvantages of, 110
 gated imaging *versus*, 135
 gated SPECT, 112
 technical aspects of, 111–112
Fission, 7

Index 279

Flow tracers.
 See also Radionuclides; specific agents
  PET versus SPECT, 2, 38
Flow velocity testing, 68–69
Fluorescence molecular tomography, 275
Fluorine-18, 2, 3
18-Fluorodeoxyglucose, 131, 182–183, 190, 266–267
Fourier transform, 16
Functional disability, 173

G
Gamma cameras, 37.
 See also Scintillation cameras
Gamma rays, 2, 4, 37
Gated imaging
 assumptions in, 119
 blood pool, 112, 118
 in cardiac function assessment, 109, 131–138
 SPECT blood pool, 128
 SPECT myocardial perfusion, 23, 131–138
Gender
 myocardial blood flow and, 90
Gene expression
 ventricular dysfunction and, 184
Generators, 7–9
Geometric response, 12
Glucose utilization, 185, 191
Glucose-lowering therapy, 104

H
Half-life, 3
Heart failure
 imaging priorities in, 202
 myocardial innervation imaging in, 250–251
 overview of, 201
 prevention of, 202–210
 prognosis in, 251
Hibernating myocardium, 211, 214–216
Hispanic population
 cardiovascular disease in, 177–178
HMG-CoA reductase inhibitors, 102–103
Horizontal long-axis imaging, 17
Hurricane sign, 42
Hyperemia, 86, 89–91, 99
Hypertrophic cardiomyopathy, 100–101, 221
Hypoperfusion indices, 143

I
Image filtering, 15–16
Image reconstruction, 15–16
Indium-111 oxine, 261
Inflammation
 in atherosclerosis, 257, 262, 265, 276
Innervation
 myocardial, 243–255
Insulin, 91
Integrin expression imaging, 207–208

Intravascular ultrasound, 259
Intravital fluorescence microscopy, 27, 2763
Intrinsic uniformity flood field, 29
Inverse square law, 3
Iodine-133, 7
Iodine-123 metaiodobenzylguanidine, 248–253
Ischemia
 myocardial, 159–161, 175, 178–179, 222, 252
Ischemic cardiomyopathy, 219
Ischemic memory, 194, 231
Isobars, isotones, and isotopes, 2
Iterative reconstruction, 19

L
Left to right shunt, 114–115
Left ventricular ejection fraction
 in coronary artery disease, 213–214
 doxorubicin and, 122
 gated imaging in measurement of, 121, 132
 in myocardial infarction, 213
Left ventricular end-diastolic volume calculation, 121
Left ventricular function
 ECG-gated SPECT assessment of, 132
 prognostic value of, 160
Left ventricular remodeling, 205, 209, 218
Left ventricular volume curve, 119–120
Levophase analysis, 112
Linear attenuation coefficients, 5
List mode acquisition, 118–119
Long-axis imaging, 17
Lung radiotracer uptake, 44

M
Magnetic resonance imaging, 216–217, 263, 268
Maximum likelihood expectation maximization, 19
Medical decision making, 159–160, 226, 230
ß-Methyl-p-[^{123}I]iodophenyl pentadecanoic acid, 182, 188
Mitral regurgitation, 123
Molecular imaging
 in atherosclerosis, 261–276
Molybdenum-99, 7–9
Molybdenum-99–technetium-99m generator, 8–9
Monocytes and macrophages
 in molecular imaging, 263–266, 269
Multidetector SPECT systems, 13
Multiheaded cameras, 13
Myocardial biopsies, 54
Myocardial blood flow quantitation.
 See also Myocardial perfusion imaging
 animal models of, 83
 base-to-apex, 95–96
 in cardiovascular disease, 97–100
 cold pressor testing in, 86–87, 91–96, 98–101, 103–104

 coronary anatomy and, 39, 80
 in hyperemia, 86, 89–91, 99
 monitoring of therapy with, 102–104
 normal findings in, 81, 85–96
 PET imaging of, 79–104
 prognostic value of, 100–102
 reproducibility of, 85–88
 stress testing in, 86, 89, 95–96
 technical aspects of, 81–84
Myocardial infarction
 abnormal wall motion in, 137
 in diabetes, 174
 investigational approaches to, 238
 neurohumoral upregulation after, 204
 non-ST segment elevation, 239–241
 post-treatment, 235–237
 size estimation in, 237
 SPECT prediction of, 149
 ST segment elevation, 233–239
 stress testing after, 73
Myocardial innervation, 243–255
 in cardiac transplantation, 254–255
 in diabetes, 254
 in heart failure, 250–251
 in ischemic heart disease, 252
 overview of, 243
 physiology of, 244–246, 248–250
 radiotracers in imaging of, 246–247
 in ventricular arrhythmias, 253
Myocardial ischemia, 159–161, 175, 178–179, 222, 234–235, 252
Myocardial necrosis, 238
Myocardial neuropathy, 254
Myocardial oxygen supply and demand imbalance, 212
Myocardial perfusion
 ventricular function and, 113
Myocardial perfusion imaging, 38–59.
 See also Myocardial blood flow quantitation
 in acute coronary syndromes, 225–241
 coronary flow velocity study versus, 69
 ECG and angiography and, 23, 50
 extracardiac activity and, 44
 indications for, 44
 normal findings in, 134
 overview of, 37
 PET in, 37–40, 56–59
 PET versus SPECT, 57
 prognostic value of, 46, 49, 51
 quantitative analysis in, 41
 radionuclides used in, 38, 52
 of reversible and irreversible defects, 43, 49
 in risk stratification, 141–165
 risk stratification in, 45
 segmental anatomy in, 41
 sensitivity and specificity of, 44, 50
 in special populations, 169–179
 SPECT in, 23, 37–55, 131–138, 141–165
Myocardial scarring, 217
Myocardial stunning, 195–196, 211, 215–216
Myocardial thickening, 134

Myocardial viability.
  See also Myocardial perfusion imaging
  assessment of, 201, 211–222
  SPECT underestimation of, 55
Myocyte metabolic pathways, 189–190
Myofibroblasts, 206–207

N

Near infrared fluorescence imaging, 263–264, 272, 274, 276
Necrotic core of plaque, 259
Neurohumoral antagonists, 209–210
Neurotransmitter synthesis, 245–246
Nitrate administration, 55
Nitric oxide synthase, 91–92, 95
Nitrogen-13 ammonia, 38, 58–59, 81–83
Noise level, 25
Non-ST segment elevation myocardial infarction, 239–241
Nuclear cardiology imaging.
  See also specific techniques and principles
  of acute coronary syndromes, 225–241
  of atherosclerosis, 257–276
  cardiac function assessment in, 109–138
  of cardiac metabolism, 181–199
  of heart failure, 201–210
  of myocardial blood flow, 79–104
  of myocardial innervation, 243–255
  of myocardial perfusion, 37–59
  of myocardial viability, 211–222
  of noncardiac conditions, 70
  overview of, 1, 37
  patient management and, 141–165
  principles of, 1–34, 37
  radionuclides used in, 8
  risk stratification in, 141–165
  in stress testing, 61–75
Nuclear reactors, 7
Nuclear stability, 2

O

Obesity, 100, 171, 184
Oblique angle reorientation, 17
Oblique imaging, 17
Ordered-subsets expectation maximization, 19
Oxidation
  contractile stimulation and, 183
Oxygen-15 water, 57–58, 82, 86

P

Pair annihilation, 2
Pair production, 4
Parathyroid adenoma, 44
Partial volume effect, 22, 132–134
Patient management
  nuclear imaging in, 159–165
  risk stratification and, 141–165
Patient motion artifact, 32

Patient selection
  for stress testing, 62, 148
Perfusion-metabolism mismatch, 194
Pericardial tamponade, 126
Perioperative event predictors, 71
Peripheral vascular disease, 70
Peroxisome proliferation activated receptor-α, 187
PET. See Positron emission tomography
Pharmacologic stress testing, 61–75.
  See also specific agents
  accuracy of, 69, 73
  cost-to-benefit data on, 74
  drug side effects in, 68
  exercise and, 67
  of flow velocity, 68–69
  guidelines for, 75
  hemodynamic responses to, 65–67
  indications for, 62
  mechanisms in, 64–65
  methods used in, 62
  in myocardial blood flow quantitation, 86, 89, 95–96
  overview of, 61, 79
  patient selection for, 62
  in perioperative event prediction, 71
  in preoperative risk assessment, 72–73
  prognostic value of, 70, 73–74
  protocols for, 65–66
  in risk stratification, 70
  SPECT canine models of, 53
Phase analysis, 126–128
Photoelectric effect, 4
Photoelectrons, 6
Photomultiplier tubes, 9–10
Photons, 4, 5
Pixel value, 24
Planar imaging, 29, 117
Plaque
  atherosclerotic, 258–261
Point spread function, 11–12
Polar maps, 84, 103, 136–137
Positron emission tomography
  in atherosclerosis, 264, 266–268
  attenuation correction in, 27
  in blood pool imaging, 110–111
  in cardiac metabolism imaging, 182, 187, 189–197
  collimation in, 26
  coronary calcium score and, 164
  hybrid SPECT systems and, 33
  mismatch and match patterns in, 191–192
  in myocardial blood flow quantitation, 79–104
  in myocardial perfusion imaging, 37–40, 56–59
  prognostic value of, 100–102
  radionuclides in, 2, 8, 38, 182, 246–247
  SPECT image fusion with, 33
  SPECT technology versus, 37
  two- versus three-dimensional systems of, 26

Positron particle range, 6
Pressure overload mechanism, 185–186
Prognostic adenosine score, 156–157
Prognostic value
  of cardiac imaging in women, 173
  of myocardial blood flow quantitation, 100–101
  of myocardial perfusion imaging, 46, 49, 51, 142, 146, 150, 152–154, 156–157, 160
  of stress testing, 70, 73–74, 146, 150, 152
Protease activity imaging, 272–273

Q

Quality control, 29, 33
Quantitative analysis and assessment
  in myocardial perfusion imaging, 41, 135–136

R

Radiation, 2, 4, 6
Radiation losses, 6
Radioactive decay law, 3
Radioactivity, 1, 3
Radionuclide angiography, 122–123
Radionuclides, 2, 6–8. See also specific agents
  blood clearance of, 40
  for innervation imaging, 246–247
  myocardial blood flow and uptake of, 40
  SPECT versus PET, 2, 38, 182
Radiotracers. See Radionuclides
Recoil electrons, 4, 6
Reconstruction
  filtered backprojection, 15–16
  half–time acquisition in, 34
  iterative, 19
  PET versus SPECT, 37
Regadenoson, 63–64, 66–68
Regurgitant index, 125
Renal failure, 198–199
Renin-angiotensin system, 204–205
Repeatability coefficient, 88
Reproducibility
  of myocardial blood flow quantitation imaging, 85–88
Resolution, 11–12, 24
Resolution and linearity test, 29
Resolution recovery, 22
Rest-redistribution thallium-201 SPECT, 49, 51
Revascularization
  in coronary artery disease, 141
  myocardial viability testing before, 195
  risk stratification for, 141, 159–162
Risk stratification
  in acute coronary syndromes, 225–241
  in elderly population, 177
  nuclear test results and, 142–165, 169
  patient management and, 141–165
  rationale for, 141–142, 225

Rubidium-82, 56–57
  overview of, 38, 56
Ruptured plaque, 261

S

Scatter correction, 21
Scintillation, 10
Scintillation cameras
  center of rotation in, 31
  in SPECT system, 10, 13–14
  uniformity of, 29
Segmental myocardial anatomy, 41
Sensitivity, 12, 44
Sensitivity tests, 29
Short-axis imaging, 17
Signal, 1, 9–10
Single-photon emission computed tomography
  after myocardial infarction, 210
  artifacts in, 42
  in atherosclerosis, 263, 271, 275
  in blood pool imaging, 110–111, 128–130
  cameras in, 10, 13–14
  in cardiac metabolism imaging, 182, 188, 194, 199
  coronary calcium score and, 162–165
  cost effectiveness of, 148
  gated, 23, 128–138
  hybrid PET systems and, 33
  indications for, 44
  in myocardial perfusion imaging, 37–55, 131–138, 141–165
  PET image fusion with, 33
  PET technology *versus*, 37
  physical factors affecting, 18
  prognostic value of, 146, 150
  quality control for, 33
  radionuclides in, 2, 8, 38, 52, 182
  in risk stratification, 141–165, 169
  sensitivity and specificity of, 44, 55
  in special populations, 169–179
Sinogram, 32
Smokers, 98
Spatial resolution, 11

Special populations
  stress myocardial perfusion imaging in, 169–179
Specificity, 44
SPECT. *See* Single-photon emission computed tomography
ST segment elevation myocardial infarction, 233–239
Stress testing
  in acute coronary syndromes, 225
  cardiac events in, 149
  cost-effectiveness of, 74, 147–148
  gated first pass blood pool imaging, 113–114
  in myocardial blood flow quantitation, 85
  options for, 63
  overview of, 61, 79
  pharmacologic.
    See Pharmacologic stress testing
  prognostic value of, 150, 156–157
  in special populations, 169–179
  SPECT myocardial perfusion, 45–55, 135–136, 144–149, 225, 230
Strontium-82-rubidium-82 generator, 9
Stunned myocardium, 195–196, 211, 215–216
Substrate oxidation rates, 183
Summed projections, 32
Summed stress score, 143, 151, 153, 157
Surgery, 70–73, 244–246, 251–253
Sympathetic nervous system, 244–246, 251–253

T

Technetium-99m
  decay curve of, 3
  formation of, 8–9
  in myocardial perfusion imaging, 38, 52–55, 134–135, 237
  overview of, 2, 38
Technetium-99m-labeled sestamibi, 52–55, 134, 151, 153
Technetium-99m-labeled teboroxime, 52
Technetium-99m-labeled tetrofosmin, 52, 55, 151

Temporal resolution, 24
Thallium-201
  decay curve of, 3
  in myocardial perfusion imaging, 38, 45–55, 135, 153
  in myocardial viability imaging, 212, 218
  overview of, 38
  in preoperative stress testing, 72–73
Thiazolidinedione, 104
Thrombolytic therapy, 235
Thymoma, 44
Transaxial imaging, 17
Triglyceride overload, 184

U

Ultrasound, 259, 268
Uniformity and uniformity artifact, 29–30
Unstable angina, 239–241

V

Valvular heart lesions, 123–125
Vascular cell adhesion molecule-1, 268
Vascular surgery, 70, 72–73
Vasodilators, 63–75, 86–87. *See also*
  Pharmacologic stress testing; specific agents
Ventricular arrhythmias, 253
Ventricular dysfunction, 184
Ventricular function assessment, 110–130
Ventricular tachycardia, 197
Verapamil, 120
Vertical long-axis imaging, 17
Voxel value, 25

W

Wall motion assessment, 136–138
Women, 172–173, 175–176, 178–179

X

Xenon-133, 7
X-rays, 2, 4

282 Atlas of Nuclear Cardiology